Alzheimer's Disease: A Clinical Guide

Alzheimer's Disease: A Clinical Guide

Edited by Trevor Cornfield

AMERICAN
MEDICAL PUBLISHERS
www.americanmedicalpublishers.com

American Medical Publishers,
41 Flatbush Avenue,
1st Floor, New York,
NY 11217, USA

Visit us on the World Wide Web at:
www.americanmedicalpublishers.com

ISBN: 978-1-63927-435-2

Cataloging-in-Publication Data

Alzheimer's disease : a clinical guide / edited by Trevor Cornfield.
p. cm.
Includes bibliographical references and index.
ISBN 978-1-63927-435-2
1. Alzheimer's disease. 2. Alzheimer's disease--Guidebooks. 3. Dementia.
4. Brain--Diseases. I. Cornfield, Trevor.
RC523 .A49 2022
616.831--dc23

Table of Contents

Preface

Alzheimer's disease (AD) is a progressive neurodegenerative disorder, and a common cause of dementia. The most noticeable symptom is short term memory loss, witnessed as an inability to acquire new information and remember new events. As the disease progresses, symptoms such as language difficulties, mood swings, behavioral issues, disorientation, inability to manage self care, etc. start to occur. With time, the person's condition declines and body functions are lost. The typical life expectancy following the diagnosis of Alzheimer's is between 3-9 years. Physical and mental exercise, and managing a healthy body weight can decrease the risk of AD. Medications and supplements are generally ineffective in decreasing the risk of AD, nor can they stop or reverse disease progression. However, exercise programs can improve outcomes, while antipsychotics can treat behavioral problems or psychosis. This book contains some path-breaking studies on Alzheimer's disease. It provides comprehensive insights into its management. This book is a resource guide for all students as well as experts.

Significant researches are present in this book. Intensive efforts have been employed by authors to make this book an outstanding discourse. This book contains the enlightening chapters which have been written on the basis of significant researches done by the experts.

Finally, I would also like to thank all the members involved in this book for being a team and meeting all the deadlines for the submission of their respective works. I would also like to thank my friends and family for being supportive in my efforts.

Editor

1

Dissecting the role of non-coding RNAs in the accumulation of amyloid and tau neuropathologies in Alzheimer's disease

Ellis Patrick[1,2,3], Sathyapriya Rajagopal[1,2,3], Hon-Kit Andus Wong[5], Cristin McCabe[3], Jishu Xu[1,2,3], Anna Tang[1,3], Selina H. Imboywa[5], Julie A. Schneider[4], Nathalie Pochet[1,2,3], Anna M. Krichevsky[5], Lori B. Chibnik[1,2,3], David A. Bennett[4] and Philip L. De Jager[1,2,3*]

Abstract

Background: Given multiple studies of brain microRNA (miRNA) in relation to Alzheimer's disease (AD) with few consistent results and the heterogeneity of this disease, the objective of this study was to explore their mechanism by evaluating their relation to different elements of Alzheimer's disease pathology, confounding factors and mRNA expression data from the same subjects in the same brain region.

Methods: We report analyses of expression profiling of miRNA (n = 700 subjects) and lincRNA (n = 540 subjects) from the dorsolateral prefrontal cortex of individuals participating in two longitudinal cohort studies of aging.

Results: We confirm the association of two well-established miRNA (miR-132, miR-129) with pathologic AD in our dataset and then further characterize this association in terms of its component neuritic β-amyloid plaques and neurofibrillary tangle pathologies. Additionally, we identify one new miRNA (miR-99) and four lincRNA that are associated with these traits. Many other previously reported associations of microRNA with AD are associated with the confounders quantified in our longitudinal cohort. Finally, by performing analyses integrating both miRNA and RNA sequence data from the same individuals (525 samples), we characterize the impact of AD associated miRNA on human brain expression: we show that the effects of miR-132 and miR-129-5b converge on certain genes such as EP300 and find a role for miR200 and its target genes in AD using an integrated miRNA/mRNA analysis.

Conclusions: Overall, miRNAs play a modest role in human AD, but we observe robust evidence that a small number of miRNAs are responsible for specific alterations in the cortical transcriptome that are associated with AD.

Keywords: Alzheimer's disease, microRNA, lincRNA, Neuritic β-amyloid plaques and neurofibrillary tangles

Background

Late onset Alzheimer's disease (AD) is an age-dependent neurodegenerative disorder characterized clinically by cognitive decline and pathologically by the accumulation of neuritic β-amyloid plaques (NP) and neurofibrillary tangles (NFT) in the brain. Currently genetic [1], epigenomic [2] and transcriptomic studies [3, 4] coupled with advances in imaging techniques [5, 6] have begun to sketch the sequence of events in the causal chain linking risk factors to a syndromic diagnosis of AD dementia. One of these events may be the dysregulation of gene expression by alterations in the expression of microRNA (miRNA) and long intergenic non-coding RNA (lincRNA) molecules.

miRNA are a class of small regulatory RNA that modulate gene expression via a multiprotein complex which facilitates the interaction between an miRNA and its complementary elements in the 3'UTR of target mRNAs to initiate transcript degradation and repression of protein production [7, 8]. Aberrant expression of miRNA and/or its target mRNAs have been implicated in abnormal neuron function [9] and in several neurodegenerative disorders [10, 11]. Recently, certain miRNA,

* Correspondence: pdejager@rics.bwh.harvard.edu
[1]Departments of Neurology and Psychiatry, Brigham and Women's Hospital, Program in Translational NeuroPsychiatric Genomics, Institute for the Neurosciences, 77 Avenue Louis Pasteur, NRB 168C, Boston, MA 02115, USA
[2]Harvard Medical School, Boston, MA, USA
Full list of author information is available at the end of the article

such as miR-132 have been associated with pathologic AD [12–16]. However, these studies were conducted in a modest number of subjects with limited phenotypic information, and few results are consistent across these studies [17].

lincRNA are RNA that are longer than 200 nucleotides and do not code for proteins [18]. As with most long non-coding RNA and unlike miRNA there is no clear common functional mechanism for lincRNA [18]; some may have a structural role in protein/RNA complexes. There is still debate over what percentage of lincRNA may be functional at all [19]. However, focusing on the lincRNA that lie in the same locus as protein coding genes may provide insight into their functional correlates. Given the reported association of the long non-coding RNA BACE1-AS [20] with AD and the lack of investigation of this class of non-coding RNAs in a large sample size, we investigated the potential role of long non-coding RNA in AD and its component pathologies.

We first evaluated the role of miRNAs previously associated with AD with measures of both neuritic amyloid plaque (NP) and neurofibrillary tangles (NFT) since these are key neuropathologic features of AD and allow us to explore the mechanism by which an AD-associated non-coding RNA contributes to disease. We secondarily expanded this effort to evaluate other miRNAs and lincRNAs to discover new associations. In addition, we leveraged transcriptome-wide RNA sequencing profiles, generated from the same RNA samples that were used to generate the miRNA profiles, to identify the functional consequences of altered miRNA expression on protein-coding genes in the human dorsolateral prefrontal cortex (DLPFC) and to identify additional cases where miRNA and mRNA AD associations converge in the human cortex.

Methods

Total RNA, including miRNA, was extracted from approximately 100 mg sections of frozen postmortem brain tissue from the dorsolateral prefrontal cortex (BA 9/46) of subjects from two previously described longitudinal cohorts of aging, Religious Order Study (ROS) and Rush Memory Aging Project (MAP) [2, 21–23]. Tissue was thawed partially on ice and between 50 and 100 mg of gray matter was dissected from the section then transferred immediately to 1 mL of Trizol. The tissue was then quickly homogenized using the Qiagen TissueLyser and a 5 mm stainless steel bead, for 30 s at 30 Hz. The foam was settled with a quick spin, and the sample incubated for a minimum of 5 mins at room temperature. Debris was pelleted at 4 °C at 12,000 g for 10 min and Trizol was transferred to a new 1.5 mL tube. We continued preparation of samples following the instructions of Qiagen's miRNeasy Mini kit, with volumes adjusted for 1 mL instead of 700uL of Trizol until wash steps. RNA was eluted from the miRNeasy spin columns in 75uL of elution buffer, and quality tested by Nanodrop and Bioanalyzer RNA 6000 Nano Agilent chips. RNA yields averaged about 25μg and RIN scores ranged from 2 to 9 with an average of 6.5. RNA was normalized to 33 ng/ul and plated into 96w plates for Nanostring processing using the nCounter Human miRNA Expression assay kit version 1 with reporter library file: NS_H_miR_1.2.rlf. The data collection from 733 post mortem brain samples was done at the Broad Institutes Genomics Platform (Broad Institute of Harvard and MIT, Cambridge, USA). Subjects from different diagnostic categories were distributed across experimental batches to reduce batch effects. To minimize variability at the ligation step, processing of the annealing and ligation steps was performed on the same thermocycler. Two thermocyclers were used for the purification steps, but all samples were placed in the same thermocycler for denaturation and hybridization steps. Two nCounter Prep Stations were utilized, but all samples were then scanned on the same Digital Analyzer. The data was collected in 8 batches of 96 samples and a single sample technical replicate was introduced as control in every single 96 well plates and sometimes twice in one single plate in two different cartridges.

Quality control and dataset pre-processing

All data is available at https://www.synapse.org/#!Synapse:syn3219045. The miRNA from the Nanostring RCC files were re-annotated to match the definitions from the miRBase v19. The raw data from the Nanostring RCC files were accumulated and the probe-specific backgrounds were adjusted according to the Nanostring guidelines with the corrections provided with the probe sets. After correcting for the probe-specific backgrounds, a three-step filtering of miRNA and sample expressions was performed. First, miRNA that had less than 95% of samples with a missing expression level were removed. This is followed by removing samples that had less than 95% of miRNAs with missing expressions. Thus, the call-rates for the samples and the miRNA are set at 95%. Finally, all miRNA whose absolute value is less than 15 in at least 50% of the samples were removed to eliminate miRNA that had negligible expression in brain samples. After the miRNA and sample filtering, the dataset consisted of 309 miRNAs and 700 samples. A combination of quantile normalization and Combat [24], specifying the cartridges as batches for the miRNA data, was used to normalize the data sets. The strong association observed between miRNA expression and RNA-integrity was validated via qRT-PCR (Additional file 1: Figure S3) and verified not to be specific to the Nanostring platform.

The mRNA sequencing data have been described elsewhere [25]. For the lincRNA analysis, a non-gapped aligner Bowtie [26] was used to align reads to a hg19 lincRNA reference [27] and then RSEM [28] applied to estimate expression levels for all lincRNA. A combination of quantile normalization and Combat [24] to account for batch was used for normalization. After filtering out lowly expressed lincRNA with an expected count less than 5, a final dataset of 454 lincRNA measured in 540 samples was used.

Identifying differentially expressed miRNA or lincRNA

Simple linear regression analysis was used to associate the expression levels of miRNA and lincRNA to several variables that measured the neuropathology in the AD brain. These included either the numbers of neuritic plaques, neurofibrillary tangles or a binary variable representing the pathologic diagnosis of AD on autopsy according to the NIA Reagan criteria [29]. All the associations were adjusted for age, sex, study (ROS or MAP), the proportion of neurons in the tissue [2], RNA Integrity number (RIN) and post-mortem interval (PMI). The proportion of neurons in the tissue is estimated from DNA methylation data available from the same brain region of each individual, as described in our recent study [2]. A Bonferroni corrected significance threshold of 0.05 was used to account for multiple comparisons.

Constructing micro-RNA and linc-RNA networks

Linear models were used to identify miRNA or lincRNA that were associated with either NP, NFT or AD. To do this the models included age, neuronal composition (NNLS), sex, study of origin (Study, ROS or MAP), post-mortem interval (PMI), RNA integrity number (RIN), NP, NFT and AD., NP, NFT and AD as covariates. Using these models a miRNA or lincRNA were included in the networks if there was evidence that any of effects sizes of NP, NFT or AD were non-zero (nominal *p*-value from an F-test from less than 0.05). For each of the included miRNA or lincRNA, forward stepwise variable selection was used with a Bayesian information criteria (BIC) to select which edges between miRNA or lincRNA and explanatory variables should be included in the network. As RIN is associated with all the miRNA and lincRNA its edges are excluded from the networks.

Pathway analysis

Our approach for pathway analysis of the miRNA data using pMim [30] involved analyses of the miRNA and mRNA data on the 525 samples which had both miRNA and gene expression data. The mRNA analyses are designed to focus on sets of genes that are co-expressed and are predicted to be a target of one of the tested miRNAs. Targetscan v6.2 [31] was used for prediction of miRNA targets and the GO biological processes [32] were used for pathway annotation. Figure 3a outlines how pMim is used to construct and test "miR-pathways", where a miR-pathway consists of genes that are targeted by a miRNA and lie in a common pathway. Specifically, pMim identifies sets of genes that (1) are predicted to be targeted by an miRNA associated with AD, (2) lie in a common biological pathway and (3) are also associated with AD diagnosis themselves in terms of mRNA expression. All 309 miRNA and their corresponding miR-pathways (sets of genes that are targeted by the same miRNA and share a common biological process) were tested; a joint statistic summarizes and ranks the evidence for both the miRNA and mRNA analyses testing if both a miRNA and one of its corresponding miR-pathways are associated with AD. This joint statistic is calculated with two significance combination methods. Within a miR-pathway, Stouffer's method was used to combine significance of genes associated with AD. A one-sided Pearson's method was used to combine the significance between the miR-pathway gene summary statistic and the association of its miRNA with AD. Under very strict assumptions these joint statistics could be considered as *p*-values, however due to the large amount of correlation within an annotated pathway they are highly inflated. Hence we consider these joint statistics for ranking purposes only.

Results

Demographic features and nature of our non-coding RNA data

The NanoString nCounter assay was used to measure miRNA expression from the DLPFC of each subject. At the conclusion of a rigorous quality control and preprocessing pipeline, expression measures from 309 miRNAs in 700 subjects were retained for downstream analysis. The subjects profiled in this study are participants in one of two prospective cohort studies of aging, the Religious Order Study (ROS) and Memory and Aging Project (MAP) which are designed to be merged for joint analyses [33, 34]. These studies enroll non-demented individuals and include detailed, annual ante-mortem characterization of each subject's cognitive status as well as prospective brain collection and a structured neuropathologic examination at the time of death. The study design of ROS and MAP yields an autopsy sample that includes a range of syndromic diagnoses and neuropathologic findings that are common in the older population. While this is not a true population-based sample, it captures the diversity of the older population at the time of death and is different than the collection of subjects typically used for age-matched case-control studies [12, 13, 15, 16]. The subjects in the study have an average age of 88 at death, 61% meet criteria for pathologic AD by NIA Reagan criteria [29] and 64% are female (Additional file 1: Table S1). To evaluate the nature of our data in relation to published results, we first assessed whether the expression of miRNAs are associated with a pathological diagnosis of AD according to the NIA Reagan criteria [29], focusing on an evaluation of previously reported miRNA associations [12, 13, 15, 16].

miRNA associated with a pathologic diagnosis of AD

We used a linear regression model controlling for age, sex, study, proportion of neuronal cells, post-mortem interval and a measure of RNA quality (RNA integrity (RIN) score) to evaluate associations of miRNA with pathologic AD. In this analysis of the human DLPFC, two previously reported associated miRNAs are significantly associated with pathologic AD, exceeding a threshold defined using a Bonferroni correction for the number of miRNA tested, $p < 1.6 \times 10^{-4}$ (Table 1, Fig. 1). Specifically, miR-132 ($P = 2 \times 10^{-8}$) and miR-129-5p ($P = 3.9 \times 10^{-6}$) were found to be diminished in expression in subjects with AD, consistent with prior studies [12, 13]. Thus, our data confirm well-validated miRNA associations with AD. To provide perspective on effect size, miR-132 explains 6.7% of the variance in AD, which is similar to the 6.1% variance explained by *APOE* ε4 in our data and 6% in previous literature [35]. In contrast, the miRNA effect is more than the <1% of variance explained by genetic susceptibility variants in *ABCA7, CD33,* and *CR1* that were originally discovered in genome-wide association studies [35].

We next systematically reviewed our results for those miRNA that have previously been associated with AD in various brain regions [13, 15, 16]: they are catalogued in Table 2. Figure 1 illustrates the strength of the association of miRNAs with pathologic AD in our cohort, highlighting 11 miRNAs that were deemed to be significantly associated with AD in a prior study of moderate sample size (n = 49 subjects) [12]. Of the 11 miRNA previously reported to be associated with AD in the prefrontal cortex, only miR-132 and miR-129-5p replicated. In addition, miR-129-3p (P = 0.0013), miR-200a (P = 0.018), miR-30e (P = 0.0048), miR-100 (P = 0.011), let-7i (P = 0.045) and miR-185 (P = 0.013) display suggestive association and may warrant further investigation. The Bonferroni threshold ($p < 0.00016$) that we employed may be overly conservative, but it provides a useful way to distinguish the most robustly associated miRNA. Given our large sample size (n = 700), we have good power to confirm results with small effect sizes: we have 80% power to detect an effect small enough to only explain 2.2% of the variance in relation to AD (which is much smaller than the effect of mi132 described above). Thus, if other miRNAs that we tested have a role in AD, they are more in line with the magnitude of effect found with AD SNPs.

The role of confounding variables in miRNA expression

There is a substantial lack of concordance in behavior between the previously reported AD miRNA signatures and their level of association in our cohort (Table 2, Additional file 1: Figure S1). While this could be explained, in part, by differences in the brain regions that have been assayed and the technologies used in the different studies, many of these miRNAs are highly associated with age, sex, the proportion of neurons in the profiled tissue sample, post-mortem interval and/or RIN score (Table 2, Additional file 2: Table S2). Thus, explicitly accounting for all of these factors is essential in brain miRNA studies, and the RIN score appears to play an especially significant role.

Identifying miRNA associated with amyloid and tau neuropathologies

Having described the nature of our data in relation to prior reports, we proceeded to our main goal of investigating the relationship of miRNA expression with specific features of AD neuropathology: namely, we investigated whether miRNA are associated with the accumulation of neuritic amyloid plaques (NP) and/or neurofibrillary tangles (NFT) that are defined by the presence of Tau accumulation. The pathologic AD-associated miRNA, miR-132 and miR-129-5p, were

Table 1 miRNA and lincRNA associated with AD, NP or NFT

	coefficient: AD	*p*-value: AD	coefficient: NP	*p*-value: NP	coefficient: NFT	*p*-value: NFT
miR-132	−0.26	**2.00E-08**	−0.29	**1.40E-11**	−0.31	**4.10E-08**
miR-129-5p	−0.11	**3.90E-06**	−0.15	**6.90E-11**	−0.17	**2.20E-08**
miR-129-3p	−0.095	0.0013	−0.13	**1.80E-06**	−0.12	0.00085
miR-99b	0.081	0.0034	0.075	0.0037	0.14	**6.00E-05**
linc-CTSD-3	−19	0.0012	−22	**6.90E-05**	−33	**8.60E-06**
linc-BRD9–1	32	0.00025	35	**2.40E-05**	23	0.036
linc-ADC	3.8	0.18	3.8	0.15	14	**6.70E-05**
linc-RNFT2–1	3.3	0.36	3.4	0.31	18	**7.10E-05**

In bold are the tests which meet the Bonferroni correction threshold of $p < 0.00016$

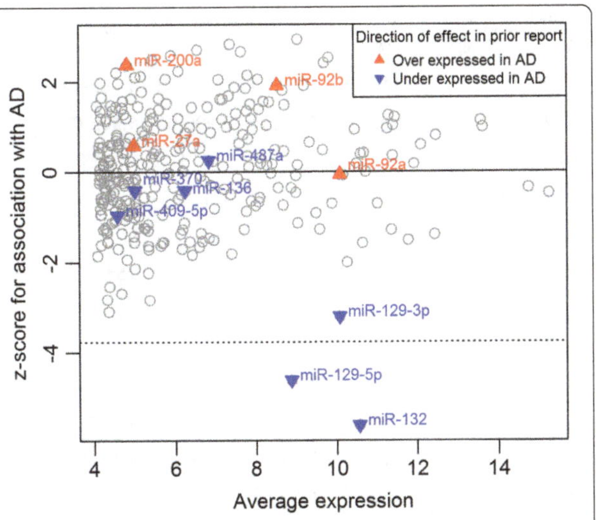

Fig. 1 Validation of miRNAs associated with AD in other studies. The relationship between average miRNA expression (x-axis) and association with pathological AD in ROSMAP (y-axis) is plotted for each miRNA. The association between a miRNA and AD is calculated as a z-score after correcting for other factors; a negative z-score denotes decreased miRNA expression in the context of AD. Previously reported miRNAs [12] are highlighted by colored triangles, with red denoting higher expression in AD and *blue* reduced expression in AD in the original publication. The *dotted* horizontal line marks the z-score threshold of significance that is equivalent to a Bonferroni *p*-value cut-off of 0.05; none of the miRNAs with positively correlated expression are significantly associated with AD. The *gray* circles represent all other miRNAs tested in our study

associated with both NP and NFT (Table 1). These two neuropathologic features of AD are strongly correlated with one another and it can be challenging to dissect the effect of one from the other unless large sample sizes are available. In addition, we found that, among the tested miRNAs, miR-129-3p ($P = 1.8 \times 10^{-6}$) was associated with NP, and miR-99b ($P = 6 \times 10^{-5}$) was associated with NFT, exceeding our significance threshold ($p < 0.00016$).

Dissecting the network of miRNA associations in AD

The complexity of the relationships between miRNA expression, the burden of NP and NFT neuropathologies, a pathologic diagnosis of AD, technical variables and demographic variables are demonstrated in Fig. 2a. Here, we consider all variables in a single model to resolve the most likely primary association between each miRNA and the neuropathologic traits. These traits are all correlated with one another (Fig. 2b, Additional file 1: Table S3), making it difficult to understand where an miRNA's primary effect may be exerted simply by looking at the univariate results: for example, while miR-132 is significantly associated with both NP and NFT in separate analyses (Table 1), it appears, in the joint network model, that its effect may be driven predominantly through NP. This is visualized by the edge linking miR-132 and NP in the network model. The effect on NFT may be secondary and result from the accumulation of NP. To elaborate a more comprehensive network model, we included all of the miRNAs with either a significant or suggestive ($p < 0.05$) association to one of the AD pathologies. Similar to miR-132, we see that many miRNAs are only associated with either NP, NFT or AD, suggesting that they may have a primary effect through one or the other pathology or some other aspect of AD not captured by these pathologic measures. On the other hand, miR-433, miR-487b and miR-485-3p are negatively associated with NP and also positively associated with AD in our joint model. This result captures the complexity and likely non-linear relationships of miRNA associations with pathology as miR-433, miR-487b and miR-485-3p are all negatively associated with AD in univariate analysis. This result highlights the need to evaluate the possibility of more complex relationships between miRNA and disease in future studies.

Evaluating the functional consequences of AD-associated miRNA in human brain

We next attempted to delineate the downstream effects of the expressed miRNAs by integrating the miRNA data with gene expression data from the same brain region and the same individuals. In fact, both the miRNA and RNA sequence data were generated from the same RNA sample. Our approach involved separate analyses of miRNA and mRNA data, with the mRNA analyses being focused on sets of genes that are co-expressed and are predicted to be a target of one of the tested miRNAs. Specifically, pMim [30] was used to identify sets of genes that (1) are predicted to be targeted by an miRNA associated with pathologic AD, (2) lie in a common biological pathway and (3) are also associated with pathologic AD themselves in terms of mRNA expression. Figure 3a outlines how pMim is used to construct and test "miR-pathways" where Targetscan v6.2 [31] was used for prediction of miRNA targets and the GO biological processes [32] were used for pathway annotation. All 309 miRNA and their corresponding miR-pathways (sets of genes that are targeted by the same miRNA and share a common biological process) were tested; a joint statistic summarizes and ranks the evidence for both the miRNA and mRNA analyses. The top eight miR-pathways in which both the miRNA and the mRNA are significantly associated with AD are presented in Table 3.

Looking more closely at the top miR-pathways, we see that, in the DLPFC, miR-132 appears to be targeting a group of five genes (*EP300, NACC2, SALL1, SREBF1* and *SIRT1*) that are related to protein acetylation. All five of these protein acetylation genes lie within the top 20 predicted miR-132 target genes whose expression is

Table 2 *P*-values from tests of association with AD and other covariates for miRNA implicated in other studies

	ROSMAP	Lau	Cogswell	Hebert	Nunez	Study	Age	Sex	NNLS	PMI	RIN	AD	AD (no covariates)
miR-132	Down	Down	Down			0.54	0.58	0.32	0.46	0.0052	7.00E-14	**2.00E-08**	**4.00E-12**
miR-129-5p	Down	Down				0.31	0.012	0.72	0.23	6.00E-04	1.70E-11	**3.90E-06**	**6.50E-07**
miR-129-3p		Down				0.59	0.089	0.063	0.73	0.0057	3.00E-08	0.0013	0.00098
miR-136		Down				0.59	0.3	0.71	0.16	0.046	0.1	0.67	0.78
miR-370		Down				0.29	0.084	0.025	0.051	0.17	0.0036	0.67	0.57
miR-409-5p		Down				0.52	0.0064	0.22	0.26	0.52	0.071	0.33	0.53
miR-487a		Down				0.89	0.1	0.78	0.79	0.53	5.90E-09	0.8	0.99
miR-92a		Up	Up			0.36	0.81	0.039	0.00056	0.43	7.50E-10	0.95	0.1
miR-27a		Up	Up			0.39	0.69	0.46	0.47	0.53	0.56	0.56	0.6
miR-92b		Up	Up			0.14	0.44	2.70E-05	0.96	0.74	2.30E-18	0.056	0.74
miR-200a		Up				0.95	0.013	0.58	0.65	0.095	2.00E-53	0.018	**0.00013**
miR-9			Down	Down		0.47	0.15	0.21	0.005	0.65	1.20E-06	0.73	0.39
miR-146b-5p			Down			0.45	0.12	0.92	0.5	0.36	0.0064	0.93	0.84
miR-425			Down			0.35	0.19	0.88	0.34	0.41	0.35	0.29	0.11
miR-30e			Up		Down	0.91	0.043	0.14	0.71	0.33	0.019	0.0048	0.0043
miR-423-5p			Up			0.5	0.023	0.78	0.42	0.076	1.80E-07	0.38	0.25
miR-27b			Up			0.19	0.57	0.84	0.66	0.16	0.08	0.48	0.38
miR-100			Up			0.13	0.99	0.0091	0.11	0.16	8.70E-05	0.011	0.0083
miR-34a			Up			0.4	0.00015	0.056	0.013	0.39	0.59	0.18	0.028
miR-145			Up			0.015	0.63	0.96	0.89	0.55	5.50E-06	0.26	0.084
miR-381			Up			0.55	0.73	0.12	0.74	0.6	0.47	0.12	0.022
miR-125b			Up			0.28	0.42	0.92	0.66	0.6	3.20E-10	0.63	0.37
miR-148a			Up			0.19	0.74	0.22	0.23	0.97	0.016	0.95	0.69
miR-15a				Down	Down	0.47	0.24	0.49	0.016	0.0053	0.031	0.51	0.48
miR-29b				Down	Down	0.98	0.27	0.15	0.99	0.057	0.00017	0.34	0.019
miR-101				Down	Down	0.77	0.24	0.013	0.21	0.099	0.96	0.3	0.15
miR-181c				Down	Down	0.13	0.49	0.24	0.038	0.23	0.42	0.34	0.3
miR-363				Down		0.2	0.027	0.13	0.2	0.072	0.096	0.92	0.54
miR-19b				Down		0.72	0.05	0.069	0.34	0.18	0.65	0.064	0.032
miR-106b				Down		0.25	0.92	0.95	0.68	0.3	0.82	0.15	0.13
miR-22				Down		0.84	0.35	0.75	0.16	0.64	0.15	0.81	0.77
miR-93				Down		0.11	0.7	0.0064	0.81	0.74	0.03	0.34	0.2
miR-26b				Down		0.34	0.36	0.25	0.94	0.76	0.67	0.13	0.21
let-7i				Down		0.46	0.79	0.79	0.58	0.93	0.39	0.045	0.036
miR-320a				Up	Up	0.44	0.24	0.26	0.78	0.38	4.60E-14	0.16	0.057
miR-197				Up		0.23	0.43	0.49	0.36	0.31	0.39	0.77	0.43
miR-29c					Down	0.87	0.36	0.43	0.089	0.0082	2.00E-06	0.35	0.31
miR-494					Down	0.61	0.4	0.94	0.5	0.044	2.50E-11	0.38	0.16
miR-598					Down	0.26	1	0.25	9.70E-05	0.1	0.0034	0.2	0.11
miR-374a					Down	0.84	0.48	0.74	0.081	0.35	0.039	0.63	0.72
miR-376a					Down	0.93	0.58	0.027	0.16	0.58	0.71	0.11	0.012
miR-148b					Down	0.89	0.15	0.69	0.12	0.6	0.92	0.72	0.75
miR-95					Down	0.51	0.76	0.33	0.0017	0.71	0.056	0.86	0.74
miR-582-5p					Down	0.6	0.86	0.94	0.012	0.89	0.00018	0.35	0.18

Table 2 *P*-values from tests of association with AD and other covariates for miRNA implicated in other studies *(Continued)*

miR-432	Up	0.59	0.32	0.99	0.16	0.084	0.53	0.12	0.1
miR-188-5p	Up	0.8	0.82	0.18	0.4	0.12	0.011	0.99	0.76
miR-382	Up	0.83	0.51	0.29	0.15	0.52	0.029	0.33	0.28
miR-185	Up	0.92	0.19	0.77	0.055	0.81	0.41	0.013	0.0044

In bold are the tests which meet the Bonferroni correction threshold of $p < 0.00016$

inversely associated with miR-132 abundance in our cortical samples (p-values <0.00018, Table 4). The miR-132 association with *EP300* expression confirms earlier reports and in vitro studies [12, 14, 36, 37], illustrating the robustness of our results and the relevance of earlier studies. As shown in Fig. 3b-d, miR-132 explains approximately a third of the association of each gene to AD, and therefore it does not appear to be the sole driver of the role of these protein acetylation genes in AD. While miR-132 may thus be influencing AD, in part, through histone acetylation and chromatin remodeling, miR-129-5p appears to be regulating genes related to the regulation of transcription. Interestingly, both miR-132 and miR-129-5p target *EP300,* which encodes the histone acetyltransferase protein E1A-associated cellular p300 transcriptional co-activator, and each miRNA explains some of the variation in *EP300* expression (adjusted R-squared 0.039 and 0.033 respectively). The role of these two miRNAs appears to be non-redundant: when they are considered together, they explain more of the variance in EP300 than either miRNA explains separately (adjusted R-squared 0.045), further illustrating the complex interactions involved in mRNA regulation by miRNAs.

In addition to these miR-pathways related to the validated miR-132 and miR-129-5p miRNAs, it is intriguing that miR-200a, which is suggestively associated to AD in our miRNA only analyses (Table 2), is the second strongest result in this pathway analysis because of the strong association of its downstream genes: this set of thirteen predicted target genes of miR-200a are all involved in anion transport. For these thirteen genes, an average of 18% of the mRNA association with AD is accounted by miR-200a. These integrated miRNA:mRNA analyses therefore report highly significant results drawn from autopsy tissue and set the stage for exploring specific downstream hypotheses; they also suggest that miRNAs

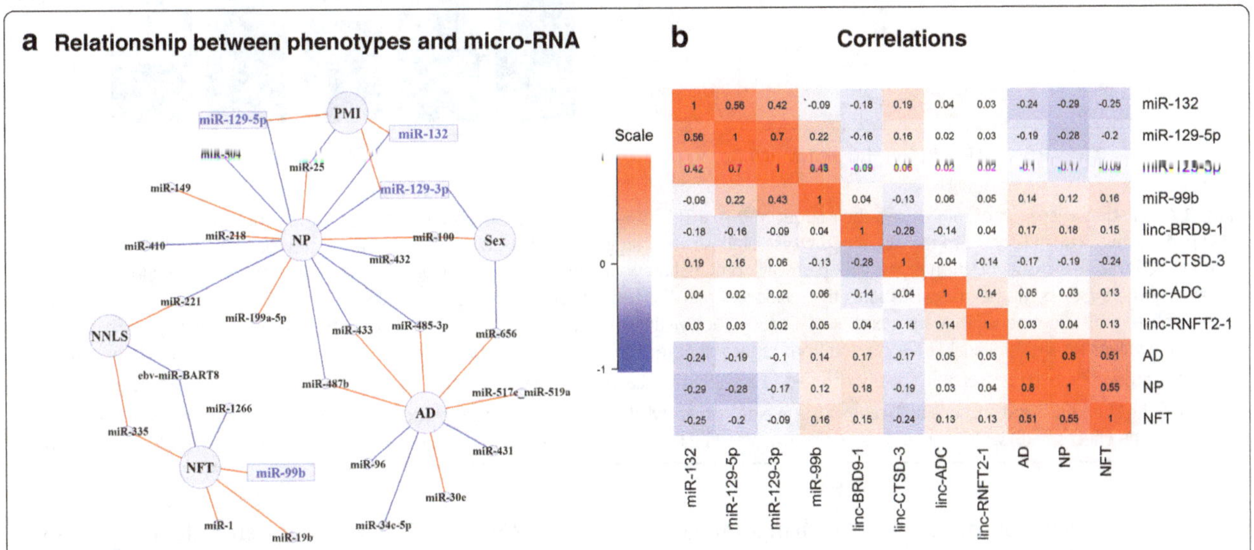

Fig. 2 Network of miRNAs associated with phenotypes. **a** The relationships between miRNA expression and various demographic and technical features as well as neuropathologic outcomes are displayed in a network diagram. All miRNA with a significant ($p < 0.00016$) or suggestive ($p < 0.05$) association are included in the network. These relationships were extracted via feature selection from linear models which explain an miRNA's expression level by using age at death (Age), neuronal composition (NNLS), sex, study of origin (Study, ROS or MAP), post-mortem interval (PMI), RNA integrity number (RIN), neuritic amyloid plaques (NP), neurofibrillary tangles (NFT) and pathological AD diagnosis (AD). Each node in the diagram represents an miRNA (small circles) or a demographic or a neuropathologic variable (*large circles*). The significantly associated miRNA (Table 1) are represented by rectangles. A red edge represents a positive association between the miRNA and trait; a blue edge denotes an inverse association. As most of the miRNAs are associated with RIN, the associations with RIN were removed from this figure for clarity. **b** The correlations between the expression levels of eight miRNA and lincRNA with significant associations in our study are shown, along with correlations with the outcome variables (NP, NFT and AD). Each of the correlations are displayed in each cell of the correlation map and is colored by the strength of correlation, red for positive associations and blue for negative associations

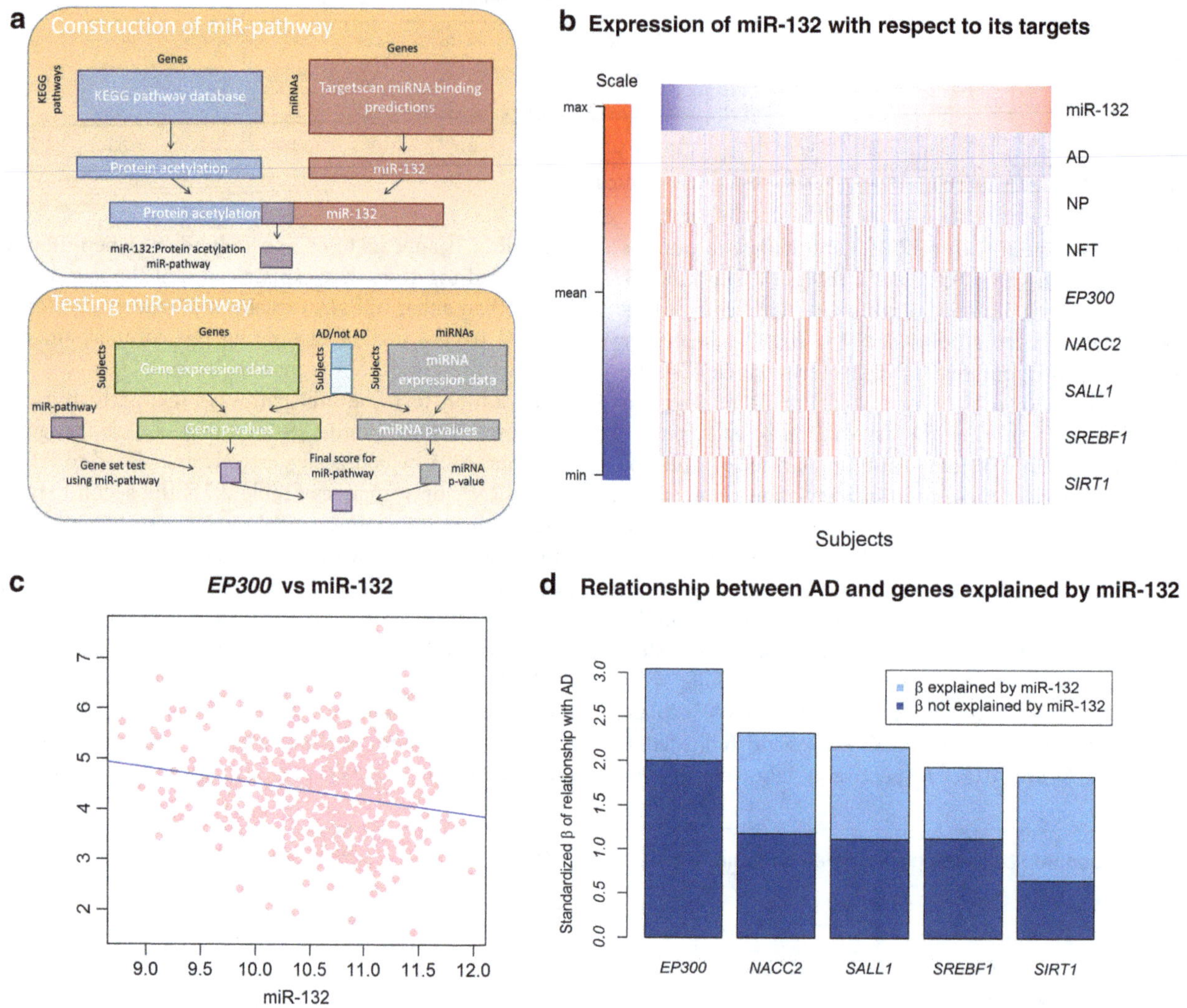

Fig. 3 An integrated analysis of miRNA and their target mRNA. **a** This diagram presents an overview of (1) how the miR-132:Protein acetylation miR-pathway was constructed from the KEGG pathways database and Targetscan miRNA binding target prediction database and (2) how a score was derived to assess the association of this miR-pathway combination with pathological AD diagnosis. The approach is described in greater detail elsewhere [30]. **b** This heatmap illustrates the relation of miR-132 with the outcome measures (AD, NP, and NFT) and the mRNA expression levels of five of its target genes that are member of a protein acetylation miR-pathway. Each column presents data from one subject. Scaled expression values for a given variable are colored from red (to denote high expression) to blue (low expression). **c** The relationship between miR-132 and one of its targets, EP300, is demonstrated in a scatterplot. Each dot represents one subject. **d** The standardized effect sizes ($\frac{\beta}{SE(\beta)}$) capturing the strength of the relationship between the five protein acetylation genes and AD are plotted in this panel. We highlight the relative amount of the effect size (β) which can and cannot be explained by miR-132 expression, as miR-132 is predicted to be regulating each of these genes

are just one element contributing to the changes in gene expression found in AD since most of the variance of the affected genes – such EP300 and the miR200a targeted genes – remains unexplained at this time.

Deregulation of lincRNA expression in relation to AD neuropathology

Our RNA sequencing data was also used to measure lincRNA expression from the DLPFC in the ROSMAP cohorts. At the conclusion of a rigorous quality control and preprocessing pipeline, expression measures from 454 lincRNAs in 540 subjects were retained for downstream analysis. The subjects with lincRNA expression are primarily a subset of the subjects with miRNA expression; 525 subjects have both miRNA and lincRNA expression data.

To investigate the relationships between lincRNA expression and the available neuropathologic measures, we used the strategy deployed in studying miRNA: we fit three independent linear models using age, sex, study, an estimate of the proportion of neuronal cells, postmortem interval and RNA integrity number and either

Table 3 Integrated analysis of miRNA and their target mRNA identifies miR:target combinations that are associated with AD

miRNA	Pathways	Direction	Score	Genes in pathway targeted by miRNA
miR-132	protein deacetylation; protein deacylation; macromolecule deacylation	Down	1.17E-09	*EP300, NACC2, SALL1, SREBF1, SIRT1*
miR-200a	anion transport	Up	1.07E-07	*SLC20A1, SLC25A3, RIMS1, SLC35A1, SLC35D1, GLS, ATP8A2, ATP8A1, IRS2, SLC38A9, CXCL12, SLC16A7, SLC18A2*
miR-129-5p	regulation of transcription, DNA-templated	Down	1.19E-07	*EP300, NCOA1, ZBTB20, PBX3, LMNA, ZBTB5, ETS1, CHD7, CBX4, WWC2, YWHAB, CBX7, PKNOX1, ZBTB10, CBX6, PHIP, ZFY*
miR-129-5p	cell migration; cell motility; localization of cell	Down	1.19E-07	*SUN2, DLC1, LMNA, TMEM201, ETS1, RPS6KB1*
miR-129-5p	positive regulation of transcription, DNA-templated; positive regulation of transcription from RNA polymerase II promoter; positive regulation of RNA metabolic process; positive regulation of RNA biosynthetic process; positive regulation of nucleic acid-templated transcription	Down	1.19E-07	*EP300, NCOA1, LMNA, ETS1, PKNOX1, PHIP*
miR-129-5p	regulation of RNA metabolic process; regulation of nucleic acid-templated transcription; regulation of RNA biosynthetic process	Down	1.19E-07	*EP300, NCOA1, ZBTB20, PBX3, LMNA, ZBTB5, ETS1, CHD7, CBX4, WWC2, YWHAB, ACTN1, CBX7, PKNOX1, ZBTB10, CBX6, PHIP, ZFY*
miR-129-5p	cardiovascular system development; circulatory system development	Down	1.19E-07	*EP300, DLC1, LMNA, ETS1, CHD7, PKNOX1, TIPARP*
miR-129-5p	single-organism organelle organization	Down	1.19E-07	*SUN2, EP300, DLC1, NCOA1, LMNA, VAMP1, WHAB, SNX9, ACTN1, PAPD5, PHIP*

NP, NFT or pathological AD as covariates to explain lincRNA expression. The lincRNA that were significantly associated with NP, NFT or AD are shown in Table 1 and Additional file 3: Table S4. No lincRNA is significantly associated with AD after Bonferroni correction. However, two are associated with NP (linc-CTSD-3 and linc-BRD9–1) and three with NFT (linc-CTSD-3, linc-ADC and linc-RNFT2–1); none of these lincRNAs have sequences that overlap the exons of protein coding genes.

We then repeated our network-building strategy to illustrate the primary associations among lincRNAs and the various demographic and pathological variables (Fig. 4a). We use linc-CTSD-3 to illustrate the fact that the pathologic AD-associated non-coding RNAs can also be independently influenced by confounding variables, highlighting the need to include them in the modeling (Fig. 4a, b, Additional file 1: Figure S2). As in the miRNA network, no lincRNA maintains a relationship between both NP and NFT after feature selection.

We have therefore investigated two different types of non-coding RNAs, miRNA and lincRNA, which may play a role in regulating gene expression in AD. Interestingly, while the expression level of different pathologic AD-associated miRNAs are fairly strongly correlated to one another, they are not strongly associated with lincRNAs, and the lincRNAs are only modestly correlated with one another (Fig. 2d). This suggests that, while related, the molecular mechanisms to which these non-coding RNAs contribute in the context of AD may be largely different, with greater coordination among miRNA effects.

Discussion

The number of individuals profiled in our cohorts and the prospective nature of the brain collection in these longitudinal studies of aging make our dataset a valuable resource for exploring, in greater detail, the role of miRNAs that have previously been associated with pathologic AD: our analysis meets a need for studies in larger datasets [17, 38] and offers a potentially less biased perspective of the disease than the comparison of AD cases and controls that are pulled from a brain bank to fit certain diagnostic criteria and were not collected prospectively. We see that the role of miRNAs in AD begins to be resolved in terms of AD's component pathologies: linking a specific miRNA with either NP or NFT. These associations with a pathologic feature relating to either amyloid or tau

Table 4 Predicted target genes that are negatively associated with miR-132 expression in the human cortex

Gene	*P*-value: association with miR-132	*P*-value: association with AD	In protein acetylation pathway
CLMN	1.00E-14	0.0016	
TJAP1	1.60E-12	0.00059	
ANKRD40	9.30E-11	0.023	
CXorf36	1.00E-10	0.0082	
CDK19	2.60E-10	0.019	
SSH2	6.10E-09	0.39	
SEMA6A	4.90E-08	0.013	
HIP1R	5.50E-08	0.0017	
EP300	9.60E-08	0.0024	✓
DYNC1LI2	1.30E-07	0.023	
NACC2	1.60E-07	0.021	✓
SOX5	1.60E-07	0.22	
SIRT1	1.70E-07	0.069	✓
SALL1	5.10E-07	0.031	✓
MAPK3	4.10E-06	0.15	
BCAN	2.00E-05	0.034	
EPB41	0.00017	0.8	
CTGF	0.00033	0.68	
MEX3C	0.00038	0.53	
SREBF1	0.00051	0.058	✓

pathology are important to generate hypotheses that can be tested in future studies, particularly in mouse models that may recapitulate only one of these pathologies. Aside from the two validated miRNAs, we found suggestive evidence of association (*p*-values <0.05) for 8 of the 48 previously proposed pathologic AD-associated miRNAs, demonstrating that additional miRNAs may have smaller effects on AD. While all of the other studies age-matched their subjects, none explicitly modeled sex or other technical covariates in their analysis. In particular, we observe strong associations with RIN score, a technical measure capturing the quality of the RNA sample that led to spurious associations when not accounted for in the analysis. One study [12] reports the overall RIN scores for their hippocampal and prefrontal cortex samples; however, they do not provide a description of how this measure correlates with AD, and the incomplete RIN score data reported by another study [13] shows some potential differences between AD and controls. By accounting for the covariates that we have measured, we not only enhance confidence in the miRNA reported as being associated with AD pathology but also provide an opportunity to speculate on the reason why some miRNA may not have been validated due to the technical, clinical and demographic differences among subjects selected for different studies.

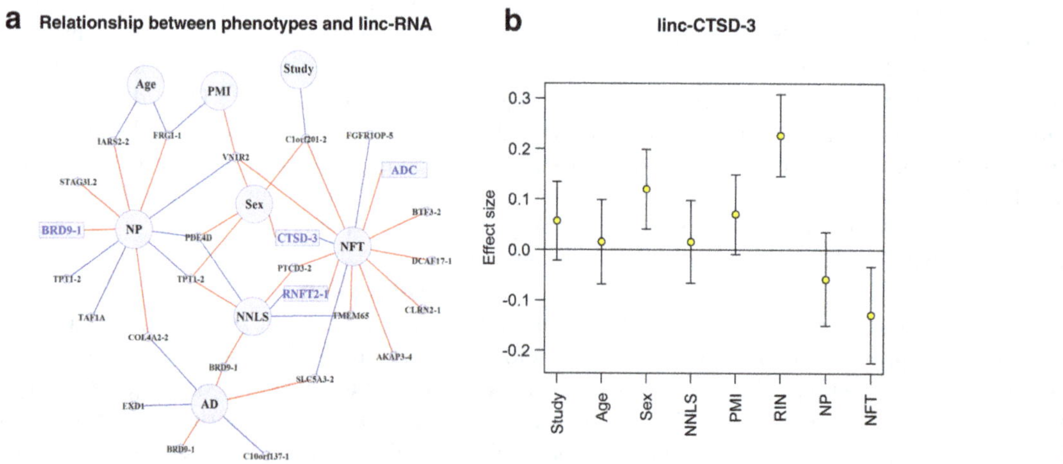

Fig. 4 Network of lincRNAs associated with phenotypes. **a** The relationships between lincRNA expression and various demographic and technical features as well as neuropathologic outcomes are displayed in a network diagram. All lincRNA with a significant ($p < 0.00016$) or suggestive ($p < 0.05$) association are included in the network. These relationships were extracted via feature selection from linear models which explain an lincRNA's expression level by using age at death (Age), neuronal composition (NNLS), sex, study of origin (Study, ROS or MAP), post-mortem interval (PMI), RNA integrity number (RIN), neuritic amyloid plaques (NP), neurofibrillary tangles (NFT) and pathological AD diagnosis (AD). Each node in the diagram represents a lincRNA (small circles) or a demographic or a neuropathologic variable (*large circles*). The significantly associated lincRNA (Table 1) are represented by rectangles. A red edge represents a positive association between the lincRNA and trait; a blue edge denotes an inverse association. As most of the lincRNAs are associated with RIN, the associations with RIN were removed from this figure for clarity. **b** The association of linc-CTSD-3 expression with each variable is plotted after fitting a model including all variables. The standardized effect size of each of these explanatory variables and 95% confidence intervals are shown. This illustrates the fact that non-coding RNAs significantly associated with AD pathology can be strongly influenced by confounding variables, but that these effects are independent

Our study has certain limitations, including the advanced average age at death (88 years) in these cohorts and the fact that they are representative of the older population but are not truly population-based, which limit the generalizability of our results. However, the high rate of autopsy (>90%) among study subjects ensures that our results are representative for the entire study population, which consists of subjects who are non-demented at the beginning of the study. Further, the data that we analyzed was generated from the cortex (gray matter). This is a practical compromise to attain large sample sizes, but it presents a challenge for future work as it is not clear which cell type may be driving a particular association. While accounting for the proportion of neurons in the tissue addresses some of the concerns that relate to the role of changes in the relative frequency of cell populations, future work in purified cell populations will be needed to resolve these questions more fully. The Nanostring technology used to measure miRNA expression could also introduce a technical bias in the replication of previously reported miRNA, and the use of probes to measure miRNA with Nanostring and of a predefined reference for aligning lincRNA data will limit the discovery of unannotated non-coding RNAs. Finally, we cannot comment on causality since we have a performed a cross-sectional analysis of brain tissue.

The availability of transcriptome-wide mRNA data from the same RNA samples in a large (n = 540) subset of the ROSMAP subjects profiled for miRNA also provides a rare opportunity to directly explore the relation of miRNA with their putative target mRNAs and of miRNAs with a different class of non-coding RNAs, lincRNAs, in human tissue. Some of the lincRNAs are associated with AD pathology but their expression appears to be largely independent of the miRNAs. On the other hand, our large autopsy-derived mRNA sequence data has identified several different molecular pathways whose component genes have mRNA levels that are associated with AD and are targeted by AD-associated miRNA. The robustness of these results is nicely demonstrated by our lead miRNA, miR-132, which has been validated to be associated with AD in prior targeted studies [12, 13, 39] and for which selected putative target genes have been evaluated in brain samples, including *EP300* and *SIRT1* [12, 14]. Here, we not only refine earlier observations by showing that the effect of miR-132 is mediated by the accumulation of amyloid pathology but also expand prior targeted studies of downstream effects by organizing the target genes in pathways to highlight cellular functions, such as protein acetylation that appear to be targeted by alterations in miR-132.

The functional consequences of lincRNAs remain poorly understood, and we therefore could not repeat our pathway analysis with this subset of non-coding RNAs. Since lincRNAs may influence the coding RNAs found in the same locus, we did evaluate the association of the neighboring protein-coding genes with AD and the neuropathologic outcomes, but none of the coding transcripts were significantly associated. We also note that the previously reported BACE1-AS lincRNA [20] was not in the reference used in this study, and therefore could not be evaluated in our study. The positive association of *BACE1* mRNA expression with AD was not replicated in our cohort (P = 0.63).

With our analyses, we have therefore begun to use autopsy data from a large set of well-characterized human subjects that capture the heterogeneity of older human brains to resolve which aspect of AD-related pathology is influenced by each miRNA of interest. The two well-validated miRNAs in AD illustrate this well: while miR-132 and mir-129-5p are strongly associated with the correlated amyloid and tau pathology measures, both miRNAs are more strongly associated with amyloid pathology than with the accumulation of Tau pathology when the pathologies are included in the same model. This leads to very different experimental paths to further dissect the mechanism of these miRNAs in AD. In addition, using these quantitative pathologic traits that are more precise than a categorical diagnosis of AD, we find that some new miRNAs, such as miR-99b, that may have a stronger effect on a specific pathology, such as Tau/NFT. lincRNAs also appear to be involved, but the downstream consequences of these non-coding RNAs remain unclear. Nonetheless, the lincRNA associations bring another dimension to the broad narrative that emerges from our report: that molecular changes associated with AD include an important alteration in the regulation of cortical transcription, which is consistent with prior reports of epigenomic changes in certain model systems such as *Drosophila melanogaster* DNA methylation profiles and the involvement of REST in AD [40, 41]. This narrative is also illustrated by miR-200 where the simple analysis of the miRNA alone is suggestive but not convincing of association with AD; however, an integrated analysis that also considers alterations of miR-200 target genes prioritizes this miRNA and downstream transcriptional changes in anion transporters for further evaluation. Such integrated analyses of complementary data may be helpful to resolve the broader perspective on alterations in cellular function in AD. With this manuscript, we therefore provide a robust foundation of detailed neuropathologic associations that set the stage for a new generation of integrative analyses that consider different molecular measures generated from the same subjects and allows for the direct modeling of the complex phenotypic and molecular heterogeneity of the aging population at risk of AD and other dementia.

Conclusions

By studying cortical levels of non-coding RNA in a large prospectively recruited cohort of well-characterized human subjects we had a unique opportunity to explore their associations with measures of both neuritic plaques and neurofibrillary tangles as well as the target mRNAs that they may be regulating. This work provides a robust foundation for future hypothesis-driven work to further dissect the mechanism of the reported associations to specific neuropathologic features of AD.

Additional files

Additional file 1: Table S1. Demographic information. **Table S3.** A table of the correlations between each of the pertinent covariates, Study, Age, Sex, NNLS, PMI, RIN, NP, NFT and AD. **Figure S1.** Behavior of miRNAs implicated in other experiments. **Figure S2.** Differentially expressed miRNAs and lincRNAs. **Figure S3.** Validation of RIN association.

Additional file 2: Table S2. A table to assess whether the various demographic and neuro-pathological variables may be confounding the relationship between miRNA expression and pathological AD. A linear model is used to model miRNA expression by Study, Age at death, Sex, neuronal proportion (NNLS), post-mortem interval (PMI), RNA Integrity number (RIN) and pathological AD. The effect of pathological AD on the miRNA is reported (coef.AD) as well as the probability of observing this effect or something more extreme assuming that it should be zero (pval.AD). Then for each of the covariates a model is fit without including this covariate in the model and the effect of AD on miRNA expression is calculated again; e.g. pval.AD (−Age) is from the model not including Age at death. (CSV 28 kb)

Additional file 3: Table S4. Reported are the *p*-value and beta coefficient for the association of each lincRNA with AD, NP and NFT from a series of linear models which include Study, Age at death, Sex, neuronal proportion (NNLS), post-mortem interval (PMI) and RNA Integrity number (RIN) as covariates. (CSV 69 kb)

Abbreviations

AD: Alzheimer's disease; BIC: Baysian information criterion; DLPFC: Dorsolateral prefrontal cortex; lincRNA: Long intergenic non-coding RNA; MAP: Rush memory aging project; miRNA: micro-RNA; NFT: Neurofibrillary tangle pathologies; NNLS: Proportion of neurons; NP: Neuritic β-amyloid plaques; PMI: Post-mortem interval; RIN: RNA integrity number; ROS: Religious order study

Acknowledgements

We would like to thank the participants of the ROS and MAP studies for their participation in these studies. Support for this research was provided by grants from the US National Institutes of Health (R01 AG036042, R01 AG036836, R01 AG17917, RF1 AG15819, R01 AG032990, R01 AG18023, RC2 AG036547, P30 AG10161, U01 AG46152, P50 AG016574, U01 ES017155, K25 AG041906-01) and the Rainwater Foundation/Tau Consortium.

Authors' contributions

CM, AT, AMK and SI collected, prepared and generated data from the samples. EP, JX, NP and SR performed analyses on the resulting data. PLD and DAB designed the study. EP, PLD and SR wrote the manuscript. All of the authors critically reviewed the manuscript.

Competing interests

The authors declare that they have no competing interests.

Author details

[1]Departments of Neurology and Psychiatry, Brigham and Women's Hospital, Program in Translational NeuroPsychiatric Genomics, Institute for the Neurosciences, 77 Avenue Louis Pasteur, NRB 168C, Boston, MA 02115, USA. [2]Harvard Medical School, Boston, MA, USA. [3]Program in Medical and Population Genetics, Broad Institute, Cambridge, MA, USA. [4]Rush Alzheimer's Disease Center, Rush University Medical Center, Chicago, IL, USA. [5]Departments of Neurology, Brigham and Women's Hospital, Boston, MA, USA.

References

1. Lambert JC, Ibrahim-Verbaas CA, Harold D, Naj AC, Sims R, Bellenguez C, et al. Meta-analysis of 74,046 individuals identifies 11 new susceptibility loci for Alzheimer's disease. Nat Genet. 2013;45:1452–8.
2. De Jager PL, Srivastava G, Lunnon K, Burgess J, Schalkwyk LC, Yu L, et al. Alzheimer's disease: early alterations in brain DNA methylation at ANK1, BIN1, RHBDF2 and other loci. Nat Neurosci. 2014;17:1156–63.
3. Berchtold NC, Coleman PD, Cribbs DH, Rogers J, Gillen DL, Cotman CW. Synaptic genes are extensively downregulated across multiple brain regions in normal human aging and Alzheimer's disease. Neurobiol Aging. 2013;34:1653–61.
4. Rhinn H, Fujita R, Qiang L, Cheng R, Lee JH, Abeliovich A. Integrative genomics identifies APOE epsilon4 effectors in Alzheimer's disease. Nature. 2013;500:45–50.
5. Oh H, Mormino EC, Madison C, Hayenga A, Smiljic A, Jagust WJ. β-amyloid affects frontal and posterior brain networks in normal aging. NeuroImage. 2011;54:1887–95.
6. Sperling RA, Laviolette PS, O'Keefe K, O'Brien J, Rentz DM, Pihlajamaki M, et al. Amyloid deposition is associated with impaired default network function in older persons without dementia. Neuron. 2009;63:178–88.
7. Guo H, Ingolia NT, Weissman JS, Bartel DP. Mammalian microRNAs predominantly act to decrease target mRNA levels. Nature. 2010;466:835–40.
8. Bartel DP. MicroRNAs: target recognition and regulatory functions. Cell. 2009;136:215–33.
9. Cohen JE, Lee PR, Chen S, Li W, Fields RD. MicroRNA regulation of homeostatic synaptic plasticity. Proc Natl Acad Sci U S A. 2011;108: 11650–5.
10. Chen-Plotkin AS, Unger TL, Gallagher MD, Bill E, Kwong LK, Volpicelli-Daley L, et al. TMEM106B, the risk gene for frontotemporal dementia, is regulated by the microRNA-132/212 cluster and affects progranulin pathways. J Neurosci. 2012;32:11213–27.
11. Johnson R, Zuccato C, Belyaev ND, Guest DJ, Cattaneo E, Buckley NJ. A microRNA-based gene dysregulation pathway in Huntington's disease. Neurobiol Dis. 2008;29:438–45.
12. Lau P, Bossers K, Janky R, Salta E, Frigerio CS, Barbash S, et al. Alteration of the microRNA network during the progression of Alzheimer's disease. EMBO Mol Med. 2013;5:1613–34.
13. Cogswell JP, Ward J, Taylor IA, Waters M, Shi Y, Cannon B, et al. Identification of miRNA changes in Alzheimer's disease brain and CSF yields putative biomarkers and insights into disease pathways. Journal of Alzheimer's disease : JAD. 2008;14:27–41.
14. Wong H-KAK, Veremeyko T, Patel N, Lemere CA, Walsh DM, Esau C, et al. De-repression of FOXO3a death axis by microRNA-132 and -212 causes neuronal apoptosis in Alzheimer's disease. Hum Mol Genet. 2013;22:3077–92.
15. Hébert SSS, Horré K, Nicolaï L, Papadopoulou AS, Mandemakers W, Silahtaroglu AN, et al. Loss of microRNA cluster miR-29a/b-1 in sporadic Alzheimer's disease correlates with increased BACE1/beta-secretase expression. Proc Natl Acad Sci U S A. 2008;105:6415–20.
16. Nunez-Iglesias J, Liu C-CC, Morgan TE, Finch CE, Zhou XJ. Joint genome-wide profiling of miRNA and mRNA expression in Alzheimer's disease cortex reveals altered miRNA regulation. PLoS One. 2010;5
17. Lau P, Frigerio CS, De Strooper B. Variance in the identification of microRNAs deregulated in Alzheimer's disease and possible role of lincRNAs in the pathology: the need of larger datasets. Ageing Res Rev. 2014;17:43–53.
18. Ulitsky I, Bartel DP. lincRNAs: genomics, evolution, and mechanisms. Cell. 2013;154:26–46.
19. Kowalczyk MS, Higgs DR, Gingeras TR. Molecular biology: RNA discrimination. Nature. 2012;482:310–1.
20. Faghihi MA, Modarresi F, Khalil AM, Wood DE, Sahagan BG, Morgan TE, et al. Expression of a noncoding RNA is elevated in Alzheimer's disease and

drives rapid feed-forward regulation of beta-secretase. Nat Med. 2008;14:723–30.

21. Bennett DA, Schneider JA, Arvanitakis Z, Kelly JF, Aggarwal NT, Shah RC, et al. Neuropathology of older persons without cognitive impairment from two community-based studies. Neurology. 2006;66:1837–44.
22. Yu L, De Jager PL, Yang J, Trojanowski JQ, Bennett DA, Schneider JA. The TMEM106B locus and TDP-43 pathology in older persons without FTLD. Neurology. 2015;84:927–34.
23. Yu L, Chibnik LB, Srivastava GP, Pochet N, Yang J, Xu J, et al. Association of Brain DNA methylation in SORL1, ABCA7, HLA-DRB5, SLC24A4, and BIN1 with pathological diagnosis of Alzheimer disease. JAMA neurology. 2015;72:15–24.
24. Johnson WE, Li C, Rabinovic A: Adjusting batch effects in microarray expression data using empirical Bayes methods. Biostatistics (Oxford, England) 2007, 8:118–127.
25. Lim AS, Srivastava GP, Yu L, Chibnik LB, Xu J, Buchman AS, et al. 24-hour rhythms of DNA methylation and their relation with rhythms of RNA expression in the human dorsolateral prefrontal cortex. PLoS Genet. 2014;10
26. Langmead B, Trapnell C, Pop M, Salzberg SL. Ultrafast and memory-efficient alignment of short DNA sequences to the human genome. Genome Biol. 2009;10
27. Cabili MN, Trapnell C, Goff L, Koziol M, Tazon-Vega B, Regev A, et al. Integrative annotation of human large intergenic noncoding RNAs reveals global properties and specific subclasses. Genes Dev. 2011;25:1915–27.
28. Li B, Dewey CN. RSEM: accurate transcript quantification from RNA-Seq data with or without a reference genome. BMC bioinformatics. 2011;12:323.
29. Group TN-RW: Consensus recommendations for the postmortem diagnosis of Alzheimer's disease. The National Institute on Aging, and Reagan Institute Working Group on Diagnostic Criteria for the Neuropathological Assessment of Alzheimer's Disease. Neurobiol Aging 1997, 18:2.
30. Patrick E, Buckley M, Müller S, Lin DM, Yang JYH: Inferring data-specific micro-RNA function through the joint ranking of micro-RNA and pathways from matched micro-RNA and gene expression data. Bioinformatics. 2015:btv220.
31. Garcia DM, Baek D, Shin C, Bell GW, Grimson A, Bartel DP. Weak seed-pairing stability and high target-site abundance decrease the proficiency of lsy-6 and other microRNAs. Nat Struct Mol Biol. 2011;18:1139–46.
32. Ashburner M, Ball CA, Blake JA, Botstein D, Butler H, Cherry JM, Davis AP, Dolinski K, Dwight SS, Eppig JT, et al: Gene ontology: tool for the unification of biology. The Gene ontology consortium. Nat Genet 2000, 25:25–29.
33. Bennett DA, Schneider JA, Arvanitakis Z, Wilson RS. Overview and findings from the religious orders study. Curr Alzheimer Res. 2012;9:628–45.
34. Bennett DA, Schneider JA, Buchman AS, Barnes LL, Boyle PA, Wilson RS. Overview and findings from the rush memory and aging project. Curr Alzheimer Res. 2012;9:646–63.
35. Ridge PG, Mukherjee S, Crane PK, Kauwe JS. Alzheimer's disease genetics C: Alzheimer's disease: analyzing the missing heritability. PLoS One. 2013;8
36. Lagos D, Pollara G, Henderson S, Gratrix F, Fabani M, Milne RS, et al. miR-132 regulates antiviral innate immunity through suppression of the p300 transcriptional co-activator. Nat Cell Biol. 2010;12:513–9.
37. Ni B, Rajaram MV, Lafuse WP, Landes MB, Schlesinger LS: Mycobacterium tuberculosis decreases human macrophage IFN-γ responsiveness through miR-132 and miR-26a. Journal of immunology (Baltimore, Md: 1950). 2014, 193:4537–4547.
38. Goodall EF, Heath PR, Bandmann O, Kirby J, Shaw PJ. Neuronal dark matter: the emerging role of microRNAs in neurodegeneration. Front Cell Neurosci. 2013;7:178.
39. Salta E, Sierksma A, Vanden Eynden E, De Strooper B. miR-132 loss de-represses ITPKB and aggravates amyloid and TAU pathology in Alzheimer's brain. EMBO molecular medicine. 2016;
40. Frost B, Hemberg M, Lewis J, Feany MB. Tau promotes neurodegeneration through global chromatin relaxation. Nat Neurosci. 2014;17:357–66.
41. Lu T, Aron L, Zullo J, Pan Y, Kim H, Chen Y, et al. REST and stress resistance in ageing and Alzheimer's disease. Nature. 2014;507:448–54.

2

Cerebrospinal fluid Presenilin-1 increases at asymptomatic stage in genetically determined Alzheimer's disease

Aitana Sogorb-Esteve[1,2], María-Salud García-Ayllón[1,2,3*], Juan Fortea[2,4,5], Raquel Sánchez-Valle[6], Alberto Lleó[2,4], José-Luis Molinuevo[6] and Javier Sáez-Valero[1,2*]

Abstract

Background: Presenilin-1 (PS1), the active component of the intramembrane γ-secretase complex, can be detected as soluble heteromeric aggregates in cerebrospinal fluid (CSF). The aim of this study was to examine the different soluble PS1 complexes in the lumbar CSF (CSF-PS1) of individuals with Alzheimer's disease (AD), particularly in both symptomatic and asymptomatic genetically determined AD, in order to evaluate their potential as early biomarkers.

Methods: Western blotting, differential centrifugation and co-immunoprecipitation served to determine and characterize CSF-PS1 complexes. We also monitored the assembly of soluble PS1 into complexes in a cell model, and the participation of Aβ in the dynamics and robustness of the stable PS1 complexes.

Results: There was an age-dependent increase in CSF-PS1 levels in cognitively normal controls, the different complexes represented in similar proportions. The total levels of CSF-PS1, and in particular the proportion of the stable 100–150 kDa complexes, increased in subjects with autosomal dominant AD that carried *PSEN1* mutations (eight symptomatic and six asymptomatic ADAD) and in Down syndrome individuals (ten demented and ten non-demented DS), compared with age-matched controls ($n = 23$), even prior to the appearance of symptoms of dementia. The proportion of stable CSF-PS1 complexes also increased in sporadic AD ($n = 13$) and mild-cognitive impaired subjects ($n = 12$), relative to age-matched controls ($n = 17$). Co-immunoprecipitation demonstrated the association of Aβ oligomers with soluble PS1 complexes, particularly the stable complexes.

Conclusions: Our data suggest that CSF-PS1 complexes may be useful as an early biomarker for AD, reflecting the pathology at asymptomatic state.

Keywords: Presenilin-1, Cerebrospinal fluid, Biomarker, Pre-symptomatic, Autosomal dominant Alzheimer's disease, Down syndrome, Mild-cognitive impairment

Background

Alzheimer's disease (AD) is a progressive neurodegenerative disorder that involves a gradual decline in memory and other cognitive functions, representing the most common cause of dementia in the elderly. Apart from the common late-onset forms of sporadic AD (sAD), rare mutations in the genes encoding the β-amyloid precursor protein (*APP*; chromosome 21q21), presenilin-1 (*PSEN1*; chromosome 14q24.3) and presenilin-2 (*PSEN2*; chromosome 1q31-q42) cause autosomal dominant AD (ADAD; also named as familial AD or FAD) [1]. ADAD exhibits similar phenotype as sAD but with an earlier clinical onset. The *APP* gene encodes a large type I transmembrane protein that upon proteolytic processing [2] can generate the β-amyloid peptide (Aβ), the major constituent of senile plaques and the triggering effector of AD. In the amyloidogenic pathway the Aβ peptide is generated by sequential cleavage of APP, starting with the cleavage of the large extracellular domain by the β-secretase cleaving enzyme (BACE1), which is followed by the successive action of γ-secretase at the membrane-spanning domain [3]. This γ-secretase is an intramembrane

* Correspondence: ms.garcia@umh.es; j.saez@umh.es
[1]Instituto de Neurociencias de Alicante, Universidad Miguel Hernández-CSIC, 03550, Av. Ramón y Cajal s/n, Sant Joan d'Alacant E-03550, Spain
Full list of author information is available at the end of the article

protease complex composed of presenilin-1 (PS1), nicastrin, APH1 (anterior pharynx-defective 1) and PEN2 (presenilin enhancer 2) [4]. PS1 is the catalytic subunit of the γ-secretase complex [5]. Duplications of APP and neighboring sequences are also linked to an early age of AD onset [6]. As such, Down's syndrome (DS) is also associated with the development of AD since the APP gene lies on chromosome 21, and the extra copy leads to Aβ over-expression. Accordingly, most DS patients who live beyond the age of 40 years develop typical brain neuropathology AD and a significant proportion develop additional cognitive decline [7–9]. Thus, both these disease conditions, ADAD and DS, can be considered as early-onset forms of genetically determined AD [10].

Classic biomarkers, total and phospho-tau, as well as Aβ42, have shown diagnostic accuracy for incipient AD [11]. However total and phospho-tau also increased as a result of other neurological processes; while levels of the pathological Aβ42 species, which increased in the AD brain, resulted decreased in CSF due to increasing deposition, hindering the interpretation of changes in their soluble levels in early stages. Thus, there is still a need to identify additional early biomarkers. We recently demonstrated the presence of heteromeric PS1 complexes in human CSF (CSF-PS1) and serum, and that increases in the proportion of stable CSF-PS1 complexes served to discriminate sAD from non-disease controls [12]. PS1 is known to undergo endoproteolytic cleavage as part of its maturation, generating N- and C-terminal fragments (NTF and CTF) of about 29 and 20 kDa, respectively [13]. Both, the NTF and CTF of PS1 contain several transmembrane domains [14]; and our earlier data indicated that PS1 fragments might be highly unstable in CSF and serum, and that they spontaneously form complexes due to the large number of hydrophobic regions. Indeed, we demonstrated the presence of stable 100–150 kDa heteromeric complexes in CSF that contained the NTF and CTF of PS1 (maybe also involving other γ-secretase components), as well other large complexes. Some of these complexes were unstable under denaturing conditions and resolved as ~50 kDa heterodimers upon electrophoresis [12]. Moreover, an increase in the proportion of stable 100–150 kDa complexes appears to be a good marker to discriminate pathological AD samples from controls.

As such, we set out to further characterize these soluble PS1 complexes and the involvement of oligomeric Aβ in the formation of these complexes. We also evaluated the possibility that the proportions and nature of the CSF-PS1 complexes may vary during aging. The main interest was to investigate the levels of CSF-PS1 complexes in ADAD, sAD and DS, particularly in AD and DS subjects who had not yet developed dementia, including also mild-cognitive impaired (MCI) subjects. Thereby, we attempt to determine whether alterations to the levels of these complexes might reflect the pathological state at early, asymptomatic stages. Using a collection of well-characterized CSF samples from sAD PS1 complexes were also analyzed. Genetically determined AD offers unique opportunities to analyze diagnostic biomarkers at asymptomatic stages, particularly given that only in this group is a diagnosis guaranteed for the early comparison of biomarkers.

Methods

Patients

Lumbar CSF samples were obtained from ADAD subject that were all carriers of *PSEN1* mutations and who were part of the Genetic Counseling Program (PICOGEN) at the Hospital Clínic, Barcelona [15]. This group included 14 subjects carrying PSEN1 mutations (including six asymptomatic mutation carriers), and eight age-matched non-mutation carriers from the same families (younger non-disease controls: yNC). The clinical and CSF data of some of these patients has been reported previously [16, 17]. We also included lumbar CSF samples from 10 DS subjects with Alzheimer's type dementia (dDS) and 10 DS subjects without signs of memory decline (ndDS) obtained at the Hospital Sant Pau, Barcelona, along with 15 additional age-matched yNC obtained from both hospitals. In addition, 15 patients with dementia due to sAD, 12 subjects with MCI and 17 age-matched elderly controls (eNC) were also obtained from the Hospital Sant Pau, Barcelona. See Table 1 for details of clinical and demographic data. All AD patients fulfilled the 2011 NIA-AA criteria for dementia or MCI due to AD [18, 19], while discrimination between the dDS subjects and those without dementia was assessed using the modified Cued Recall Test and the CAMDEX-DS battery [20, 21]. All the control subjects had no history or symptoms of neurological or psychiatric disorders, or memory complaints. This study was approved by the ethics committee at the Miguel Hernandez University and it was carried out in accordance with the Declaration of Helsinki.

PS1 over-expressing cells silencing by siRNA

CHO cells (400,000 cells/well) were grown in DMEM® (Gibco) containing 10 % Fetal Bovine Serum (Gibco) and 1 % Penicillin/Streptomycin (Sigma-Aldrich), and they were transfected with a construct encoding full-length PS1 (2 μg cDNA) [22] or with the pcDNA3 expression plasmid alone (Invitrogen), using Lipofectamine 2000® (Invitrogen). To reduce the PS1 gene expression we used CHO cells stably over expressing wild-type human PS1 and APP (CHO-PS1/APP) [23]. CHO-PS1/APP cells (350,000 cells/well) were grown in DMEM® containing 10 % Fetal Bovine Serum, 0,1 % Puromicin (Sigma-

Table 1 Clinical, demographic data and classic CSF biomarker levels

Group	Age (years)	n (Gender)	MMSE score	CSF Aβ42 (pg/mL)	CSF T-tau (pg/mL)	CSF P-tau (pg/mL)
yNC {yNC member of the same ADAD families}	45 ± 2 [25–60] {37 ± 3 [25–47]}	n = 23 (15 F/8 M) {6 F/2 M}	29 ± 1 [25–30] {29 ± 1 [28–30]}	809 ± 44 {791 ± 84}	207 ± 15 {231 ± 29}	43 ± 3 {45 ± 11}
syADAD	45 ± 3 [31–59]	n = 8 (5 F/3 M)	21 ± 2* [11–28]	300 ± 54*	899 ± 186*	164 ± 60*
psADAD	36 ± 3 [24–41]	n = 6 (4 F/2 M)	30 ± 1 [29, 30]	1120 ± 252	222 ± 26	49 ± 5
dDS	55 ± 2 [43–61]	n = 10 (5 F/5 M)	ND	411 ± 24*	788 ± 125*,a	106 ± 14*,a
ndDS	43 ± 2 [33–49]	n = 10 (5 F/5 M)	ND	570 ± 51*	232 ± 53	45 ± 8
eNC	67 ± 1 [61–80]	n = 17 (11 F/6 M)	29 ± 1 [26–30]	753 ± 30	197 ± 12	42 ± 2
sAD	68 ± 2 [54–83]	n = 13 (9 F/4 M)	20 ± 1** [18–24]	351 ± 17**	833 ± 87**	135 ± 18**
MCI due to AD	66 ± 1 [61–72]	n = 12 (5 F/7 M	26 ± 1** [20–30]	422 ± 31	618 ± 66**	81 ± 8**

In the yNC group (younger controls), the values for the control subgroup of non-mutation carriers from the same families as the carriers of *PSEN1* mutations are also indicated; the rest of cases correspond to subject without family history of ADAD. The *PSEN1* mutations included in this study from syADAD cases ("symptomatic" autosomal dominant AD subjects) corresponded to 3 carriers of L286P, and one of I439S, S169P, L173F, L235R and L282R. Those psADAD subjects (pre-symptomatic subjects carrying mutations in *PSEN1*) were 3 carriers of M139T, and one of I439S, R220G and K239N. Patients with (dDS) or without (ndDS) signs of clinical dementia were also compared with yNC; sporadic AD (sAD) and mild-cognitive impaired (MCI) subjects were compared with elderly controls (eNC). Levels of Aβ42, T-tau and P-tau were determined by ELISA; the intra-assay coefficient of variability (CV) was below 5 % and inter-assay CV below 15 % for all the classical AD biomarkers, in agreement with previous reports [36]. The number of samples "n" for female (F) and male (M) subjects is indicated. The data represent the means ± SEM, and for age and MMSE (Minimental State Examination), the range of values is also indicated. *Significantly different (p <0.05) from the yNC group, [a]and from the ndDS group; **Significantly different (p <0.05) from the eNC group

Aldrich) and 0,2 % G418 disulfate salt (Sigma-Aldrich), were transfected with BLOCK iT™ Alexa Fluor® Red Fluorescent Oligo (Invitrogen) as control, or siRNA (50 nM) targeting human PS1 (Santa Cruz Biotechnology, INC). Without removing the cell media, 24 h after the first transfection cells were transfected with the same siRNA (30 nM) and incubated for an additional 18 h.

Western blotting and immunoprecipitation

Although the denaturation temperature prior to electrophoresis has not been standardized, we found that high temperature sample preparation for electrophoresis (98 °C) produced an overall loss of CSF-PS1 immunoreactivity [24]. Hence, all analyses of in this study PS1 avoided freeze-thaw cycles (samples were aliquoted), and denaturation prior to electrophoresis was conducted at 50 °C.

Samples (30 μL for CSF) were resolved by sodium dodecyl sulfate-polyacrylamide gel electrophoresis (SDS-PAGE) under reducing conditions. The proteins were then transferred to nitrocellulose membranes (Schleicher and Schuell Bioscience GmbH) that were probed with PS1 antibodies directed against the N-terminal amino acids 1–20 (antibody 98/1) [24]. GAPDH (Abcam) served as a loading control for cellular extracts. Membranes were incubated with the corresponding horseradish peroxidase conjugated secondary antibody and the immunoreactive signal was detected in a Luminescent Image Analyzer LAS-1000 Plus (FUJIFILM) using SuperSignal West Dura Extended Duration Substrate (Thermo Scientific). A control CSF sample was used to normalize the immunoreactive signal, and for semi-quantitative studies the intensity of the immunoreactive bands was measured by densitometry using Science Lab Image Gauge v 4.0 software provided by FUJIFILM. Aβ peptides in CSF immunoprecipitates (see below) were resolved by 16 % Tris-tricine SDS-PAGE and detected with the 6E10 antibody (Covance Research).

For immunoprecipitation, samples were precleared for 2 h at 4 °C by incubation with protein A-Sepharose (Sigma-Aldrich). Immunoprecipitations were performed at 4 °C by incubating 150 μL of CSF or cell media, overnight with the primary PS1 C-terminal antibody 00/2 (raised against residues 301–317) [23] previously coupled to protein A-Sepharose using Dimethyl pimelimidate dihydrochloride (Sigma-Aldrich Co). Precipitated proteins were washed with PBS and eluted with 0.1 M glycine buffer at pH 2.5. After pH neutralization, supernatants were denatured in Laemmli sample buffer at 50 °C for 15 min and subjected to SDS-PAGE. The membranes were then probed with anti-PS1 (98/1) and anti-Aβ (6E10) antibodies.

Sucrose gradients

PS1 complexes were analyzed by ultracentrifugation for 4 h at 4 °C on a continuous sucrose density gradient (5–20 %) at 250,000 × *g*. CSF aliquots (65 μL) were carefully loaded onto the top of the gradient containing 2 mL of 0.15 M NaCl, 50 mM $MgCl_2$ and 0.5 % Brij 97 in 50 mM Tris-HCl (pH 7.4). After centrifugation, ~14 fractions were collected gently from the top of the tubes. Enzyme markers of known sedimentation coefficient, β-galactosidase, catalase and alkaline phosphatase were used in the gradients to determine the approximate sedimentation coefficients. The sucrose fractions containing highly stable and unstable PS1 complexes were pooled separately, dialyzed against Tris buffer and concentrated by ultrafiltration (Amicon Ultra 10,000 MWCO, Millipore Corporation, Bedford, MA). The PS1 complexes were then immunoprecipitated with anti-PS1 00/2 as described.

Measurement of T-tau, P-tau and Aβ42 by ELISA

The CSF levels of total tau (T-tau), phosphorylated tau (P-tau) and Aβ1-42 (Aβ42) were determined using specific enzyme-linked immunosorbent assays (ELISA: Fujirebio Europe, Ghent, Belgium).

Statistical analysis

All data were analyzed using SigmaStat (Version 3.5; Systac Software Inc.), applying a one-way analysis of variance or a Kruskal-Wallis test when the hypothesis of equality of sample variances was rejected. Pairwise group comparisons were then sustained using Student t test (two-tailed) or Mann-Whitney U test, and the exact p values determined. The results are presented as the means ± SEM, and correlations between the variables were assessed by linear regression analyses, with p values <0.05 considered statistically significant.

Results

The increase in CSF-PS1 with age

Since the main aim of the present study was to determine the changes in CSF-PS1 associated with ADAD and DS, and given that both ADAD and DS exhibits earlier clinical onset, we first assessed whether the amount and nature of the soluble PS1 complexes varies with age. The PS1 complexes in samples from control subjects (NC) from 25 to 80 years-of-age were detected with the 98/1 antibody, which predominantly recognized complexes of approximately 100 and 150 kDa, together with a less abundant 50 kDa band (Fig. 1a). The identity of these bands as complexes involving NTF- and CTF-PS1 was demonstrated in a previous study [12]. This soluble 50 kDa PS1 band may represent a NTF and CTF-PS1 aggregate, as the holoprotein had a mass of ~43 kDa and it differs in its electrophoretic migration [12]. PS1-NTF monomers are not detectable in human CSF samples. Since ADAD starts prior to 60 years of age [1], we sub-grouped young and elderly NC below and above this threshold. The sum of the immunoreactivity for the major 100 and 150 kDa PS1 complexes was significantly higher (~58 %) in the elderly NC (eNC; $n = 18$) than in the young NC samples (yNC; $n = 19$; p <0.001: Fig. 1b). No differences were found between values obtained from the two center of sample collection. In all the NC samples, the major 100 and 150 kDa PS1 complexes were positively correlated with age ($r = 0.54$; p <0.001: Fig. 1c). Therefore, this age-dependent increase in PS1 complexes must be taken into account when comparing the different pathological groups with non-disease subjects, defining appropriate age-matched controls.

We also attempted to assess potential differences in the class of the PS1 complexes in the NC sub-groups based on the direct analysis of the Western blots. As such, we defined the (100 + 150 kDa)/50 kDa quotient for each sample. No change was observed in the (100 + 150 kDa)/50 kDa quotient evaluated in CSF from yNC and eNC subjects (Fig. 1b).

Higher PS1 levels in symptomatic and asymptomatic ADAD

To assess whether the amount of CSF-PS1 is altered in ADAD, the levels in the age-matched yNC group were compared with those in the CSF from symptomatic (syADAD) and asymptomatic (pre-symptomatic: psADAD) subjects carrying mutations in *PSEN1* in Western blots (see Table 1 and Fig. 2a). Stronger immunoreactivity for the 100 and 150 kDa complexes was evident in syADAD (~119 %; p <0.001) and in psADAD (~87 %; p <0.001) subjects compared to the yNC, with no differences between the two pathological groups (Fig. 2b). Indeed, the levels in these AD subjects were significantly higher than in the yNC sub-group, composed by non-mutation carriers from the same ADAD families (p <0.001). The previously defined quotient of CSF-PS1 complexes (see above) also discriminated between the yNC and the two ADAD groups, both individually ($p = 0.007$ for syADAD; $p = 0.027$ for psADAD) or when considered as a unique pathological group ($p = 0.007$). Thus, a higher proportion of 100 + 150 kDa CSF-PS1 complexes appears to be associated with ADAD even at pre-symptomatic stages (Fig. 2b).

PS1 complexes can be also characterized by gradient ultracentrifugation [24], followed by Western blotting under denaturing conditions, which served to illustrate the existence of different CSF-PS1 complexes [12]. When, CSF-PS1 complexes from yNC and syADAD subjects were characterized by sedimentation analysis on sucrose density gradients (Fig. 2c), 100–150 kDa PS1 complexes were identified close to the alkaline phosphatase marker (~140–160 kDa), along with larger complexes that sedimented in regions closer to the catalase marker (~232 kDa). These latter complexes were unstable and resolved as 50 kDa peptides by SDS-PAGE/Western blot analysis (Fig. 2c). In good agreement with results with the CSF-PS1 complex quotient obtained for direct Western blot analysis, samples separated by ultracentrifugation revealed higher abundance of the highly stable 100–150 kDa PS1 complexes in the syADAD samples than in the yNC samples, more so than the complexes of the 50 kDa fragments that sedimented in the denser fractions. This difference was clearly evident with the determination of a refined quotient, the "stability" quotient, reflecting the differences between the

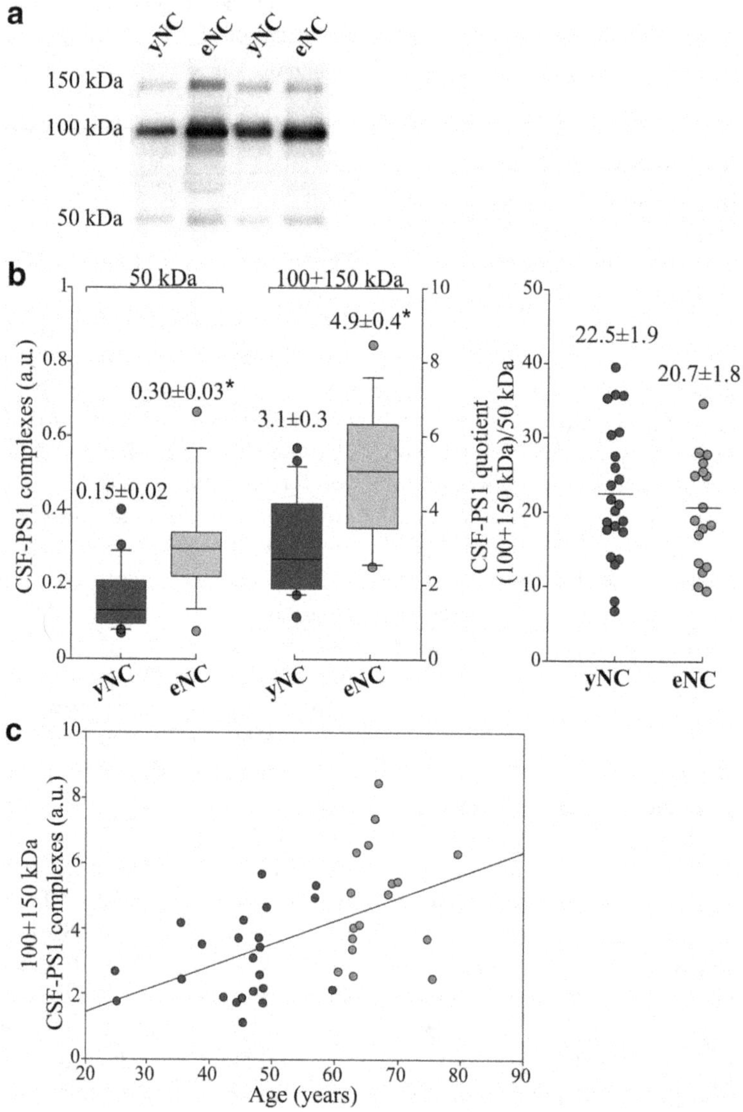

Fig. 1 Characterization of the CSF-PS1 complexes in younger and elderly NC subjects, and their correlation with age. **a** Representative Western blots of human CSF samples from non-demented control (NC) subjects arbitrarily categorized as young (yNC; ≤60 years; $n = 23$) and elderly (eNC; >60 years; $n = 17$), and probed with an anti-NTF-PS1 antibody. **b** Densitometric quantification of the major 100 and 150 kDa CSF-PS1 complexes (the sum of the 100 + 150 kDa CSF-PS1 bands) and the quotient derived from the immunoreactivity for the 100 and 150 kDa bands relative to that for the minor 50 kDa band in each sample [(100 + 150 kDa)/50 kDa]. The data represent the means ± SEM and they were compared using a paired Students t test: $^*p < 0.001$. **c** Correlation between the levels of the 100 + 150 kDa CSF-PS1 complexes with age

highly stable complexes (the 100–150 kDa heterodimers that sediment close to the internal marker of similar molecular mass) and the unstable complexes (the 50 kDa complexes that sediment closer to catalase), this quotient allowing us to discriminate syADAD ($p = 0.004$) from yNC samples (Fig. 2d).

Highly stable CSF-PS1 complexes are elevated in sAD and MCI

In sAD no notable differences in total PS1 were observed between patients with dementia due to sAD, MCI due to AD, or age-matched eNC subjects (Fig. 3a, b). However, the highly stable PS1 complexes were again more abundant in probable sAD cases compared to elderly eNCs when the CSF-PS1 complexes quotient was calculated ($p = 0.006$; Fig. 3b). Sucrose density centrifugation profiles (Fig. 3c) and the subsequent estimation of the "stability" quotient confirmed the greater abundance of highly stable PS1 complexes in sAD compared to eNC ($p = 0.02$; Fig. 3d), as well as indicating that the highly stable complexes were particularly increased in MCI subjects ($p = 0.008$; Fig. 3d).

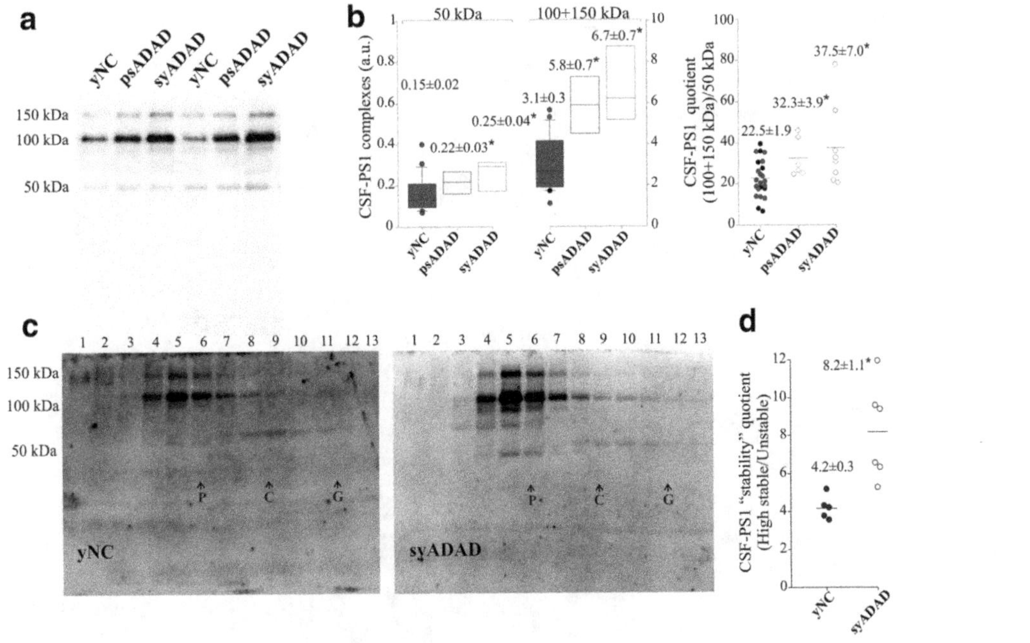

Fig. 2 The increase in the CSF-PS1 complexes in ADAD. **a** Representative blot of the PS1 complexes in the CSF samples from eight symptomatic ADAD (syADAD), six presymptomatic mutation carriers (psADAD) and 23 younger NC controls (yNC), eight of which were from the same families a the ADAD subjects but that did not carry mutations (black symbol; see also Table 1). **b** Densitometric quantification of the accumulative immunoreactivity from the sum of the higher molecular mass PS1 complex (100 + 150 kDa). A quotient was calculated for each sample defined as the sum of (100 + 150 kDa) immunoreactivity relative to the 50 kDa immunoreactivity: (100 + 150 kDa/50 kDa). **c** Six syADAD and five yNC samples were fractionated on 5–20 % sucrose density gradients to further characterize the PS1 complexes. The fractions (collected from the top of each tube) were immunoblotted under denaturing conditions and probed for PS1, as in (**a**). β-Galactosidase (G, 16.0S; ~540 kDa), catalase (C, 11.4S; ~232 kDa) and alkaline phosphatase (P, 6.1S; ~140–160 kDa) were used as internal markers. Representative blots are shown. **d** The "stability" quotient was defined as the sum of the stable immunoreactive bands that sediment close to alkaline phosphatase (~140–160 kDa; fractions 2–7), mainly the 100 and 150 kDa bands, relative to the large unstable complexes that sediment closer to catalase (~232 kDa; fractions 8–12), and resolve mainly as 50 kDa immunoreactive bands in Western blots. The data are the means ± SEM: *Significantly different (p <0.005) from the yNC group as assessed by the Student t or Mann-Whitney U tests

Higher PS1 levels in demented and non-demented DS

DS is considered a pre-symptomatic AD [10]. To assess whether an increase in the CSF-PS1 complexes is also associated with DS, we analyzed CSF samples from DS patients with (dDS) or without (ndDS) signs of clinical dementia, comparing these to age-matched yNC (Fig. 4a). The cumulative immunoreactivity of the major 100 and 150 kDa bands was significantly higher in both dDS (p <0.001) and ndDS ($p = 0.007$) CSF than in that from yNC subjects (Fig. 4b). Remarkably, the CSF-PS1 complexes quotient also revealed consistent changes in the proportion of the different complexes for both dDS (p <0.001) and ndDS subjects ($p = 0.04$) relative to yNC (Fig. 4b).

The formation of stable CSF-PS1 complexes is favored by β-amyloid

Although PS1 clearly forms native complexes in CSF, there is little knowledge about the dynamics of soluble PS1 fragment assembly into heteromeric complexes. Thus, we monitored the assembly of soluble PS1 into complexes in a cell model, CHO cells over-expressing wild-type human PS1. An increase in the 29 kDa NTF of PS1 in extracts from CHO cells transfected with human PS1 corroborated that these cells over-expressed the protein (Additional file 1: Figure S1A). Immunoblotting of the cell-conditioned medium revealed predominant bands of approximately 100 and 150 kDa, and a weaker ~70 kDa band. The amounts of these soluble PS1 complexes increased in conditioned media from CHO cells transfected with PS1 (Additional file 1: Figure S1A). CHO cells stably transfected with PS1 and APP showed similar soluble PS1 complexes with additional 50 kDa band and monomeric NTF (Additional file 1: Figure S1A). To ascertain the identity of the soluble PS1 complexes in the cellular model, we reduced PS1 expression in CHO cells stably over expressing wild-type human PS1 with siRNA PS1. Cells transfected with siRNA PS1 displayed decrease in cellular PS1-NTF, but also in soluble PS1 complexes identified in cell media (Additional file 1: Figure S1A).

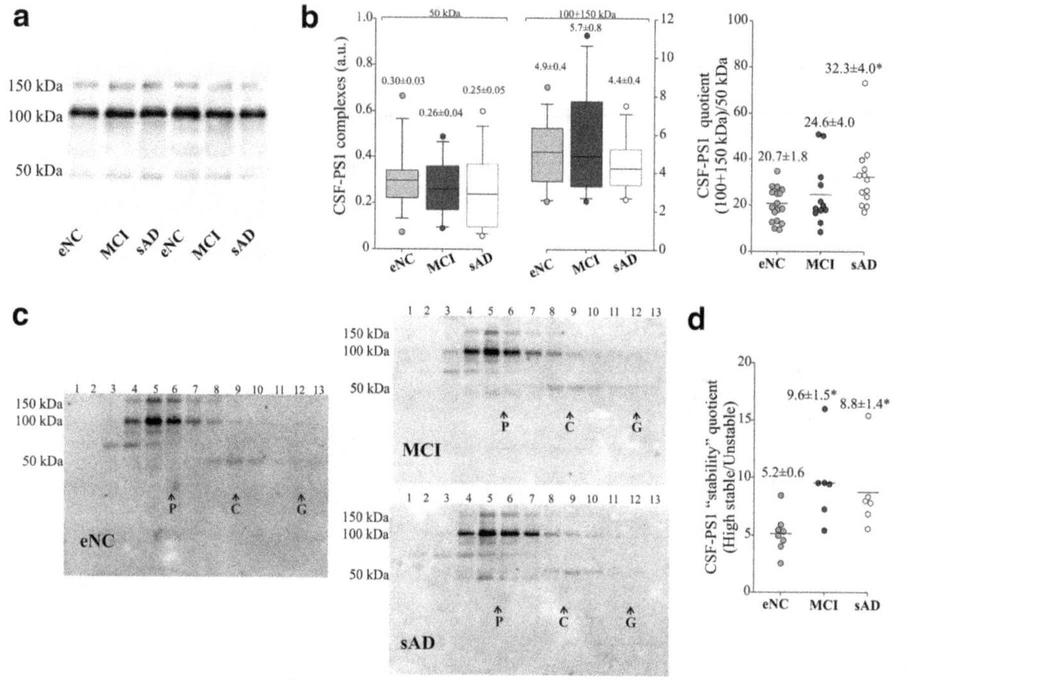

Fig. 3 Increase in the stable PS1 complexes in AD and MCI CSF. **a** Representative blot and (**b**) densitometric quantification of the accumulative immunoreactivity from the sum of stable higher molecular mass PS1 complexes (100 + 150 kDa) in CSF samples from 13 sAD, 12 MCI and 17 age-matched eNC subjects. A quotient calculated as the sum of (100 + 150 kDa) immunoreactivity relative to the 50 kDa immunoreactivity: (100 + 150 kDa/50 kDa) is also shown. **c** Six AD and MCI individuals, and 8 eNC subjects were fractionated on 5–20 % sucrose density gradients, and probed with the PS1 antibody under denaturing conditions. The internal markers were β-galactosidase (G), catalase (C) and alkaline phosphatase (P), as in Fig. 3. **d** The values for the "stability" quotient reflecting the highly stable complexes (100 + 150 kDa immunoreactive bands sedimenting in fractions 2–7) relative to the unstable complexes (50 kDa immunoreactive bands sedimenting in fractions 8–12) is also shown. **p* <0.05, ***p* <0.01 as assessed by the Student *t* or Mann-Whitney U tests

We also analyzed the soluble PS1 complexes in the conditioned medium of PS1-transfected CHO cells and CHO cells over-expressing PS1 and APP, using sucrose-density gradient fractionation followed by Western blotting under denaturing conditions (Additional file 1: Figure S1B). The majority of the soluble PS1 in the CHO cell-conditioned medium accumulated close to the alkaline phosphatase marker (~140–160 kDa) and resolved as 70 kDa complexes after denaturation, with only faint bands at 100 kDa. However, some 29 kDa monomeric PS1 was also evident, probably released from the complexes (Additional file 1: Figure S1B). By contrast, in the medium of CHO cells over-expressing PS1 and APP there was virtually no 29 kDa NTF immunoreactivity, indicating that in the context of β-amyloid over-expression, most of the soluble PS1 is stably incorporated into complexes (Additional file 1: Figure S1B).

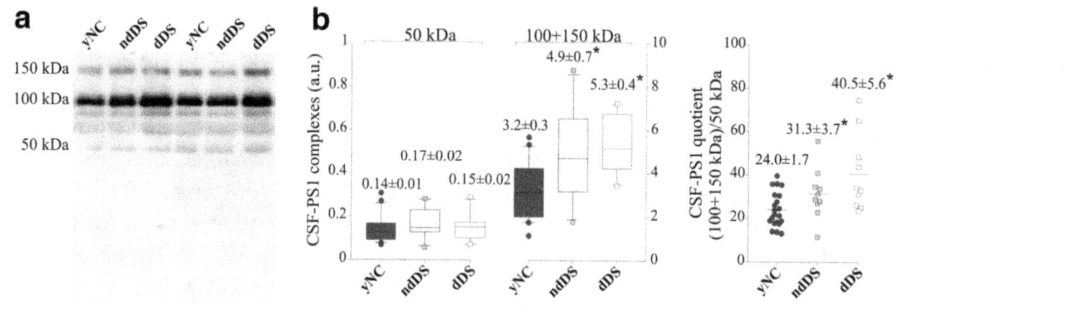

Fig. 4 An increase in PS1 stable complexes in DS CSF. **a** Representative blot of PS1 complexes in CSF from 10 DS subjects with dementia of the Alzheimer's type (dDS), 10 DS without any sign of memory decline (ndDS) and 23 yNC. **b** Densitometric quantification of the accumulated immunoreactivity from the sum of the higher molecular mass PS1 complex (100 + 150 kDa), and the quotient of the (100 + 150 kDa) immunoreactivity relative to the 50 kDa immunoreactivity (100 + 150 kDa/50 kDa). The means ± SEM are shown: **p* <0.005, ***p* <0.005, Student *t* test

We further tested the possible interaction between soluble PS1 complexes and Aβ. PS1 was immunoprecipitated from the medium of CHO cells over-expressing PS1 and APP with the 00/2 antibody that recognizes the PS1 CTF. Immunoprecipitation of heteromeric PS1 complexes was confirmed in Western blots probed with the anti-N-terminal 98/1 antibody (Additional file 1: Figure S1C). Considerable amounts of Aβ oligomers were also detected in these immunoprecipitates by the 6E10 antibody (Additional file 1: Figure S1C), while no immunoreactivity was resolved by a C-terminal APP antibody (not shown); indicating that oligomers of Aβ, but not C-terminal fragments, interact with the soluble PS1 complexes.

To confirm that Aβ oligomers favors the formation of stable PS1 complexes in human CSF we examined the Aβ peptides in PS1 complexes immunoprecipitated from CSF samples from sAD and eNC subjects. Again, CSF samples immunoprecipitated with 00/2 antibody were probed in immunoblots with the 98/1 and 6E10 antibodies (Fig. 5a), demonstrating that Aβ oligomers co-immunoprecipitated with heteromeric PS1 complexes from both eNC and sAD CSF samples. We further tested the involvement of Aβ on the formation of the highly stable PS1 complexes. After CSF-PS1 complexes were fractioned by sucrose density gradients and the peak fractions of the highly stable and unstable complexes were isolated, they were immunoprecipitated with the 00/2 antibody (Fig. 5b). Aβ oligomers were clearly present in the fractions rich in stable 100–150 kDa complexes from both eNC and sAD samples, whereas

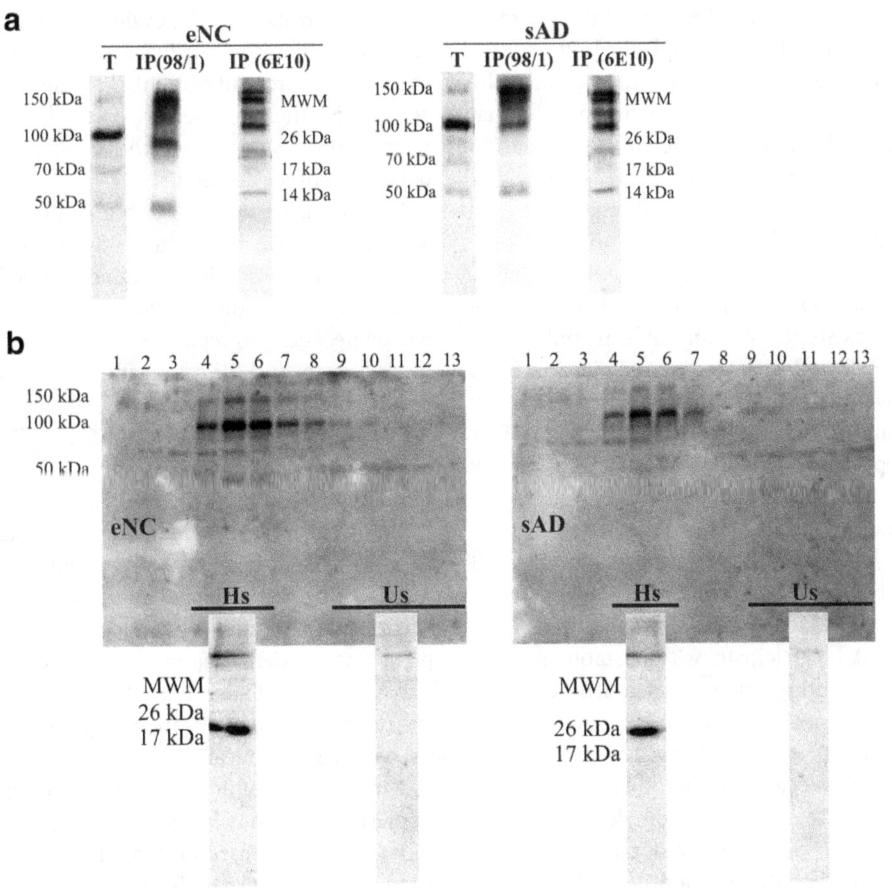

Fig. 5 Aβ oligomers are present in highly stable CSF-PS1 complexes. **a** CSF samples from eNC and sAD subjects were precleared with protein A-Sepharose (T: total), and then immunoprecipitated with the anti CTF-PS1 00/2 antibody. The precipitated proteins (IP) were probed in immunoblots with the antibody indicated (98/1 for NTF-PS1 and 6E10 for Aβ). Note that oligomeric Aβ species co-immunoprecipitate and interact with CSF-PS1 complexes in both eNC and sAD. None immunoreactivity was resolved in negative controls incubated with beads in the absence of antibody (not shown). **b** CSF-PS1 complexes were fractionated by sucrose gradient centrifugation, and the fractions containing highly stable (Hs) or unstable (Us) PS1 complexes were pooled, dialyzed and concentrated by ultrafiltration. Representative sedimentation profiles illustrate the fractions selected for peak isolation. The enriched CSF-PS1 complexes were then immunoprecipitated with the 00/2 antibody and assayed in immunoblots probed with the 6E10 antibody against Aβ (insert). Representative blots reveal that Aβ oligomers are mainly present in peak fractions containing highly stable PS1 complexes (illustrative examples from two different experiments)

virtually no Aβ immunoreactivity was detected in the pooled fractions of 50 kDa PS1 complexes (Fig. 5b). Hence, oligomers of Aβ appear to mainly associate with the highly stable PS1 complexes.

Discussion

The detection of soluble PS1 in CSF and serum [12] was a somewhat unexpected finding, particularly since PS1 is a multi-pass transmembrane protein with several hydrophobic regions [14]. Indeed, the presence of soluble PS1 has been reported in the medium of primary neurons [25] and confirmed in human serum [26]. Here, we corroborated the existence of different PS1 complexes in human CSF and we revealed their potential utility as a biomarker for AD. Like many membrane proteins, PS1 has a tendency to aggregate under non-native conditions [27, 28]. Thus, CSF-PS1 complexes probably represent non-specific aggregates of PS1 NTF and CTF distinct to the active γ-secretase membrane-complexes [12].

How PS1 complexes become soluble and appear in the CSF is yet to be determined. However, it appears that Aβ oligomers can probably contribute to the formation of stable CSF-PS1 complexes which are particularly abundant in AD. Indeed, it is remarkable that when we follow the formation of PS1 complexes in the cell-conditioned media, the co-expression of APP and PS1 favored the accumulation of complexes and not soluble monomeric PS1 is existent. We were able to pull down oligomeric Aβ species by PS1 immunoprecipitation from the medium, as well as from human CSF, in which Aβ oligomers are mainly associated to the highly stable PS1 complexes. Aβ peptides are chemically "sticky", gradually building up into fibrils and aggregates; although the mechanism of how can Aβ stabilize CSF-PS1 is yet to be determined. Also in this context, levels of soluble Aβ peptide assessed by ELISA determinations appear consistently decreased in AD CSF [11]. The possibility that some amounts of Aβ participate within stable protein complexes in CSF, resulting underestimated by conventional ELISA protocols, may deserve consideration.

In CSF samples from NC subjects we observe an age-related increase in the total amount of PS1, while the relative proportion of the different complexes remains unaltered. No changes were observed comparing NC samples from different center of sample collection or gender. However, the relative proportion of stable PS1 complexes does appear to increase in the AD condition.

We propose that the most significant phenomenon related to the potential use of CSF-PS1 to discriminate the pathological state is the change in the proportion of PS1 complexes, rather than the estimates of the total PS1 levels. Accordingly, we focused our analysis on the highly stable 100–150 kDa PS1 complexes in CSF. The highly stable CSF-PS1 complexes co-exist with unstable complexes, sedimenting after differential centrifugation in regions closer to 200–250 kDa, but mainly resolved as 50 kDa components by reducing SDS-PAGE. We found that a quotient of PS1 complexes can discriminate all pathological groups from age-matched controls. We suggest that these quotients reflect differences in the properties of the PS1 complexes formed under pathological conditions. Screening large numbers of samples by sucrose gradient ultracentrifugation is difficult. As a reliable alternative, we addressed the discrimination of samples using a complementary parameter, a quotient of CSF-PS1 complexes calculated directly from Western blot analysis [(100 + 150 kDa)/50 kDa], thereby simplifying the analysis. This alternative quotient is useful to discriminate ADAD and DS subjects from age-matched yNC, as well as sAD from eNC. In our analysis, this quotient of PS1 complexes only failed to adequately discriminate MCI subjects, maybe indicating a lack of sensibility with respect to the evaluation of the complexes after separation by ultracentrifugation in sucrose density gradients. The inherent uncertainty in clinical diagnosis may also account for these differences, particularly for MCI group in which some subjects maybe remained MCI stable or develop to other dementias.

Anyhow, large overlap is observed between groups when assessment of the relative amount of CSF-PS1 complexes is estimated by a quotient obtained directly from Western blot analysis, without fractioning by ultracentrifugation. It will be necessary to replicate these finding using other techniques, such as ELISA specific for stable CSF-PS1 complexes, to evaluate their true potential as biomarkers.

Interestingly, altered levels of CSF-PS1 are detectable in both symptomatic and asymptomatic ADAD subjects. Similarly, alterations to CSF-PS1 levels occur in DS subjects with and without dementia. The analysis of CSF samples from DS subjects is of particular interest since it is well known that almost all adults with DS over 40 years of age display AD neuropathology [29, 30], although the prevalence of dementia in these individuals varies considerably [31–34]. Thus, there is no association between the age of onset of AD neuropathology in DS subjects and the appearance of clinical dementia [35], and we cannot predict the number of ndDS that will develop future cognitive impairment. In the view of the consistent changes in CSF-PS1 in ndDS we assume that this biomarker is more related to the brain pathological status than the occurrence of dementia and cognitive decline.

Conclusions

In conclusion, our present findings demonstrate that CSF-PS1 complexes are altered in genetically determined AD, as well as in sAD. Together, our results indicate that the increase in stable PS1 complexes in CSF is an early phenomenon associated to AD pathology and may constitute an asymptomatic biomarker.

Additional file

Additional file 1: Figure S1. Aβ affects the dynamics and stability of the soluble PS1 complexes. (**A**) CHO cell were transfected with human PS1 or with the pcDNA3 expression plasmid as a control (Ø). CHO cells stably over-expressing PS1 and APP were also transfected with PS1 siRNA. PS1 in the cell extracts and soluble PS1 complexes in the medium were assayed in Western blots using a NTF-PS1 antibody (equivalent amounts of protein of the cell extracts and equal volumes of medium were loaded in each lane). GAPDH served as a loading control for cellular extracts. (**B**) Soluble PS1 complexes from the medium conditioned by CHO cells transfected with PS1 (CHO-PS1), or CHO cells over-expressing PS1 and APP (CHO-PS1/APP), characterized by ultracentrifugation on 5–20 % sucrose density gradients. Fractions were collected from the top of each tube and they were analyzed by SDS-PAGE under denaturing conditions. Enzymes of known sedimentation coefficient were used as internal markers: β-galactosidase (G, 16.0S; molecular mass ~540 kDa), catalase (C, 11.4S; ~232 kDa) and alkaline phosphatase (P, 6.1S; ~140–160 kDa). Note that both PS1 complexes and 29 kDa monomers were identified in CHO-PS1 cells, while the 29 kDa monomers are mostly absent from the CHO-PS1/APP cells. (**C**) Cell medium conditioned by CHO-PS1/APP cells was precleared with protein A-Sepharose and the soluble PS1 complexes were immunoprecipitated with the anti-PS1 antibody 00/2 raised against the CTF. The immunoprecipitated proteins (IP) were probed with the 98/1 antibody against the NTF of PS1 and the 6E10 antibody against Aβ (T: total). The PS1 antibody confirms the immunoprecipitation of heteromeric complexes of PS1 and the 6E10 confirms that these PS1 complexes contain or interact with small Aβ oligomers. Illustrative examples from three different experiments are shown. (TIF 2441 kb)

Abbreviations

AD: Alzheimer's disease; ADAD: Autosomal dominant AD; APP: β-amyloid precursor protein; Aβ: β-amyloid peptide; CSF: Cerebrospinal fluid; CTF: C-terminal fragment of PS1; dDS: DS patients with dementia; DS: Down syndrome; eNC: Elderly NC; MCI: Mild-cognitive impairment; NC: Normal control subjects; ndDS: DS patients without dementia; NTF: N-terminal fragment of PS1; PS1: Presenilin-1; psADAD: Pre-symptomatic ADAD; P-tau: Phosphorylated tau; sAD: Sporadic Alzheimer's disease; syADAD: Symptomatic ADAD; T-tau: Total tau; yNC: Young NC samples

Acknowledgements

We thank Drs J. Culvenor and G. Evin (Department of Pathology, The University of Melbourne, Australia) for the generous gift of the PS1 antibodies; and Dr D. Selkoe, Brigham and Women's Hospital, Boston for providing CHO cells over-expressing human PS1. We also thank Dr J. F. Hernández-Sánchez (Servicio de Análisis Clínicos, Hospital General Universitario de Elche) for assistance in the preliminary assays.

Funding

This study was funded in part by the EU BIOMARKAPD-Joint Programming on Neurodegenerative Diseases (JPND) project, by the Instituto de Salud Carlos III (ISCIII grants PI11/03026 to JSV, PI11/02425 and PI14/01126 to JF, PI11/03035 and PI14/1561 to AL, PI08/0036 and PI12/00013 to RSV, and PI11/03023 to JLM), co-financed by the Fondo Europeo de Desarrollo Regional, under the aegis of JPND, and through CIBERNED, ISCIII. This work was also supported by the Fundació Catalana de Síndrome de Down and by a "Marató TV3" grant (20141210 to JF) and a grant from the Griffols Foundation. The funding bodies played no role in the study design, data collection and analysis, the decision to publish, or the preparation of the manuscript. We also acknowledge the support for the publication fee to the CSIC Open Access Publication Support Initiative through its Unit of Information Resources for Research (URICI).

Authors' contributions

JSV, MSGA, AL and JLM were involved with the conception, design, and interpretation of data. ASE and MSGA performed the experiments. JSV, ASE and MSGA were involved with data analysis. JLM, AL, RSV and JF collected the clinical material. JSV, JLM, AL, RSV and JF provided general overall supervision of the study, and acquired funding. All authors contributed to the drafting and critical revision of the manuscript and have given final approval of the version to be published.

Competing interests

All the authors contributed to this work and are in agreement with the findings presented. MSGA and JSV have submitted a patent application for the use of PS1 complexes as a biomarker for AD, as described herein. Appropriate procedures were followed to obtain approval from local ethics committees.

Author details

[1]Instituto de Neurociencias de Alicante, Universidad Miguel Hernández-CSIC, 03550, Av. Ramón y Cajal s/n, Sant Joan d'Alacant E-03550, Spain. [2]Centro de Investigación Biomédica en Red sobre Enfermedades Neurodegenerativas (CIBERNED), Sant Joan d'Alacant & Barcelona, Spain. [3]Unidad de Investigación, Hospital General Universitario de Elche, FISABIO, 03203 Elche, Spain. [4]Memory Unit, Neurology Department, Hospital de la Santa Creu i Sant Pau, 08026 Barcelona, Spain. [5]Down Medical Center, Fundació Catalana Síndrome de Down, 08029 Barcelona, Spain. [6]Alzheimer's Disease and Other Cognitive Disorders Unit, Neurology Service, Hospital Clinic; Institut d'Investigacions Biomèdiques Agust Pi i Sunyer, 08036 Barcelona, Spain.

References

1. Tanzi RE. The genetics of Alzheimer disease. Cold Spring Harb Perspect Med. 2012;2. doi: 10.1101/cshperspect.a006296.
2. Beyreuther K, Dyrks T, Hilbich C, Mönning U, König G, Multhaup G, Pollwein P, Masters CL. Amyloid precursor protein (APP) and beta A4 amyloid in Alzheimer's disease and Down syndrome. Prog Clin Biol Res. 1992;379:159–82.
3. Thinakaran G, Koo EH. Amyloid precursor protein trafficking, processing, and function. J Biol Chem. 2008;283:29615–9.
4. Kaether C, Haass C, Steiner H. Assembly, trafficking and function of gamma-secretase. Neurodegener Dis. 2006;3:275–83.
5. Yu G, Chen F, Levesque G, Nishimura M, Zhang DM, Levesque L, Rogaeva E, Xu D, Liang Y, Duthie M, St George-Hyslop PH, Fraser PE. The presenilin 1 protein is a component of a high molecular weight intracellular complex that contains beta-catenin. J Biol Chem. 1998;273:16470–5.
6. Guerreiro RJ, Gustafson DR, Hardy J. The genetic architecture of Alzheimer's disease: beyond APP, PSENs and APOE. Neurobiol Aging. 2012;33:437–56.
7. Glenner GG, Wong CW. Alzheimer's disease and Down's syndrome: sharing of a unique cerebrovascular amyloid fibril protein. Biochem Biophys Res Commun. 1984;122:1131–5.
8. Mann DM, Yates PO, Marcyniuk B. Alzheimer's presenile dementia, senile dementia of Alzheimer type and Down's syndrome in middle age form an age related continuum of pathological changes. Neuropathol Appl Neurobiol. 1984;10:185–207.
9. Wisniewski KE, Wisniewski HM, Wen GY. Occurrence of neuropathological changes and dementia of Alzheimer's disease in Down's syndrome. Ann Neurol. 1985;17:278–82.
10. Dubois B, Feldman HH, Jacova C, Hampel H, Molinuevo JL, Blennow K, DeKosky ST, Gauthier S, Selkoe D, Bateman R, Cappa S, Crutch S, Engelborghs S, Frisoni GB, Fox NC, Galasko D, Habert MO, Jicha GA, Nordberg A, Pasquier F, Rabinovici G, Robert P, Rowe C, Salloway S, Sarazin M, Epelbaum S, de Souza LC, Vellas B, Visser PJ, Schneider L, Stern Y, Scheltens P, Cummings JL. Advancing research diagnostic criteria for Alzheimer's disease: the IWG-2 criteria. Lancet Neurol. 2014;13:614–29.
11. Blennow K, Hampel H. CSF markers for incipient Alzheimer's disease. Lancet Neurol. 2003;2:605–13.
12. García-Ayllón MS, Campanari ML, Brinkmalm G, Rábano A, Alom J, Saura CA, Andreasen N, Blennow K, Sáez-Valero J. CSF Presenilin-1 complexes are increased in Alzheimer's disease. Acta Neuropathol Commun. 2013;1:46.
13. Thinakaran G, Borchelt DR, Lee MK, Slunt HH, Spitzer L, Kim G, Ratovitsky T, Davenport F, Nordstedt C, Seeger M, Hardy J, Levey AI, Gandy SE, Jenkins NA, Copeland NG, Price DL, Sisodia SS. Endoproteolysis of presenilin 1 and accumulation of processed derivatives in vivo. Neuron. 1996;17:181–90.
14. Laudon H, Hansson EM, Melén K, Bergman A, Farmery MR, Winblad B, Lendahl U, von Heijne G, Näslund J. A nine-transmembrane domain topology for presenilin 1. J Biol Chem. 2005;280:35352–60.
15. Fortea J, Lladó A, Clarimón J, Lleó A, Oliva R, Peri J, Pintor L, Yagüe J, Blesa R, Molinuevo JL, Sánchez-Valle R. PICOGEN: five years experience with a genetic counselling program for dementia. Neurologia. 2011;26:143–9.

16. Fortea J, Lladó A, Bosch B, Antonell A, Oliva R, Molinuevo JL, Sanchez-Valle R. Cerebrospinal fluid biomarkers in Alzheimer's disease families with PSEN1 mutations. Neurodegener Dis. 2010;8:202–7.
17. Pera M, Alcolea D, Sánchez-Valle R, Guardia-Laguarta C, Colom-Cadena M, Badiola N, Suárez-Calvet M, Lladó A, Barrera-Ocampo AA, Sepulveda-Falla D, Blesa R, Molinuevo JL, Clarimón J, Ferrer I, Gelpi E, Lleó A. Distinct patterns of APP processing in the CNS in autosomal-dominant and sporadic Alzheimer disease. Acta Neuropathol. 2013;125:201–13.
18. McKhann GM, Knopman DS, Chertkow H, Hyman BT, Jr Jack CR, Kawas CH, Klunk WE, Koroshetz WJ, Manly JJ, Mayeux R, Mohs RC, Morris JC, Rossor MN, Scheltens P, Carrillo MC, Thies B, Weintraub S, Phelps CH. The diagnosis of dementia due to Alzheimer's disease: recommendations from the National Institute on Aging-Alzheimer's Association workgroups on diagnostic guidelines for Alzheimer's disease. Alzheimers Dement. 2011;7:263–9.
19. Albert MS, DeKosky ST, Dickson D, Dubois B, Feldman HH, Fox NC, Gamst A, Holtzman DM, Jagust WJ, Petersen RC, Snyder PJ, Carrillo MC, Thies B, Phelps GH. The diagnosis of mild cognitive impairment due to Alzheimer's disease: recommendations from the National Institute on Aging-Alzheimer's Association workgroups on diagnostic guidelines for Alzheimer's disease. Alzheimers Dement. 2011;7:270–9.
20. Benejam B, Fortea J, Molina-López R, Videla S. Patterns of performance on the modified cued recall test in Spanish adults with down syndrome with and without dementia. Am J Intellect Dev Disabil. 2015;120:481–9.
21. Esteba-Castillo S, Dalmau-Bueno A, Ribas-Vidal N, Vilà-Alsina M, Novell-Alsina R, García-Alba J. Adaptation and validation of CAMDEX-DS (Cambridge Examination for Mental Disorders of Older People with Down's Syndrome and others with intellectual disabilities) in Spanish population with intellectual disabilities. Rev Neurol. 2013;57:337–46.
22. Culvenor JG, Maher F, Evin G, Malchiodi-Albedi F, Cappai R, Underwood JR, Davis JB, Karran EH, Roberts GW, Beyreuther K, Masters CL. Alzheimer's disease-associated presenilin 1 in neuronal cells: evidence for localization to the endoplasmic reticulum-Golgi intermediate compartment. J Neurosci Res. 1997;49:719–31.
23. Xia W, Zhang J, Kholodenko D, Citron M, Podlisny MB, Teplow DB, Haass C, Seubert P, Koo EH, Selkoe DJ. Enhanced production and oligomerization of the 42-residue amyloid beta-protein by Chinese hamster ovary cells stably expressing mutant presenilins. J Biol Chem. 1997;272:7977–82.
24. Evin G, Sharples RA, Weidemann A, Reinhard FB, Carbone V, Culvenor JG, Holsinger RM, Sernee MF, Beyreuther K, Masters CL. Aspartyl protease inhibitor pepstatin binds to the presenilins of Alzheimer's disease. Biochemistry. 2001;40:8359–68.
25. Benussi L, Alberici A, Mayhaus M, Langer U, Ghidoni R, Mazzoli F, Nicosia F, Barbiero L, Frisoni G, Zanetti O, Gasparini L, Nitsch RM, Binetti G. Detection of the presenilin 1 COOH-terminal fragment in the extracellular compartment: a release enhanced by apoptosis. Exp Cell Res. 2001;269:256–65.
26. Luciano R, Barraco GM, Muraca M, Ottino S, Spreghini MR, Sforza RW, Rustico C, Morino GS, Manco M. Biomarkers of Alzheimer disease, insulin resistance, and obesity in childhood. Pediatrics. 2015;135:1074–81.
27. Kovacs DM, Fausett HJ, Page KJ, Kim TW, Moir RD, Merriam DE, Hollister RD, Hallmark OG, Mancini R, Felsenstein KM, Hyman BT, Tanzi RE, Wasco W. Alzheimer-associated presenilins 1 and 2: neuronal expression in brain and localization to intracellular membranes in mammalian cells. Nat Med. 1996;2:224–9.
28. De Strooper B, Beullens M, Contreras B, Levesque L, Craessaerts K, Cordell B, Moechars D, Bollen M, Fraser P, George-Hyslop PS, Van Leuven F. Phosphorylation, subcellular localization, and membrane orientation of the Alzheimer's disease-associated presenilins. J Biol Chem. 1997;272:3590–8.
29. Mann DMA. Alzheimer's disease and Down's syndrome. Histopathology. 1988;13:125–27.
30. Teipel SJ, Hampel H. Neuroanatomy of Down syndrome in vivo: a model of preclinical Alzheimer's disease. Behav Genet. 2006;36:405–15.
31. Lai F, Williams RS. A prospective study of Alzheimer disease in Down syndrome. Arch Neurol. 1989;46:849–53.
32. Zigman W, Schupf N, Haveman M, Silverman W. The epidemiology of Alzheimer's disease in mental retardation: results and recommendations from an international conference. J Intellect Disabil Res. 1997;41:76–80.
33. Oliver C, Crayton L, Holland A, Hall S, Bradbury J. A four year prospective study of age-related cognitive change in adults with Down's syndrome. Psychol Med. 1998;28:1365–77.
34. Holland AJ, Hon J, Huppert FA, Stevens F, Watson P. Population-based study of the prevalence and presentation of dementia in adults with Down's syndrome. Br J Psychiatry. 1998;172:493–8.
35. Head E, Powell D, Gold BT, Schmitt FA. Alzheimer's disease in down syndrome. Eur J Neurodegener. 2012;1:353–64.
36. Alcolea D, Martínez-Lage P, Sánchez-Juan P, Olazarán J, Antúnez C, Izagirre A, Ecay-Torres M, Estanga A, Clerigué M, Guisasola MC, Sánchez Ruiz D, Marín J, Calero M, Blesa R, Clarimón J, Carmona-Iragui M, Morenas-Rodríguez E, Rodríguez-Rodríguez E, Vázquez Higuera JL, Fortea J, Lleó A. Amyloid precursor protein metabolism and inflammation markers in preclinical Alzheimer disease. Neurology. 2015;85:626–33.

3

Aβ accumulation causes MVB enlargement and is modelled by dominant negative VPS4A

Katarina Willén[1], James R. Edgar[2,3], Takafumi Hasegawa[4], Nobuyuki Tanaka[5], Clare E. Futter[3] and Gunnar K. Gouras[1*]

Abstract

Background: Alzheimer's disease (AD)-linked β-amyloid (Aβ) accumulates in multivesicular bodies (MVBs) with the onset of AD pathogenesis. Alterations in endosomes are among the earliest changes associated with AD but the mechanism(s) that cause endosome enlargement and the effects of MVB dysfunction on Aβ accumulation and tau pathology are incompletely understood.

Methods: MVB size and Aβ fibrils in primary neurons were visualized by electron microscopy and confocal fluorescent microscopy. MVB-dysfunction, modelled by expression of dominant negative VPS4A (dnVPS4A), was analysed by biochemical methods and exosome isolation.

Results: Here we show that AD transgenic neurons have enlarged MVBs compared to wild type neurons. Uptake of exogenous Aβ also leads to enlarged MVBs in wild type neurons and generates fibril-like structures in endocytic vesicles. With time fibrillar oligomers/fibrils can extend out of the endocytic vesicles and are eventually detectable extracellularly. Further, endosomal sorting complexes required for transport (ESCRT) components were found associated with amyloid plaques in AD transgenic mice. The phenotypes previously reported in AD transgenic neurons, with net increased intracellular levels and reduced secretion of Aβ, were mimicked by blocking recycling of ESCRT-III by dnVPS4A. DnVPS4A further resembled AD pathology by increasing tau phosphorylation at serine 396 and increasing markers of autophagy.

Conclusions: We demonstrate that Aβ leads to MVB enlargement and that amyloid fibres can form within the endocytic pathway of neurons. These results are consistent with the scenario of the endosome-lysosome system representing the site of initiation of Aβ aggregation. In turn, a dominant negative form of the CHMP2B-interacting protein VPS4A, which alters MVBs, leads to accumulation and aggregation of Aβ as well as tau phosphorylation, mimicking the cellular changes in AD.

Keywords: Alzheimer's disease, Amyloid, Endocytosis, Multivesicular body, Tau

Background

Alzheimer's disease (AD) is characterized by progressive decline in cognitive function, anatomical selective loss of synapses and neurons, and aggregation of the β-amyloid peptide (Aβ) in amyloid plaques and hyperphosphorylated tau in neurofibrillary tangles (NFTs). Although plaques are extracellular aggregates of Aβ, accumulation of Aβ42, the most pathogenic Aβ peptide, begins within neurons in AD [1–3] and in AD transgenic mouse models [4–6]. In AD transgenic mice, cognitive, physiological and structural impairments appear prior to plaques [7–9] and are accompanied by intraneuronal Aβ peptide accumulation, supporting that accumulation of intraneuronal Aβ peptides is one of the earliest events in AD pathogenesis [10].

Abnormalities in the endocytic pathway are also among the earliest pathological features reported in AD, preceding the classical pathological markers of Aβ plaques and NFTs [11]. Specifically, enlargement of Rab5-positive early endosomes and Rab7-positive late endosomes were reported in AD [12, 13], as well as progressive accumulation

* Correspondence: gunnar.gouras@med.lu.se
[1]Department of Experimental Medical Science, Lund University, 221 84 Lund, Sweden
Full list of author information is available at the end of the article

of multivesicular bodies (MVBs), lysosomes and autophagic vacuoles [14]. The amyloidogenic cleavage of APP occurs predominantly in endosomes [15–19]. Proteins in the amyloidogenic pathway (APP, the β-site APP cleaving enzyme (BACE1) and the γ-secretase that generates the Aβ peptides) are transmembrane proteins that traffic through the secretory pathway as well as the endocytic pathway. Immuno-electron microscopy revealed that particularly the limiting membrane of MVBs are the normal location of Aβ42 in neurons of the brain and are the sites of Aβ accumulation during AD pathogenesis [20], especially at synapses [5]. Sorting of EGFR via the MVB pathway was impaired by endosomal Aβ accumulation in cultured AD transgenic neurons [21]. Translocation into MVBs appeared particularly affected, suggesting Aβ dependent dysfunction of the late endosomal sorting complexes required for transport (ESCRT) pathway in AD.

The ESCRTs are a set of proteins conserved from yeast to mammals that regulate and drive formation of the intraluminal vesicles of MVBs. They assemble into distinct subcomplexes: ESCRT-0, ESCRT-I, ESCRT-II and ESCRT-III. Their sequential action directs the sorting of ubiquitinated transmembrane proteins and the inward budding of intraluminal vesicles (ILVs) into the lumen of endosomes, thereby generating MVBs that then either deliver membrane-associated cargo to the lysosome for degradation, release the intraluminal vesicles (then called exosomes) via fusion with the plasma membrane or traffic cargo back to the Golgi apparatus. ESCRT-III subunits, among them CHMP2B, are inactive monomers in the cytoplasm [22] that assemble on endosomal membranes in an ordered manner to generate the transient ESCRT-III complex. CHMP2B, linked genetically to frontotemporal dementia (FTD) and AD [23, 24], directly interacts with and recruits the VPS4 AAA–ATPase complex that disassembles ESCRT-III, and genome-wide association studies for late onset AD identified an association with VPS4B [25].

Given the cumulative genetic, biological and pathological evidence implicating Aβ in AD, and the early accumulation of Aβ in MVBs in AD, we set out to test our first hypothesis (1) that Aβ can cause the abnormal endosomal phenotype seen in AD. To determine this, we investigated the effects of Aβ on MVB size and Aβ aggregation in late endosomes. Since Aβ accumulates particularly at the outer limiting membrane of MVBs where ESCRTs reside and since ESCRT dysfunction leads to endosomal enlargement we also tested our second hypothesis (2) that Aβ causes dysfunction of the ESCRT pathway. This was investigated by examining changes in ESCRT proteins in primary neurons, as well as modulating the late ESCRT pathway to examine how this influences Aβ accumulation.

Here we provide experimental evidence of Aβ-dependent MVB enlargement as well as Aβ aggregation within late endocytic compartments of neurons. Consistent with the scenario of MVBs representing the site of initiation of Aβ aggregation, the accumulation of neuronal ESCRT components was evident in amyloid plaques. Moreover, dysfunction of ESCRT-III, modelled by dominant negative VPS4A (dnVPS4A) mimicked the Aβ accumulation and aggregation in MVBs as well as the enlarged late endosomal size seen in AD. These results support a novel scenario where a vicious cycle of ESCRT-dependent late endosomal dysfunction causes further Aβ accumulation as well as AD-pathogenic tau phosphorylation.

Methods

Cell culture

Primary neuronal cultures were generated from B6.Cg-Tg (APPswe, PSEN1dE9)85Dbo/Mmjax mice (APP/PS1) AD transgenic (tg) and wild-type (wt) mouse embryos. The APP sequence in APP/PS1 encodes a chimeric mouse/human APP (Mo/HuAPP695swe) that was humanized by modifying three amino acids, and introducing the Swedish AD mutation. The PS1 sequence encodes human presenilin 1 lacking exon 9 (dE9) that models AD-associated mutations in PS1. Both APPswe and PS1 are independently controlled by the prion protein promoter. Primary neuronal cultures were prepared from cortices and hippocampi of embryonic day 15 embryos as previously described [9]. In brief, E15 brain tissue was dissociated by trypsinization and trituration in DMEM with 10% fetal bovine serum (Gibco). Dissociated neurons were cultured on poly-D-lysine (Sigma) coated plates or glass coverslips (Bellco Glass Inc.) and were maintained until 12 and 19 DIV in neurobasal medium (Gibco), B27 supplement (Gibco), glutamine (Invitrogen) and antibiotics (ThermoScientific).

Wild type mouse N2a neuroblastoma cells (N2a) or N2a cells stably transfected with the 670/671 Swedish mutation human APP (Swe) [26] or wild-type α-synuclein with HA-Tag (α-syn) were grown on 10 cm dishes or coverslips.

Electron microscopy

Cells were grown on Thermanox coverslips (Nalgene, Nunc) and fixed with 2% PFA, 2.5% glutaraldehyde in 0.1 M cacodylate. Cells were then secondarily fixed with 1% osmium tetroxide followed by incubation with 1% tannic acid to enhance contrast. Cells were dehydrated using increasing percentages of ethanol before being embedded onto Epoxy resin (Agar scientific, UK) stubs. Coverslips were cured overnight at 65 °C. Ultrathin sections were cut using a diamond knife mounted to a Reichert ultracut S ultramicrotome and sections were collected onto copper grids. Grids were post-stained with drops of lead citrate. Sections were viewed on a FEI Tecnai transmission electron microscope (Eindhoven, The Netherlands) at a working voltage of 80 kV. BSA-gold was prepared as previously described [27]. For quantification of MVB diameter, MVBs were defined as organelles containing intraluminal vesicles and monomeric rather than flocculated BSA-gold.

Aβ1-42 peptides (Sigma) were incubated at 37 °C for 1 h to induce fibril formation in vitro. Grids were inverted onto the drops of Aβ1-42, negatively stained with 2% uranyl acetate, washed with water and dried on filter paper before being viewed by EM.

Transfection and constructs

Cells were transfected using Lipofectamine 2000 (Invitrogen) for N2a cells or Lipofectamine 3000 (Invitrogen) for primary neurons. N2a cells were transfected in Opti-MEM while primary neurons were transfected directly in their growth medium. The plasmids p3xFLAG-CMV-10-hVPS4A-wt and p3xFLAG-CMV-10-hVPS4A-dn E228Q were generated as described [28]. The control plasmids p3xFLAG-CMV-7-BAP Control Plasmid was purchased from Sigma-Aldrich and pcDNA3-CMV-GFP from Addgene. pcDNA3-synapsin-FLAG-wtVPS4 and pcDNA3-synapsin-FLAG-dnVPS4 were constructed from pcDNA3-synapsin-FLAG and PCR products from the p3xFLAG-CMV-10-hVPS4A-wt and p3xFLAG-CMV-10-hVPS4A-dn respectively. Control plasmid pAAV-synapsin-GFP was purchased from Addgene.

Antibodies and reagents

The following antibodies were used (see also Additional file 1: Table S1): 369 [29] (Buxbaum et al., 1990) for Western blot (WB) 1:1000; 6E10 (BioLegend, previously Covance SIG-39320) IF: 1:500, WB 1:1000; 12F4 (BioLegend, previously Covance SIG-39142) for immunofluorescence (IF) 1:250; Amyloidβ (1-42) (IBL, 18,582); Amyloidβ (1-42) (Invitrogen, 700,254) IF 1:1000; beta-actin (Sigma, A 5316) WB 1:2000; CD63 (ThermoFisher Scientific, MAI-19281) WB 1:1000; CHMP2B (Abcam, ab33174) IF 1:250, WB 1:1000; Clavestin-1 + 2 (Bioss, bs-6569R-A647) IF 1:250; DAPI (Sigma, D9542) IF 1:2000; drebrin (Abcam, ab11068) IF 1:1000; FLAG (Biolegend, 637,302) IF 1:1000, (Sigma, F1804) WB 1:1000; Flotillin-1 (BD Biosciences, 610,821) IF 1:400; GM130 (BD Biosciences, 610,822) IF: 1:500; GSK3β (Cell Signaling Technology, 12,456) IF 1:400; pGSKα/β (Cell Signaling Technology, 9331S) WB 1:1000; HA-Tag (Cell Signaling Technology, 3724) WB 1:1000; Hrs and Hrs-2 (Enzo, ALX-804-382-C050) IF 1:100; LAMP1 (Abcam, ab24170) IF 1:1000; LAMP1 (Abcam, ab25245) IF: 1:1500; LC3β (Cell Signaling Technology, 2775) WB 1:1000; Amyloid fibrils OC (Merck Millipore, AB2286) IF 1:1000; P2:1 (ThermoFisher Scientific, OMA1-03132) IF 1:500; Phospho-tau pSer396 (ThermoFisher, 44-752G); Rab7 (Abcam, ab50533) IF 1:500; Synaptophysin (Merck Millipore, MAB5258) IF 1:1000; Tsg101 (Genetex, GTX70255) IF 1:250, WB 1:1000; VPS4 (SantaCruz, sc-133,122) IF 1:100, WB 1:1000; secondary antibodies conjugated to Alexa Fluor-488, −546, −647 (IF 1:500; Invitrogen) or to HRP (WB 1:2000; R&D Systems, Minneapolis, MN).

Bafilomycin A (Sigma), torin 1 (Tocris) or rapamycin (Fisher BioReagents) were added to pre-warmed culture media at appropriate concentrations. Starvation media for induction of autophagy was 33% Opti-MEM in Hank's Balance Salt solution (HBSS). Aβ1-40 or Aβ1-42 peptides (Tocris) were reconstituted in DMSO to 250 μM, sonicated for 10 min and followed by 15 min of centrifugation at 12 k rpm before adding the supernatant to the culture media for the depicted times. All experiments used 0.5 μM of Aβ1-40 or Aβ1-42, except for EM and LAMP-1 positive vesicle size experiments that used 5 μM and 1 μM respectively.

Cell immunofluorescence

Cultured neurons at 12 DIV or N2a cells were fixed in 4% paraformaldehyde (PFA) in phosphate buffered saline (PBS) with 0.12 M sucrose for 20 min, permeabilized and blocked in PBS containing 2% normal goat serum (NGS), 1% bovine serum albumin (BSA), and 0.1% saponin at room temperature (RT) for 1 h, and then immunolabelled in 2% NGS in PBS overnight at 4 °C. After appropriate washing, coverslips were mounted with SlowfadeGold (Invitrogen). Immunofluorescence was examined by confocal laser scanning microscopy (Leica TCS SP8 or Zeiss LSM 510). In multiple label experiments, channels were imaged sequentially to avoid bleed-through. Images were taken with Leica Confocal Software or Zeiss ZEN software and analysed with ImageJ or Imaris 7.6. LAMP1-positive vesicles in pyramidal neurons were quantified by measuring the diameter of the five largest LAMP1-positive vesicles per cell, imaged by confocal microscopy in z-stacks, (n= >45 LAMP1-positive vesicles). All fluorescent labelling of cells was performed $n \geq 3$; and in the case of primary neurons from different embryos.

Brain immunofluorescence

Mice were anesthetized with isoflurane and perfused transcardially with saline followed by 4% PFA in 0.1 M PBS (pH 7.4) at RT. After dissection, brains were postfixed by immersion in 4% PFA in 0.1 M PBS (pH 7.4) at 4 °C for 2 h or overnight. After fixation, brains were cut in 40 μm thick sections with a sliding microtome. Sections were kept in storage buffer composed of 30% sucrose and 30% ethylene glycol in PBS at −20 °C. Free-floating sections were blocked for 1 h in RT with serum and triton-X and then incubated in primary antibodies overnight at 4 °C, followed by appropriate fluorescent Alexa secondary antibodies for 1 h at RT.

Western blot

Medium was collected and centrifuged and cells were washed twice, harvested in ice cold PBS, and centrifuged. Cell pellets were lysed with 6% sodium dodecyl sulfate

(SDS) containing 10 μl/ml β-mercaptoethanol, sonicated, and then heated at 95 °C for 6 min. After centrifugation, supernatants and medium were mixed with loading buffer, heated at 95 °C for 5 min and loaded into 10–20% Tricine gels (Invitrogen). Samples were subjected to electrophoresis and transferred to polyvinylidine difluoride membranes (Millipore). Membranes were blocked in PBS containing 0.1% Tween-20 (PBST) and 5% milk, and incubated in primary antibodies overnight and then with HRP-conjugated secondary antibodies for 1 h diluted in PBS containing 0.1% Tween-20 (PBST) and 5% milk. The immunoreaction was visualized by a chemiluminescence system (Pierce or BioRad). Bands were quantified using Image Lab (Bio-Rad Laboratories). For visualization of Aβ, membranes were boiled in PBS for 5 min prior to blocking. For analysis of exosomes, WB was performed as above but without β-mercaptoethanol in the 6% SDS lysis buffer.

For analysis of LC3β cells were lysed in RIPA buffer (Thermo Fisher Scientific) with protease inhibitor and phosphatase inhibitor (Thermo Fisher Scientific). Lysates with NuPAGE LDS sample buffer and NuPAGE reducing agent were loaded on NuPAGE 4-12% BisTris gels and run with NuPAGE MES SDS buffer (Invitrogen).

For analysis of α-synuclein in medium, total protein was extracted using a trichloroacetic acid (TCA)/acetone precipitation protocol. Briefly, freshly collected samples were cleared by centrifugation at 10000 rpm for 10 min to pellet debris and intact cells. The supernatant was transferred to a new tube and added with ¼ volume of ice-cold 20% TCA followed by incubation on ice for 3 h. The proteins were pelleted by centrifugation at 14000 rpm and washed twice with cold acetone.

For native conditions, cell pellets were lysed on ice in NativePAGE sample buffer (1X, Life Technologies) containing 1% digitonin (Life Technologies) and Halt proteinase inhibitor cocktail (1X, Thermo Scientific) by pipetting up and down and incubating on ice for 15 min. Lysates were centrifuged at 20000 x g for 30 min at 4 °C and protein concentrations of the supernatants were determined with BCA assay. Equal amounts of protein were loaded on a 3-12% NativePAGE Novex Bis-Tris gel (Life Technologies).

Exosome isolation and analysis

Exosomes were purified from cell culture medium by differential ultracentrifugation as described previously [30]. Briefly, Swe N2a cells were cultured and transfected for 48 h in exosome-free medium. Collected medium was depleted of cells and cellular debris by sequential low speed centrifugation. Exosomes were then isolated by centrifugation of the collected supernatant at 100,000×g at 4 °C for 70 min. The resultant pellet was washed in PBS and centrifuged for 70 min at 100,000×g at 4 °C.

Statistical analysis

Statistical analysis was performed with PRISM 6 software (Graph-Pad Software, San Diego, CA, USA) by using unpaired t-test or ANOVA with Tukey's multiple comparisons test or ANOVA with Dunnett's multiple comparisons test. All data are expressed as the mean ± SD. Differences were considered significant at $^{*}p < 0.05$, $^{**}p < 0.01$, $^{***}p < 0.001$, $^{****}p < 0.0001$.

Results

Aβ-dependent MVB enlargement

Endogenous Aβ42 is present in both dendrites and axons of cultured primary APP transgenic neurons and localizes especially with markers of late endosomes/MVBs [21]. In order to examine whether increased levels of Aβ can lead to the enlarged endosomal phenotype seen in AD, MVB size was compared between APP/PS1 transgenic and wt primary mouse neurons. Cells were incubated with BSA-gold 2 h (h) before fixation to confirm identity of the endocytic compartments. Remarkably, electron micrographs showed a significantly greater MVB diameter (52% increase; $p < 0.001$) in APP/PS1 transgenic compared to wt neurons at 12 days in vitro (DIV) (Fig. 1a and b) consistent with the larger diameter of endosomes described in human AD. Since full length APP, β-CTFs, Aβ and the presenilin mutation in the APP/PS1 transgenic neurons potentially all could be the cause of this effect, wt neurons at 12 DIV were treated with freshly prepared human synthetic Aβ1-40 or Aβ1-42 for 48 h, to test if Aβ was sufficient to induce the endosomal enlargements. The neurons demonstrated a 69% and 114% increase in the diameter of MVBs with Aβ1-40 or Aβ1-42 treatment, respectively ($p < 0.001$; Fig. 1c and d) as measured on EM images compared to controls. Further, an increased size by 165% of LAMP1-positive late endosomes/lysosomes was already evident by immunofluorescent labelling at 3 h in pyramidal neurons treated with Aβ1-42 ($p < 0.0001$, Fig. 1e and f). LAMP1-changes at different time points of Aβ1-42 treatment, ranging from 30 s to 48 h, are shown in Additional file 2: Figure S1B. Taken together, our results indicate that enlarged MVBs, one of the earliest pathological features in AD, can be caused by Aβ, which however does not rule out important contributions also of other APP components such as β-CTFs.

Fibril-like structures in endocytic organelles of wild-type neurons treated with Aβ

Interestingly, fibril-like structures were apparent by EM in endocytic organelles of wt primary neurons incubated with synthetic human Aβ1-42 for 48 h that were not seen in untreated neurons (Fig. 2a), and were more prominent in neurons treated with Aβ1-42 than Aβ1-40. For comparison, Aβ1-42 fibrilized in vitro showed similar size and morphology of fibrils on EM as in the endocytic vesicles

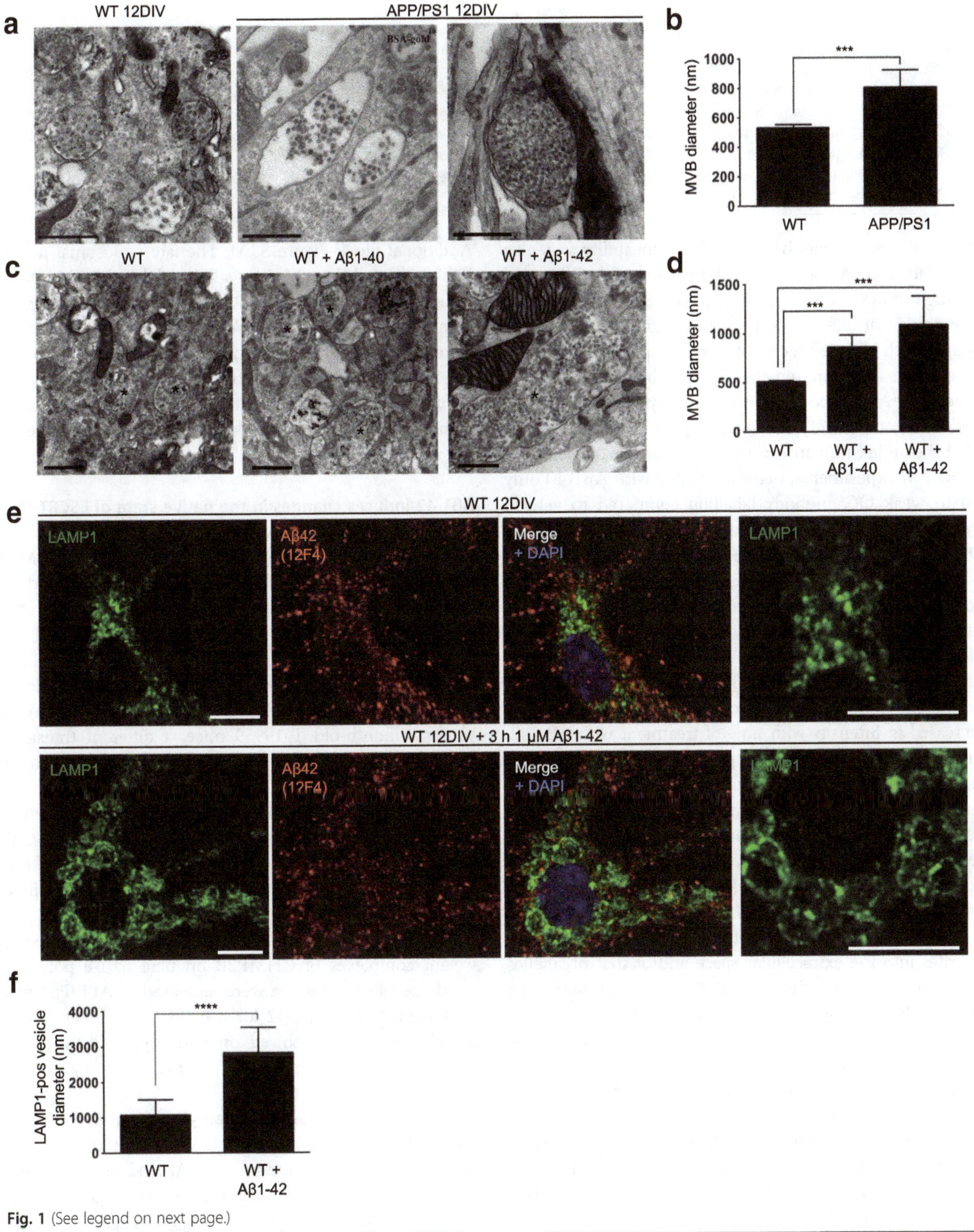

Fig. 1 (See legend on next page.)

(See figure on previous page.)
Fig. 1 Aβ increases MVB diameter in primary neurons. **a** Electron microscopy reveals that APP/PS1 AD transgenic compared to wt mouse primary neurons have significantly larger MVBs at 12 DIV. Scale bar 500 nm. **b** Quantification of A shows an increase of 52% in MVB diameter in Tg compared to wt neurons, $n > 94$ MVBs per group; *** $p < 0.001$. **c** Exogenously added monomeric Aβ1-40 or Aβ1-42 to wt primary neurons at 12 DIV leads to increased MVB diameter at 48 h on EM images. MVBs are marked with an asterisk. Scale bar 500 nm. **d** Quantification of C, $n > 45$ MVBs per group; *** $p < 0.001$. **e** Shorter time-points of exogenously added monomeric Aβ1-42 already leads to increased size of LAMP1-positive vesicles 3 h after treatment in wt mouse neurons at 12 DIV; 3D-rendering with Imaris from confocal z-stack. High magnification image of LAMP1 labelling from a single focal plane to the right. Scale bar 10 μm. **f** Quantification of E shows significant increase in diameter of LAMP1-positive vesicles after addition of Aβ. The diameters of the five largest LAMP1-positive vesicles per pyramidal neuron were measured in the z-stacks; $n > 10$ neurons per treatment; **** $p < 0.0001$

(Fig. 2b). Loss of endolysosomal impermeability was also seen with Aβ1-42 treatment of neurons with BSA-gold leaking out into the cytoplasm (Fig. 2c). To further investigate the fibril-like structures, wt murine neurons were treated with elevated levels of human Aβ1-42 at different time points and immunolabelled with the conformational dependent Aβ antibody OC to label amyloid fibrils and fibrillar oligomers [31] and antibody 6E10 to specifically label the added human Aβ. Using the same parameters as in the EM experiments, neurons treated with Aβ1-40 only led to weak OC antibody labelling compared to vehicle treated cells, while Aβ1-42 treated neurons showed robust OC labelling (Additional file 3: Figure S2).

Already at 45 min of treatment with 0.5 μM Aβ1-42 (Fig. 2d) and up to 24 h of incubation, antibodies OC and 6E10 revealed an almost completely overlapping vesicular pattern of labelling, indicating that the amyloid fibrils and/or fibrillar oligomers consisted of Aβ1-42, which was particularly prominent along neuronal processes. Of note, OC labelling increased in intensity with time of treatment with Aβ1-42. Interestingly, at 48 h the OC positive structures were enlarged and elongated, displaying a part that was human Aβ antibody 6E10 positive and an extension that was 6E10 negative (Fig. 2e). Surface labelling of non-permeabilized cells revealed that the elongated OC labelling at 48 h was now to a certain extent extracellular, whereas the punctate OC and 6E10 co-labelling at 24 h was generally intracellular (Fig. 2f). This suggests that with time, fibrils extend out of neurites into the extracellular space and/or that organelles containing the fibrils fuse with the plasma membrane. To better define the subcellular site of Aβ aggregation, cells were double labelled with OC antibody and the late endosomal/lysosomal marker LAMP1. At 45 min colocalization with OC was evident in small LAMP1-positive vesicles in the processes but not in the larger LAMP1-positive vesicles in the cell soma (Additional file 4: Figure S3A). Since lysosomes normally do not localize to axons and dendrites, other than their very proximal part, this suggests that Aβ42 starts to aggregate in late endosomes/MVBs of neurites. At 48 h, OC and LAMP1 still colocalized mainly in neuronal processes, but in LAMP1-positive structures that now appeared somewhat enlarged and irregular in their shape. Elongated OC-positive structures could be seen extending out from the more punctate LAMP1 labelling (Fig. 2g and Additional file 4: Figure S3A). The late endosomal marker Rab7 indicated that at least a subset of the vesicular OC labelling at 24 h colocalized with Rab7 positive late endocytic compartments in neurites (Additional file 4: Figure S3C). Taken together these data indicate that Aβ1-42 can be taken up by neurons in culture and forms amyloidogenic fibrils and/or fibrillar oligomers in late endocytic compartments particularly within neuronal processes that eventually appear to extend extracellularly.

Aβ1-42 induces changes in the native state of ESCRT-III complex component CHMP2B

Given prior evidence supporting that sorting via the MVB pathway was impaired by Aβ accumulation in cultured AD transgenic neurons and that Aβ dependent translocation into MVBs seemed affected [21], we next investigated possible dysfunction of the ESCRT pathway in models of AD. In APP/PS1 transgenic primary neurons Aβ42 was found associated with CHMP2B-positive vesicles (Fig. 3a). In young 3-month-old Tg19959 mice, a different transgenic mouse model of β-amyloidosis harbouring the Swedish and Indiana APP mutations, CHMP2B immunolabelling was most prominent in the area of hippocampus and entorhinal cortex that also expressed increased levels of Aβ/APP (Additional file 5: Figure S4A-B). Although levels of total CHMP2B and VPS4 were not significantly changed in wt compared to APP/PS1 primary neurons lysed in 6% SDS (Additional file 5: Figure S4C), levels of high molecular weight complexes of CHMP2B on blue native polyacrylamide gel electrophoresis were increased in APP/PS1 neurons treated with Aβ1-42 for 3 h (Fig. 3b). Other ESCRT proteins were not resolved on native gels, likely due to masking of antibody epitopes under native conditions.

ESCRT components localize to amyloid plaques

Since AD transgenic neurons showed an increased diameter of MVBs and treatment with Aβ1-42 led to prominent fibril-like structures in late endocytic organelles, and as prior immuno-EM work has indicated early Aβ accumulation in dystrophic neurites [10], we next examined whether aggregating Aβ42 in endosomes might lead to the presence of ESCRT components in amyloid plaques. Indeed, APP/PS1 transgenic mice with plaque pathology demonstrated that the ESCRT-III associated protein VPS4

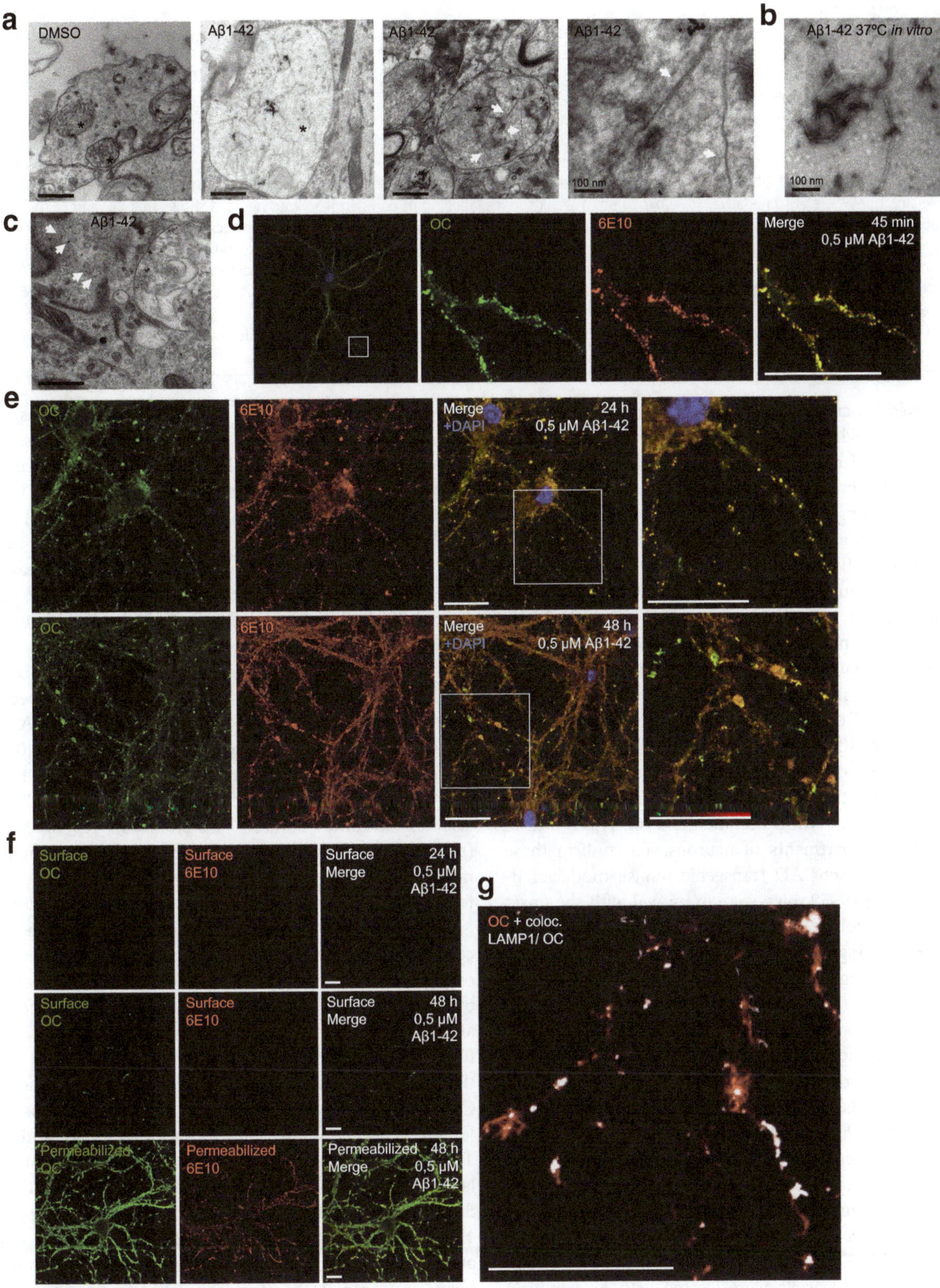

Fig. 2 (See legend on next page.)

(See figure on previous page.)

Fig. 2 Fibril-like structures in endocytic organelles of wild-type neurons treated with Aβ1-42. **a** Wt primary neurons treated at 12 DIV with Aβ for 48 h induced fibril-like structures in endocytic organelles with Aβ1-42. BSA-gold was added to cells 2 h before fixation to delineate endocytic organelles (*marked with asterisk*). Scale bar 500 nm. High magnification image to the right, scale bar 100 nm. **b** Aβ1-42 peptides incubated in vitro at 37 °C for 1 h to induce fibril formation, imaged with EM. Scale bar 100 nm. **c** BSA-gold (white arrows) was found in the cytosol in Aβ1-42 treated neurons, indicating loss of endolysosomal impermeability due to Aβ1-42. Scale bar 500 nm. **d** OC antibody labelling for fibrillar oligomers and/or fibrils is seen in a vesicular pattern in processes after 45 min treatment with 0.5 μM of Aβ1-42 and colocalizes with human Aβ antibody 6E10 confirming that fibrils consist of the added human Aβ1-42. Scale bar 10 μm. **e** Feeding 0.5 μM of Aβ1-42 to wt primary neurons at 12 DIV at 24 h vs 48 h. At 24 h most of the OC labelling was also antibody 6E10 positive. At 48 h the outer aspects of OC positive structures were 6E10 negative. Scale bar 20 μm. **f** Weak surface labelling of non-permeabilized neurons shows that OC and 6E10 antibody positive structures were intracellular after 24 h of treatment with Aβ1-42 (*upper panel*). At 48 h extracellular OC antibody labelling was now more visible consistent with penetration of the plasma membrane by the elongated OC positive fibrils (*middle panel*). Strong OC and 6E10 antibody labelling of permeabilized cells after fixation but before immunolabelling, shows that the vast majority of added human Aβ1-42 (antibody 6E10) and OC antibody positive fibrils and/or fibrillar oligomers are inside neurons (*lower panel*). Scale bar 20 μm. **g** After 48 h of treatment with 0.5 μM Aβ1-42, OC antibody labelling was seen extending out from LAMP1-positive structures in the processes. The image shows OC with the superimposed colocalizing channel for LAMP1 and OC. For the complete image with separate channels see Additional file 3: S2A. Scale bar 20 μm

was markedly increased in plaques (Fig. 3c and Additional file 5: Figure S4D), where it partially colocalized with Aβ42. ESCRT–I component Tsg101, a marker of MVBs, also showed increased labelling in plaques (Fig. 3d). In contrast, labelling of CHMP2B and the earlier ESCRT-0 component Hrs appeared decreased in plaques compared to surrounding brain parenchyma (Additional file 5: Figure S4E-F). Brain sections were also co-labelled with an antibody against clavestin-1 and 2 (Fig. 3d), which are neuron-specific proteins in the endo-lysosomal pathway [32]. The strong colocalization between Tsg101 and clavesin-1 and 2 in amyloid plaques supports the neuronal origin of ESCRT components in plaques. Moreover, much of the strong Aβ42 labelling outside of plaques in AD transgenic brain occurred in vesicle-like structures of dystrophic neurites that also contained clavesin-1 and 2 and Tsg101, consistent with accumulation of Aβ42 within endosomal compartments of neurons. To confirm these results in a different AD transgenic mouse model of β-amyloidosis, Tg19959 mice were examined with the onset of plaque pathology. In early plaques of 3-month-old Tg19959 mice Tsg101 (Fig. 3e) and VPS4 (not shown) also colocalized strongly with Aβ42.

Blocking VPS4A increases intracellular accumulation and decreases secretion of Aβ

In order to model the effect of dysfunctional ESCRT-dependent MVBs on Aβ accumulation, a dominant negative, E228Q ATPase-deficient form of VPS4A (dnVPS4A) was expressed for 24 h in N2a neuroblastoma cells harbouring stably transfected human Swedish mutant APP. N2a cells were used here because of their high transfection efficiency compared to primary neurons. To assess that N2a cells react to Aβ1-42 in a similar manner as primary neurons, N2a cells were treated with exogenously added Aβ1-42 for different time points. N2a cells treated with Aβ1-42 also exhibited increased size of LAMP1-positive vesicles (Additional file 6: Figure S5). The ATPase VPS4 is a key component of the ESCRT machinery as it is the only energy-consuming enzyme, promotes disassembly and recycling of ESCRT-III oligomers, and is recruited to the ESCRT-III complex by direct interaction with CHMP2B. We found that the expression of dnVPS4A markedly increased the intracellular pool of Aβ by 424% ($p < 0.001$, Fig. 4a and d) while concurrently decreasing the amounts of Aβ secreted into the medium by 87% ($p < 0.0001$, Fig. 4c and d). DnVPS4A also increased higher molecular weight bands between 17 kDa and 34 kDa that might represent Aβ oligomers within cells (Fig. 4a) as they were not seen with C-terminal specific APP antibody 369 (Fig. 4b). In addition, dnVPS4A increased the levels of APP within cells by 149% ($p < 0.05$) and secreted APPα in conditioned media by 149% ($p < 0.05$). Overexpression of wild type VPS4A (wtVPS4A) also significantly reduced secretion of Aβ by 72% ($p < 0.001$), although not to the extent of the dominant negative construct. Such a partially dominant negative effect of over-expressing wtVPS4 has been described [28].

Confocal immunofluorescence microscopy of Swe N2a cells transfected with dnVPS4A confirmed the increase of Aβ and full-length APP (Fig. 4e). Increased labelling by immunofluorescent microscopy with the conformational antibody OC in dnVPS4A-transfected cells confirmed the increase in Aβ oligomers and showed that the fibrillar oligomers and/or fibrils labelled by antibody OC colocalized with enlarged vesicles labelled positive for dnVPS4A protein and flotillin-1 (Fig. 4f and g). Triple labelling revealed that Aβ42 accumulated in enlarged vesicles positive for the MVB marker Tsg101 in dnVPS4A expressing cells labelled by the FLAG-tag (Fig. 4h). Thus, dysfunctional MVBs accumulate Aβ42 that, at least in part, is in an oligomeric and/or fibrillar form. In contrast to effects on Aβ and in agreement with a prior report [28], dnVPS4A increased secretion of α-synuclein in α-syn N2a cells without altering the total pool of intracellular α-synuclein (Additional file

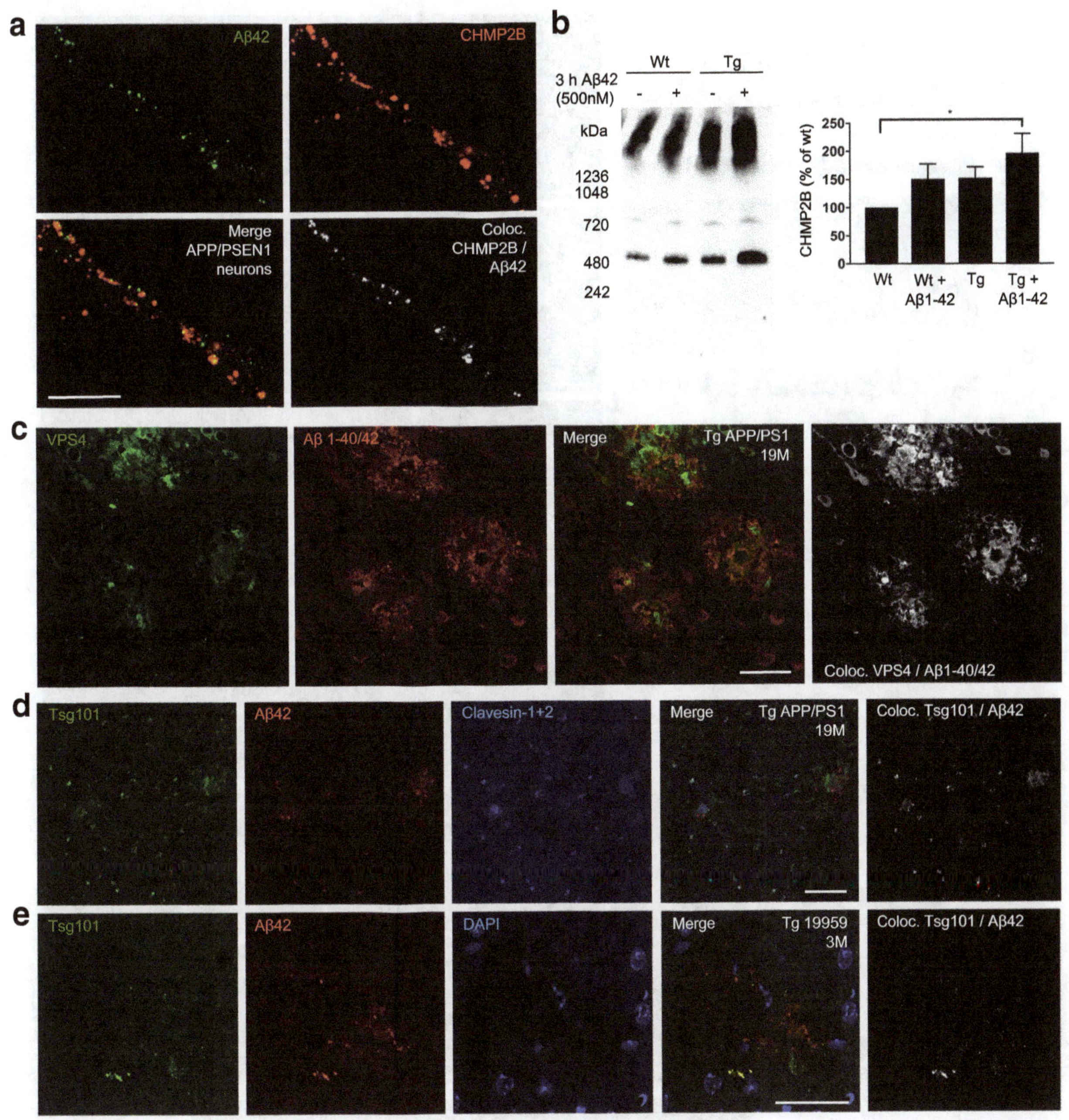

Fig. 3 Aβ42 increases high molecular weight complexes of CHMP2B and ESCRT proteins accumulate in amyloid plaques. **a** Immunolabelling of APP/PS1 transgenic primary neurons shows Aβ42 colocalizing with CHMP2B-positive vesicles. Scale bar 10 μm, $n = 3$. **b** A trend for increased high molecular weight complexes of CHMP2B, a 24 kDa ESCRT-III component, in APP/PS1 transgenic compared to wt neurons is seen on native gel. Treatment with 0.5 μM of Aβ1-42 for 3 h further increases these high molecular weight complexes. However only APP/PS1 transgenic neurons treated with Aβ1-42 show a statistically significant increase in high molecular weight complexes compared to wt. Equal amounts of total protein were loaded into the wells, $n = 6$; $^*p < 0.05$. **c** VPS4 colocalizes with Aβ42 in amyloid plaques of 19-month-old APP/PS1 mice. Scale bar 40 μm, $n = 4$. **d** Tsg101 colocalizes with both Aβ42 and the neuronal-specific endo-lysosomal marker clavesin 1 and 2 in amyloid plaques of 19-month-old APP/PS1 mice. Scale bar 40 μm, $n = 3$. **e** In early plaques present in the 3-month-old Tg19959 mice Tsg101 also colocalized with Aβ42. Scale bar 40 μm, $n = 3$

7: Figure S6). Since the CMV-FLAG-dnVPS4A induced toxicity in primary neurons, we constructed a plasmid under the weaker synapsin promoter. Expressing dnVPS4A under this synapsin promoter in wt or APP/PS1 primary neurons showed increased labelling of Aβ42 (Fig. 4i), supporting that dysfunctional ESCRT-dependent MVB formation leads to increased levels of Aβ within neurons.

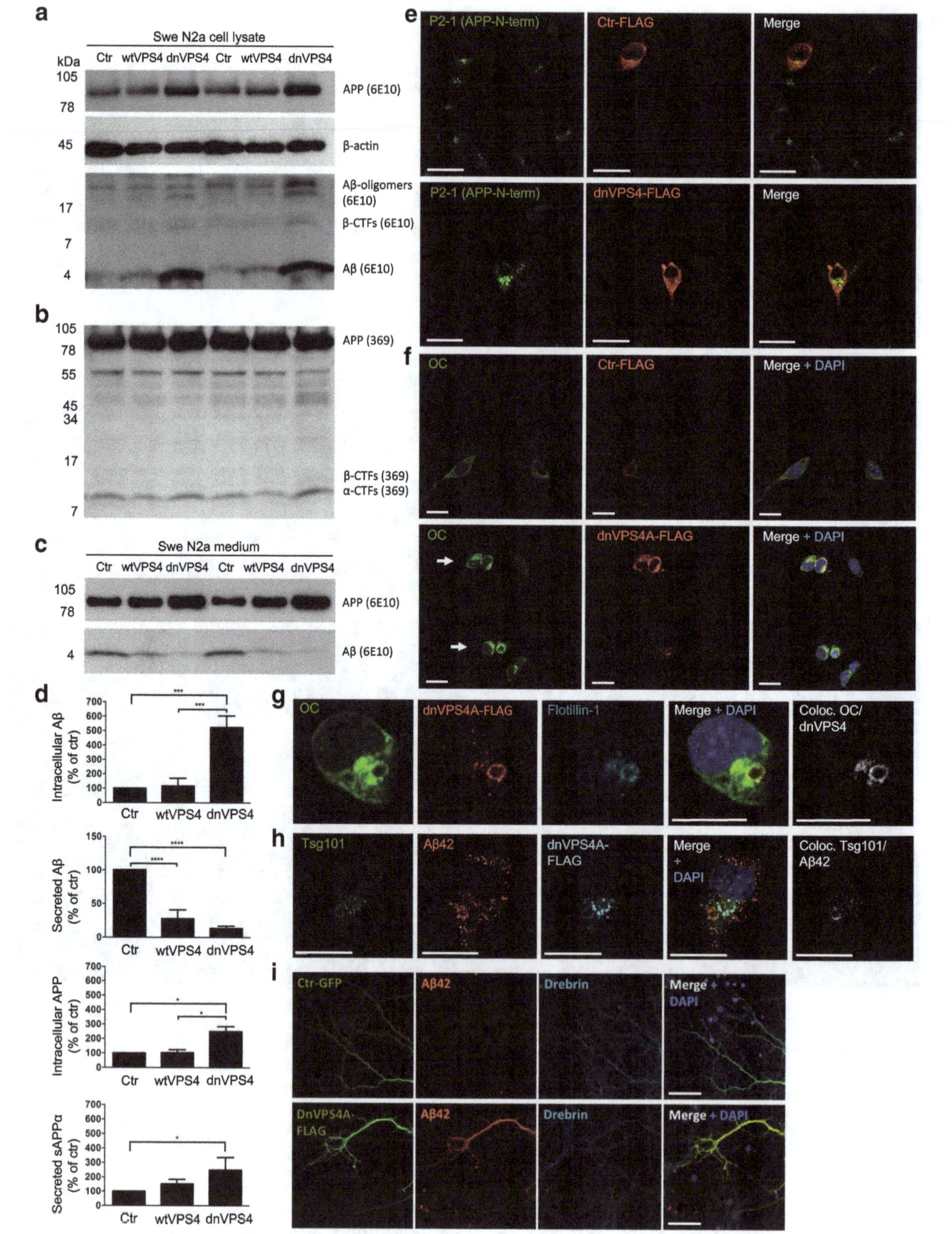

Fig. 4 (See legend on next page.)

(See figure on previous page.)
Fig. 4 DnVPS4A causes increased accumulation and reduced secretion of Aβ42. Expression of control plasmid (ctr), wtVPS4A (wtVPS4) or the ATP hydrolysis deficient mutant dnVPS4A (dnVPS4) in Swe N2a cells (A-H) or wt primary mouse neurons (I) for 24 h. **a** Representative Western blot of APP, SDS-stable oligomeric Aβ species, β-CTFs and monomeric Aβ in cell lysate probed with antibody 6E10, and β-actin for protein normalization. **b** Western blot analysis of full length APP, β-CTFs and α-CTFs in cell lysate probed with the C-terminal specific APP antibody 369. **c** Western blot analysis of secreted αAPP (sAPPα) and Aβ in cell medium with antibody 6E10. **d** Densitometric quantification of A and C demonstrates that expression of dnVPS4, but not wtVPS4, increases intracellular Aβ compared to ctr. On the other hand, both wtVPS4A and dnVPS4A reduces secreted Aβ compared to ctr, although to a greater extent with dnVPS4A. DnVPS4 increases both cellular and secreted APP. Values are normalized against actin and expressed as percentage of control, $n > 3$; $*p < 0.05$, $**p < 0.01$, $***p < 0.001$, $****p < 0.0001$. **e** Cellular full length APP is increased in cells transfected with dnVPS4A-FLAG (lower panel) compared to control plasmid Ctr-FLAG (*upper panel*). Scale bar 25 μm. **f** Antibody OC labelling of fibrillar oligomers and fibrils is increased in cells transfected with dnVPS4A (*arrows*) compared to control plasmid. Scale bar 25 μm. **g** Antibody OC labelling in dnVPS4-transfected cells is associated with enlarged vesicles positive for flotillin-1. Scale bar 15 μm. **h** Aβ42 accumulation in vesicles positive for ESCRT protein Tsg101 in dnVPS4A-transfected cells. Scale bar 25 μm. **i** Wt primary neurons at 12 DIV transfected with synapsin-dnVPS4A-FLAG or control synapsin-GFP plasmid for 24 h, immunolabelled for Aβ42 and the post-synaptic protein drebrin shows that Aβ42 labelling is increased with expression of dnVPS4A but not with control plasmid. Scale bar 50 μm

Increased cellular levels of Aβ with dysfunctional MVBs is mimicked by inhibiting lysosomal degradation

The increased intracellular levels of Aβ with dnVPS4A could be due to changes in the production of Aβ, reduced secretion and/or reduced fusion of MVBs with the lysosome for degradation. In order to investigate the turnover of APP and Aβ, Swe N2a were treated with the protein synthesis inhibitor cycloheximide (Additional file 8: Figure S7A-B and Additional file 9: Figure S8D). This revealed a rapid turnover of APP in cell lysates with a half-life of about 45 min, while cellular Aβ had a half-life of about 4 h. In contrast, the degradation of APP and Aβ in conditioned media was slower, not reaching 50% of control levels within 6 h of cycloheximide treatment. To investigate the role of lysosomal degradation, Swe N2a cells were treated for 24 h with 5 nM bafilomycin A1 (BafA1), which inhibits the vacuolar H+ ATPase. BafA1 treatment had the same effects on Aβ as dnVPS4A, markedly increasing intracellular levels of Aβ and reducing the secretion of Aβ (Fig. 5a-b and Additional file 9: Figure S8A-D). These results suggest that dnVPS4A blocks MVBs with Aβ on route to lysosomes for degradation. Consistently, when the endo-lysosomal pH gradient was blocked with BafA1, dnVPS4A transfected cells no longer showed higher cellular levels of Aβ than the wtVPS4A or GFP transfected cells (Fig. 5c). Hence, when the ability of lysosomes to degrade Aβ is abolished, blocking Aβ on route to the lysosomes via dnVPS4 does not lead to further Aβ accumulation.

To investigate the secretion of Aβ via fusion of MVBs with the plasma membrane and concomitant release of exosomes, exosomes from dnVPS4A-transfected Swe N2a cells were isolated and analysed (Fig. 5d). Secretion of exosomes was not prevented but instead increased by dnVPS4A in Swe N2a cells, possibly due to upregulation of ESCRT independent (CD63 dependent) MVB formation [33–35].

Blocking ESCRT dependent ILV formation increases pathological tau phosphorylation

A major question in AD is how Aβ links to tau pathology. MVBs are necessary for the sequestration of GSK3 [36] which phosphorylates tau at serine 396 (S396). Both elevated tau phosphorylation at S396 [37] and hyperactive GSK3 is implicated in AD [38, 39]. Therefore, we examined the effects of dnVPS4A on tau phosphorylation. Tau phosphorylation at residue S396 was significantly increased by 56% with dnVPS4A ($p < 0.05$; Fig. 6a and b), suggesting increased activation of GSK3β and increased GSK3β dependent phosphorylation of tau caused by dysfunctional ESCRT dependent MVBs. Immunofluorescence microscopy revealed increased GSK3β labelling of cells upon dnVPS4A transfection (Additional file 10: Figure S9A), although changes in total GSK3β or phosphorylated GSK3α/β (S21/9) levels were not detected by Western blot in cell lysates of Swe N2a cells transfected with dnVPS4A (Additional file 10: Figure S9B). One possible explanation for this apparent discrepancy is that the active GSK3β in the cytosol and early endosomes (facing the cytosol) is easier to visualize with immunofluorescence than the sequestered GSK3β inside the ILVs of MVBs.

Autophagy induction partially rescues the intracellular accumulation of Aβ

Since autophagic organelles are markedly increased in AD and autophagy is thought to be impaired in the disease [14], we next examined LC3β-II and p62, markers of autophagy, in dnVPS4A transfected cells accumulating intracellular Aβ. Expression of dnVPS4A in Swe N2a cells showed increased levels of LC3β-II, which correlate with increased numbers of autophagosomes in the cell, by 35% ($p < 0.05$, Fig. 7a) and increased levels of p62 by 52% ($p < 0.05$, Fig. 7b). Inducing autophagy by 1 μM Rapamycin ($p < 0.01$, Fig. 7c), 250 nM Torin1 or starvation (Fig. 7d) reduced the dnVPS4A-induced increase in intracellular Aβ. Thus, in the setting of dysfunctional MVBs with Aβ that is inefficiently trafficked to

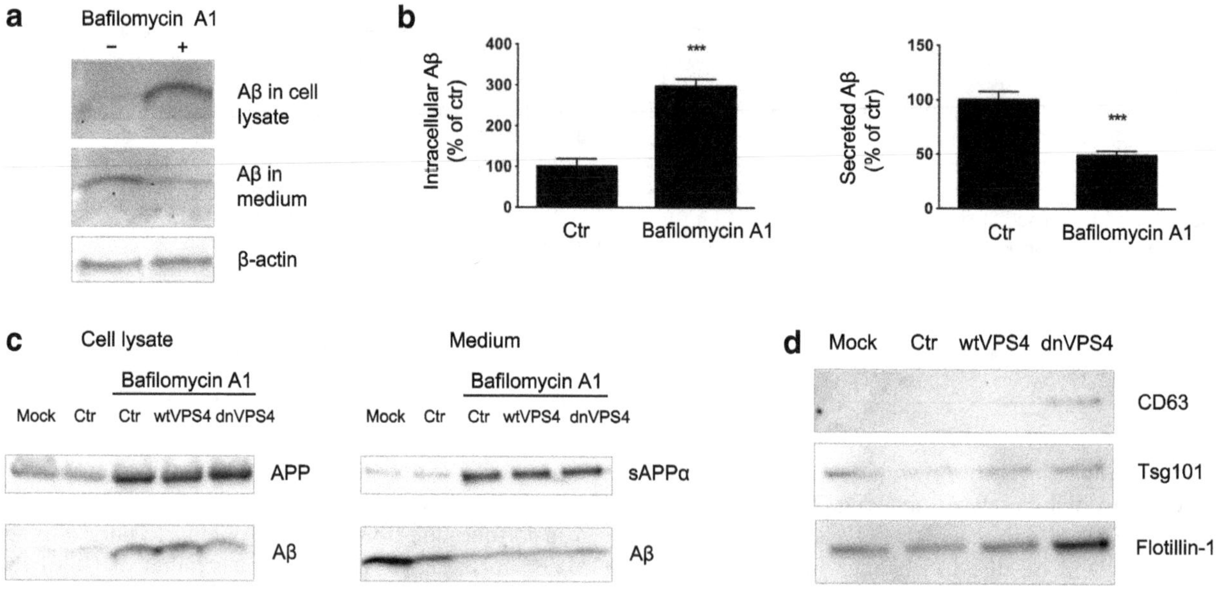

Fig. 5 Increased cellular levels of Aβ with dnVPS4A expression is consistent with decreased lysosomal degradation. **a** Bafilomycin A1 (BafA1) treatment had similar effects on Aβ as dnVPS4a, markedly increasing intracellular levels of Aβ and reducing Aβ secretion. Representative Western blot analysis of cell lysates and cell medium from Swe N2a cells treated with 5 nM BafA1 for 24 h and blotted for 6E10 for Aβ and β-actin. **b** Densitometric quantification of A. Values are normalized against actin and expressed as percentage of untreated control, $n = 3$, *** $p < 0.001$. **c** When the ability of lysosomes to degrade Aβ is abolished by BafA1, blocking Aβ on route to the lysosomes via dnVPS4 does not lead to further Aβ accumulation. Representative Western blots are shown of lysates (*left*) and medium (*right*) from Swe N2a cells treated with 5 nM BafA1 6 h after transfection with mock (no plasmid), control plasmid ctrGFP, wtVPS4A or dnVPS4A. Cells were collected 24 h post-transfection, $n = 3$. **d** Western blot analysis of isolated exosomes secreted from Swe N2a cells transfected with mock (no plasmid), ctrGFP, wtVPS4 or dnVPS4 for 48 h. Representative blots demonstrate that exosome secretion is not reduced with dnVPS4. Instead, increased amounts of CD63, an exosomal marker postulated to be involved in ESCRT independent ILV formation, is seen in the exosomal fraction from dnVPS4 transfected cells. Flotillin-1, an exosomal marker associated with cholesterol-enriched lipid rafts is also increased in the exosomal fraction from dnVPS4 transfected cells, while the ESCRT-I protein and exosomal marker Tsg101 is not changed, $n = 3$

lysosomes for degradation and/or inefficiently secreted, stimulation of autophagy is associated with decreased cellular Aβ.

Discussion

Over the past years, the view of the role of Aβ in the pathogenesis of AD has been changing. Rather than merely aggregation of extracellular Aβ, a complex and interrelated biology of intra- and extra-cellular pools of Aβ has emerged. Progressive intraneuronal Aβ accumulation and impaired secretion of Aβ were reported in AD transgenic neurons with time in culture [9, 40] and plaque-independent, Aβ-dependent synapse damage and memory impairment correlated with this intracellular pool of Aβ but not plaques in AD-transgenic mice [41]. Our working hypothesis is that dystrophic neurites with accumulating intraneuronal Aβ, initially within MVBs, are a nidus of plaque formation [10], with an important contribution of secreted Aβ originating also from hyperactive neurons.

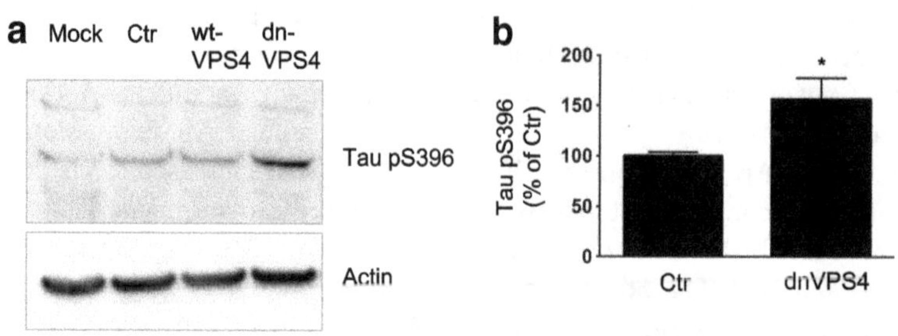

Fig. 6 Blocking ESCRT dependent ILV formation increases tau phosphorylation at serine 369 (S396). **a** Western blot of transfected N2a Swe cells demonstrates increased tau phosphorylation at S396 with expression of dnVPS4A. **b** Quantification of A shows a 56% increase in levels tau phosphorylated at S396 with dnVPS4A; values are normalized against actin and expressed as percentage of ctrGFP, ($n = 5$, *$p < 0.05$)

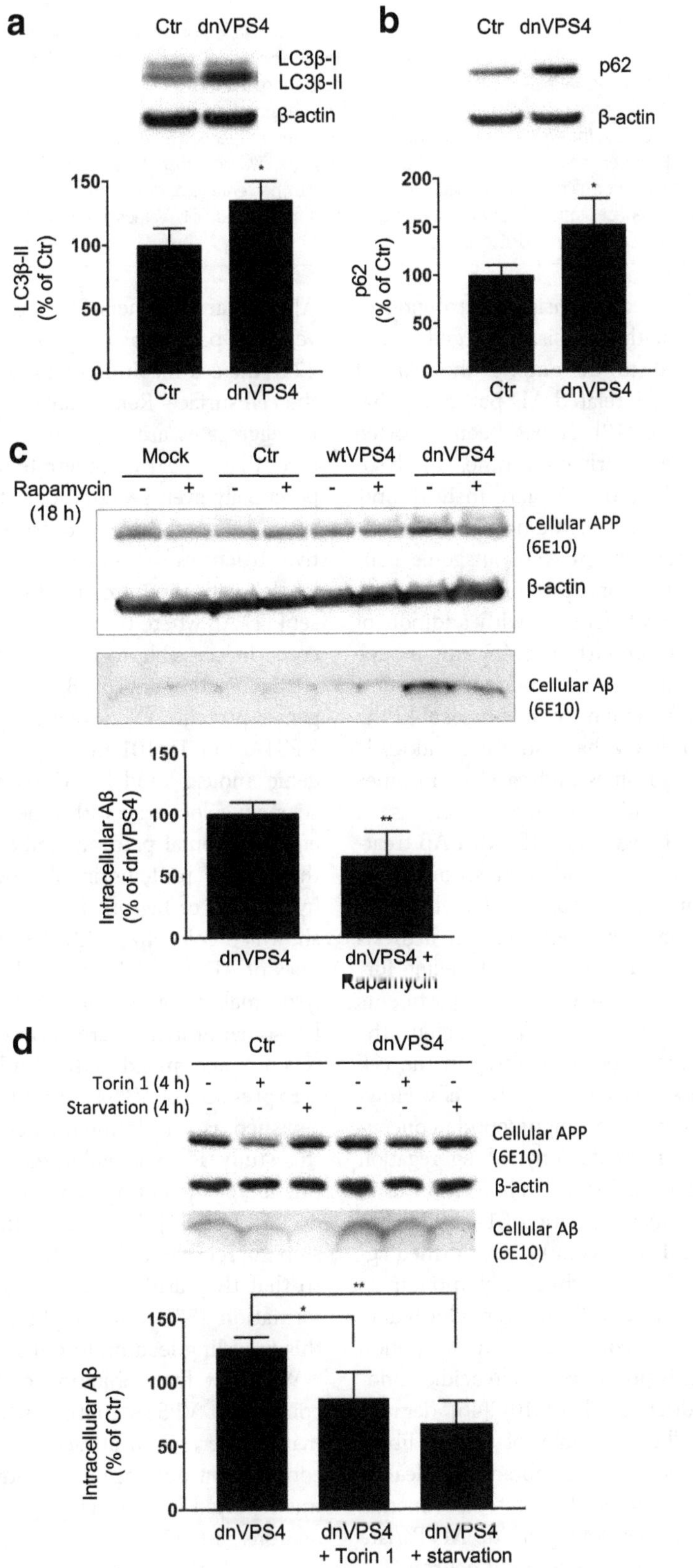

Fig. 7 (See legend on next page.)

(See figure on previous page.)

Fig. 7 Induction of autophagy partially rescues dnVPS4A induced intracellular accumulation of Aβ. **a** Expression of dnVPS4A increases levels of LC3β-II, an indicator of autophagy, by 35% ($n = 3$, $^*p < 0.05$). Representative blot (above) and quantification (below); values are normalized against actin and expressed as percentage of ctrGFP. **b** dnVPS4A increases levels of p62, an indicator of autophagy, by 52% ($n = 3$, $^{**}p < 0.01$). Representative blot (above) and quantification (below); values are normalized against actin and expressed as percentage of ctrGFP. **c** Chemically induced autophagy by Rapamycin partially rescues the increase in intracellular Aβ from dnVPS4A. 6 h after transfection Swe N2a cells were treated with 1 μM Rapamycin and harvested 24 h post-transfection. Representative blot (above) and quantification (below) demonstrating 35% reduction in intracellular Aβ by Rapamycin on dnVPS4 transfected cells. Values are normalized against actin and expressed as percentage of dnVPS4 ($n = 6$, $^{**}p < 0.01$). **d** Induced autophagy by torin 1 or by starvation significantly reduces intracellular Aβ to levels in dnVPS4 transfected cells. Values are normalized against actin and expressed as percentage of control transfected cells ($n = 3$, $^*p < 0.05$, $^{**}p < 0.01$)

Here we provide novel molecular insights into endosomal alterations with AD pathogenesis. Enlarged endosomes have been observed to be among the earliest cellular changes in AD and the related AD pathology that develops in Down syndrome [12]. It has been reported that the enlarged phenotype in early endosomes and lysosomes in AD is independent of Aβ and instead only dependent on APP β-CTFs [42, 43]. We now provide evidence that MVB size is increased in AD transgenic neurons, and that this phenotype of increased late endosomal size can be recapitulated in wt neurons with addition of exogenous Aβ. These data support that Aβ can induce endosomal enlargement, but do not exclude an important role also for APP β-CTFs. Although we only measured the size of MVBs with EM, it is likely that also other endocytic compartments including lysosomes and early endosomes were affected. The large LAMP1-positive vesicles seen and measured on confocal images (Fig. 1f) with Aβ treatment, likely also include lysosomes and autolysosomes.

We show by EM fibrillar-like structures inside abnormal MVBs/late endocytic/lysosomal compartments in neurons treated with Aβ1-42, and immunofluorescent labelling further indicates that MVBs/late endocytic compartments contain aggregated Aβ1-42. We cannot fully exclude the possibility that these aggregates begin to form in the cell culture medium and then are taken up by the cells. However, the acidic pH environment and high peptide concentration in a limited space promote amyloid aggregation [44], a milieu that is found inside MVBs. In line with this, it was shown in SHSY5Y cells that synthetic Aβ1-42 added to cell culture medium at 1 μM was taken up and formed aggregates of Aβ inside these cells, while only monomers could be found in the cell culture medium even after 5 days [45]. Overall, these results are consistent with the notion that aggregation of Aβ1-42 is promoted inside acidic endocytic compartments. Friedrich et al. (2010) [46] demonstrated in a macrophage cell line, bundles of Aβ1-40 fibrils in MVBs that penetrated the MVB membrane and leaked into the cytoplasm. We now present the first experimental evidence of Aβ42 aggregates developing inside MVBs/late endocytic/lysosomal compartments of cultured neurons.

We also found evidence of loss of endolysosomal impermeability with Aβ1-42 treatment of neurons, in line with reports in non-neuronal cells [47]. Further, we show that Aβ fibrillar oligomers/fibrils are visible inside neurons in a vesicular pattern as early as 45 min after addition of Aβ1-42 to the cell medium, that are not seen when only labelling the cell surface. Remarkably, at later time points intracellular aggregates are larger and extend into elongated structures that appear to penetrate the plasma membrane or are potentially even secreted or extruded into the extracellular space. Of note, the part of the elongated OC antibody positive structures that developed with time and no longer colabeled with the human Aβ specific antibody, might represent (1) Aβ where the N-terminal antibody binding sites become inaccessible to the antibody, (2) endogenous mouse Aβ aggregation and/or (3) incorporation of other amyloidogenic proteins. We demonstrate the ESCRT proteins VPS4A and Tsg101 in plaques of two different AD transgenic mouse models. Moreover, these ESCRT proteins strongly colocalized with a neuronal specific marker of the endo-lysosomal pathway, indicating the neuronal origin of the ESCRT proteins in plaques. Previously the lysosomal hydrolases cathepsin D and β-hexosaminidase A were shown to colocalize with Aβ in a subgroup of diffuse plaques of AD and DS patients [48] consistent with an endolysosomal origin of aggregated Aβ. However, whether these lysosomal proteins were derived from glial cells or neurons was not determined in that study.

Expression of VPS4 mutants deficient in ATP hydrolysis, such as the dominant negative VPS4 E228Q used in this study, leads to enlarged vesicles defined as a class E phenotype, resulting from disruption of ESCRT-III recycling [49–51]. VPS4 acts after the membrane scission step to recycle ESCRT-III proteins back to monomers, so that they are available to start a second wave of ILV formation [52]. One might speculate that Aβ disturbs this recycling leading to enlarged endocytic vesicles.

We show that inhibition of the late ESCRT machinery component VPS4A mimics AD pathogenesis by causing a marked increase in intracellular accumulation of Aβ and a concomitant decrease in secreted Aβ, consistent with what was reported in cultures of AD-transgenic compared to wt neurons [40]. Choy et al., 2012, reported that depletion of Hrs and Tsg101 in HEK293 cells stably expressing APP695 reduced Aβ secretion [53] and Edgar et al. (2015) found reduced Aβ40 secretion and increased intracellular Aβ when depleting APP overexpressing N2a cells of Hrs or Tsg101

[54], consistent with a role for the ESCRT machinery in preventing intracellular Aβ accumulation. However, in contrast to reduced Aβ secretion on depletion of early ESCRTs, Choy et al. found increased Aβ40 secretion upon VPS4A depletion with siRNA [53]. The difference with our demonstration of reduced Aβ secretion upon expression of dnVPS4 might be explained by the different cell types and methods of altering VPS4A that were used.

We provide evidence that the reduced secretion of Aβ with dnVPS4 was not due to reduced exosome secretion, since total exosome secretion was increased with dnVPS4A. Multiple mechanisms of ILV formation have been identified, but the relationship between different populations of ILVs and MVBs remains unclear. Both ESCRT-dependent and ESCRT-independent mechanisms of MVB biogenesis exist in mammalian cells. A competitive relationship between ESCRT-dependent and -independent mechanisms of ILV formation within single MVBs has been suggested, with upregulation of CD63-dependent ILV formation from ESCRT depletion [33–35]. It was shown in HeLa-CIITA-OVA cells that depletion of VPS4B increased the secretion of CD63 positive exosomes [55], in line with our results of increased amounts of CD63 positive exosomes with dnVPS4A. It is interesting to note that in our EM data from APP/PS1 neurons and in wt neurons treated with Aβ1-42, we saw both enlarged MVBs with many ILVs as well as enlarged MVBs with few ILVs. One can speculate that these might represent two different subsets of MVBs; it is possible that ESCRT-dependent ILV formation is disturbed by Aβ/APP, resulting in enlarged and empty MVBs, and potentially subsequent up-regulation of CD63 dependent ILVs formation resulting in MVBs filled with many ILVs. Others have reported that formation of ILVs destined for exosomal release was not ESCRT dependent, while ESCRTs were necessary for ILVs destined for degradation in the lysosome [56].

The intraneuronal pool of Aβ can have a dual origin, namely the production of Aβ from APP inside neurons and uptake of Aβ from the extracellular space that is secreted by other cells and/or the same neuron. Although we saw a net increase in intracellular Aβ levels with the expression of dnVPS4A supporting impaired degradation of Aβ and APP, we can not rule out that the production of Aβ from APP inside neurons was unaffected. In the OC antibody positive dnVPS4A-transfected cells, the enlarged vesicles also colocalized with increased labelling of flotillin-1 (Fig. 4g), hence associating with cholesterol-enriched lipid microdomains. Interestingly, ATPase-defective mammalian VPS4 was reported to localize to aberrant late endosomes accumulating cholesterol, due to impaired cholesterol trafficking [50] and retention of cholesterol in late endosomal/lysosomal compartments was reported to be associated with alterations in APP processing [57].

Our data also demonstrate that defective MVBs, modelled by dnVPS4A, leads to increased tau phosphorylation at serine 396 (S396). This site is phosphorylated by GSK3β; hence the increased tau phosphorylation could be due to impaired GSK3β sequestration into MVBs. Immunofluorescent labelling of GSK3β was increased with dnVPS4A (Additional file 10: Figure S9A), although total levels of GSK3β or GSK3α/β phosphorylated at serine 21/9 were not changed by Western blot. Hence, we cannot fully conclude that defective sequestration of GSK3β into MVBs is responsible for the increased levels of tau phosphorylation that we see with dnVPS4. However, consistent with our results, Tg APP-V7171 mice with the London mutation were found to have increased phosphorylation of tau at S396 and increased GSK3β activity, but no change in total levels of GSK3β and GSK3β phosphorylated at serine 9 [58].

We show that Aβ aggregation can initiate inside nerve cells from vesicular accumulation of Aβ. Aberrant endosomal trafficking has been linked genetically and biologically to a number of neurodegenerative diseases. Proteins involved in endocytosis are also prominent among genes linked to AD [11]. Interestingly, CD2AP, which is genetically linked to late onset AD and has been reported to affect MVB biogenesis and ILV formation [59], was recently reported to elevate levels of intracellular Aβ in dendrites [60]. While the ESCRT-III protein CHMP2B was first genetically linked to FTD [23], copy number variation in CHMP2B has since been reported in a family with familial Alzheimer's disease [24] and genome-wide association studies for late onset AD identified an association with VPS4B [25]. Moreover, Immunoreactivity for CHMP2B is increased in neurons of hippocampus in another characteristic neuropathology of AD, granulovacuolar degeneration (GVD) [61]. CHMP2B-positive GVDs were reported to colocalize to a greater extent with the late endosomal/lysosomal marker LAMP1 than to the lysosomal marker cathepsin D or to the autophagic markers LC3 and p62, suggesting a late endosomal origin of GVDs or that they accumulate at the nexus of autophagic and endocytic pathways [62]. It is interesting to note that we found CHMP2B immunoreactivity particularly in hippocampus and medial temporal lobe of 3-month-old Tg19959 mice before plaque pathology, the two areas that are the first to have GVD-affected neurons in AD [63].

Conclusions

Neuropathological studies have pointed to an early and aberrant accumulation and aggregation of Aβ within neurons in AD, in particular in dystrophic neurites. Cell biological studies that model this aggregation in neurons are valuable in delineating the molecular mechanisms of Aβ-related synaptic dysfunction. We propose a model where elevated levels of Aβ42 cause enlarged and defective MVBs, possibly via effects on ESCRT-III components. Alternatively, MVB dysfunction, as modelled by the expression of dnVPS4A, can lead to accumulation of Aβ in enlarged endocytic compartments. These results support a scenario where disturbances in the MVB pathway caused by Aβ42, or vice versa, could turn into a vicious cycle where more Aβ42 accumulates and oligomeric and fibrillar aggregates form. Our findings that ESCRT components colocalize with Aβ42 in amyloid plaques in two different mouse models of AD support the scenario that aggregated Aβ42 in MVBs/late endocytic compartments, potentially together with ESCRT-components could serve as seeds for plaques.

Additional files

Additional file 1: Table S1. List of antibodies.

Additional file 2: Figure S1. (A) EM image of an enlarged MVB in wt neurons treated with Aβ1-42. This image shows an example of an enlarged MVB with very few ILVs. (B) Confocal analysis of changes in size of LAMP1-positive structures in Aβ1-42 treated wt primary neurons with time. Scale bar 40 μm.

Additional file 3: Figure S2. (A) Confocal analysis of wt primary neurons show that untreated (DMSO) cells have no OC labelling, while cells incubated with Aβ1-40 for 48 h have low levels of OC labelling. However, cells incubated with Aβ1-42 display very strong OC labelling.

Additional file 4: Figure S3. (A) The early relatively weak OC labelling at 45 min of Aβ1-42 treatment colocalizes with LAMP1 labelling in the neurites, but not with the large LAMP1-positive structures in the cell soma. Confocal analysis of wt primary neurons treated with Aβ1-42 for 45 min. Scale 20 μm. (B) After 48 h of Aβ1-42 treatment, OC labelling is stronger and colocalizes partly with LAMP1-positive structures that appear enlarged and irregular in their shape. Elongated OC-positive structures extend out from such punctate LAMP1 labelling in the neuronal processes. Scale 20 μm. (C) At high magnification, antibody OC labelling can be seen colocalizing with the late endocytic marker Rab7 in neuronal processes of wt neurons treated for 24 h with Aβ1-42. Scale bar 5 μm.

Additional file 5: Figure S4. ESCRT proteins in primary neurons and plaques. (A-B) In young 3-month-old Tg19959 mice, CHMP2B immunolabelling is increased in areas of hippocampus (a) and entorhinal cortex (b) that also have increased labelling of APP/Aβ (6E10). Scale bar 40 μm, $n = 4$. (C) Western blot analysis of APP/PS1 compared to wt primary neurons at 12 DIV lysed in 6% SDS shows that protein levels of CHMP2B and VPS4 are not significantly changed, although there is a trend for increased levels of CHMP2B in APP/PS1 neurons, $n > 6$. Protein levels are expressed as percentage of control and are corrected against actin. (D) VPS4 colocalizes with Aβ42 in a vesicular pattern in 19-month-old wt mice (upper panel), $n = 3$. In 19-month-old APP/PS1 mice VPS4 accumulates in and around amyloid plaques (lower panel, white arrows). Scale bar 40 μm, $n = 4$. (E) Decreased labelling of CHMP2B in plaques (white arrows) in 19-month-old APP/PS1 mice. Some colocalization of CHMP2B is seen in Aβ/APP (6E10) positive cells (grey arrows). Scale bar 40 μm, $n = 3$. (F) Labelling of early ESCRT-0 component Hrs is decreased in amyloid plaques compared to surrounding brain parenchyma. Scale bar 40 μm, $n = 2$.

Additional file 6: Figure S5. Aβ1-42 increases the diameter of LAMP-1 positive vesicles in N2a cells. Confocal images of exogenously added monomeric Aβ1-42 incubated for different time points, ranging from 15 min to 48 h, in N2a cells. 3D-rendering with Imaris from confocal z-stack. Colocalization of OC labelling and LAMP1 labelling can be seen from 45 min of Aβ treatment. The last image is from a single focal plane showing OC labelling inside an enlarged LAMP1-positive structure as well as OC labelling that appears to localize at the cell surface. Scale bar 10 μm.

Additional file 7: Figure S6. DnVPS4A increases secretion but does not change levels of intracellular α-syn. (A) Western blot analysis of α-syn N2a cells transfected with dnVPS4A shows increased levels of extracellular α-synuclein without altering the total pool of intracellular α-synuclein. (B) Quantification of A. Values are normalized against actin and expressed as percentage of control, $n = 3$; $*p < 0.05$, $**p < 0.01$. (C) Overexposed WB membrane for secreted α-synuclein (same as above) with increased intensity to better visualize the bands.

Additional file 8: Figure S7. (A) Western blot analysis of APP and Aβ in Swe N2a cells treated with 40 μg/ml cycloheximide (CHX) at different times in hours (h) before harvest. Cell culture media was replaced with fresh media 24 h before harvest. For quantification, values are normalized against actin and expressed as percentage of control, $n = 3$; $*p < 0.05$, $**p < 0.01$, $***p < 0.001$, $****p < 0.0001$ (ANOVA with Dunnett's multiple comparisons test, compared to ctr). (B) Confocal images of 6E10 and Golgi marker GM130 in Swe N2a cells treated with 40 μg/ml CHX for the depicted times.

Additional file 9: Figure S8. (A) Western blot analysis of APP and Aβ in Swe N2a cells treated with 5 nM bafilomycin A1 (BafA1) at different time points (h) before harvest. Cell culture media was replaced with fresh media 24 h before harvest. (B) Quantification of A. Values are normalized against actin and expressed as percentage of control, $n = 3$; $*p < 0.05$, $**p < 0.01$, $***p < 0.001$, $****p < 0.0001$ (ANOVA with Dunnett's multiple comparisons test, compared to ctr). (C) Confocal images of 6E10 and LAMP1 labelling in Swe N2a cells treated with 5 nM bafilomycin A1 for the depicted times. At 24 h there is a build up of both 6E10 labelling and punctate LAMP1-positive structures. (D) Western blot analysis of APP and Aβ in Swe N2a cells treated with 5 nM bafilomycin A1 (BafA1) 24 h before harvest and 40 μg/ml cycloheximide (CHX) at different time points (h) before harvest. Cell culture media was replaced with fresh media 24 h before harvest, before the addition of Baf A1.

Additional file 10: Figure S9. (A) 3D images show increased GSK3β labelling in dnVPS4-expressing N2a Swe compared to cells transfected with control plasmid. Rab7 labelling is also increased in dnVPS4 expressing cells. Scale bar 15 μm. (B) Western blot analysis of cell lysates of Swe N2a cells transfected with dnVPS4A showing no changes in total GSK3β or phosphorylated GSK3α/β (serine 21/9).

Abbreviations

AD: Alzheimer's disease; APP: Amyloid precursor protein; APP/PS1: B6.Cg-Tg (APPswe,PSEN1dE9)85Dbo/Mmjax mice; BACE1: Beta-secretase 1; BafA1: Bafilomycin A1; BSA: Bovine serum albumin; DIV: Days in vitro; dnVPS4A: Dominant negative VPS4A; EM: Electron microscopy; ESCRT: Endosomal sorting complexes required for transport; FTD: Frontotemporal dementia; ILV: Intraluminal vesicle; MVB: Multivesicular bodies; NFTs: Neurofibrillary tangles; NGS: Normal goat serum; PBS: Phosphate buffered saline; PBST: PBS containing 0.1% Tween-20; PFA: Paraformaldehyde; PS1: Presenilin 1; RT: Room temperature; SDS: Sodium dodecyl sulfate; TCA: Trichloroacetic acid; tg: AD transgenic; wtVPS4A: Wild type VPS4A

Acknowledgements

We thank Drs. Gopal Thinakaran and Sangram Sisodia at the University of Chicago for sharing their stably transfected human APP N2a cells. We also thank Bodil Israelsson at Lund University for technical support.

Funding

This study was supported by MultiPark, Parkinsonsfonden and the Swedish Research Council.

Authors' contributions

KW and GKG conceived the study; KW performed and analysed all experiments except for the EM imaging, which was performed and analysed by JRE and CEF; TH and NT supplied the p3xFLAG-CMV-10-hVPS4A-wt and p3xFLAG-CMV-10-hVPS4A-dn plasmids; KW wrote the paper, with input and editing provided by GKG, JRE and CEF. All authors read and approved the final manuscript.

Competing interests
The authors declare that they have no competing interests.

Author details
[1]Department of Experimental Medical Science, Lund University, 221 84 Lund, Sweden. [2]Cambridge Institute for Medical Research, University of Cambridge, Cambridge CB2 0XY, UK. [3]UCL Institute of Ophthalmology, London EC1V 9EL, UK. [4]Division of Neurology, Department of Neuroscience and Sensory Organs, Tohoku University Graduate School of Medicine, Sendai 980-8574, Japan. [5]Division of Cancer Biology and Therapeutics, Miyagi Cancer Center Research Institute, Natori 981-1293, Japan.

References

1. Cataldo AM, Petanceska S, Terio NB, Peterhoff CM, Durham R, Mercken M, Mehta PD, Buxbaum J, Haroutunian V, Nixon RA. Abeta localization in abnormal endosomes: association with earliest Abeta elevations in AD and down syndrome. Neurobiol Aging. 2004;25:1263–72.
2. D'Andrea MR, Nagele RG, Wang HY, Peterson PA, Lee DHS. Evidence that neurones accumulating amyloid can undergo lysis to form amyloid plaques in Alzheimer's disease. Histopathology. 2001;38:120–34.
3. Gouras GK, Tsai J, Naslund J, Vincent B, Edgar M, Checler F, Greenfield JP, Haroutunian V, Buxbaum JD, Xu H, Greengard P, Relkin NR. Intraneuronal Ab42 accumulation in human brain. Am J Pathol. 2000;156:15–20.
4. Oakley H, Cole SL, Logan S, Maus E, Shao P, Craft J, Guillozet-Bongaarts A, Ohno M, Disterhoft J, Van Eldik L, Berry R, Vassar R. Intraneuronal beta-amyloid aggregates, neurodegeneration, and neuron loss in transgenic mice with five familial Alzheimer's disease mutations: potential factors in amyloid plaque formation. J Neurosci. 2006;26:10129–40.
5. Takahashi RH, Milner TA, Li F, Nam EE, Edgar MA, Yamaguchi H, Beal MF, Xu H, Greengard P, Gouras GK. Intraneuronal Alzheimer Abeta42 accumulates in multivesicular bodies and is associated with synaptic pathology. Am J Pathol. 2002;161:1869–79.
6. Wirths O, Multhaup G, Czech C, Blanchard V, Moussaoui S, Tremp G, Pradier L, Beyreuther K, Bayer TA. Intraneuronal Abeta accumulation precedes plaque formation in beta-amyloid precursor protein and presenilin-1 double-transgenic mice. Neurosci Lett. 2001;306:116–20.
7. Billings LM, Oddo S, Green KN, McGaugh JL, LaFerla FM. Intraneuronal Abeta causes the onset of early Alzheimer's disease-related cognitive deficits in transgenic mice. Neuron. 2005;45:675–88.
8. Chapman PF, White GL, Jones MW, Cooper-Blacketer D, Marshall VJ, Irizarry M, Younkin L, Good MA, Bliss TV, Hyman BT, Younkin SG, Hsiao KK. Impaired synaptic plasticity and learning in aged amyloid precursor protein transgenic mice. Nat Neurosci. 1999;2:271–6.
9. Takahashi RH, Almeida CG, Kearney PF, Yu F, Lin MT, Milner TA, Gouras GK. Oligomerization of Alzheimer's beta-amyloid within processes and synapses of cultured neurons and brain. J Neurosci. 2004;24:3592–9.
10. Gouras GK, Tampellini D, Takahashi RH, Capetillo-Zarate E. Intraneuronal beta-amyloid accumulation and synapse pathology in Alzheimer's disease. Acta Neuropathol. 2010;119:523–41.
11. Peric A, Annaert W. Early etiology of Alzheimer's disease: tipping the balance toward autophagy or endosomal dysfunction? Acta Neuropathol. 2015;129:363–81.
12. Cataldo AM, Peterhoff CM, Troncoso JC, Gomez-Isla T, Hyman BT, Nixon RA. Endocytic pathway abnormalities precede amyloid beta deposition in sporadic Alzheimer's disease and down syndrome: differential effects of APOE genotype and presenilin mutations. Am J Pathol. 2000;157:277–86.
13. Cataldo AM, Mathews PM, Boiteau AB, Hassinger LC, Peterhoff CM, Jiang Y, Mullaney K, Neve RL, Gruenberg J, Nixon RA. Down syndrome fibroblast model of Alzheimer-related endosome pathology: accelerated endocytosis promotes late endocytic defects. Am J Pathol. 2008;173:370–84.
14. Nixon RA, Wegiel J, Kumar A, Yu WH, Peterhoff C, Cataldo A, Cuervo AM. Extensive involvement of autophagy in Alzheimer disease: an immuno-electron microscopy study. J Neuropathol Exp Neurol. 2005;64:113–22.
15. Small SA, Gandy S. Sorting through the cell biology of Alzheimer's disease: intracellular pathways to pathogenesis. Neuron. 2006;52:15–31.
16. De Strooper B, Vassar R, Golde T. The secretases: enzymes with therapeutic potential in Alzheimer disease. Nat Rev Neurol. 2010;6:99–107.
17. Rajendran L, Annaert W. Membrane trafficking pathways in Alzheimer's disease. Traffic. 2012;13:759–70.
18. Sannerud R, Declerck I, Peric A, Raemaekers T, Menendez G, Zhou L, Veerle B, Coen K, Munck S, De Strooper B, Schiavo G, Annaert W. ADP ribosylation factor 6 (ARF6) controls amyloid precursor protein (APP) processing by mediating the endosomal sorting of BACE1. Proc Natl Acad Sci U S A. 2011; 108:E559–68.
19. Sannerud R, Esselens C, Ejsmont P, Mattera R, Rochin L, Tharkeshwar AK, De Baets G, De Wever V, Habets R, Baert V, Vermeire W, Michiels C, Groot AJ, Wouters R, Dillen K, Vints K, Baatsen P, Munck S, Derua R, Waelkens E, Basi GS, Mercken M, Vooijs M, Bollen M, Schymkowitz J, Rousseau F, Bonifacino JS, Van Niel G, De Strooper B, Annaert W. Restricted location of PSEN2/γ-Secretase determines substrate specificity and generates an intracellular Aβ pool. Cell. 2016;166:193–208.
20. Langui D, Girardot N, El Hachimi KH, Allinquant B, Blanchard V, Pradier L, Duyckaerts C. Subcellular topography of neuronal Abeta peptide in APPxPS1 transgenic mice. Am J Pathol. 2004;165:1465–77.
21. Almeida C, Takahashi H, Gouras GK. Beta-amyloid accumulation impairs multivesicular body sorting by inhibiting the ubiquitin-proteasome system. J Neurosci. 2006;26:4277–88.
22. Babst M, Katzmann DJ, Estepa-Sabal EJ, Meerloo T, Emr SD. Escrt-III: an endosome-associated heterooligomeric protein complex required for mvb sorting. Dev Cell. 2002;3:271–82.
23. Skibinski G, Parkinson NJ, Brown JM, Chakrabarti L, Lloyd SL, Hummerich H, Nielsen JE, Hodges JR, Spillantini MG, Thusgaard T, Brandner S, Brun A, Rossor MN, Gade A, Johannsen P, Sørensen SA, Gydesen S, Fisher EM, Collinge J. Mutations in the endosomal ESCRTIII-complex subunit CHMP2B in frontotemporal dementia. Nat Genet. 2005;37:806–8.
24. Hooli BV, Kovacs-Vajna ZM, Mullin K, Blumenthal MA, Mattheisen M, Zhang C, Lange C, Mohapatra G, Bertram L, Tanzi RE. Rare autosomal copy number variations in early-onset familial Alzheimer's disease. Mol Psychiatry. 2014;19:676–81.
25. Jones L, Holmans PA, Hamshere ML, Harold D, Moskvina V, Ivanov D, Pocklington A, Abraham R, Hollingworth P, Sims R, Gerrish A, Pahwa JS, Jones N, Stretton A, Morgan AR, Lovestone S, Powell J, Proitsi P, Lupton MK, Brayne C, Rubinsztein DC, Gill M, Lawlor B, Lynch A, Morgan K, Brown KS, Passmore PA, Craig D, McGuinness B, Todd S, Holmes C, Mann D, Smith AD, Love S, Kehoe PG, Mead S, Fox N, Rossor M, Collinge J, Maier W, Jessen F, Schürmann B, Heun R, Kölsch H, van den Bussche H, Heuser I, Peters O, Kornhuber J, Wiltfang J, Dichgans M, Frölich L, Hampel H, Hüll M, Rujescu D, Goate AM, Kauwe JS, Cruchaga C, Nowotny P, Morris JC, Mayo K, Livingston G, Bass NJ, Gurling H, McQuillin A, Gwilliam R, Deloukas P, Al-Chalabi A, Shaw CE, Singleton AB, Guerreiro R, Mühleisen TW, Nöthen MM, Moebus S, Jöckel KH, Klopp N, Wichmann HE, Rüther E, Carrasquillo MM, Pankratz VS, Younkin SG, Hardy J, O'Donovan MC, Owen MJ, Williams J. Genetic evidence implicates the immune system and cholesterol metabolism in the aetiology of Alzheimer's disease. PLoS One. 2010;5:e13950.
26. Thinakaran G, Teplow DB, Siman R, Greenberg B, Sisodia SS. Metabolism of the "Swedish" amyloid precursor protein variant in neuro2a (N2a) cells. Evidence that cleavage at the "beta-secretase" site occurs in the golgi apparatus. J Biol Chem. 1996;271:9390–7.
27. Slot JW, Geuze HJ. A new method of preparing gold probes for multiple-labeling cytochemistry. Eur J Cell Biol. 1985;38:87–93.
28. Hasegawa T, Konno M, Baba T, Sugeno N, Kikuchi A, Kobayashi M, Miura E, Tanaka N, Tamai K, Furukawa K, Arai H, Mori F, Wakabayashi K, Aoki M, Itoyama Y, Takeda A. The AAA-ATPase VPS4 regulates extracellular secretion and lysosomal targeting of α-synuclein. PLoS One. 2011;6:e29460.
29. Buxbaum JD, Gandy SE, Cicchetti P, Ehrlich ME, Czernik AJ, Fracasso RP, Ramabhadran TV, Unterbeck AJ, Greengard P. Processing of Alzheimer beta/A4 amyloid precursor protein: modulation by agents that regulate protein phosphorylation. Proc Natl Acad Sci U S A. 1990;87:6003–6.
30. Théry C, Amigorena S, Raposo G, Clayton A. Isolation and characterization of exosomes from cell culture supernatants and biological fluids. Curr Protoc Cell Biol. 2006;30(3.22):3.22.1–3.22.29.
31. Kayed R, Head E, Sarsoza F, Saing T, Cotman CW, Necula M, Margol L, Wu J, Breydo L, Thompson JL, Rasool S, Gurlo T, Butler P, Glabe CG. Fibril specific, conformation dependent antibodies recognize a generic epitope common to amyloid fibrils and fibrillar oligomers that is absent in prefibrillar oligomers. Mol Neurodegener. 2007;2:18.
32. Katoh Y, Ritter B, Gaffry T, Blondeau F, Höning S, McPherson PS. The clavesin family, neuron-specific lipid- and clathrin-binding sec14 proteins regulating lysosomal morphology. J Biol Chem. 2009;284:27646–54.

33. Stuffers S, Sem Wegner C, Stenmark H, Brech A. Multivesicular endosome biogenesis in the absence of ESCRTs. Traffic. 2009;10:925–37.
34. van Niel G, Charrin S, Simoes S, Romao M, Rochin L, Saftig P, Marks MS, Rubinstein E, Raposo G. The tetraspanin CD63 regulates ESCRT-independent and -dependent endosomal sorting during melanogenesis. Dev Cell. 2011;21:708–21.
35. Edgar JR, Eden ER, Futter CE. Hrs- and CD63-dependent competing mechanisms make different sized endosomal intraluminal vesicles. Traffic. 2014;15:197–211.
36. Taelman VF, Dobrowolski R, Plouhinec JL, Fuentealba LC, Vorwald PP, Gumper I, Sabatini DD, De Robertis EM. Wnt signaling requires sequestration of glycogen synthase kinase 3 inside multivesicular endosomes. Cell. 2010;143:1136–48.
37. Kimura T, Whitcomb DJ, Jo J, Regan P, Piers T, Heo S, Brown C, Hashikawa T, Murayama M, Seok H, Sotiropoulos I, Kim E, Collingridge GL, Takashima A, Cho K. Microtubule-associated protein tau is essential for long-term depression in the hippocampus. Philos Trans R Soc Lond Ser B Biol Sci. 2013;369:20130144.
38. Hooper C, Killick R, Lovestone S. The GSK3 hypothesis of Alzheimer's disease. J Neurochem. 2008;104:1433–9.
39. Dunning CJ, McGauran G, Willén K, Gouras GK, O'Connell DJ, Linse S. Direct high affinity interaction between Aβ42 and GSK3α stimulates hyperphosphorylation of tau. A new molecular link in Alzheimer's disease? ACS Chem Neurosci. 2016;7:161–70.
40. Tampellini D, Rahman N, Lin MT, Capetillo-Zarate E, Gouras GK. Impaired beta-amyloid secretion in Alzheimer's disease pathogenesis. J Neurosci. 2011;31:15384–90.
41. Tampellini D, Capetillo-Zarate E, Dumont M, Huang Z, Yu F, Lin MT, Gouras GK. Effects of synaptic modulation on beta-amyloid, synaptophysin, and memory performance in Alzheimer's disease transgenic mice. J Neurosci. 2010;30:14299–304.
42. Kim S, Sato Y, Mohan PS, Peterhoff C, Pensalfini A, Rigoglioso A, Jiang Y, Nixon RA. Evidence that the rab5 effector APPL1 mediates APP-βCTF-induced dysfunction of endosomes in down syndrome and Alzheimers disease. Mol Psychiatry. 2016;21:707–16.
43. Lauritzen I, Pardossi-Piquard R, Bourgeois A, Pagnotta S, Biferi MG, Barkats M, Lacor P, Klein W, Bauer C, Checler F. Intraneuronal aggregation of the β-CTF fragment of APP (C99) induces Aβ-independent lysosomal-autophagic pathology. Acta Neuropathol. 2016;132:257–76.
44. Burdick D, Soreghan B, Kwon M, Kosmoski J, Knauer M, Henschen A, Yates J, Cotman C, Glabe C. Assembly and aggregation properties of synthetic Alzheimer's A4/beta amyloid peptide analogs. J Biol Chem. 1992;267:546–54.
45. Hu X, Crick SL, Bu G, Frieden C, Pappu RV, Lee JM. Amyloid seeds formed by cellular uptake, concentration, and aggregation of the amyloid-beta peptide. Proc Natl Acad Sci U S A. 2009;1(106):20324–9.
46. Friedrich RP, Tepper K, Rönicke R, Soom M, Westermann M, Reymann K, Kaether C, Fändrich M. Mechanism of amyloid plaque formation suggests an intracellular basis of Aβ pathogenicity. Proc Natl Acad Sci U S A. 2010;107:1942–7.
47. Yang AJ, Chandswangbhuvana D, Margol L, Glabe CG. Loss of endosomal/lysosomal membrane impermeability is an early event in amyloid Abeta1-42 pathogenesis. J Neurosci Res. 1998;52:691–8.
48. Cataldo AM, Barnett JL, Mann DM, Nixon RA. Colocalization of lysosomal hydrolase and beta-amyloid in diffuse plaques of the cerebellum and striatum in Alzheimer's disease and Down's syndrome. J Neuropathol Exp Neurol. 1996;55:704–15.
49. Babst M, Wendland B, Estepa EJ, Emr SD. The Vps4p AAA ATPase regulates membrane association of a Vps protein complex required for normal endosome function. EMBO J. 1998;11:2982–93.
50. Bishop N, Woodman P. ATPase-defective mammalian VPS4 localizes to aberrant endosomes and impairs cholesterol trafficking. Mol Biol Cell. 2000; 11:227–39.
51. Dores MR, Chen B, Lin H, Soh UJ, Paing MM, Montagne WA, Meerloo T, Trejo J. ALIX binds a YPX(3)L motif of the GPCR PAR1 and mediates ubiquitin-independent ESCRT-III/MVB sorting. J Cell Biol. 2012;197:407–19.
52. Wollert T, Wunder C, Lippincott-Schwartz J, Hurley JH. Membrane scission by the ESCRT-III complex. Nature. 2009;458:172–7.
53. Choy RW, Cheng Z, Schekman R. Amyloid precursor protein (APP) traffics from the cell surface via endosomes for amyloid β (Aβ) production in the trans-Golgi network. Proc Natl Acad Sci U S A. 2012;109:E2077–82.
54. Edgar JR, Willén K, Gouras GK, Futter CE. ESCRTs regulate amyloid precursor protein sorting in multivesicular bodies and intracellular amyloid-β accumulation. J Cell Sci. 2015;128:2520–8.
55. Colombo M, Moita C, van Niel G, Kowal J, Vigneron J, Benaroch P, Manel N, Moita LF, Théry C, Raposo G. Analysis of ESCRT functions in exosome biogenesis, composition and secretion highlights the heterogeneity of extracellular vesicles. J Cell Sci. 2013;126:5553–65.
56. Trajkovic K, Hsu C, Chiantia S, Rajendran L, Wenzel D, Wieland F, Schwille P, Brügger B, Simons M. Ceramide triggers budding of exosome vesicles into multivesicular endosomes. Science. 2008;319:1244–7.
57. Runz H, Rietdorf J, Tomic I, de Bernard M, Beyreuther K, Pepperkok R, Hartmann T. Inhibition of intracellular cholesterol transport alters presenilin localization and amyloid precursor protein processing in neuronal cells. J Neurosci. 2002;22:679–89.
58. Terwel D, Muyllaert D, Dewachter I, Borghgraef P, Croes S, Devijver H, Van Leuven F. Amyloid activates GSK-3beta to aggravate neuronal tauopathy in bigenic mice. Am J Pathol. 2008;172:786–98.
59. Kim JM, Wu H, Green G, Winkler CA, Kopp JB, Miner JH, Unanue ER, Shaw AS. CD2-associated protein haploinsufficiency is linked to glomerular disease susceptibility. Science. 2003;300:1298–300.
60. Ubelmann F, Burrinha T, Salavessa L, Gomes R, Ferreira C, Moreno N, Guimas AC. Bin1 and CD2AP polarise the endocytic generation of beta-amyloid. EMBO Rep. 2017;18:102–22.
61. Yamazaki Y, Takahashi T, Hiji M, Kurashige T, Izumi Y, Yamawaki T, Matsumoto M. Immunopositivity for ESCRT-III subunit CHMP2B in granulovacuolar degeneration of neurons in the Alzheimer's disease hippocampus. Neurosci Lett. 2010;477:86–90.
62. Funk KE, Mrak RE, Kuret J. Granulovacuolar degeneration (GVD) bodies of Alzheimer's disease (AD) resemble late-stage autophagic organelles. Neuropathol Appl Neurobiol. 2011;37:295–306.
63. Thal DR, Del Tredici K, Ludolph AC, Hoozemans JJ, Rozemuller AJ, Braak H, Knippschild U. Stages of granulovacuolar degeneration: their relation to Alzheimer's disease and chronic stress response. Acta Neuropathol. 2011; 122:577–89.

4

Multiscale network modeling of oligodendrocytes reveals molecular components of myelin dysregulation in Alzheimer's disease

Andrew T. McKenzie[1,2,3], Sarah Moyon[4,13], Minghui Wang[1,2], Igor Katsyv[1,2,3], Won-Min Song[1,2], Xianxiao Zhou[1,2], Eric B. Dammer[5], Duc M. Duong[6,7], Joshua Aaker[8], Yongzhong Zhao[1,2], Noam Beckmann[1,2], Pei Wang[1,2], Jun Zhu[1,2], James J. Lah[9,10], Nicholas T. Seyfried[6,7,9], Allan I. Levey[9,10], Pavel Katsel[11], Vahram Haroutunian[2,11,12], Eric E. Schadt[1,2], Brian Popko[8], Patrizia Casaccia[2,4,13*] and Bin Zhang[1,2*]

Abstract

Background: Oligodendrocytes (OLs) and myelin are critical for normal brain function and have been implicated in neurodegeneration. Several lines of evidence including neuroimaging and neuropathological data suggest that Alzheimer's disease (AD) may be associated with dysmyelination and a breakdown of OL-axon communication.

Methods: In order to understand this phenomenon on a molecular level, we systematically interrogated OL-enriched gene networks constructed from large-scale genomic, transcriptomic and proteomic data obtained from human AD postmortem brain samples. We then validated these networks using gene expression datasets generated from mice with ablation of major gene expression nodes identified in our AD-dysregulated networks.

Results: The robust OL gene coexpression networks that we identified were highly enriched for genes associated with AD risk variants, such as *BIN1* and demonstrated strong dysregulation in AD. We further corroborated the structure of the corresponding gene causal networks using datasets generated from the brain of mice with ablation of key network drivers, such as *UGT8*, *CNP* and *PLP1*, which were identified from human AD brain data. Further, we found that mice with genetic ablations of *Cnp* mimicked aspects of myelin and mitochondrial gene expression dysregulation seen in brain samples from patients with AD, including decreased protein expression of *BIN1* and *GOT2*.

Conclusions: This study provides a molecular blueprint of the dysregulation of gene expression networks of OL in AD and identifies key OL- and myelination-related genes and networks that are highly associated with AD.

Keywords: Alzheimer's disease, Oligodendrocyte, Myelin, co-expression network, Causal network, RNA sequencing, Proteomics, Differential expression, CNP, BIN1

* Correspondence: Patrizia.Casaccia@mssm.edu; patrizia.casaccia@asrc.cuny.edu; bin.zhang@mssm.edu
Sarah Moyon, Patrizia Casaccia and Bin Zhang are Co-senior authors.
Andrew T. McKenzie and Sarah Moyon contributed equally to this work.
[2]Icahn Institute of Genomics and Multiscale Biology, Icahn School of Medicine at Mount Sinai, One Gustave L. Levy Place, New York, NY 10029, USA
[1]Department of Genetics and Genomic Sciences, Icahn School of Medicine at Mount Sinai, One Gustave L. Levy Place, 1470 Madison Avenue, Room S8-111, New York, NY 10029, USA
Full list of author information is available at the end of the article

Background

Alzheimer's disease (AD) causes a progressive dementia that affects approximately 1/6th of people in the US age 75 and above [1]. Although the number one risk factor for AD is advanced age, the reason for this remains unknown [2, 3]. A wealth of evidence has emerged over the past decade to support the role of non-neuronal cells, especially astrocytes and microglia, in amyloid beta (Aβ) processing and AD pathogenesis [4–6]. While less well studied, several lines of evidence have suggested that dysregulation of oligodendrocytes (OLs) and associated dysmyelination might be important in AD pathology. For example, human neuroimaging studies have shown that white matter changes occur early in AD and are predictive of disease status [7–9]. In particular, MRI studies have detected white matter volume atrophy in multiple brain regions prior to changes in gray matter in AD progression [10–12]. Further, post-mortem human pathological studies have demonstrated that the pattern of neurofibrillary tangle deposition in AD is highly correlated with the developmental pattern of myelination, with late-myelinated axonal tracts substantially more vulnerable to degeneration in AD [13, 14]. Recent reports have highlighted the importance of OLs and myelin metabolic function for axonal health and transport capacity [15–20], thereby suggesting the possibility that OL-driven axonal damage could precede a secondary demyelination in the pathogenesis of AD. In particular, there are several mouse models of ablation of the OL-associated myelin genes *Ugt8* [21], *Cnp* [22, 23], and *Plp1* [24, 25], in which axonal degeneration occurs in the presence of minimal ultrastructural myelin alterations and therefore are well suited to study altered OL gene expression, presumably leading to myeling dysfunction preceding the onset of neurodegeneration. To investigate the hypothesis that OL dysregulation in AD may be part of the underlying mechanism leading to neurodegeneration, we sought to employ a detailed molecular and systems-level analysis to provide a molecular substrate for the potential role of OLs in mediating the initial axonal damage.

In this study, we systematically examined and validated OL-enriched gene networks to uncover key genes and molecular signaling circuits of OLs in AD. We built upon AD-associated and OL-enriched networks constructed in a previous study of genetic, gene expression, and pathophysiologic data in late-onset AD [26]. We constructed a union of the three OL-enriched modules from a multi-tissue AD co-expression network and found that it was strongly enriched for AD risk factor genes. Our OL-enriched consensus module includes genes encoding proteins associated with Aβ-production *PSEN1* and *BACE1*, as well as the AD risk factor genes *BIN1*, *PSEN1*, *PICALM*, and *UNC5C* [27–30]. We next built co-expression networks from a large-scale proteomics data set, identifying a strong loss of coordination among proteins in the most OL-enriched network, an interaction of this dysregulation and dementia status, as well as a down-regulation of key OL network genes, including *BIN1*. We then used the OL modules to construct regulatory networks and found that the topological structures of our OL-enriched networks were validated through in vitro and in vivo perturbations of the predicted key regulatory genes in the networks. Further, transcriptomic analysis of brain tissue isolated from mice with a genetic ablation of three top key driver genes (*Ugt8*, *Cnp*, and *Plp1*) recapitulated key aspects of the dysregulation in gene pathways related to myelination that are seen in human AD brains. We chose to profile the mice with these genetic ablations at an early stage of development (postnatal day 20), in order to detect alterations in gene pathways occurring during the process of myelination and prior to the onset of widespread axon degeneration in *Cnp*-KO [22] or *Plp1*-KO [24] mice. This approach allowed us to define alterations in OL gene expression occurring during the "pre-symptomatic" or prodromal phase of the disease, as opposed to reactive changes that might be consequent to axonal degeneration. We found that differentially expressed gene (DEG) signature in the *Cnp* knockout (KO) mouse mimicked gene expression changes detected in AD brains at the early stages of the pathology, both at the gene pathway and individual protein level, thereby suggesting that dysregulation of OLs in general and *CNP* in particular may play a key role in driving AD-associated gene expression changes.

Methods

Oligodendrocyte network construction from AD data and key driver analysis

We re-analyzed data from the Harvard Brain Tissue Resource Center (HBTRC) consisting of 376 late-onset Alzheimer's disease brain samples as well as 173 non-demented brain samples, harvested from the cerebellum (CBM), dorsolateral prefrontal cortex (Brodmann area 9; henceforth, PFC), and visual cortex (Brodmann area 7; VC), which has been previously described [26] (GEO: GSE44772). Based upon the HBTRC AD data, we previously built up a multi-tissue weighted gene co-expression network using WGCNA [26, 31]. In order to find the AD OL-specific modules, we tested the enrichment of each module for the gene signatures specifically expressed in OLs. To do this, we employed datasets on cell enrichment and identified the genes most highly expressed in myelinating OLs compared to the non-OL cell types [32]. Three modules, one with probes primarily derived from each of the three investigated brain regions were found to be the most enriched for the OL gene signature. We therefore refer to these as the "region-specific oligodendrocyte co-expression network" modules. We further inferred an interaction network for each OL-enriched and region-specific gene module by integrating gene expression and DNA genotypic data, as previously described [26]. Specifically, relationships between genes in each co-expression module were inferred based on conditional independence tests of gene expression in a Bayesian framework, and the presence of more expression single nucleotide polymorphisms (eSNPs) associated with a gene were used as priors to break Markov equivalence [33]. We refer to each of these networks as the "region-specific OL-enriched Bayesian interaction networks". For robustness, we combined the genes in the three region-specific co-expression networks into a core OL gene set (COLGS), merged the three brain region-specific Bayesian interaction networks by a set union of directed links into a core OL-enriched Bayesian interaction network (COLBN). The gene symbols from this previous study were updated to current Hugo Gene Nomenclature Committee (HGNC) standards using the R package HGCNhelper (v. 0.3.1), and the two gene symbols in the OL-enriched networks that were still mapped to multiple symbols were mapped to the more common symbol (*MARCH1* and *LPAR1*) for legibility. In order to identify key regulatory genes in this interaction network, we then performed key driver analysis on COLBN [34, 35], which uses network connectivity to infer regulatory importance scores for genes.

Enrichment of brain co-expression modules in AD GWAS risk factor genes

In order to find the enrichment of COLGS and other co-expression modules in Alzheimer's risk factor genes, we converted the International Genomics of Alzheimer's Project (IGAP) GWAS SNP-level data set [28] to gene-level *p*-value calls using VEGAS2 [36], and used the genes with significant association at a nominal $p < 0.05$ for further analysis. We then measured the enrichment of this 543 AD GWAS risk factor gene set in the 62 overall qualifying multiscale AD modules with at least 50 genes using Fisher's Exact Test (FET).

Proteomics data analysis from PFC human postmortem brain samples

Grey matter brain samples in 50 mg aliquots were harvested from the prefrontal cortex (PFC; Brodmann Area 10) from the autopsied brains of persons with a wide range of cognitive status at the time of death, ranging from no cognitive impairment to dementia, as well as a wide range of Braak scores, from 0 to 6. Liquid chromatography-tandem mass spectrometry (LC-MS/MS) was used to measure the abundance of peptides in each brain sample, from which a protein-level quantitation was estimated using MaxQuant (v1.5.3.30). We used WGCNA to define modules of proteins in the proteomics data, with a soft-thresholding power coefficient of 3. We next annotated these modules based on their relative FET enrichment in the human homologues of genes specifically expressed in each of the five major mouse brain cell types (see "Estimating brain cell type enrichment").

Within this OL-enriched module, we performed modular differential connectivity analysis in order to assess the overall difference in between samples classified as non-AD (Braak 0–2) and AD (Braak 5–6), calculated using the mean difference in z-scores option in DGCA [37] (v. 1.0.1), with 10,000 permutation samples to assess significance. We used a Student's t-test to measure differences in average expression between conditions, using the q value R package [38] to estimate false discovery rates in the context of the multiple hypothesis tests.

Generating in vivo mouse genetic perturbation signatures

Animals

Use of animals in this research was strictly compliant with the guidelines set forth by the US Public Health Service in their policy on Humane Care and Use of Laboratory Animals, and in the Guide for the Care and Use of Laboratory Animals. All animal procedures received prior approval from the Institutional Animal Care and Use Committee at Icahn School of Medicine at Mount Sinai.

Tissue collection

For each of the control and knockout model mice of the three key drivers (*Cnp*, *Ugt8*, and *Plp1*), mice of either sex were sacrificed at postnatal day 20 and tissue was flash-frozen in liquid nitrogen vapors. The frontal cortex and cerebellum were dissected on ice and immediately processed for RNA isolation. Integrity of the RNA was confirmed by measuring RNA Integrity Number (RIN) and only samples with RIN > 8.5 were used for RNA sequencing.

RNA isolation and reverse transcription

RNA was isolated using Trizol reagent (Invitrogen, CA) and cleaned using RNeasy Mini kit (Qiagen, CA). Ribosomal RNA was removed from the samples using Ribo-Zero rRNA Removal Kit (Illumina, CA). Approximately 500 nanograms of total RNA was used in cDNA library construction with the TruSeq RNA Sample Prep Kit (Illumina, CA), followed by RNA sequencing using an Illumina HiSeq2000.

Read mapping and quantification of RNAseq data

RNA-sequencing reads were mapped to the mouse genome (mm10, UCSC assembly) using Bowtie (version

2.2.3.0), TopHat (version 2.0.11), and SamTools (version 0.1.19.0) using a read length of 100. For RNAseq knockout experiments, reads were converted to counts at the gene level using HTSeq [39] on the BAM files from TopHat2 using the UCSC known genes data set. For each key driver knockout and brain region, genes that mapped less than 100 counts in 80% or more of the samples were filtered out from downstream analysis, because these genes are likely to have especially high variance in expression calls.

Compartmental approach to compare of mouse key driver perturbation signatures with human postmortem AD gene expression signatures

We found the enrichment of both mouse key driver knockout DEG signatures, aggregated across significant DEGs ($p < 0.05$, FDR < 0.3) from both the frontal cortex and cerebellum, as well as two human AD gene expression signatures in the gene ontology pathways. The prefrontal cortex (PFC) human AD DEG signature was estimated from the HBTRC cohort. We used the list of genes identified as previously identified as having significantly different RNA levels in brain samples from persons with high levels of Alzheimer's neuropathology (Braak = 5–6) compared brain samples from persons with low levels of Alzheimer's neuropathology (Braak = 0–2) via a Student's t-test [26]. The second human AD DEG signature is from a previous study that identified genes with a significant trend in RNA expression changes across the severity spectrum of AD (control, incipient, moderate, and severe) in the hippocampus (HIPP) [40]. In this data set, we selected the genes as having an increasing or decreasing trend in expression across AD severity stages and an ANOVA p-value <0.05 as the HIPP AD DEG signature. We used the moduleGO function in DGCA [37] (version 1.0.1) to perform gene ontology (GO) enrichment analysis on these DEG sets, which leverages the GOstats (version 2.34) [41] and org.Hs.eg.db GO annotation (version 3.1.2) R packages. We filtered for those GO terms with less than 800 and greater than 100 gene symbols. We adjusted the enrichment p-values for all GO terms in each DEG set using the Benjamani-Hochberg method. In order to determine whether there was a similar pattern of dysregulation in the mouse key driver knockout models as in human AD, we next found the degree to which the compartment overlaps intersected, using the R package SuperExactTest (version 0.99.2) [42].

In vivo validation of gene expression

Animals

The *Cnp-cre* knock-in mouse line has been described previously [23]. For the sake of clarity, in this manuscript, $Cnp^{+/+}$ mice are called *Cnp*-WT and $Cnp^{cre/cre}$ mice are called *Cnp*-KO.

Western blot

Mice of either sex were sacrificed at postnatal day 60 and brains were cut into 1 mm coronal sections using a refrigerated brain matrix. Corpus callosum (CC) was dissected from coronal sections on ice using a light microscope. The tissue was then immediately processed for protein extraction. Protein lysates (50 μg) were separated by sodium dodecyl sulfate–polyacrylamide gel electrophoresis (SDS–PAGE) and transferred onto a PolyVinylidene DiFluoride (PVDF) (Millipore, Billerica, MA, USA) membrane using a buffer containing 25 mM Tris base, pH 8.3, 192 mM glycine, 20% (vol/vol) methanol for 1 h at 100 V at 4 °C. Membranes were blocked for 1 h in 10% Milk/0.1% Tween/TBS, then incubated overnight at 4 °C with the primary antibody diluted 1:1000 in 5% BSA/ 0.02% sodium azide/0.1% Tween/TBS. Antibodies used are: mouse anti-CNPase (Sternberger Inc., SMI-91, 1:5,00), mouse anti-alpha-TUBULIN (Calbiochem, CP06, 1:5000), rabbit anti-BIN1 (Abcam, ab185950, 1:2500), rabbit anti-GOT2 (Abcam, ab171739, 1:2500). After rinsing with 0.1% Tween/TBS, membranes were incubated 2 h at room temperature with the secondary light-chain specific antibody (Jackson Immunoresearch, 1:10,000) in 10% Milk/0.1% Tween/TBS. After rinsing, membranes were incubated with ECL (Amersham) for 3 min and then revealed. Quantification was carried out on three biological and technical replicates per genotype, using ImageJ. Protein expressions were normalized to alpha-TUBULIN expression, then compared to their respective expression levels in *Cnp*-WT samples.

Immunohistochemistry

Mice were perfused with 4% paraformaldehyde and post-fixed overnight in the same solution at 4 °C. Tissue samples were then transferred to 70% ethanol, sequentially dehydrated and embedded in paraffin. Four-micrometer sections were cut, deparaffinized and rehydrated. Antigen retrieval was performed by incubating slides in sub-boiling (94 °C) citrate buffer (pH 6.0) for 15 min. Slides were incubated in blocking buffer (20% Normal Goat Serum / 1% BSA / PBS 1X) for 1 h at room temperature and then incubated overnight at 4 °C with the primary antibodies in 1% BSA / PBS 1X. Antibodies used are: mouse anti-OLIG2 (Millipore, MABN50, 1:200), mouse anti-NeuN (Millipore, MAB377, 1:200), mouse anti-GFAP (Sternberger Inc., SMI-22, 1:200), rabbit anti-BIN1 (Abcam, ab185950, 1:200), rabbit anti-GOT2 (Abcam, ab171739, 1:200). After rinsing with Tris-buffer / 2% milk, sections were processed with he appropriate Alexa Fluor conjugated secondary antibodies (1:1000 in 1% BSA / PBS 1X, Invitrogen), washed with Tris-buffer, and mounted using Fluoromount-G with DAPI. All images were acquired using a Zeiss Observer A1 fluorescent microscope or

Zeiss LSM780 upright Confocal. Quantification was carried out on two-three sections per mouse and three-four mice for each genotype evaluated using ImageJ.

Results

A robust myelination- and oligodendrocyte-enriched gene module is strongly associated with genetic data in late-onset AD

The primary goal of this study was to interrogate OL-enriched multiscale gene networks constructed from human AD postmortem brain samples (Fig. 1). We first identified co-expressed human gene modules, that were built from data obtained from three regions [e.g. prefrontal cortex (PFC), visual cortex (VC), and cerebellum (CBM)] from postmortem late-onset AD human brains samples from a large cohort of patients [26]. We further annotated these gene modules with additional gene sets to investigate their associations with OLs and AD. We then constructed Bayesian gene regulatory networks for the OL-enriched co-expression modules, identified key regulatory genes in the regulatory networks, and systematically validated the topological structures of the regulatory networks based on a series of gene perturbation experiments in vitro and in vivo. Specifically, in order to identify OL co-expression networks in AD, we tested each of the 62 co-expression modules with at least 50 genes for the enrichment of genes expressed specifically in each of five major brain cell types, i.e., astrocytes, endothelial cells, microglia, neurons, and myelinating OLs [32] (Fig. 2). We identified three co-expression modules with the strongest enrichment of OL genes (Fig. 2), which we subsequently combined, leading to a set of 1631 unique gene symbols,

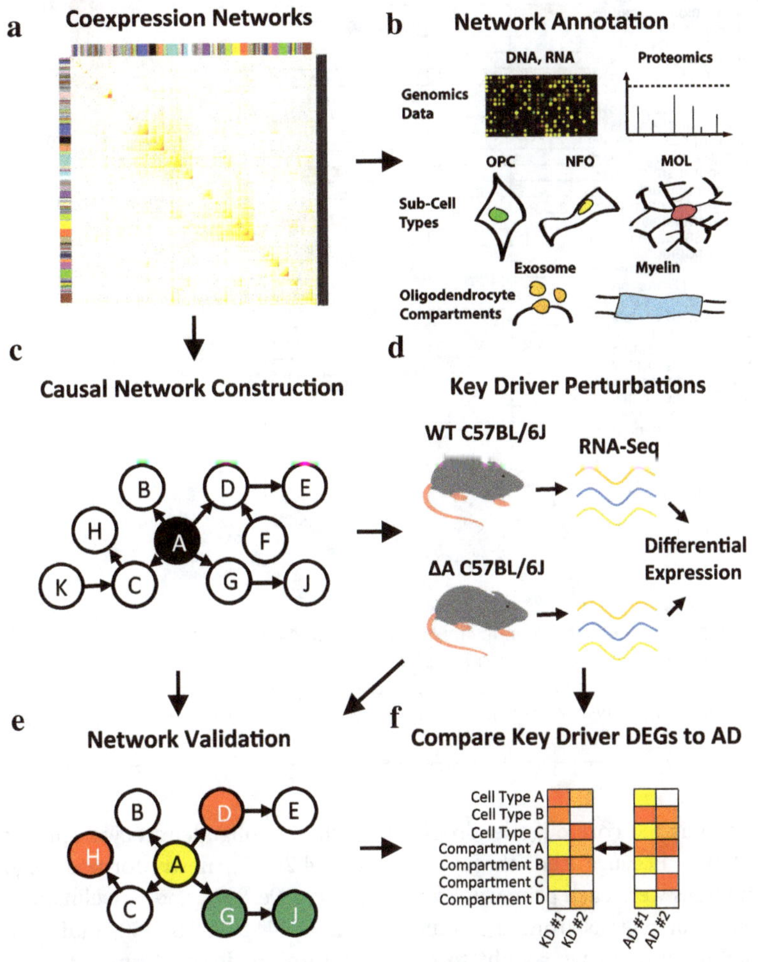

Fig. 1 Workflow of the analyses performed in this study. Human postmortem AD brain tissue samples from multiple brain regions were used to construct coexpression networks (**a**) using Weighted Gene Coexpression Network Analysis (WGCNA). The oligodendrocyte/myelination enriched coexpressed gene modules from WGCNA were annotated by a variety of external data sets including DNA, RNA, proteomic, cell type, and proteome compartment data (**b**). Next, Bayesian gene regulatory networks were constructed based on the DNA and RNA postmortem human AD data (**c**). The Bayesian networks were used to identify key driver genes and several key drivers were perturbed in mouse models to identify their downstream targets (**d**). The gene signatures in response to the perturbations of the key driver genes were used to validate the network structure (**e**) and to compare with the differential expression patterns in human AD postmortem brains (**f**)

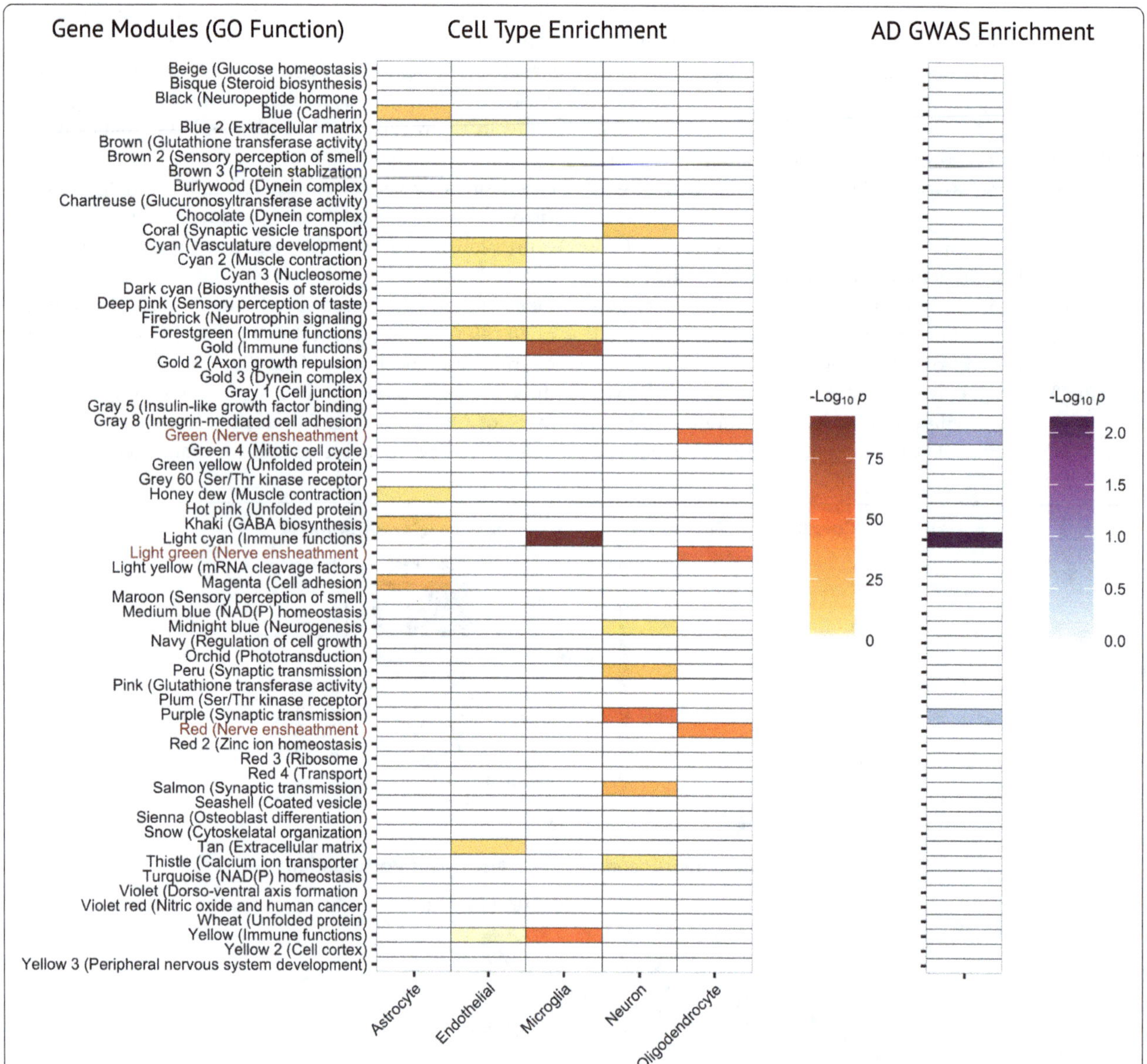

Fig. 2 A myelination/oligodendrocyte enriched module in the multi-tissue AD coexpression network is enriched for AD GWAS genes. The left panel shows a heatmap of the enrichments (BH-adjusted -$\log_{10}$ p-values) of multiscale modules with at least 50 members in marker genes from each of the five major brain cell types, i.e. astrocytes, endothelial cells, microglia, neurons, and myelinating oligodendrocytes, derived from a previous study in mice [32]. The bottom panel shows the enrichment (BH-adjusted -$\log_{10}$ p-values) of each corresponding module in the 543 AD risk genes derived from the IGAP AD GWAS study

which we henceforth refer to as the core oligodendrocyte gene set (COLGS). Notably, because the three OL-enriched co-expression modules were each primarily identified in one of the three brain regions from the multi-tissue experiment, by combining them we sought to obtain a more sensitive measure of genes whose expression is associated with OLs in the context of AD across brain regions. COLGS is highly enriched for genes encoding proteins identified in the myelin proteome [43] (Fold Enrichment (FE) = 1.92, Fisher's Exact Test (FET) p = 2.4e-15), and is also enriched for genes specifically expressed in each of oligodendrocyte precursor cells (FE = 2.8, p = 4.2e-17), newly formed oligodendrocytes (FE = 6.2, p = 1.0e-84), and myelinating oligodendrocytes [32] (FE = 7.4, p = 2.5e-87), indicating that genes in COLGS capture a wide spectrum of OL functions.

To systematically evaluate the AD genetics of COLGS, we identified 543 genes with nominally significant ($p < 0.05$) gene-level associations with AD based on a meta-analysis of AD genome-wide association study (GWAS) data by the International Genomics of Alzheimer's Project (IGAP) [28]. We identified a significant enrichment of the AD risk genes in COLGS (FE = 1.71, *p*-value = 0.0004), due to the presence of *BIN1, PICALM, NME8, SNX1,* and other genes. Of all the individual co-expression modules, one OL-enriched module had the second strongest enrichment for AD GWAS risk genes, second only to an immune- and microglia-enriched module (Fig. 2, Table 1). We further highlighted the specific genes in COLGS that were also identified as AD risk genes (Fig. 3, Table 2). These results suggest that the COLGS contains a relatively large proportion of AD risk genes.

Next, we sought to examine the robustness of COLGS to a variety of sources of variance. We first used data from an independent study that also identified coexpression modules in human AD postmortem brain RNA expression samples [44]. Despite originating from a different brain region (the hippocampus), we found that 83% of the genes in the module with the strongest OL-enrichment in this data set overlapped with the members of COLGS (FE = 18.3, p = 9.1e-79). In order to measure the robustness of the co-expression network with respect to an alternative gene expression modality, we utilized a large AD proteomic data set from the prefrontal cortex (PFC; Brodmann area 10), which we corrected for batch, age of death, and sex. We used WGCNA [31] to identify gene modules in this proteomic data set, and found that the module with the strongest OL-enrichment (FE = 1.7, p = 0.0053), has 50% overlap with COLGS (FE = 10.7, p = 6.6e-58), including the AD risk factor *BIN1* (Additional file 1: Figure S1, Additional file 2). These results suggest a robust co-regulation of the COLGS genes at both the transcript and protein levels in AD.

Dysregulation of an oligodendrocyte-associated module in AD at the protein level

Our previous analysis showed that the three OL-enriched modules were each among the modules with the strongest loss of connectivity in AD samples on the RNA expression level [26]. We sought to extend these results by interrogating gene expression dysregulation in the OL-enriched proteomics module, which includes 150 proteins and is the most OL-enriched module. We found that this module has a significant decrease in correlation in AD samples (mean difference in z-transformed correlation = –0.466, empirical *p*-value = 0.0489; Fig. 4a), thus validating the

Table 1 The region-specific oligodendrocyte-enriched gene networks are among the top associated functional coexpression modules with the 543 significant Alzheimer's disease GWAS hits

Module Name	Enriched Cell Type	Enriched GO Term	Size	Shared	P-Value	Adjusted P-Value
Light cyan	Microglia	Immune functions	559	23	1.91e-05	0.00118
Green	Oligodendrocyte	Nerve ensheathment	1098	32	0.000389	0.0121
Purple	Neuron	Synaptic transmission	847	26	0.000636	0.0131
Gold	Microglia	Immune functions	400	14	0.00352	0.0546
Salmon	Neuron	Synaptic transmission	750	21	0.00582	0.0722
Burlywood	Ependymal Cell	Dynein complex	114	6	0.008	0.0806
Magenta	Astrocyte	Cell adhesion	841	22	0.0103	0.0806
Gray 1	None	Cell junction	56	4	0.0104	0.0806
Light green	Oligodendrocyte	Nerve ensheathment	474	14	0.0145	0.0998
Seashell	None	Coated vesicle	313	10	0.0222	0.127
Black	None	Neuropeptide hormone	1067	25	0.0226	0.127
Tan	Mural Cell	Extracellular matrix	734	18	0.033	0.171
Blue	Astrocyte	Cadherin	1508	31	0.0557	0.247
Yellow	Microglia	Immune functions	1174	25	0.058	0.247
Honey dew	Astrocyte	Muscle contraction	139	5	0.0613	0.247
Medium blue	None	NAD(P) homeostasis	233	7	0.066	0.247
Red 4	Ependymal Cell	Transport	62	3	0.0682	0.247
Red	Oligodendrocyte	Nerve ensheathment	1089	23	0.0717	0.247
Gold 3	Ependymal Cell	Dynein complex	71	3	0.0936	0.294
Peru	Neuron	Synaptic transmission	408	10	0.095	0.294

The 20 modules with the strongest Fisher's Exact Test enrichment in AD GWAS genes from the IGAP data set of the 62 multiscale coexpression modules with at least 50 members were considered. P-values were adjusted via the Benjamini-Hochberg method. Size = the number of genes in the module, Shared = the number of overlaps between the IGAP AD GWAS genes and the coexpression modules, GO = Gene Ontology

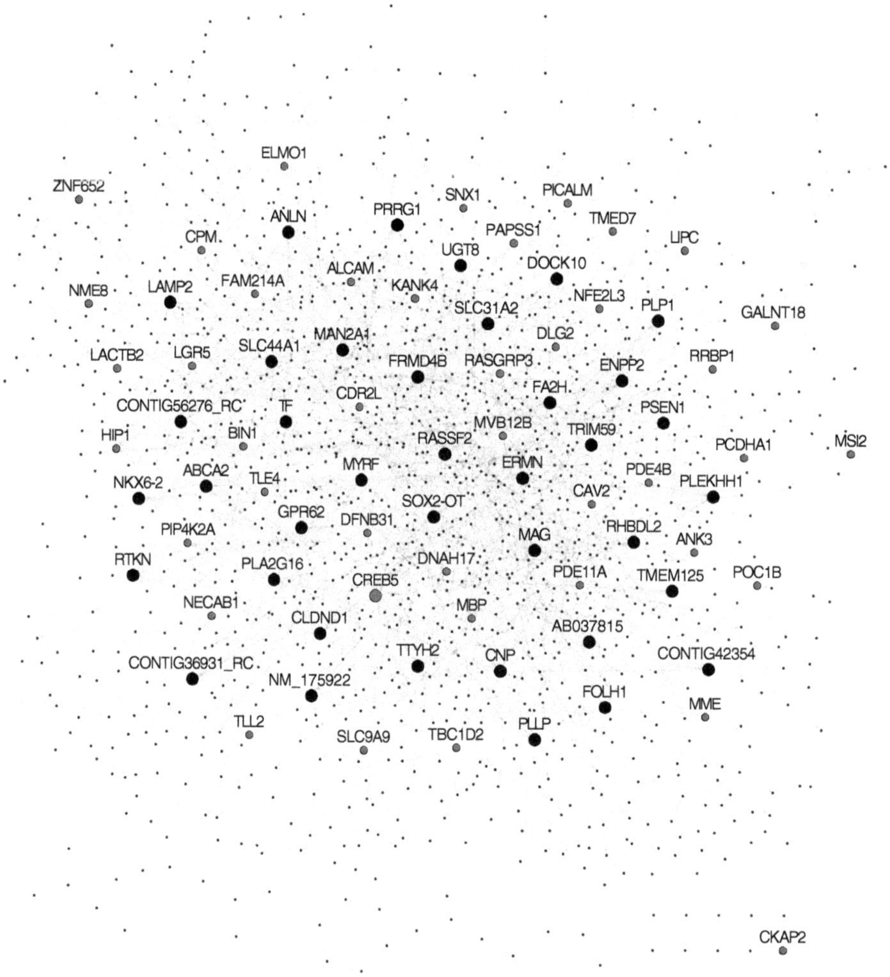

Fig. 3 Key drivers and AD GWAS risk genes in the AD oligodendrocyte regulatory network. Visualization of the core oligodendrocyte Bayesian regulatory network (COLBN), where arrows refer to the predicted direction of interaction in the AD sample-derived network. Nodes corresponding to genes that are called as one of the top 40 key drivers in the network are larger sized, while nodes corresponding to genes that are one of the AD GWAS risk factors are colored pink

loss of coordination among OL network genes in AD at the protein level. To further explore gene expression changes in this module in AD, we measured differences in protein expression of the module members, identifying 17 proteins up-regulated in AD and 7 proteins down-regulated in AD at FDR < 0.3 and p-value <0.05 (Additional file 3). Notably, we found that a BIN1 protein isoform was down-regulated in AD (t = −2.4, p = 0.019, FDR = 0.19), as well as an MBP protein isoform (t = −2.3, p = 0.023, FDR = 0.19). Therefore, we found that there are both variable changes in expression levels for individual proteins as well as a loss of overall coordination of OL network protein expression in AD.

Construction and validation of an oligodendrocyte gene regulatory network in AD

We next sought to predict the gene-gene regulatory relationships among the COLGS genes in the RNA expression data, which profiles a wider set of genes than the proteomics data. Specifically, we constructed a Bayesian gene regulatory network for each of the three OL-enriched co-expression modules we identified by integrating RNA expression and genotype data from autopsied brain samples of persons with AD. As detailed in our previous studies [33, 34], Bayesian networks are a type of probabilistic causal network, providing a natural framework for integrating highly dissimilar genetic and gene expression data to predict regulatory relationships. We then combined the three OL Bayesian networks by a set union of directed links, leading to a more robust core oligodendrocyte-enriched Bayesian network (COLBN), and performed key driver analysis on COLBN to identify master regulatory OL genes in the context of AD (Fig. 1b; Table 3).

To interrogate the topology of the COLBN as well as how the dysregulation of COLBN key drivers could

Table 2 The members of the core oligodendrocyte gene set (COLGS) that are identified as significant ($p < 0.05$) AD GWAS hits in the IGAP data set

Gene	Chromosome	Top SNP	Top SNP *P*-value
BIN1	2	rs35114168	1.05e-25
PICALM	11	rs639012	4.87e-19
NME8	7	rs2060712	6.30e-07
SNX1	15	rs138194169	2.72e-06
CPM	12	rs10878881	1.48e-05
DLG2	11	rs422267	2.09e-05
RASGRP3	2	rs10200743	2.76e-05
GALNT18	11	rs11021857	4.511e-05
DNAH17	17	rs117779187	7.04e-05
LIPC	15	rs17269397	8.32e-05
ZNF652	17	rs12948660	0.000119
MVB12B	9	rs887656	0.000145
CAV2	7	rs75396674	0.000157
CREB5	7	rs42711	0.000158
NFE2L3	7	rs73281529	0.000224
CDR2L	17	rs117639581	0.000299
PIP4K2A	10	rs11013051	0.000390
TLL2	10	rs11594430	0.000542
RRBP1	20	rs6080757	0.000873
KANK4	1	rs114648128	0.00118
SLC9A9	3	rs10804689	0.00141
HIP1	7	rs10259351	0.00165
CKAP2	13	rs58655347	0.00168
TLE4	9	rs62569297	0.00172
NECAB1	8	rs7003020	0.00194
TBC1D2	9	rs73488713	0.00222
LGR5	12	rs75928881	0.00278
PDE4B	1	rs12138629	0.00374
PDE11A	2	rs4893975	0.00380
PAPSS1	4	rs62313402	0.00387
DFNB31	9	rs10817615	0.00450
MBP	18	rs8095585	0.00484
LACTB2	8	rs10097463	0.00545
ALCAM	3	rs114219776	0.00628
TMED7	5	rs10069695	0.00691
CAT	11	rs494024	0.00849
MSI2	17	rs12450585	0.00849
MME	3	rs61758192	0.00885
POC1B	12	rs770369	0.0117
PCDHA1	5	rs2879086	0.0151
ANK3	10	rs117641222	0.0185
FAM214A	15	rs8030871	0.0241
ELMO1	7	rs1420423	0.0333

The p-value column shows the smallest p-value of any associated SNP for each gene

relate to AD, we identified an in vitro experiment that perturbed a key driver gene in the COLBN, *MYRF*, and examined how the predicted network structures correspond to its identified experimental targets. Specifically, we used data from a previous study that performed transcriptional profiling of cultured mouse OLs with a deletion of the myelination transcription factor *Myrf* (also known as *C11orf9*) [45]. The set of genes differentially expressed in the cells with a *Myrf* deletion compared with the control was significantly enriched in the 5-layer downstream neighborhood of *MYRF* in the COLBN (FE = 2.5, p = 7.5e-33; Fig. 5a, Fig. 6a-b), thus validating the topology of the subnetwork regulated by *MYRF*. The validated downstream targets of *MYRF* include *PLD1*, which encodes a protein that regulates the shuttling of *APP* and is associated with *APP* in AD brains [46, 47], as well as *APLP1*, which encodes a protein that has been shown to accumulate within neuritic plaques [48].

Next, we validated the network structure of COLBN in vivo using knockout mouse models of three of the top 40 key drivers in COLBN, *Ugt8*, *Cnp*, and *Plp1*, each of which have been found to cause axon pathology without substantial myelin structural alterations [21, 23, 49]. We performed RNAseq (GEO: GSE80437) on tissue samples of postnatal day 20 mice from the frontal cortex (FC) and cerebellum (CBM) in these three mouse models to determine their KO DEG gene signatures at FDR < 0.3 (Additional files 4 and 5, Additional file 1: Figure S2). We profiled RNA from the FC and CBM because these two regions were also profiled in the human AD postmortem brain tissue study, from which the COLBN was generated. We selected this time point because we wanted to focus on gene changes that occurred prior to the development of axonal pathology and therefore more directly would allow us to determine gene changes characteristic of the prodromic stage of the disease.We identified no DEGs for Δ*Cnp* in the CBM and Δ*Plp1* in the FC, while we found that all of the other DEG signatures were significantly enriched in the downstream neighborhoods of their corresponding driver genes (Fig. 6c-d). *UGT8* encodes an enzyme that transfers galactose to ceramide to generate galactosylceramide, which makes up approximately one-fourth of myelin lipid dry mass [50]. *UGT8*'s 5-layer neighborhood is most enriched for the *Ugt8* KO signature in the CBM (FE = 2.1, p = 2.4e-9). One validated downstream target of *UGT8* is *LIPA*, which encodes a lysosomal cholesterol-metabolizing enzyme associated with genetic polymorphisms that affect plasma 24S–hydroxycholesterol/cholesterol levels in AD patients [51] (Fig. 5d). The key driver *CNP* encodes a protein that plays a role in OL process outgrowth and promoting axon survival [23, 52]. *CNP*'s 5-layer neighborhood is significantly enriched for the *Cnp* KO signature in the FC (FE = 1.7, p = 6.4e-6). One of the

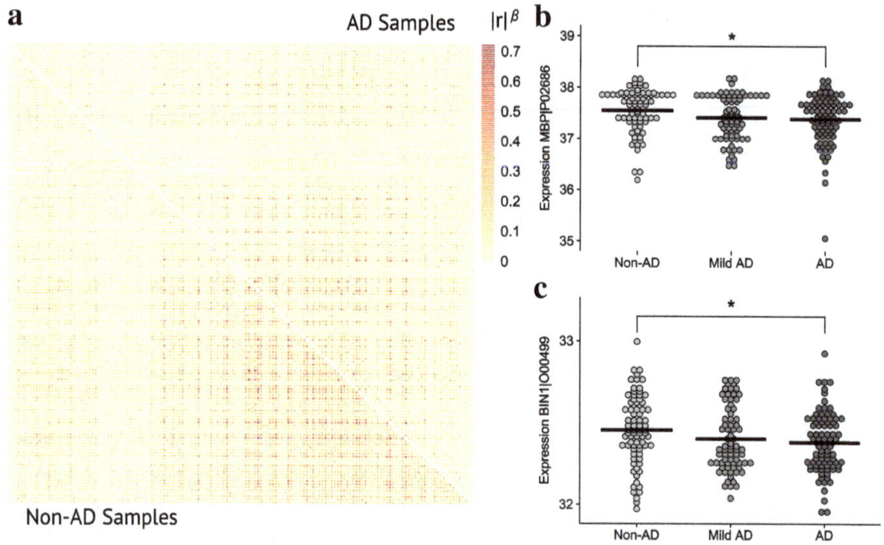

Fig. 4 An oligodendrocyte-enriched protein coexpression module is dysregulated in AD. **a** Heatmap of transformed correlations in non-AD samples (Braak <= 2; lower left) and AD samples (Braak > = 5; upper right) in the OL-enriched module consisting of 150 proteins. The transformation consists of taking the absolute value of Pearson correlation coefficients raised to the power of β, i.e., the soft-thresholding power coefficient of 3 used in coexpression network construction. **b, c** Expression levels for MBP (**b**) and BIN1 (**c**) in samples classified as non-AD (Braak <= 2), mild AD (Braak 3–4), and AD samples (Braak > = 5). Significance assessed using Student's t-tests (* = p-value <0.05)

validated downstream targets of *CNP* is *SEC14L5*, which has been previously found to be down-regulated in CA1 in AD [53] (Fig. 5c). Finally, the key driver *PLP1* encodes a protein that is the most abundant protein in CNS myelin sheaths [54], regulates OPC process outgrowth [55], and promotes axonal integrity [56]. *PLP1*'s 5-layer neighborhood is significantly enriched for the *Plp1* KO signature in the CBM (FE = 2.0, p = 1.2e-4). A validated downstream target of *Plp1* is *Fgf1* (Fig. 5b), which encodes a protein that has been found to stimulate neuronal growth and promote remyelination [57] and has been found to have increased levels in the CSF in AD [58].

Overall, as with the in vitro perturbation data, the in vivo perturbation experiments strongly support the network structure of COLBN and pinpoint specific downstream targets to explain how dysregulation of the key drivers may help mediate AD pathology.

Perturbations of key OL network drivers in mice mimic aspects of dysregulation in human AD brain samples

Since the key drivers of COLBN are predicted to orchestrate the expression of a network with a strong genetic association with AD, we hypothesized that the KO signatures of COLBN key drivers in vivo would mimic their gene expression dysregulation in human AD brains. In order to test this hypothesis, we performed gene ontology analysis on DEG signatures from postmortem brain tissue from both key driver KO mice and patients with AD. The DEG signatures in AD were derived based on samples from the PFC in the Harvard Brain Tissue Resource Center cohort [26] and samples from the hippocampus (HIPP) in the University of Kentucky Brain Bank cohort [40], because these regions are among those with the strongest AD pathology. Overall, the enrichment of DEGs from the human AD cases in these gene compartments show several similar dysregulation patterns as that seen in the key driver knockouts (Fig. 7a). For example, we identified a strong enrichment for genes in the gene ontology (GO) category "mitochondrial protein complex" in the down-regulated Δ*Cnp* signature (FE = 10.6, p = 8.2e-22) and the down-regulated AD HIPP signature (FE = 6.7, p = 7.5e-11). We next found that the down-regulated Δ*Cnp* and AD HIPP signatures intersected along with the mitochondrial gene set substantially more than expected due to chance (FE = 34, p = 2.1e-9; Fig. 7b), suggesting that the actual genes dysregulated in the mitochondria are similar between *Cnp*-KO mice and in the hippocampus of AD patients. For example, *COX6A1*, a mitochondrial-associated gene in which mutations are causative of peripheral neuropathy [59], was found to be down-regulated in both *Cnp*-KO mice and in the hippocampus of AD patients. We also identified a strong enrichment for genes in the GO category "ribosome" in the down-regulated Δ*Cnp* signature (FE = 4.8, p = 3e-11), the down-regulated Δ*Plp1* signature (FE = 8.1, p = 4e-18), and the down-regulated AD PFC signature (FE = 3.0, p = 0.002). We identified a significant overlap of all three of these down-regulated signatures and the ribosomal

Table 3 Of the 40 top-ranked key drivers from the core oligodendrocyte-enriched Bayesian network (COLBN), 4 have a type of perturbation signature that we used to validate the network, either in vitro or in vivo

Gene Symbol	Major Annotated Roles of Gene Product	Myelin	OL Exosome	Lipid-Binding	AD Risk	Perturbation
ERMN	Myelination	Yes				
UGT8	Galactocerebroside production			Yes		In vivo; this study
CNP	Myelination; Axon interaction	Yes	Yes			In vivo; this study
ENPP2	LPA production					
FRMD4B	?					
PLEKHH1	?					
SLC44A1	Choline transporter	Yes				
TRIM59	?					
PLLP	Myelination	Yes		Yes		
PRRG1	?					
SOX2-OT	lncRNA					
CONTIG36931_RC	?					
CLDND1	?					
ANLN	Actin cytoskeleton	Yes				
TTYH2	Chloride channel					
MYRF	OL differentiation					In vitro; [49]
FA2H	Ceramide hydroxylation			Yes		
CARNS1	Carnosine production					
RNLS	Alpha-NAD(P)H oxidase					
RASSF2	Apoptosis					
PRR18	?					
RTKN	Rho pathway					
DOCK10	Rho pathway					
LPAR1	LPA receptor	Yes		Yes		
MAG	Myelination	Yes				
TF	Iron transport					
TMEM125	?					
PLP1	Myelination; Axon interaction	Yes	Yes	Yes		In vivo; this study
RHBDL2	Protease activity					
NKX6–2	OL differentiation					
FOLH1	Folate hydrolase	Yes				
PSEN1	Protease activity				Yes	
MAN2A1	Glycosylation					
PLA2G16	Phospholipase			Yes		
CONTIG56276_RC	?					
ABCA2	Sterol transport				Yes	
CREB5	?				Yes	
GPR62	?					
SLC31A2	Copper transport					
LAMP2	Glycosylation					

The Major Annotated Roles of Gene Product column is based on a literature review for the major known role(s) of that gene's product in oligodendrocytes, for which a question mark indicates that no major role is known, to the best of our knowledge. The Myelin column indicates whether or not that gene encodes a protein found in in the myelin proteome [43], the OL Exosome column indicates whether or not that gene encodes a protein found in the OL exosome proteome [97], and the lipid-binding column indicates whether or not that gene encodes a protein found in the set of lipid-binding proteins [98]. The AD risk indicates whether a variant associated with the gene has been previously associated with AD risk, and the Perturbation column indicates whether there is a perturbation signature that we used to corroborate the downstream neighborhood topology for that key driver

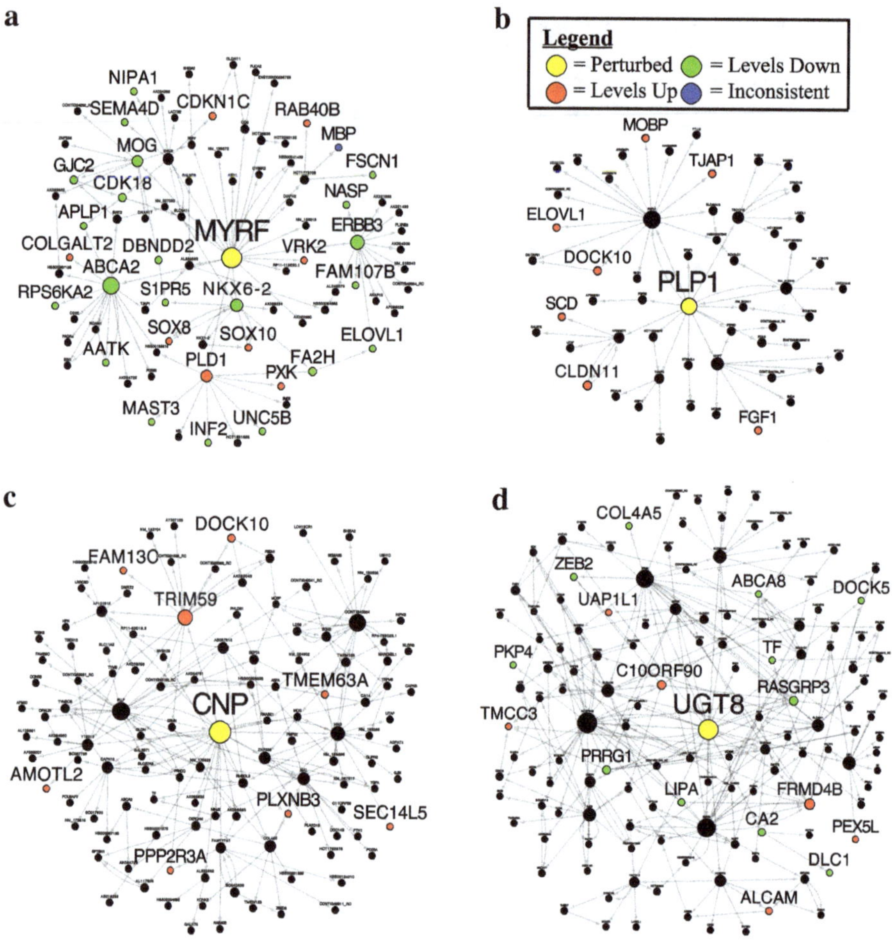

Fig. 5 In vitro and in vivo perturbations of key driver genes in the AD myelin/oligodendrocyte networks validated a number of predicted downstream targets. In these network plots, arrows refer to the predicted direction of interaction in the AD sample-derived core oligodendrocyte Bayesian regulatory network (COLBN). The presence of multiple arrows between two genes is because COLBN was constructed by a union of directed links of three networks from three brain regions. In each plot, the perturbed (i.e., knocked-down or knocked-out) gene is colored yellow, the genes significantly down-regulated in the samples with the driver perturbed are colored green, the genes up-regulated are colored red, and the genes with inconsistent expression changes (i.e., multiple probes corresponding to the same gene show opposite directions of changes in expression) are colored blue. The size of the node is proportional to the number of downstream nodes in the subnetwork. **a** Validation of the two-layer subnetwork regulated by *MYRF* using the differentially expressed genes (FDR < 0.3, $p < 0.05$) derived from a *Myrf* knockout experiment in cultured mouse oligodendrocytes. **b**, **c**, **d** Validation of the two-layer subnetworks regulated by *PLP1*, *CNP*, and *UGT8* using the differentially expressed gene signatures (FDR < 0.3, $p < 0.05$) from the RNAseq data derived from our knockout experiments in mice

gene set (FE = 76, $p = 0.013$; Fig. 7c), which has limited power due to the small size of the overall ribosomal gene set. Since the *Cnp* and *Plp1* knockout RNAseq profiling occurred prior to the typical age of onset of axon degeneration in these mice, the mitochondrial and ribosomal gene set dysregulation seen is suggestive of "presymptomatic" pathways that precede subsequent axonal and neuronal degeneration.

Finally, we also detected that there was a significant enrichment for genes in myelin sheath GO category in the up-regulated Δ*Plp1* signature (FE = 4.3, p = 3e-8), the down-regulated Δ*Cnp* signature (FE = 2.5, p = 0.002), and the down-regulated AD HIPP signature (FE = 5.2, p = 2e-9). However, the myelin sheath GO signature only contains 161 genes, which makes overlap analysis difficult. In order to use a more well-powered gene set, we utilized a larger set of 1778 genes that have been previously reported to be present in the myelin proteome [43]. In this gene set, we found a strong enrichment for the intersection of genes in the myelin proteome with down-regulated genes in *Cnp*-KO mice and human AD hippocampus (FE = 6.0, p = 2.1e-8; Fig. 7d). This shared set of down-regulated myelin genes includes *CDK5*, which encodes an enzyme whose activity is associated with tau pathology [60] and is essential for myelination [61]. Both *Cnp*-KO mice and patients with AD undergo axon damage in the absence dramatic ultrastructural changes in myelin structure [62], and our data

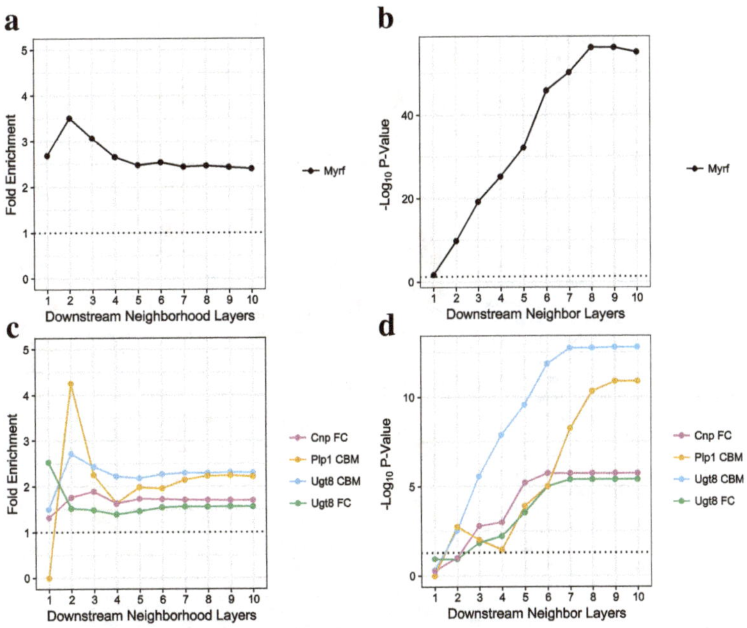

Fig. 6 Gene signatures from in vitro and in vivo perturbations of key driver genes in the AD myelin/oligodendrocyte network are significantly enriched in the predicted subnetworks regulated by the driver genes. **a, b** Fold-enrichment (**a**) and BH-adjusted -$\log_{10}$ enrichment *p*-values (**b**) for the overlap between the *Myrf* in vitro perturbation signature and each n-layer network neighborhood regulated by *MYRF* in the core oligodendrocyte Bayesian regulatory network (COLBN). **c, d** Fold-enrichment (**c**) and -$\log_{10}$ enrichment p-values (**d**) for the overlap between each in vivo perturbation signature and each n-layer network neighborhood regulated by the corresponding driver gene. The result was based on the in vivo knockout differentially expressed gene signatures experiments for *Cnp*, *Plp1*, and *Ugt8* from the cerebellum (CBM) and/or the frontal cortex (FC)

shows that both conditions share a down-regulation of myelin-associated genes that may be associated with dysmyelination [22] and subsequent axon damage.

In order to validate the decreased expression of key myelin and mitochondrial genes in *Cnp*-KO mice, we measured the protein expression of BIN1 and GOT2 in *Cnp*-KO mice compared to WT mice. BIN1 is primarily expressed in mature OLs and white matter in AD patients [63]. Interestingly, the longer, central nervous system (CNS)-specific isoform of *Bin1* has decreased expression levels in AD, although overall *Bin1* transcript levels show increased expression [64]. This may reflect a proliferation of monocyte lineage cells in AD and a concomitant decrease in expression of *Bin1* in other cell types, including OLs. BIN1 protein expression has been found to decrease in the myelin proteome of *Cnp*-KO mice compared to WT mice, but not in *Plp*-KO, *Mag*-KO, or *Sept8*-KO mice [65]. Consistent with this previous data, we found a significant down-regulation of BIN1 expression in the corpus callosum in *Cnp*-KO mice compared to WT mice ($p = 0.0041$ and $p = 0.0007$, Fig. 8a-b). We selected to profile the corpus callosum because it is an OL- and myelin-rich tissue, and therefore we reasoned that protein expression in this region more accurately would reflect the effect of *Cnp*-KO on OLs protein expression. No changes in the subcellular distribution of BIN1 were detected in *Cnp*-KO mice, which was primarily expressed in the cytoplasm of cells that were also stained by antibodies specific for the nuclear pan-OL lineage marker OLIG2 (Fig. 8c-e). Next, we measured the protein expression of GOT2, which is a mitochondrial protein that has been shown to be down-regulated in many AD gene expression studies [66], and has down-regulated transcript levels in *Cnp*-KO mice in our RNAseq expression profiles. Consistent with this data, we found a down-regulation of GOT2 protein levels in *Cnp*-KO mice ($p = 0.0332$; Fig. 8a-b). Although GOT2 has been identified in the myelin proteome, we found that it was primarily co-expressed with neurons (Fig. 8f–h), suggesting that the loss of *Cnp* expression may also affect mitochondrial gene expression within neurons. Taken together, these results validate that *Cnp*-KO mice have gene dysregulation in key myelin and mitochondrial proteins that is similar to that seen in AD brain samples.

Discussion

In this study, we employed an unbiased systems biology approach to characterize OL-enriched and AD-associated co-expression and regulatory molecular networks. We derived a core OL-enriched gene set (COLGS) that was highly enriched in AD GWAS genes. We found that this set of genes strongly overlapped with the corresponding genes from a protein co-expression

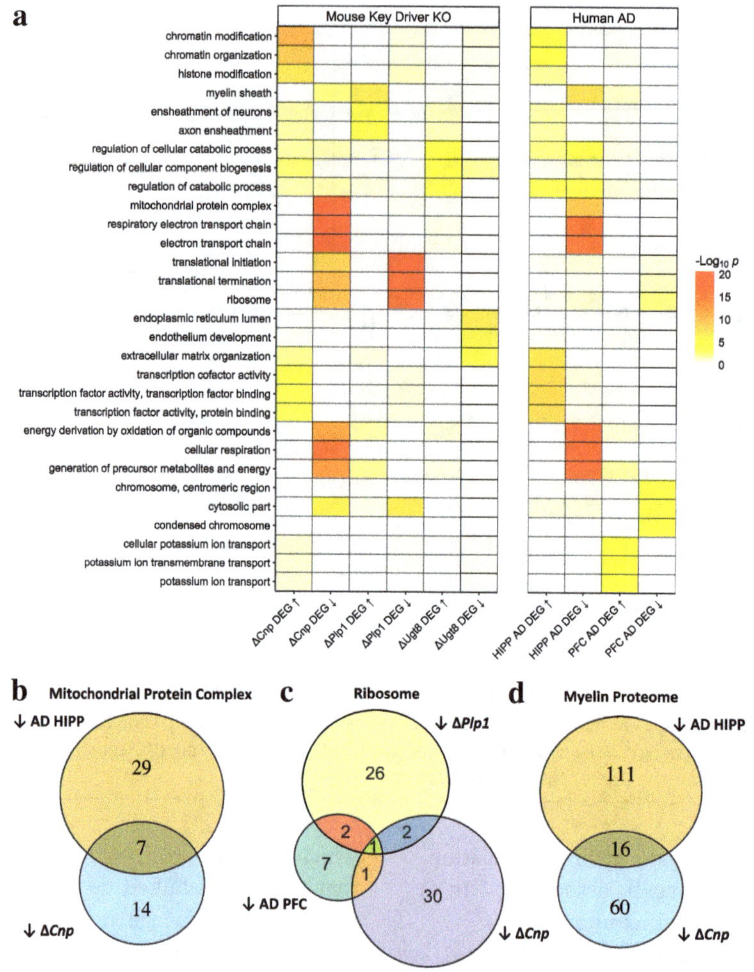

Fig. 7 Perturbation of oligodendrocyte network key drivers in mice recapitulates key gene expression changes in human AD brain samples. **a** A heatmap of the $-\log_{10}$ gene ontology (GO) enrichment p-values of core oligodendrocyte Bayesian regulatory network key driver knockout differentially expressed gene (DEG) signatures (left panel) and AD DEG signatures from the hippocampus and prefrontal cortex (right panel). The top 3 GO terms with between 100 and 800 gene symbols most enriched in each of the DEG signatures are shown. The p-values for each tested signature were adjusted using the Benjamini-Hochberg method. **b, c, d** Venn diagrams showing the intersections of genes encoding proteins associated with the GO terms "mitochondrial protein complex" (**b**), "ribosome" (c), and genes in the myelin proteome (**d**) with genes downregulated in various DEG signatures are shown

module, which we found to be highly dysregulated in AD. We next constructed a core OL Bayesian regulatory network (COLBN) to dissect the causal relationships among the genes in COLGS. By employing a series of in vitro and in vivo perturbations of key driver genes in COLBN, we validated the predicted network structures in COLBN. We further showed that the knockouts of key drivers of COLBN in mice mimic the dysregulation of OL-associated compartments of genes in human postmortem AD brains. In particular, our data revealed a surprisingly strong, convergent gene expression effect of the knockouts *Cnp* and *Plp1* on organelle-associated gene expression pathways, specifically in genes annotated for mitochondrial and ribosome functions. These organelles have also been reported to be dysregulated in axons in AD brains [17, 67–69], suggesting that altered OL-axon communication may lead to dysregulated expression of ribosomal and mitochondrial genes and possibly play a role in contributing to AD axonal pathology. It is difficult to study prodromal changes in late-onset AD brains, because we are not able to determine a priori the individuals who would progress to AD. However, in mice with well-defined ablation of myelin genes also detected as key drivers of human gene network in AD, it is possible to define alterations that occur in OL and that precede frank neurodegeneration. For this reason the detection of similar gene changes in brain tissue samples of *Cnp*-KO and *Plp1*-KO mice prior to the development of any axonal pathology [22, 24], allowed us to infer that the dysregulated expression of similar genes in murine samples and in human AD brains is suggestive of similar events occurring during the early part of the

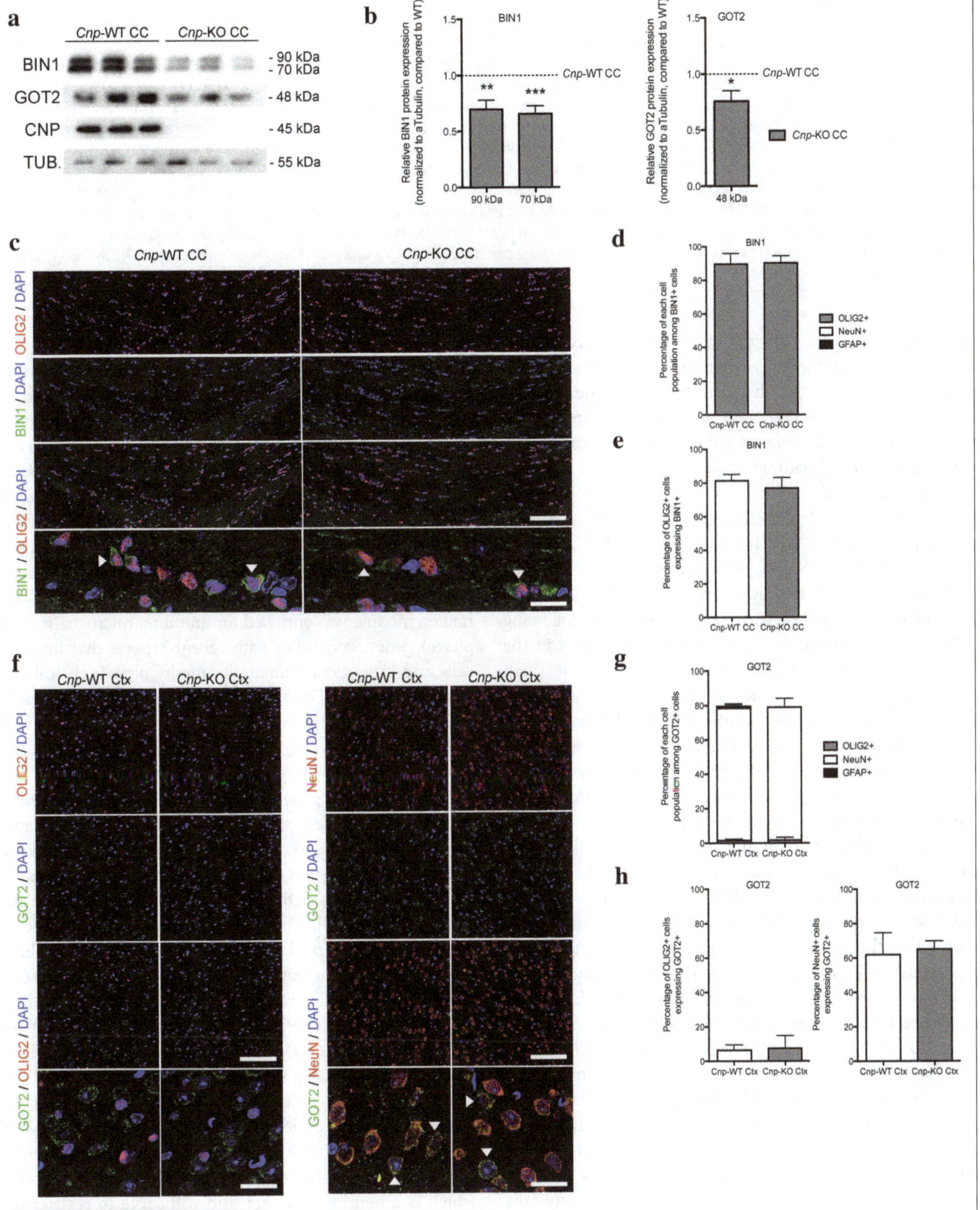

Fig. 8 (See legend on next page.)

(See figure on previous page.)
Fig. 8 Downregulation of AD-associated proteins in mice lacking the oligodendrocyte network key driver *Cnp*. **a** Representative western blots of BIN1, GOT2, CNP and alpha-TUBULIN stainings on *Cnp*-WT and *Cnp*-KO corpus callosum (CC) tissues ($n = 3$). **b** Quantification of BIN1 and GOT2 protein expression in *Cnp*-KO corpus callosum compared to *Cnp*-WT corpus callosum (protein expression normalized to alpha-TUBULIN expression for each sample, n = 3 per condition; $p = 0.0041$, $p = 0.0007$, $p = 0.032$). **c** Representative confocal image of post-natal day 60 sections of *Cnp*-WT and *Cnp*-KO corpus callosum, stained for OLIG2 (red), BIN1 (green) and DAPI (blue), scale bar = 300 μm. The bottom panel shows higher magnification of the double stainings (white arrowheads indicate double positive for BIN1 and OLIG2), scale bar = 50 μm. **d** Quantification of the proportion of each cell types expressing BIN1 in *Cnp*-WT and *Cnp*-KO corpus callosum (oligodendrocytes – OLIG2+ in gray, neurons – NeuN+ in white, astrocytes – GFAP+ in black; n = 3–4). **e** Quantification of the percentage of OLIG2+ cells expressing BIN1 in *Cnp*-WT and *Cnp*-KO corpus callosum (n = 3–4). **f** Representative confocal image of post-natal day 60 sections of *Cnp*-WT and *Cnp*-KO cortex, stained for OLIG2 or NeuN (red), GOT2 (green) and DAPI (blue), scale bar = 300 μm. The bottom panel shows magnification of the double stainings (white arrowheads indicate double positive for GOT2 and OLIG2 or NeuN, respectively), scale bar = 50 μm. **g** Quantification of the proportion of each cell types expressing GOT2 in *Cnp*-WT and *Cnp*-KO cortex (oligodendrocytes – OLIG2+ in gray, neurons – NeuN + in white, astrocytes – GFAP+ in black; n = 3–4). **h** Quantification of the percentage of OLIG2+ cells and of NeuN+ cells expressing GOT2 in *Cnp*-WT and *Cnp*-KO corpus callosum (n = 3–4). * $p < 0.05$, ** $p < 0.01$, *** $p < 0.001$

pathological cascade. Overall, this study improves our understanding of the molecular underpinnings of myelination and OLs in AD by identifying biologically relevant pathways, dissecting the causal relationships among the OL- and myelin-related genes, and implicating key driver genes in AD pathogenesis.

At the individual gene level, many of the genes in COLGS have been described as genetic risk factors associated with late-onset AD, including *BIN1* [28], *PICALM* [28], *NME8* [28], *UNC5C* [30], and *PSEN* [27]. Notably, *BIN1* is the nearest protein-coding gene to the SNP with the second-strongest GWAS signal for AD, following *APOE* [28]. Histologically, BIN1 is primarily found in the brain at the nodes of Ranvier, consistent with its high RNA expression in OLs and its presence in the myelin proteome [43, 70, 71]. In COLBN, *BIN1* is downstream of *ABCA2*, a cholesterol transporter that has been associated with the risk of AD in many study populations [28, 72–75]. Much of the literature about the role of *BIN1* in AD has focused on its roles in neurons and microglia [76], but our data, in addition to another recent study [63], suggest that its role in OLs should be explored further. In addition to genetic risk factors, our AD OL network also contains many genes encoding proteins that have been associated with AD pathophysiology (e.g., via Aβ production) including *PSEN1* [77], *BACE1* [77], *PLD1* [46, 78], and *APLP1* [79]. Consistent with the important role of *BACE1* in OLs suggested by our network, *BACE1* has been shown to play a key role in myelination [80, 81]. The role of *BACE1* in OLs is of high relevance to AD, as mutations in the *BACE1*-cleaving region of APP have been associated with a decreased risk of AD [82], and β-secretase inhibitors intended to treat AD may have side-effects of myelin defects [83]. A focus on the interaction targets of both *PSEN1* and *BACE1* within OLs using regulatory networks may be a fruitful avenue to identify treatment modalities that decrease deleterious Aβ production without causing off-target effects.

At the gene set level, our enrichment analysis of the AD co-expression modules shows that the three modules significantly enriched for AD risk genes are associated with three different cell types, i.e., microglia, OLs, and neurons (Table 1). Note that gene modules were identified based on the correlation between gene expression profiles in postmortem human AD brains, and they don't necessarily correspond to any particular known cell types or biological processes due to interactions among cell types and biological processes. Therefore, we denote the co-expression modules by randomly selected color names in addition to their most enriched gene ontology term, to emphasize their multifaceted and highly context-dependent functions. The top ranked module was enriched for immune (microglia/macrophage) genes, consistent with recent reports that immune cells and in particular innate immunity plays a critical role in promoting AD [76, 84–86]. However, it is imprudent to focus on a single cell type and ignore the interactions with other cells. For example, *TREM2*, an established AD risk factor that is primarily expressed in immune cells [87, 88], is also the causative gene of Nasu-Hakola disease, an early-onset subcortical dementia that presents with white matter demyelination [89]. Mice lacking *Trem2* have been shown to have delayed myelin debris clearance, which may lead to increased microglia activation and thus demyelination and neuronal death [90]. The dysregulation of myelin proteome genes that we observed in AD may contribute to pathologic inflammation, by increasing the available lipid pool for scavenging by microglia, which can activate microglia into a pro-inflammatory state [91, 92]. Further investigation of cell type interactions in AD via network biology is a promising approach in addressing the underlying causes of AD.

Existing mouse models of AD tend to focus on Aβ and/or neuronal deficits in AD. For example, several mouse models of AD express genes with familial AD-causative mutations under the *Thy1* promoter [93–95], which is a neuronal marker and will serve to restrict the pathologic changes to neurons. However, the data presented in this study and others suggest that the dysregulation of other cell types, including OLs, may play a role in AD. This opens up a need for mouse models of AD that can recapitulate the OL- and myelin-associated dysregulation in AD. In this study, we found that a mouse knockout model of one of the key drivers in the OL network, *Cnp*, demonstrates a strikingly similar myelin and mitochondrial dysregulation pattern as is seen in brain samples of patients with AD. Notably, we did expression profiling prior to the onset of axon degeneration in *Cnp*-KO mice [22], to minimize the possibility that the myelin gene expression changes observed would be reactive to as opposed to premonitory for axon damage. Taken together, our data suggest that the *Cnp*-KO mice may be a good model of the OL network gene dysregulation and dysmyelination that occurs in the brains of patients with AD. Therefore, therapeutic agents that are able to mitigate and/or prevent the dysmyelination and axon degeneration seen in *Cnp*-KO mice are worthwhile of investigation as potential therapeutic agents for ameliorating cognitive deficits in patients with AD.

In this study, we focused on the molecular networks in AD in a brain cell type, OLs, which have not been widely studied in AD. Our network modeling approach uncovered a network of OL-associated genes that is enriched for AD GWAS genes, pathways through which dysregulation of this OL network may promote AD pathology, and key driver genes that orchestrate these pathways. Further work on our model for the role of OLs in AD may help to address why aging is the major risk factor for AD, since myelin maintenance and plasticity are known to become progressively less robust in normal aging [62, 96]. In particular, preventing or reversing the dysregulation of key OL driver genes such as *CNP* and downstream targets such as *BIN1* deserve further research as interventions to help to alleviate the progression of cognitive deficits in AD.

Conclusions

This study systematically identifies and validates a comprehensive molecular blueprint of OLs in the context of AD. Our gene network analysis of large-scale genetic and genomic data from AD brains reveals that OL/myelin-enriched subnetworks in multiple brain regions are strongly associated with clinical and neuropathologic traits in AD. These OL/myelin-enriched subnetworks harbor not only Aβ production-related genes, but also several genes involved in myelin biology. Our network analysis further identifies key causal regulators of the OL/myelin-enriched networks, including *UGT8*, *CNP*, *MYRF*, and *PLP1*. These predicted network structures can be validated by gene perturbation signatures of these drivers. Mice with genetic ablations of *Cnp* mimicked components of organelle and myelin sheath gene expression dysregulation seen in brain samples from patients with AD, including decreased protein expression of BIN1 and GOT2. Overall, our network models of OLs in AD and the comprehensive validation experiments reveal details of the molecular mechanisms of OL dysregulation in AD and thus pave a way for the development of novel AD therapies.

Additional files

Additional file 1: Supplementary Experimental Procedures. **Figure S1.** The topological overlap matrix plot of the protein co-expression network constructed from the proteomics data from the autopsied brains in the MSBB cohort, along with the dendrogram showing the tree cutting process used to define modules (above). **Figure S2.** Confirmation that the key driver knockouts abrogate gene expression of the key driver in the RNA-seq experiments. For each of the key driver knockouts whose genome-wide gene expression was profiled in this study using RNA-seq, we plotted the $\log_{10}$ counts overlapping that gene in both the wildtype (WT) and knockout (KO) samples. Notably, one of the matched samples from *Cnp* was detected as an outlier in both the CBM and FC brain regions (red), due to suspected mislabeling. These samples were removed prior to downstream differential expression analysis. (DOCX 161 kb)

Additional file 2: Module membership file for the Mount Sinai Brain Bank (MSBB) proteomic coexpression network. The module label, a randomly chosen color name, is in the 1st column, while the protein name is in the 2nd column. (TSV 34 kb)

Additional file 3: Differentially expressed proteins in the MSBB proteomics data set between AD cases and controls in the OL-enriched module (which has been randomly assigned the color name "Yellow"). (TSV 9 kb)

Additional file 4: Summary of read mapping from the three knockout mouse RNAseq experiments generated by TopHat. (XLSX 52 kb)

Additional files 5: Differentially expressed genes found the mouse knockout RNAseq analyses of *Ugt8* in the CBM (Data 1) and FC (Data 2), *Cnp* in the FC (Data 3), and *Plp1* in the CBM (Data 4). For these differential expression analyses, we mapped RNAseq reads using TopHat, converted to count space using HTSeq, used *voom* to transform the read space data to $\log_2$ counts per million, and used *limma* for differential expression analysis. We also used the Ensembl database to identify the human gene with the highest homology percentage based on protein coding region DNA divergence, and report this homology percentage for each gene. Note that the differential expression signatures of *Cnp* in the CBM and *Plp1* in the FC were not found not have any differentially expressed genes at FDR < 0.3, so they are not included here. (ZIP 358 kb)

Abbreviations

AD: Alzheimer's disease; Aβ: Amyloid beta; CBM: Cerebellum; CNS: Central nervous system; COLBN: Core oligodendrocyte-enriched Bayesian network; COLGS: Core oligodendrocyte gene set; DEG: Differentially expressed gene; eSNPs: Expression single nucleotide polymorphisms; FC: Frontal cortex; FDR: False discovery rate; FE: Fold enrichment; FET: Fisher's exact test; GEO: Gene expression omnibus; GO: Gene ontology; GWAS: Genome-wide association study; HBTRC: Harvard brain tissue resource center; HGNC: Hugo Gene nomenclature committee; HIPP: Hippocampus; IGAP: International genomics of Alzheimer's Project; KO: Knockout; MSBB: Mount Sinai Brain Bank; OL: Oligodendrocyte; PFC: Prefrontal cortex; RIN: RNA integrity number; RNAseq: RNA sequencing; VC: Visual cortex; WGCNA: Weighted gene coexpression network analysis

Acknowledgments

We would like to thank members of the Zhang and Casaccia labs for many fruitful discussions.

Funding

This work was supported by the NIH grants R01AG046170, U01AG052411, RF1AG054014, RF1AG057440, R01AG057907, U01AI111598-01, R01NS067550, P50AG025688, U01AG046161, and F30AG052261. R01AG046170 is a component of the AMP-AD Target Discovery and Preclinical Validation Project. We thank the International Genomics of Alzheimer's Project (IGAP) for providing summary results data for these analyses. The investigators within IGAP contributed to the design and implementation of IGAP and/or provided data but did not participate in analysis or writing of this report. IGAP was made possible by the generous participation of the control subjects, the patients, and their families. The i–Select chips was funded by the French National Foundation on Alzheimer's disease and related disorders. EADI was supported by the LABEX (laboratory of excellence program investment for the future) DISTALZ grant, Inserm, Institut Pasteur de Lille, Université de Lille 2 and the Lille University Hospital. GERAD was supported by the Medical Research Council (Grant n° 503,480), Alzheimer's Research UK (Grant n° 503,176), the Wellcome Trust (Grant n° 082604/2/07/Z) and German Federal Ministry of Education and Research (BMBF): Competence Network Dementia (CND) grant n° 01GI0102, 01GI0711, 01GI0420. CHARGE was partly supported by the NIH/NIA grant R01 AG033193 and the NIA AG081220 and AGES contract N01–AG–12100, the NHLBI grant R01 HL105756, the Icelandic Heart Association, and the Erasmus Medical Center and Erasmus University. ADGC was supported by the NIH/NIA grants: U01 AG032984, U24 AG021886, U01 AG016976, and the Alzheimer's Association grant ADGC–10–196,728.

Authors' contributions

Conceptualization, ATM, SM, BZ and PC; Methodology, ATM, SM, BZ and PC; Software, ATM, MW, IK, W-MS, XZ, ED, JZ and BZ; Investigation, ATM, SM, BZ and PC; Resources, ATM, SM, BP, JA, K-A N, ED, DD, JL, NS, AL, EE, B.Z and PC; Writing – Original Draft, ATM; Writing – Review & Editing All Authors; Supervision, BZ and PC; Funding Acquisition, BZ and PC. All authors read and approved the final manuscript.

Authors' information

Not applicable.

Competing interests

The authors declare that they have no competing interests.

Author details

[1]Department of Genetics and Genomic Sciences, Icahn School of Medicine at Mount Sinai, One Gustave L. Levy Place, 1470 Madison Avenue, Room S8-111, New York, NY 10029, USA. [2]Icahn Institute of Genomics and Multiscale Biology, Icahn School of Medicine at Mount Sinai, One Gustave L. Levy Place, New York, NY 10029, USA. [3]Medical Scientist Training Program, Icahn School of Medicine at Mount Sinai, One Gustave L. Levy Place, New York, NY 10029, USA. [4]Fishberg Department of Neuroscience and Friedman Brain Institute, Icahn School of Medicine at Mount Sinai, One Gustave L. Levy Place, New York, NY 10029, USA. [5]Department of Human Genetics, Emory University School of Medicine, Atlanta, GA 30322, USA. [6]Department of Biochemistry, Emory University School of Medicine, Atlanta, GA 30322, USA. [7]Integrated Proteomics Core Facility, Emory University School of Medicine, Atlanta, GA 30322, USA. [8]Department of Neurology, The University of Chicago Pritzker School of Medicine, 5841 S. Maryland Avenue, Chicago, IL 60637, USA. [9]Department of Neurology, Emory University School of Medicine, Atlanta, GA 30322, USA. [10]Center for Neurodegenerative Disease, Emory University School of Medicine, Atlanta, GA 30322, USA. [11]Department of Psychiatry, Icahn School of Medicine at Mount Sinai, New York, NY 10029, USA. [12]Mental Illness Research, Education, and Clinical Center (VISN 3), James J. Peters VA Medical Center, Bronx, NY 10468, USA. [13]Neuroscience Initiative, The City University of New York, Advanced Science Research Center, 85 St. Nicholas Terrace, New York, NY 10031, USA.

References

1. Hebert LE, Weuve J, Scherr PA, Evans DA. Alzheimer disease in the United States (2010-2050) estimated using the 2010 census. Neurology. 2013;80:1778–83.
2. Plassman BL, Langa KM, Fisher GG, Heeringa SG, Weir DR, Ofstedal MB, Burke JR, Hurd MD, Potter GG, Rodgers WL, et al. Prevalence of dementia in the United States: the aging, demographics, and memory study. Neuroepidemiology. 2007;29:125–32.
3. Jack CR, Wiste HJ, Weigand SD, Knopman DS, Vemuri P, Mielke MM, Lowe V, Senjem ML, Gunter JL, Machulda MM, et al. Age, sex, and APOE ε4 effects on memory, brain structure, and β-Amyloid across the adult life span. JAMA Neurol. 2015;72:511–9.
4. Veeraraghavalu K, Zhang C, Zhang X, Tanzi RE, Sisodia SS. Age-dependent, non-cell-autonomous deposition of amyloid from synthesis of β-amyloid by cells other than excitatory neurons. J Neurosci. 2014;34:3668–73.
5. Li C, Zhao R, Gao K, Wei Z, Yin MY, Lau LT, Chui D, Hoi Yu AC. Astrocytes: implications for neuroinflammatory pathogenesis of Alzheimer's disease. Curr Alzheimer Res. 2011;8:67–80.
6. Griciuc A, Serrano-Pozo A, Parrado AR, Lesinski AN, Asselin CN, Mullin K, Hooli B, Choi SH, Hyman BT, Tanzi RE. Alzheimer's disease risk gene CD33 inhibits microglial uptake of amyloid beta. Neuron. 2013;78:631–43.
7. Salat DH, Greve DN, Pacheco JL, Quinn BT, Helmer KG, Buckner RL, Fischl B. Regional white matter volume differences in nondemented aging and Alzheimer's disease. NeuroImage. 2009;44:1247–58.
8. Cash DM, Ridgway GR, Liang Y, Ryan NS, Kinnunen KM, Yeatman T, Malone IB, Benzinger TLS, Jack CR, Thompson PM, et al. The pattern of atrophy in familial Alzheimer disease: volumetric MRI results from the DIAN study. Neurology. 2013;81:1425–33.
9. Salat DH, Kaye JA, Janowsky JS. Prefrontal gray and white matter volumes in healthy aging and Alzheimer disease. Arch Neurol. 1999;56:338–44.
10. Hua X, Hibar DP, Lee S, Toga AW, Jack CR, Weiner MW, Thompson PM. Sex and age differences in atrophic rates: an ADNI study with n=1368 MRI scans. Neurobiol Aging. 2010;31:1463–80.
11. Lee GJ, Lu PH, Hua X, Lee S, Wu S, Nguyen K, Teng E, Leow AD, Jack CR, Toga AW, et al. Depressive symptoms in mild cognitive impairment predict greater atrophy in Alzheimer's disease-related regions. Biol Psychiatry. 2012;71:814–21.
12. Lee GJ, Lu PH, Medina LD, Rodriguez-Agudelo Y, Melchor S, Coppola G, Braskie MN, Hua X, Apostolova LG, Leow AD, et al. Regional brain volume differences in symptomatic and presymptomatic carriers of familial Alzheimer's disease mutations. J Neurol Neurosurg Psychiatry. 2013;84:154–62.
13. Braak H, Braak E. Development of Alzheimer-related neurofibrillary changes in the neocortex inversely recapitulates cortical myelogenesis. Acta Neuropathol. 1996;92:197–201.
14. Braak H, Del Tredici K. The preclinical phase of the pathological process underlying sporadic Alzheimer's disease. Brain. 2015;138((Pt 10)):2814–33.
15. Kim JY, Shen S, Dietz K, He Y, Howell O, Reynolds R, Casaccia P. HDAC1 nuclear export induced by pathological conditions is essential for the onset of axonal damage. Nat Neurosci. 2010;13:180–9.
16. Werner HB, Kuhlmann K, Shen S, Uecker M, Schardt A, Dimova K, Orfaniotou F, Dhaunchak A, Brinkmann BG, Möbius W, et al. Proteolipid protein is required for transport of sirtuin 2 into CNS myelin. J Neurosci. 2007;27:7717–30.
17. Nave K-A. Myelination and the trophic support of long axons. Nat Rev Neurosci. 2010;11:275–83.
18. Nave K-A, Werner HB. Myelination of the nervous system: mechanisms and functions. Annu Rev Cell Dev Biol. 2014;30:503–33.
19. Vossel KA, Zhang K, Brodbeck J, Daub AC, Sharma P, Finkbeiner S, Cui B, Mucke L. Tau reduction prevents Abeta-induced defects in axonal transport. Science (New York, NY). 2010;330:198.
20. Zhang B, Maiti A, Shively S, Lakhani F, McDonald-Jones G, Bruce J, Lee EB, Xie SX, Joyce S, Li C, et al. Microtubule-binding drugs offset tau sequestration by stabilizing microtubules and reversing fast axonal transport deficits in a tauopathy model. Proc Natl Acad Sci U S A. 2005;102:227–31.
21. Coetzee T, Fujita N, Dupree J, Shi R, Blight A, Suzuki K, Popko B. Myelination in the absence of galactocerebroside and sulfatide: normal structure with abnormal function and regional instability. Cell. 1996;86:209–19.
22. Edgar JM, McLaughlin M, Werner HB, McCulloch MC, Barrie JA, Brown A, Faichney AB, Snaidero N, Nave K-A, Griffiths IR. Early ultrastructural defects of axons and axon-glia junctions in mice lacking expression of Cnp1. Glia. 2009;57:1815–24.
23. Lappe-Siefke C, Goebbels S, Gravel M, Nicksch E, Lee J, Braun PE, Griffiths IR, Nave K-A. Disruption of Cnp1 uncouples oligodendroglial functions in axonal support and myelination. Nat Genet. 2003;33:366–74.
24. Edgar JM, McLaughlin M, Yool D, Zhang SC, Fowler JH, Montague P, Barrie JA, McCulloch MC, Duncan ID, Garbern J, et al. Oligodendroglial modulation of fast axonal transport in a mouse model of hereditary spastic paraplegia. J Cell Biol. 2004;166(1):121–31.
25. Griffiths I, Klugmann M, Anderson T, Yool D, Thomson C, Schwab MH, Schneider A, Zimmermann F, McCulloch M, Nadon N, et al. Axonal swellings and degeneration in mice lacking the major proteolipid of myelin. Science. 1998;280(5369):1610–3.
26. Zhang B, Gaiteri C, Bodea L-G, Wang Z, McElwee J, Podtelezhnikov AA, Zhang C, Xie T, Tran L, Dobrin R, et al. Integrated systems approach identifies genetic nodes and networks in late-onset Alzheimer's disease. Cell. 2013;153:707–20.
27. Cruchaga C, Haller G, Chakraverty S, Mayo K, Vallania FLM, Mitra RD, Faber K, Williamson J, Bird T, Diaz-Arrastia R, et al. Rare variants in APP, PSEN1 and

PSEN2 increase risk for AD in late-onset Alzheimer's disease families. PLoS One. 2012;7:e31039.
28. Lambert JC, Ibrahim-Verbaas CA, Harold D, Naj AC, Sims R, Bellenguez C, DeStafano AL, Bis JC, Beecham GW, Grenier-Boley B, et al. Meta-analysis of 74,046 individuals identifies 11 new susceptibility loci for Alzheimer's disease. Nat Genet. 2013;45:1452–8.
29. Ahmed RR, Holler CJ, Webb RL, Li F, Beckett TL, Murphy MP. BACE1 and BACE2 enzymatic activities in Alzheimer's disease. J Neurochem. 2010;112:1045–53.
30. Wetzel-Smith MK, Hunkapiller J, Bhangale TR, Srinivasan K, Maloney JA, Atwal JK, Sa SM, Yaylaoglu MB, Foreman O, Ortmann W, et al. A rare mutation in UNC5C predisposes to late-onset Alzheimer's disease and increases neuronal cell death. Nat Med. 2014;20:1452–7.
31. Zhang B, Horvath S. A general framework for weighted gene co-expression network analysis. Stat Appl Genet Mol Biol. 2005;4:Article17.
32. Zhang Y, Chen K, Sloan SA, Bennett ML, Scholze AR, O'Keeffe S, Phatnani HP, Guarnieri P, Caneda C, Ruderisch N, et al. An RNA-sequencing Transcriptome and splicing database of Glia, neurons, and vascular cells of the cerebral cortex. J Neurosci. 2014;34:11929–47.
33. Zhu J, Wiener MC, Zhang C, Fridman A, Minch E, Lum PY, Sachs JR, Schadt EE. Increasing the power to detect causal associations by combining genotypic and expression data in segregating populations. PLoS Comput Biol. 2007;3(4):e69.
34. Zhu J, Zhang B, Smith EN, Drees B, Brem RB, Kruglyak L, Bumgarner RE, Schadt EE. Integrating large-scale functional genomic data to dissect the complexity of yeast regulatory networks. Nat Genet. 2008;40:854–61.
35. Wang I-M, Zhang B, Yang X, Zhu J, Stepaniants S, Zhang C, Meng Q, Peters M, He Y, Ni C, et al. Systems Analysis of Eleven Rodent Disease Models Reveals an Inflammatome Signature and Key Drivers. Mol Syst Biol 2012, (in press).
36. Mishra A, Macgregor S. VEGAS2: software for more flexible gene-based testing. Twin Res Hum Genet. 2015;18:86–91.
37. McKenzie AT, Katsyv I, Song WM, Wang M, Zhang B. DGCA: a comprehensive R package for differential gene correlation analysis. BMC Syst Biol. 2016;10(1):106.
38. Storey J. Qvalue: Q-value estimation for false discovery rate control. 2015.
39. Anders S, Reyes A, Huber W. Detecting differential usage of exons from RNA-seq data. Genome Res. 2012;22:2008–17.
40. Blalock EM, Geddes JW, Chen KC, Porter NM, Markesbery WR, Landfield PW. Incipient Alzheimer's disease: microarray correlation analyses reveal major transcriptional and tumor suppressor responses. Proc Natl Acad Sci U S A. 2004;101:2173–8.
41. Falcon S, Gentleman R. Using GOstats to test gene lists for GO term association. Bioinformatics (Oxford, England). 2007;23:257–8.
42. Wang M, Zhao Y, Zhang B. Efficient test and visualization of multi-set intersections. Sci Rep. 2015;5:16923.
43. Dagley LF, White CA, Liao Y, Shi W, Smyth GK, Orian JM, Emili A, Purcell AW. Quantitative proteomic profiling reveals novel region-specific markers in the adult mouse brain. Proteomics. 2014;14:241–61.
44. Miller JA, Oldham MC, Geschwind DH. A systems level analysis of transcriptional changes in Alzheimer's disease and normal aging. J Neurosci. 2008;28:1410–20.
45. Emery B, Agalliu D, Cahoy JD, Watkins TA, Dugas JC, Mulinyawe SB, Ibrahim A, Ligon KL, Rowitch DH, Barres BA. Myelin gene regulatory factor is a critical transcriptional regulator required for CNS Myelination. Cell. 2009;138:172–85.
46. Cai D, Zhong M, Wang R, Netzer WJ, Shields D, Zheng H, Sisodia SS, Foster DA, Gorelick FS, Xu H, et al. Phospholipase D1 corrects impaired betaAPP trafficking and neurite outgrowth in familial Alzheimer's disease-linked presenilin-1 mutant neurons. Proc Natl Acad Sci U S A. 2006;103:1936–40.
47. Jin J-K, Ahn B-H, Na Y-J, Kim J-I, Kim Y-S, Choi E-K, Ko Y-G, Chung KC, Kozlowski PB, Min DS. Phospholipase D1 is associated with amyloid precursor protein in Alzheimer's disease. Neurobiol Aging. 2007;28:1015–27.
48. Bayer TA, Paliga K, Weggen S, Wiestler OD, Beyreuther K, Multhaup G. Amyloid precursor-like protein 1 accumulates in neuritic plaques in Alzheimer's disease. Acta Neuropathol. 1997;94:519–24.
49. Klugmann M, Schwab MH, Pühlhofer A, Schneider A, Zimmermann F, Griffiths IR, Nave KA. Assembly of CNS myelin in the absence of proteolipid protein. Neuron. 1997;18:59–70.
50. Morell P, Quarles RH. Characteristic Composition of Myelin. Philadelphia: Lippincott-Raven; 1999.
51. von Trotha KT, Heun R, Schmitz S, Lutjohann D, Maier W, Kolsch H. Influence of lysosomal acid lipase polymorphisms on chromosome 10 on the risk of Alzheimer's disease and cholesterol metabolism. Neurosci Lett. 2006;402(3):262–6.
52. Lee J. Process outgrowth in oligodendrocytes is mediated by CNP, a novel microtubule assembly myelin protein. J Cell Biol. 2005;170:661–73.
53. Miller JA, Woltjer RL, Goodenbour JM, Horvath S, Geschwind DH. Genes and pathways underlying regional and cell type changes in Alzheimer's disease. Genome Med. 2013;5(5):48.
54. de Monasterio-Schrader P, Jahn O, Tenzer S, Wichert SP, Patzig J, Werner HB. Systematic approaches to central nervous system myelin. Cell Mol Life Sci. 2012;69(17):2879–94.
55. Harlow DE, Saul KE, Culp CM, Vesely EM, Macklin WB. Expression of proteolipid protein gene in spinal cord stem cells and early oligodendrocyte progenitor cells is dispensable for normal cell migration and myelination. J Neurosci. 2014;34:1333–43.
56. Garbern JY, Yool DA, Moore GJ, Wilds IB, Faulk MW, Klugmann M, Nave K-A, Sistermans EA, van der Knaap MS, Bird TD, et al. Patients lacking the major CNS myelin protein, proteolipid protein 1, develop length-dependent axonal degeneration in the absence of demyelination and inflammation. Brain. 2002;125:551–61.
57. Mohan H, Friese A, Albrecht S, Krumbholz M, Elliott CL, Arthur A, Menon R, Farina C, Junker A, Stadelmann C, et al. Transcript profiling of different types of multiple sclerosis lesions yields FGF1 as a promoter of remyelination. Acta Neuropathol Commun. 2014;2:168.
58. Mashayekhi F, Hadavi M, Vaziri HR, Naji M. Increased acidic fibroblast growth factor concentrations in the serum and cerebrospinal fluid of patients with Alzheimer's disease. J Clin Neurosci. 2010;17(3):357–9.
59. Tamiya G, Makino S, Hayashi M, Abe A, Numakura C, Ueki M, Tanaka A, Ito C, Toshimori K, Ogawa N, et al. A mutation of COX6A1 causes a recessive axonal or mixed form of Charcot-Marie-tooth disease. Am J Hum Genet. 2014;95:294–300.
60. Piedrahita D, Hernández I, López-Tobón A, Fedorov D, Obara B, Manjunath BS, Boudreau RL, Davidson B, Laferla F, Gallego-Gómez JC, et al. Silencing of CDK5 reduces neurofibrillary tangles in transgenic alzheimer's mice. J Neurosci. 2010;30:13966–76.
61. Yang Y, Wang H, Zhang J, Luo F, Herrup K, Bibb JA, Lu R, Miller RH. Cyclin dependent kinase 5 is required for the normal development of oligodendrocytes and myelin formation. Dev Biol. 2013;378:94–106.
62. Bartzokis G. Alzheimer's disease as homeostatic responses to age-related myelin breakdown. Neurobiol Aging. 2011;32:1341–71.
63. De Rossi P, Buggia-Prevot V, Clayton BL, Vasquez JB, van Sanford C, Andrew RJ, Lesnick R, Botte A, Deyts C, Salem S, et al. Predominant expression of Alzheimer's disease-associated BIN1 in mature oligodendrocytes and localization to white matter tracts. Mol Neurodegener. 2016;11(1):59.
64. Holler CJ, Davis PR, Beckett TL, Platt TL, Webb RL, Head E, Murphy MP. Bridging integrator 1 (BIN1) protein expression increases in the Alzheimer's disease brain and correlates with neurofibrillary tangle pathology. J Alzheimers Dis. 2014;42(4):1221–7.
65. Patzig J, Erwig MS, Tenzer S, Kusch K, Dibaj P, Mobius W, Goebbels S, Schaeren-Wiemers N, Nave KA, Werner HB. Septin/anillin filaments scaffold central nervous system myelin to accelerate nerve conduction. elife. 2016;5: e17119.
66. Puthiyedth N, Riveros C, Berretta R, Moscato P. Identification of differentially expressed genes through integrated study of Alzheimer's disease affected brain regions. PLoS One. 2016;11(4):e0152342.
67. Calkins MJ, Manczak M, Mao P, Shirendeb U, Reddy PH. Impaired mitochondrial biogenesis, defective axonal transport of mitochondria, abnormal mitochondrial dynamics and synaptic degeneration in a mouse model of Alzheimer's disease. Hum Mol Genet. 2011;20:4515–29.
68. Iijima-Ando K, Sekiya M, Maruko-Otake A, Ohtake Y, Suzuki E, Lu B, Iijima KM. Loss of axonal mitochondria promotes tau-mediated neurodegeneration and Alzheimer's disease-related tau phosphorylation via PAR-1. PLoS Genet. 2012;8:e1002918.
69. González C, Couve A. The axonal endoplasmic reticulum and protein trafficking: cellular bootlegging south of the soma. Semin Cell Dev Biol. 2014;27:23–31.
70. Butler MH, David C, Ochoa GC, Freyberg Z, Daniell L, Grabs D, Cremona O, De Camilli P. Amphiphysin II (SH3P9; BIN1), a member of the amphiphysin/Rvs family, is concentrated in the cortical cytomatrix of axon initial segments and nodes of ranvier in brain and around T tubules in skeletal muscle. J Cell Biol. 1997;137:1355–67.
71. Zhang Y, Sloan Steven A, Clarke Laura E, Caneda C, Plaza Colton A, Blumenthal Paul D, Vogel H, Steinberg Gary K, Edwards Michael SB, Li G, et al. Purification and characterization of progenitor and mature human

Astrocytes reveals transcriptional and functional differences with mouse. Neuron. 2015;89:37–53.
72. Macé S, Cousin E, Ricard S, Génin E, Spanakis E, Lafargue-Soubigou C, Génin B, Fournel R, Roche S, Haussy G, et al. ABCA2 is a strong genetic risk factor for early-onset Alzheimer's disease. Neurobiol Dis. 2005;18:119–25.
73. Wollmer MA, Kapaki E, Hersberger M, Muntwyler J, Brunner F, Tsolaki M, Akatsu H, Kosaka K, Michikawa M, Molyva D, et al. Ethnicity-dependent genetic association of ABCA2 with sporadic Alzheimer's disease. Am J Med Genet B Neuropsychiatr Genet. 2006;141B:534–6.
74. Xu X, Wang Y, Wang L, Liao Q, Chang L, Xu L, Huang Y, Ye H, Xu L, Chen C, et al. Meta-analyses of 8 polymorphisms associated with the risk of the Alzheimer's disease. PLoS One. 2013;8:e73129.
75. Minster RL, DeKosky ST, Kamboh MI. No association of DAPK1 and ABCA2 SNPs on chromosome 9 with Alzheimer's disease. Neurobiol Aging. 2009;30:1890–1.
76. Karch CM, Goate AM. Alzheimer's disease risk genes and mechanisms of disease pathogenesis. Biol Psychiatry. 2015;77:43–51.
77. Karran E, Mercken M, De Strooper B. The amyloid cascade hypothesis for Alzheimer's disease: an appraisal for the development of therapeutics. Nat Rev Drug Discov. 2011;10(9):698–712.
78. Liu Y, Zhang Y-W, Wang X, Zhang H, You X, Liao F-F, Xu H. Intracellular trafficking of presenilin 1 is regulated by beta-amyloid precursor protein and phospholipase D1. J Biol Chem. 2009;284:12145–52.
79. Zhou F, van Laar T, Huang H, Zhang L. APP and APLP1 are degraded through autophagy in response to proteasome inhibition in neuronal cells. Protein & cell. 2011;2:377–83.
80. Treiber H, Hagemeyer N, Ehrenreich H, Simons M. BACE1 in central nervous system myelination revisited. Mol Psychiatry. 2012;17:237–9.
81. Hu X, Hicks CW, He W, Wong P, Macklin WB, Trapp BD, Yan R. Bace1 modulates myelination in the central and peripheral nervous system. Nat Neurosci. 2006;9:1520–5.
82. Jonsson T, Atwal JK, Steinberg S, Snaedal J, Jonsson PV, Bjornsson S, Stefansson H, Sulem P, Gudbjartsson D, Maloney J, et al. A mutation in APP protects against Alzheimer's disease and age-related cognitive decline. Nature. 2012;488:96–9.
83. Willem M, Garratt AN, Novak B, Citron M, Kaufmann S, Rittger A, DeStrooper B, Saftig P, Birchmeier C, Haass C. Control of peripheral nerve myelination by the beta-secretase BACE1. Science (New York, NY). 2006;314:664–6.
84. Miller JA, Woltjer RL, Goodenbour JM, Horvath S, Geschwind DH. Genes and pathways underlying regional and cell type changes in Alzheimer's disease. Genome Med. 2013;5:48.
85. Jones L, Lambert J-C, Wang L-S, Choi S-H, Harold D, Vedernikov A, Escott-Price V, Stone T, Richards A, Bellenguez C, et al. Convergent genetic and expression data implicate immunity in Alzheimer's disease. Alzheimers Dement. 2015;11(6):658–71.
86. Seyfried NT, Dammer EB, Swarup V, Nandakumar D, Duong DM, Yin L, Deng Q, Nguyen T, Hales CM, Wingo T, et al. A multi-network approach identifies protein-specific co-expression in asymptomatic and symptomatic Alzheimer's disease. Cell Syst. 2017;4(1):60–72 e64.
87. Jin SC, Benitez BA, Karch CM, Cooper B, Skorupa T, Carrell D, Norton JB, Hsu S, Harari O, Cai Y, et al. Coding variants in TREM2 increase risk for Alzheimer's disease. Hum Mol Genet. 2014;23:5838–46.
88. Guerreiro R, Wojtas A, Bras J, Carrasquillo M, Rogaeva E, Majounie E, Cruchaga C, Sassi C, Kauwe JSK, Younkin S, et al. TREM2 variants in Alzheimer's disease. N Engl J Med. 2013;368:117–27.
89. Paloneva J, Manninen T, Christman G, Hovanes K, Mandelin J, Adolfsson R, Bianchin M, Bird T, Miranda R, Salmaggi A, et al. Mutations in two genes encoding different subunits of a receptor signaling complex result in an identical disease phenotype. Am J Hum Genet. 2002;71:656–62.
90. Poliani PL, Wang Y, Fontana E, Robinette ML, Yamanishi Y, Gilfillan S, Colonna M. TREM2 sustains microglial expansion during aging and response to demyelination. J Clin Invest. 2015;125:2161–70.
91. Painter MM, Atagi Y, Liu CC, Rademakers R, Xu H, Fryer JD, Bu G. TREM2 in CNS homeostasis and neurodegenerative disease. Mol Neurodegener. 2015;10:43.
92. Cherry JD, Olschowka JA, O'Banion MK. Neuroinflammation and M2 microglia: the good, the bad, and the inflamed. J Neuroinflammation. 2014;11:98.
93. Oakley H, Cole SL, Logan S, Maus E, Shao P, Craft J, Guillozet-Bongaarts A, Ohno M, Disterhoft J, Van Eldik L, et al. Intraneuronal beta-amyloid aggregates, neurodegeneration, and neuron loss in transgenic mice with five familial Alzheimer's disease mutations: potential factors in amyloid plaque formation. J Neurosci. 2006;26(40):10129–40.
94. Radde R, Bolmont T, Kaeser SA, Coomaraswamy J, Lindau D, Stoltze L, Calhoun ME, Jaggi F, Wolburg H, Gengler S, et al. Abeta42-driven cerebral amyloidosis in transgenic mice reveals early and robust pathology. EMBO Rep. 2006;7(9):940–6.
95. Sturchler-Pierrat C, Abramowski D, Duke M, Wiederhold KH, Mistl C, Rothacher S, Ledermann B, Burki K, Frey P, Paganetti PA, et al. Two amyloid precursor protein transgenic mouse models with Alzheimer disease-like pathology. Proc Natl Acad Sci U S A. 1997;94(24):13287–92.
96. Krestinina O, Azarashvili T, Baburina Y, Galvita A, Grachev D, Stricker R, Reiser G. In aging, the vulnerability of rat brain mitochondria is enhanced due to reduced level of 2′,3′-cyclic nucleotide-3′-phosphodiesterase (CNP) and subsequently increased permeability transition in brain mitochondria in old animals. Neurochem Int. 2015;80:41–50.
97. Krämer-Albers E-M, Bretz N, Tenzer S, Winterstein C, Möbius W, Berger H, Nave K-A, Schild H, Trotter J. Oligodendrocytes secrete exosomes containing major myelin and stress-protective proteins: Trophic support for axons? Proteomics Clin Appl. 2007;1:1446–61.
98. Subramaniam S, Fahy E, Gupta S, Sud M, Byrnes RW, Cotter D, Dinasarapu AR, Maurya MR. Bioinformatics and systems biology of the lipidome. Chem Rev. 2011;111:6452–90.

iPSC-derived familial Alzheimer's *PSEN2* ^{N141I} cholinergic neurons exhibit mutation-dependent molecular pathology corrected by insulin signaling

Cesar L. Moreno[1,2], Lucio Della Guardia[3], Valeria Shnyder[3], Maitane Ortiz-Virumbrales[1], Ilya Kruglikov[4], Bin Zhang[5], Eric E. Schadt[5], Rudolph E. Tanzi[6], Scott Noggle[4*], Christoph Buettner[3*] and Sam Gandy[1,2*]

Abstract

Background: Type 2 diabetes (T2D) is a recognized risk factor for the development of cognitive impairment (CI) and/or dementia, although the exact nature of the molecular pathology of T2D-associated CI remains obscure. One link between T2D and CI might involve decreased insulin signaling in brain and/or neurons in either animal or postmortem human brains as has been reported as a feature of Alzheimer's disease (AD). Here we asked if neuronal insulin resistance is a cell autonomous phenomenon in a familial form of AD.

Methods: We have applied a newly developed protocol for deriving human basal forebrain cholinergic neurons (BFCN) from skin fibroblasts via induced pluripotent stem cell (iPSC) technology. We generated wildtype and familial AD mutant *PSEN2*^{N141I} (presenilin 2) BFCNs and assessed if insulin signaling, insulin regulation of the major AD proteins Aβ and/or tau, and/or calcium fluxes is altered by the *PSEN2*^{N141I} mutation.

Results: We report herein that wildtype, *PSEN2*^{N141I} and CRISPR/Cas9-corrected iPSC-derived BFCNs (and their precursors) show indistinguishable insulin signaling profiles as determined by the phosphorylation of canonical insulin signaling pathway molecules. Chronic insulin treatment of BFCNs of all genotypes led to a reduction in the Aβ42/40 ratio. Unexpectedly, we found a CRISPR/Cas9-correctable effect of *PSEN2*^{N141I} on calcium flux, which could be prevented by chronic exposure of BFCNs to insulin.

Conclusions: Our studies indicate that the familial AD mutation *PSEN2*^{N141I} does not induce neuronal insulin resistance in a cell autonomous fashion. The ability of insulin to correct calcium fluxes and to lower Aβ42/40 ratio suggests that insulin acts to oppose an AD-pathophysiology. Hence, our results are consistent with a potential physiological role for insulin as a mediator of resilience by counteracting specific metabolic and molecular features of AD.

Background

Type 2 diabetes (T2D) is associated with an increased risk for dementia in the setting of hyperinsulinemia and peripheral insulin resistance [15, 30]. There is as yet no consensus on whether the most important cause of dementia in the setting of T2D is related to Alzheimer's disease (AD), vascular cognitive impairment and dementia (VCID) or some novel form of cognitive impairment with a predilection for a shared pathogenesis with T2D [13, 22, 26]. Furthermore, there is no consensus on the nomenclature for how these phenomena are described. The only exception is stroke, where it is accepted that the brain develops insulin resistance as a result of stroke [7] but even here, the brain regions, cell types, and intracellular bases of post-stroke insulin resistance are not well-established [25]. Other reports indicate that "brain insulin signaling" is diminished in patients

* Correspondence: snoggle@nyscf.orgu; Christoph.buettner@mssm.edu; Samuel.gandy@mssm.edu
[4]New York Stem Cell Foundation Laboratories, New York, NY 10032, USA
[3]Department of Medicine, Diabetes, Obesity, and Metabolism Institute, Icahn School of Medicine at Mount Sinai, New York, NY 10029, USA
[1]Department of Neurology, NFL Neurological Care Center, Icahn School of Medicine at Mount Sinai, New York, NY 10029, USA
Full list of author information is available at the end of the article

with AD [3] and that insulin resistance and glucose hypo-metabolism seen in positron emission tomography (PET) brain scans predict cognitive outcome in humans [34]. There is substantial interest in the repurposing of intranasal insulin as a means of improving brain insulin signaling and thereby the cognitive function of both healthy individuals [4] and AD patients [6].

Given the poorly defined molecular pathology of brain insulin resistance in AD, we began by examining various potential mechanisms for the development of human brain insulin resistance as a cell autonomous phenomenon in neurons. Recently, an intriguing potential clue emerged in a report that γ-secretase hypofunction can underlie insulin resistance in adipocytes [27]. The most common mutations leading to familial Alzheimer's disease (FAD) target the presenilin 1 (*PSEN1)* gene. Mutations in *PSEN1* or its homologue *PSEN2* are associated with hypofunction of the γ-secretase leading to an increase in the amyloid β (Aβ) 42:40 ratio and Aβ42. The main aim of this study then was to test whether neuronal insulin signaling is impaired in neurons from subjects carrying FAD genes that encode hypofunctional γ-secretase and whether insulin resistance contributes to the phenotype of AD.

We analyzed the effect of insulin signaling on Aβ speciation as well as a battery of other determinations (such as electrophysiological profiling, toxin sensitivity, etc) in iPSC-derived wildtype and FAD mutant *PSEN2*^{N141I} neurons as well as their CRISPR/Cas9-corrected counterparts. We focused on a particular iPSC-derived neuronal subtype: the basal forebrain cholinergic neurons (BFCNs) [19] since these are believed to be one of the most vulnerable cells to early degeneration in AD. In many cases of early CI, the severity of the memory deficit appears to reflect the severity of the cholinergic deficiency [10, 11].

We observed that wildtype, *PSEN2*^{N141I} and CRISPR/Cas9-corrected iPSC-derived BFCNs (and their precursors) showed indistinguishable insulin signaling profiles as determined by the apparent phosphorylation stoichiometry of the canonical insulin signaling pathway molecules. Chronic insulin treatment of BFCNs of all genotypes led to a reduction in the Aβ42/40 ratio. Unexpectedly, a previously reported CRISPR/Cas9-correctable effect of *PSEN2*^{N141I} on calcium flux could be corrected by chronic exposure of BFCNs to physiologically stimulatory concentrations of insulin. Hence, the ability of insulin to correct calcium fluxes and to lower Aβ42/40 ratio suggests that insulin acts to oppose an AD-pathophysiology. Our results are consistent with a potential physiological role for insulin as a mediator of resilience by acting as an antagonist of specific metabolic and molecular features of AD.

Results

iPSC-derived neuroprecursors of BFCNs display dose-dependent insulin signaling

The cell lines used in this study are listed in Table 1. Three of these lines were derived from a cohort of siblings, two of whom carry the Volga German *PSEN2* ^{N141I} mutation [5] (AD1 and AD2) and a third who does not (fControl). Dedifferentiated fibroblasts were differentiated into iPSCs using non-incorporating modified mRNA transfer as described [21]. In addition, we also included a cell line that we have previously characterized from a healthy individual, which was reprogrammed using Sendai virus.

To characterize the insulin signaling of iPSC-derived wildtype and *PSEN2*^{N141I} neurons, we first conducted pilot studies to identify the optimal response time to achieve a maximal insulin signaling response. We found that after an overnight incubation without insulin, cells were responsive to a dose of 1000 ng/ml (~ 172 nM) after 10 and 30 min as assessed by AKT activation (see Additional file 1: Figure S1). We therefore used the 30-min incubation time to study phosphorylation of downstream molecules in the insulin signaling pathway. We next determined an insulin dose- response in neuroprecursor cells for BFCNs (Fig. 1).

Western blot analyses indicated that insulin activated all the canonical targets at the concentration employed. For reference, the dose range utilized ranged from reported physiological levels [32] (10 ng/ml is approximately 1.72 nM) to hyperphysiological levels (1000 ng/ml). Note that our highest insulin dose, 172 nM, is comparable to Kahn's standard dose of 100 nM that was used to study insulin signaling in iPSC-derived myotubes [12]. We found that the effect of insulin was most robust on the phosphorylation of AKT (Fig. 1c and d), which is a key signaling node within the PI-3 K signaling pathway. Downstream of AKT, glycogen synthase kinase-3 β (GSK3β) and ribosomal protein S6 (pS6RP), which mediates the translational regulation through insulin were activated by insulin. Similarly, insulin phosphorylated mammalian target of rapamycin complex (pMTOR) in a dose responsive fashion [31]. Importantly, insulin signaling was not reduced in neuroprecursor lines that carried the FAD-mutation. Thus, the insulin resistance effect of hypofunctional γ-secretase as reported in adipocytes [27] was not readily detectable in our iPSC-derived BFCNs harboring hypofunctional γ-secretase due to familial AD mutant *PSEN2*^{N141}.

iPSC-derived BFCNs display dose-dependent insulin signaling

Different transcriptomic signatures and protein markers are observed through the neuronal differentiation process in iPSCs, corresponding with neurodevelopmental observations seen in vivo [28]. We have detected similar processes in the differentiation of our BFCNs [19]. Since insulin/

Table 1 Nomenclature and descriptions of iPSC lines used in this study

Line	Sex	*APOE*	Genotype	Reprogramming Method
Control	Male	E3/E3	Normal	Sendai virus
fControl	Female	E3/E3	Normal	mRNA Transfection
AD1	Female	E3/E4	*PSEN2* ^{N141I}	mRNA Transfection
AD2	Female	E3/E3	*PSEN2* ^{N141I}	mRNA Transfection
iAD1	Female	E3/E4	*Normal (Corrected AD1)*	mRNA Transfection
iAD2	Female	E3/E3	*Normal (Corrected AD2)*	mRNA Transfection

insulin-like growth factor signaling exerts pleiotropic effects during neurodevelopment, we next studied whether insulin signaling differed as a function of the different developmental stages of the BFCN lineage. For this and all subsequent experiments, we compared the FAD-related lines with their engineered isogenic controls, due to the inherent variations we had observed across cell lines in our studies with the neuroprecursor cell lines (Fig. 1). We found similar molecular responses to insulin, whereby the proximal insulin cascade signatures i.e. pAKT were most robustly induced (Fig. 2). These findings demonstrated the integrity of insulin signaling via AKT and downstream signaling pathways such as s6RP in iPSC-derived BFCNs. However, we were unable to identify FAD-related differences in insulin signaling in the iPSC-derived BFCNs from *PSEN* mutation carriers.

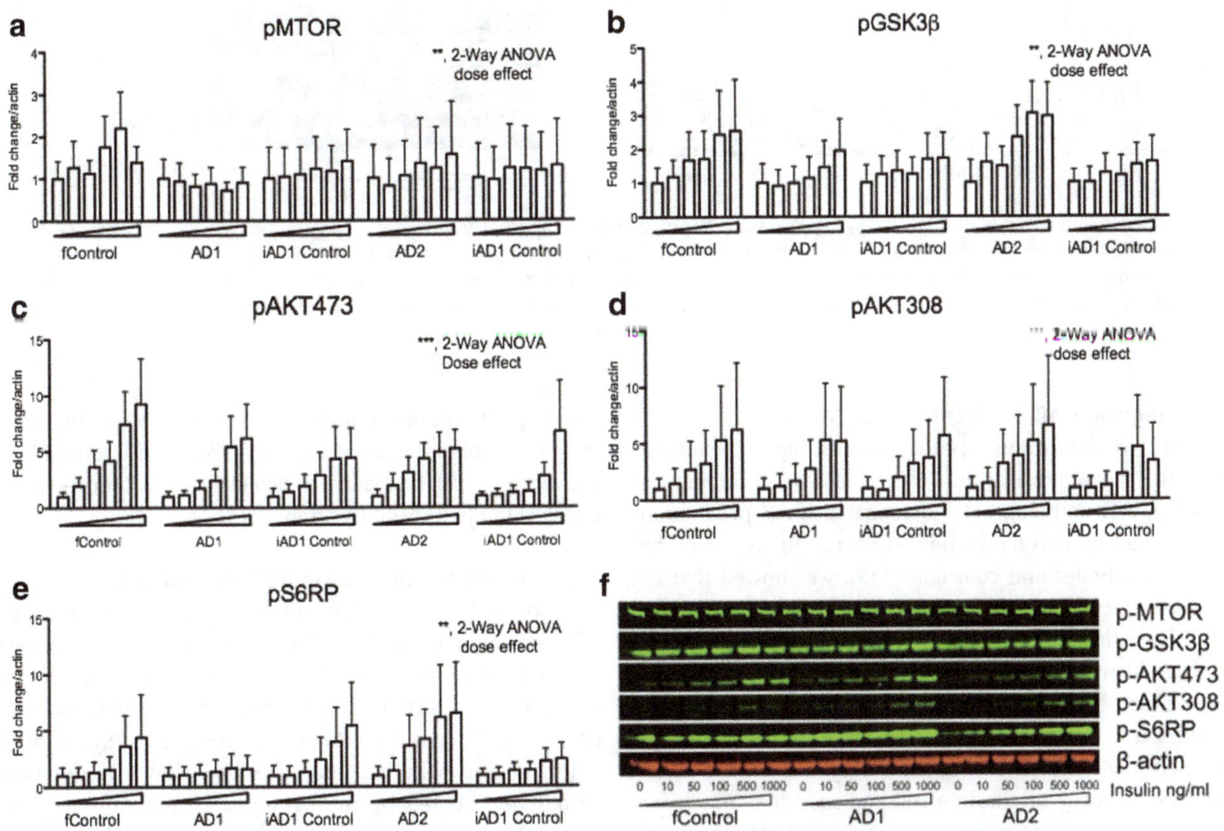

Fig. 1 Downstream insulin signaling pathway molecules display similar phosphorylation status in iPSC-derived wildtype and *PSEN2*^{N141I} basal forebrain cholinergic neuroprecursors. **a-e** Western blot analysis of insulin signaling in iPSC-derived basal cholinergic neuroprecursor cell lines. Cells were insulin deprived overnight before the addition of corresponding insulin concentrations of 0, 10, 50, 100, 500, 1000 ng/ml. Lysates were collected after a 30-min exposure to the specified insulin concentration. Quantified western blot data was normalized to an actin standard and expressed as fold change to the 0 ng/ml vehicle control. Dose dependency was detected by 2-way ANOVA where indicated. These data correspond to results of three independent experiments. ** $P < 0.01$; *** $P < .001$. **f** Representative blots from a single experiment showing three of the lines

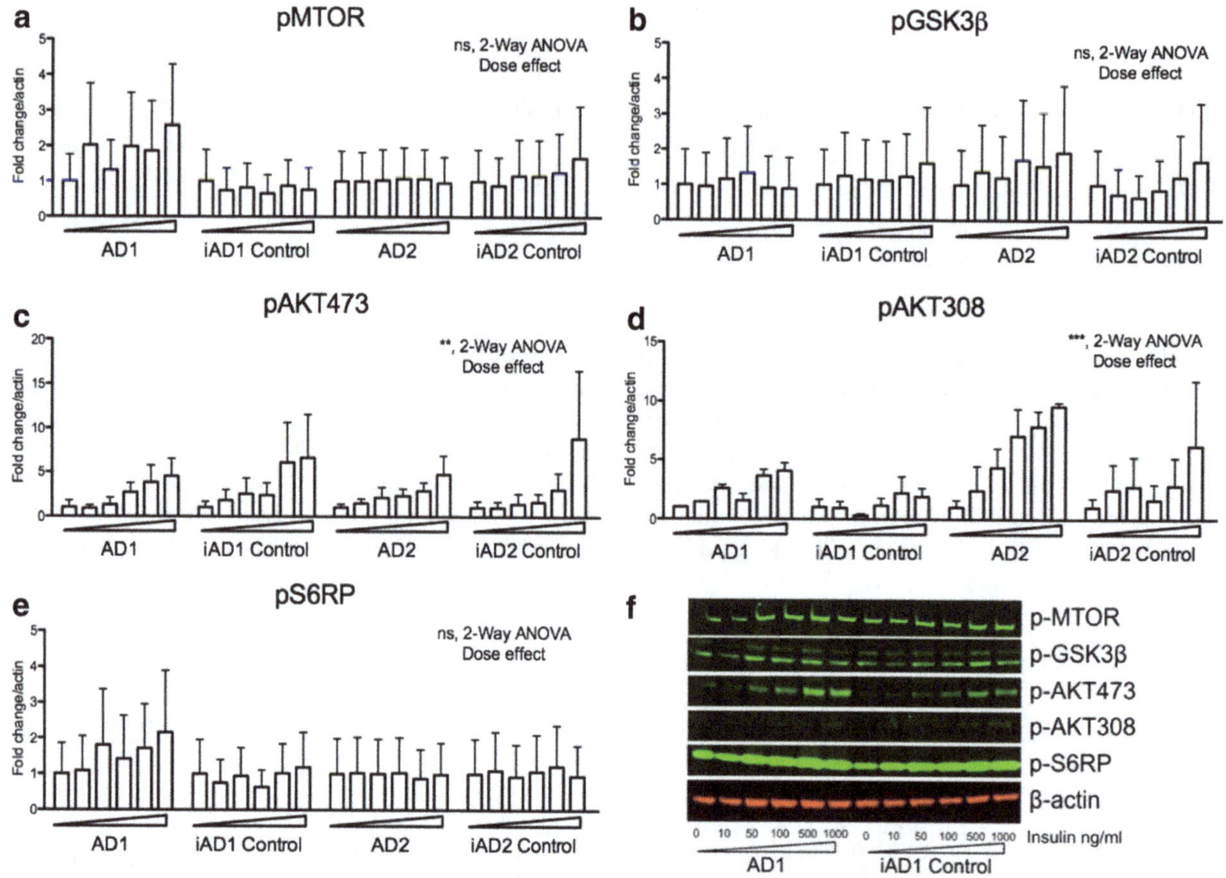

Fig. 2 Downstream insulin signaling pathway molecules display similar status of phosphorylation in iPSC-derived wildtype and *PSEN2*^{N141I} basal forebrain cholinergic neurons (BFCNs). **a-e** Western blot analysis of iPSC-derived BFCNs. Cells (DIV 34) were insulin deprived overnight before the addition of insulin at 0, 10, 50, 100, 500, 1000 ng/ml. Cells were collected after a 30-min exposure. Quantifications of western blot data is normalized over actin and expressed as fold change to vehicle treated cells. These data correspond to results of two to three independent experiments. Dose dependency was detected by 2-way ANOVA where indicated. ** $P < 0.01$; *** $P < .001$. **f** Representative blots from a single experiment showing three of the lines

Insulin regulates Aβ production by BFCNs

In order to determine whether insulin signaling could affect the metabolism of any of the hallmark proteins involved in AD pathology, we investigated if Aβ production was affected by chronic insulin exposure. In the study by Ortiz-Virumbrales and colleagues [19], we showed that by correcting the Volga German point mutation in *PSEN2*, the Aβ 42/40 ratio was normalized. We next tested whether insulin could modulate the Aβ 42/40 ratio in the cell lines that we were studying. Indeed, the Aβ 42/40 ratio that accumulated in the media being normalized in the corrected clones (e.g. AD1 vs iAD1 Control) (Fig. 3a-c). This effect was modulated by insulin in a cell-line-specific manner; for example, a significant reduction of Aβ 42/40 ratio by insulin was seen in the iAD1 control and the AD2 line. Hence, insulin tended to reduce the Aβ 42/40 ratio regardless of whether the ratio was elevated or not suggesting that insulin exerts anti-amyloidogenic effects, which in turn would be consistent with a role for insulin in preventing cerebral amyloidosis.

Using the same experimental design, we tested the status of tau phosphorylation at Ser^{202}/Thr205 (Additional file 1: Figures S2a, 2b), but failed to detect FAD mutation-related changes in tau phosphorylation.

Insulin promotes Ca^{2+} flux in iPSC-derived BFCNs

As reported by Ortiz-Virumbrales and colleagues [19], iPSC-derived BFCNs from FAD mutation carriers showed reduced excitability and decreased spike amplitudes. We tested whether insulin could stimulate Ca^{2+} activity, as a proxy for electrophysiological activity, in iPSC-derived neurons and whether any changes that we detected would be affected by the presence of the mutant FAD gene. We recorded Ca^{2+} flux as measured by relative fluorescent units (Fig. 4) and observed that insulin robustly increased Ca^{2+} mediated fluorescence in all cell lines tested (Fig. 4a), compared to vehicle treatment (Fig. 4b). We obtained additional visual corroboration of Ca^{2+} activity (Fig. 4c and Additional file 2: Video 1). In conclusion, we observed that all cell lines tested

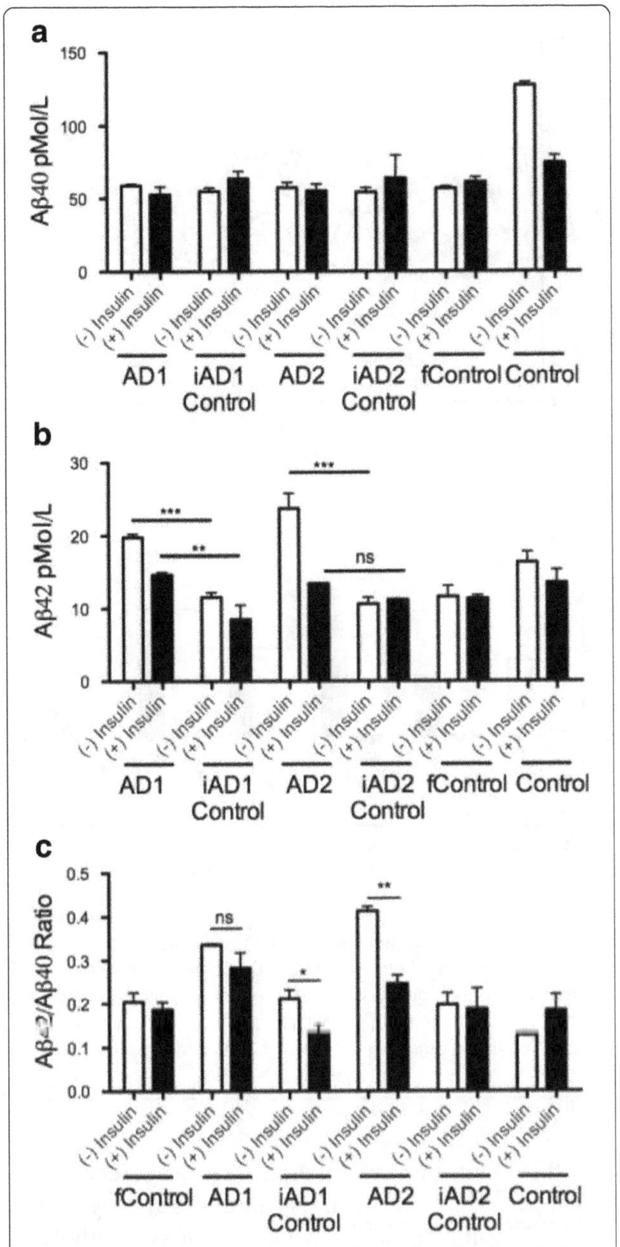

Fig. 3 Chronic insulin administration reduces the Aβ42/40 ratio in the conditioned media of BFCNs harboring FAD mutations. ELISA quantification of iPSC derived basal cholinergic neurons measuring amyloid β. Cells (DIV 34) were insulin deprived for 3 days or given 1000 ng/mL every 24 h for 3 days. Aβ 40 (**a**), Aβ 42 (**b**), and Aβ 42/40 (**c**) measured in collected media. These data correspond to results of 2 independent experiments. * $P < 0.05$; ** $P < .01$

displayed enhanced calcium-mediated fluorescence following insulin treatment.

Discussion

Alzheimer's disease (AD) pathology is characterized by synaptic and neuronal degeneration together with accumulation of extracellular plaques composed of Aβ [17], as well as neurofibrillary tangles composed of hyper-phosphorylated tau [16]. In terms of molecular pathogenesis, Aβ accumulation can be directly linked to some mutations leading to early onset FAD. However, in the vast majority of cases, i.e. in sporadic AD, the disease may begin with inflammation or lipid abnormalities and the plaques and tangles arise only later as the disease progresses [14]. Multiple co-existent pathologies (vascular, synuclein, etc.) can further complicate the picture.

The causality dilemma is illustrated by evidence linking AD to insulin resistance. An early analysis of this relationship comes from the Rotterdam study where a significant association of T2D and dementia believed to be AD was reported [20]. Additional epidemiological studies also reported similar links between T2D and dementia believed to be AD [1, 35], while others have observed that cognitively normal patients with T2D can show reduced cerebral glucose metabolism [2]. The latter observation could potentially dovetail with the fact that most dementia phenotypes are preceded by cerebral glucose hypo-metabolism [34], but it is not at all clear that all T2D patients develop cognitive decline. These studies support the notion that AD and T2D may have additive or synergistic effects on brain glucose metabolism. This hypothesis however is limited in its ability to elucidate the exact nature and molecular underpinnings of the relevant neuropathology.

At least three studies using post-mortem brains have suggested that AD (or cognitive impairment) is associated with impaired insulin signaling. In one study, AD brains were reported to display changes in the distribution of the insulin receptor as well as a reduction in IRS-1 and IRS-2, supporting the notion that insulin signaling would be impaired in those brain regions [18]. These observations complemented previous reports showing comparable reductions in mRNA levels within the insulin/IGF pathways [29]. However, none of these data substitute for a functional assessment of insulin signaling. The more definitive test of impaired insulin signaling was performed by Talbot et al.. using postmortem brain slices from subjects that were cognitively impaired or with AD, demonstrating that insulin signaling was indeed impaired in neuronal populations [32]. Taken together, these observations support the hypothesis that AD (and cognitive impairment) may be associated with disrupted insulin signaling in the brain.

Alternatively, some studies also suggest that AD is the causative or exacerbating factor for T2D [13, 35]. In this context, it is important to point out that brain insulin signaling controls systemic metabolism by regulating autonomic outflow from the brain to visceral organs such as liver and adipose tissue. The experimental induction of insulin resistance in a variety of brain regions and neuronal cell types has been found to impair metabolic control and increase the susceptibility to metabolic disease [23].

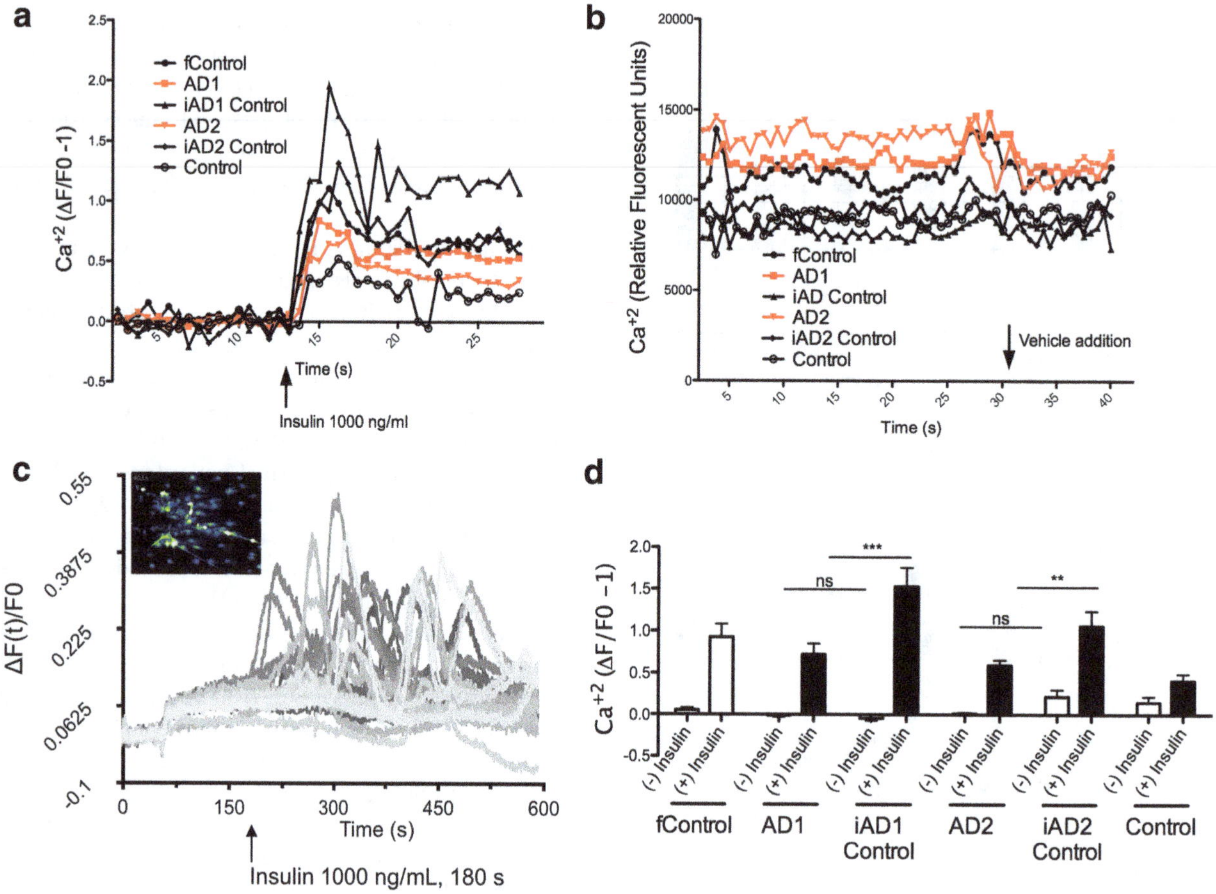

Fig. 4 Insulin promotes Ca^{2+} flux in iPSC-derived BFCNs. Cells cultured in 96-well plates were insulin deprived overnight before insulin or vehicle was added to a final concentration of 1000 ng/ml after 25 s of baseline recording (data from a total of 4 experiments). **a** Calcium response to insulin normalized to 20 s of baseline recording before insulin addition. **b** Calcium response to addition of vehicle recorded as arbitrary relative fluorescent units. **c** Visual corroboration and quantification of Ca^{2+} in individual cells. **d** Average normalized calcium responses for baseline, (–) Insulin, and response, (+) insulin, in IPSC-derived basal cholinergic neurons. An effect by insulin exposure was detected by 2-way ANOVA ($p < .0001$). Bonferroni comparisons ***, $P < .001$; ** $P < 0.01$

Hence, a disruption of insulin signaling along with AD pathology in brain regions controlling metabolism, such as the hypothalamus, can increase the susceptibility to diabetes and underpin the association of AD with T2D. For example, our group recently showed that *APP/PSEN1* amyloid-depositing mice exhibit reduced hypothalamic insulin signaling and are more susceptible to aging and over-nutrition induced prediabetes [24]. It is possible that hypothalamic amyloidosis may contribute to this phenomenon and may further potentiate T2D due to reduced brain insulin signaling [32]. A study by Calon et al summarizes this reciprocity by showing an enhanced sensitivity of triple transgenic amyloid-depositing mice to high fat diet and a reversal of memory deficits and decrease in soluble Aβ following insulin administration [33]. These observations suggest that AD and T2D pathologies may be able to set up a self-perpetuating "vicious cycle" with one another.

At this point, the key questions are: how exactly does AD impair brain and neuronal insulin signaling and if neuronal insulin resistance is induced by AD pathology, is it a cell autonomous effect or secondary to altered in-vivo – including paracrine – regulation. As an example of paracrine regulation of insulin signaling, a recent study demonstrated that ApoE4 secreted from astrocytes binds to the insulin receptor and may reduce insulin signaling by trapping the insulin receptor in the endosome [36]. FAD could similarly impair insulin signaling through altered paracrine signaling or indirect effects in the microenvironment resulting in available cytokines or metabolites. The fact that we did not find insulin signaling to be altered in neurons derived from several FAD forms supports this notion. Future studies that examine such paracrine signaling in co-culture models of astrocytes or glia cells with neurons will examine these possibilities.

In an earlier study, we generated basal cholinergic neurons from iPSC lines carrying the *PSEN2*^{N141I} mutation, along with corresponding familial and isogenic controls [19]. In the current study, we observed that both cholinergic neuroprecursors and BFCNs derived from iPSCs exhibit classic responses to insulin that are not affected by the presence of AD mutations.

We went on to test whether chronic exposure to insulin could affect the production of Aβ. Previous pulse-chase studies demonstrated that insulin reduces intracellular amyloid beta production by modulating βAPP trafficking [9]. We observed a bimodal response where chronic insulin exposure resulted in the ostensibly beneficial reduction of the Aβ42/40 ratio. These results support the existence of additional mechanisms that synergize with insulin action in its potential regulation of amyloid production. These data correlate well with results from a human clinical trial using intranasal insulin administration in patients with mild cognitive impairment and mild to moderate AD. Unbiased exploratory analyses revealed that some subtle memory benefits resulted and that the memory changes were associated with changes in Aβ42 [6]. These observations merit additional studies aimed at identifying factors that interact with insulin in modulating brain Aβ42, and to study the underpinnings generating the variabilities in Aβ42/40 that have been observed in our lab and in other labs using iPSC models of AD [8].

Finally, in our earlier study [19], we reported that electrophysiological parameters such as action potential frequency and amplitude were reduced in cells carrying the *PSEN2* ^{N141I} mutation. Therefore, we decided to assess whether insulin could modulate calcium transients as a reflection of electrophysiological effects. We found that insulin promotes Ca^{2+} mediated-fluorescence in all lines tested, and that *PSEN2* mutant lines show reduced responses compared to their isogenic control lines. These changes were normalized either when the mutation was corrected with CRISPR/Cas9 gene editing or when insulin was chronically administered, apparently leading to a physiological correction by promoting Ca^{2+} currents that enhanced synaptic transmission [37]. These observations warrant future patch-clamp studies to best illustrate the nature of Ca^{2+} deficiencies in response to insulin. Furthermore, future studies would benefit by the inclusion of corresponding isogenic controls i.e., with engineered FAD mutations. These studies would help explain if the deficiency Ca^{2+} flux in the insulin-mediated response of the unrelated control line (which was lower than in all other lines), is a result of genetic background, and if FAD mutations would further dampen such responses.

Conclusions

In summary, wildtype, *PSEN2*^{N141I} and CRISPR/Cas9-corrected iPSC-derived BFCNs (and their precursors) showed indistinguishable insulin signaling profiles as determined by the apparent phosphorylation stoichiometry of the canonical insulin signaling pathway molecules. Chronic insulin treatment of BFCNs of all genotypes led to a reduction in the Aβ42/40 ratio. Unexpectedly, a previously reported CRISPR/Cas9-correctable effect of *PSEN2*^{N141I} on calcium flux could be corrected by chronic exposure of BFCNs to physiologically stimulatory concentrations of insulin. Taking this calcium flux-correction effect of insulin together with its Aβ42/40 ratio-lowering effect suggests that insulin action at each of these steps acts to oppose an AD-related phenomenon. Our results are consistent with a potential physiological role for insulin as a mediator of resilience by acting as an antagonist of specific metabolic and molecular features of AD.

Methods

Cell derivation and maintenance

All iPSC lines utilized in these studies were originally obtained from the NYSCF Repository and were propagated according to standard guidelines [21]. The lines used were designated 28,945 (Control), 948 (AD1), 949 (fControl), and 950 (AD2). Additional clones with single point mutation corrections were generated from AD1 and AD2 using CRISPR technology as described [19]. Briefly, the CRISPR/Cas9 system was engineered to target the *PSEN2*^{N141I} locus by cloning a single guide RNA (sgRNA) into pSpCas9 (BB)-2A-GFP (PX458). Subsequently, the cells were transfected with the vector and a complementary ssODN by electroporation to serve as a correctional template via homology-directed repair (HDR). All iPSC cell lines were expanded and maintained in serum-free mTeSR1 media (Stem Cell Technologies) in a feeder-free system using Cultrex (Trevigen). Media was supplemented with 10 μM ROCK inhibitor (Y27632, Stemgent) during cell passages.

BFCN differentiation

The differentiation protocol has been described in detail in [19]. Briefly, iPSC lines grown in mTeSR1 media were dissociated using Accutase (Sigma-Aldrich) and plated onto Cultrex (Trevigen) coated 6-well plates at a density of 400,000–1,000,000 cells per well. The cells were allowed to reach full confluency in mTeSR1 media before initiating the differentiation process. At the beginning of differentiation (day 0) and continuing to day 8, cells were maintained in Custom mTeSR1 media (Stem Cell Technologies) lacking pluripotency promoters (i.e., bFGF, TGF-Beta, Li-Cl, GABA and pipecolic acid). Starting on day 2, the media was supplemented with dual SMAD inhibitors (SB431542 10 μM plus LDN193189 250 nM, Selleck Chem) as well as the ventralizing agents SAG at 500 nM (R&D) and Purmorphamine at 2 μM (Stemgent). During this period of induction, the media were changed every other day. On day 9, the media were gradually switched to Brainphys media (Stemcell Technologies) supplemented with B27 (Life Technologies). At the end of this period, neural progenitors were generated and used in subsequent assays. Alternatively, neuro-progenitors were dissociated using Accutase and seeded in plates coated with branched polyethynilimine (0.1%, Sigma-Aldrich) and laminin (10 mg/mL, Life Technology) in Brainphys media + B27 supplement with nerve growth factor (NGF) (Alamone labs, 50 ng/mL) and brain derived neurotrophic factor (BDNF) (R&D, 50 ng/mL). For this protocol, the media were changed every 2 days until analysis.

Insulin administration

Cells were cultured overnight using media supplemented with B27 without insulin (Thermofisher A1895601). After the overnight culture, insulin (Sigma Cat. 91077C) or vehicle was added to the media as indicated. Insulin was prepared fresh from frozen stocks every day before administration. For chronic studies, a daily dose of 1000 ng/ml of insulin or vehicle (PBS) was added.

Protein extraction and western blot analysis

Cells were washed with cold PBS and then lysed with cold RIPA buffer (Thermo Fisher Scientific) supplemented with a cocktail of phosphatase and protease inhibitors (Life Technologies). The cells were scraped from the plates and passed through a 23-gauge needle four times before centrifuging at 12000RPM for 20 min at 4 °C. After centrifugation, the supernatant was collected and protein concentration was measured using a BCA or a Bradford quantification assay (Thermo Fisher Scientific). Equal amounts of protein lysates were loaded into NuPage BisTris 4–12% gradient gels (Thermo Fisher Scientific) and then transferred to 0.45 μm PVDF membranes (Millipore). The membranes were blocked with TBS and Odyssey blocking buffer (LI-COR) for one hour at room temperature followed by an overnight incubation with primary antibodies at 4 °C. The following antibodies were used: phospho-mTOR (#2971), phospho-AKT (Thr308) (#4056), phospho-AKT (Ser473) (#9271), phospho-GSK-3β (Ser9) (#9323), phospho-S6-Ribosomal Protein (Ser235/236) (#2211) from Cell Signaling Technology; phospho-Tau (Ser202/Thr205) (MN1020) from Thermo Fisher Scientific; and β-Actin (sc-81,178) from Santa Cruz Biotechnology or Gapdh (g8795) from Sigma-Aldrich. After overnight incubation, membranes were washed 3X with TBS-Tween and stained for one hour with secondary antibodies IR-Dye 800 Goat Anti-rabbit (LI-COR) and Dylight 680 Goat Anti-mouse (Thermo Fisher Scientific) – diluted at room temperature in 0.01% SDS TBS-Tween. Finally, the membranes were washed 4 times and scanned using Odyssey Classic (LI-COR). Image Studio Software (LI-COR) was used to quantify bands.

Calcium image staining and microfluorimetry in response to insulin

Cells were deprived of insulin for a period of 24 h as previously described, and then incubated with a 2.5 ng/μl solution of Fluo-4, AM in 0.01% Pluronic F-127 (Life Technologies) dissolved in cell media (1:1000) for 15 min at 37 °C. The cells were then washed twice with media and cultured with a Brainphys media lacking Phenol Red (Stem Cell Technologies) for an additional 15 min before recording fluorescence. For microfluorimetry, relative fluorescent units (RFUs) were obtained using a Flexstation 2 (Molecular Devices Corp.) that was set to record RFUs in a 96-well format for a period of 70 s in 0.6 s intervals using Softmax Pro software (Molecular Devices Corp.). The wavelengths used were - excitation at 485 nm, emission at 538 nm and cut-off at 530 nm. The RFUs were exported using Softmax Pro (Molecular Devices) and after recording the baseline fluorescence, the cells were treated with 1000 ng/ml insulin or vehicle for 25 s. Visual corroboration of Ca^{2+} activity in individual cells was obtained using coverslips that were transferred to a recording chamber mounted on an upright Olympus BX61 microscope and fluorescence was recorded at 2 Hz by a cooled CCD camera (Hamamatsu Orca R2). A baseline recording of transients was obtained for the first 180 s before insulin application (1000 ng/ml) via whole chamber perfusion at room temperature for a period of 420 s. Ca^{2+} transients were expressed in a form of $\Delta F(t)/F0$, where F0 is a baseline fluorescence of a given region of interest and ΔF is a difference between current level of fluorescence F(t) and F0. Fluctuations of $\Delta F(t)/F0$ that were less than 0.05 were considered as non-responses.

Enzyme-linked immunosorbent assay (ELISA)

Cells were plated in a 24-well plate with Brainphys media supplemented with B27 (minus insulin) and treated with 1000 ng/ml of insulin or equivalent volume of PBS daily for 3 days. On the third day, the culture media were collected 30 min after insulin administration and ELISAs were performed on these aspirates using β-Amyloid 40 and 42 kits (WAKO Chemicals) according to manufacturer's instructions.

Statistical analysis

Western blot experiments, Aβ42/40 ELISAs and relative fluorescent units (RFUs) or $\Delta F(t)/F0$ were analyzed for statistical significance using 2-Way ANOVA followed by Bonferroni post hoc tests. All statistical analysis was computed using PRISM 5. *, $p < .05$; **, $p < .01$; ***, $p < .001$.

Additional files

Additional file 1: Figure S1. Western blots of iPSC-derived basal cholinergic neuroprecursors cell lines. Cells were insulin deprived overnight before the addition 1000 ng/ml of insulin (insulin was not added to time 0'). Lysates were collected at 0, 10, or 30-min exposure. Quantified western blot data was normalized over Gapdh and expressed as fold change of 0 ng/ml dose. An effect on concentration response was detected by 2-way ANOVA if indicated. These data correspond to results of three independent experiments. ** $P < 0.01$; *** $P < .001$. (H) Representative blots from a single experiment showing three of the lines. **Figure S2.** (A) Western blot quantification of iPSC derived basal cholinergic neurons (two independent experiments). Cells (DIV 34) were insulin deprived for 3 days or given 1000 ng/mL every 24 h for 3 days. (B) Representative blots from a single experiment.

Additional file 2: Video 1. Supplemental Video.

Funding

CLM, SN, CB and SG were supported by the Mount Sinai Alzheimer's Disease Research Center P50 AG05138 to Mary Sano. Scott Noggle by the Charles Evans Foundation, the Alzheimer's Drug Discovery Foundation, and The NY Community Trust. Scott Noggle and Sam Gandy were jointly supported by the Cure Alzheimer's Fund and by National Institutes of Health (NIH) grants R21AG042965 and U01AG046170 (to Eric Schadt, Bin Zhang, and Sam Gandy). Sam Gandy and Bin Zhang were also supported by R01AG057907. Sam Gandy was also supported by The Werber Family Foundation, the Scott and Jennifer Moskowitz Foundation, the Louis B. Mayer Foundation, the Georgianne and Dr. Reza Khatib Foundation, and the Sarah and Gideon Gartner Foundation. Rudolph Tanzi was supported by the Cure Alzheimer's Fund. Maitane Ortiz-Virumbrales was a NYSCF-Druckenmiller Fellow and was supported by The Werber Family Foundation and U01AG046170.

Authors' contributions

CLM, MOV, LDG, VS and CB designed, performed, analyzed and interpreted in vitro insulin signaling studies. CLM, MOV, SN, CB, and SG wrote the manuscript. CLM and IK performed electro-physiological studies. CLM and MOV cloned CRISPR/Cas9 constructs. CLM and MOV generated CRISPR/Cas9-corrected lines. RET, MOV, SN, CB and SG contributed to data interpretation and manuscript editing. The authors appreciate the critical reading and discussion of this manuscript provided by Steven E. Arnold (Massachusetts General Hospital, Harvard Medical School). All authors read and approved the final manuscript.

Competing interests

The authors declare that they have no competing interests.

Author details

[1]Department of Neurology, NFL Neurological Care Center, Icahn School of Medicine at Mount Sinai, New York, NY 10029, USA. [2]Department of Psychiatry, Alzheimer's Disease Research Center, Icahn School of Medicine at Mount Sinai, 5 E 98th St, New York, NY 10029, USA. [3]Department of Medicine, Diabetes, Obesity, and Metabolism Institute, Icahn School of Medicine at Mount Sinai, New York, NY 10029, USA. [4]New York Stem Cell Foundation Laboratories, New York, NY 10032, USA. [5]Icahn Institute and Department of Genetics and Genomic Sciences, Icahn School of Medicine at Mount Sinai, New York, NY 10029, USA. [6]Genetics and Aging Unit, Harvard Medical School, Massachusetts General Hospital, 114 16th Street, Charlestown, MA 02129, USA.

References

1. Arvanitakis Z, Wilson RS, Bienias JL, Evans DA, Bennett DA. Diabetes mellitus and risk of Alzheimer disease and decline in cognitive function. Arch Neurol. 2004;61:661–6. https://doi.org/10.1001/archneur.61.5.66161/5/661.
2. Baker LD, Cross DJ, Minoshima S, Belongia D, Watson GS, Craft S. Insulin resistance and Alzheimer-like reductions in regional cerebral glucose metabolism for cognitively normal adults with prediabetes or early type 2 diabetes. Arch Neurol. 2011;68:51–7. https://doi.org/10.1001/archneurol.2010.225.
3. Bedse G, Di Domenico F, Serviddio G, Cassano T. Aberrant insulin signaling in Alzheimer's disease: current knowledge. Front Neurosci. 2015;9:204. https://doi.org/10.3389/fnins.2015.00204.
4. Benedict C, Hallschmid M, Hatke A, Schultes B, Fehm HL, Born J, Kern W. Intranasal insulin improves memory in humans. Psychoneuroendocrinology. 2004;29:1326–34. https://doi.org/10.1016/j.psyneuen.2004.04.003.
5. Bird TD, Lampe TH, Nemens EJ, Miner GW, Sumi SM, Schellenberg GD. Familial alzheimer's disease in american descendants of the Volga germans: probable genetic founder effect. Ann Neurol. 1988;23:25–31. https://doi.org/10.1002/ana.410230106.
6. Craft S, Baker LD, Montine TJ, Minoshima S, Watson GS, Claxton A, Arbuckle M, Callaghan M, Tsai E, Plymate SR, Green PS, Leverenz J, Cross D, Gerton B. Intranasal insulin therapy for Alzheimer disease and amnestic mild cognitive impairment. Arch Neurol. 2012;69:29. https://doi.org/10.1001/archneurol.2011.233.
7. Deng X-L, Liu Z, Wang C, Li Y, Cai Z. Insulin resistance in ischemic stroke. Metab Brain Dis. 2017;32:1323–34. https://doi.org/10.1007/s11011-017-0050-0.
8. Duan L, Bhattacharyya BJ, Belmadani A, Pan L, Miller RJ, Kessler JA. Stem cell derived basal forebrain cholinergic neurons from Alzheimer's disease patients are more susceptible to cell death. Mol Neurodegener. 2014;9:3. https://doi.org/10.1186/1750-1326-9-3.
9. Gasparini L, Gouras GK, Wang R, Gross RS, Beal MF, Greengard P, Xu H. Stimulation of β-amyloid precursor protein trafficking by insulin reduces Intraneuronal β-amyloid and requires mitogen-activated protein kinase signaling. J Neurosci. 2001;21
10. Haense C, Kalbe E, Herholz K, Hohmann C, Neumaier B, Krais R, Heiss W-D. Cholinergic system function and cognition in mild cognitive impairment. Neurobiol Aging. 2012;33:867–77. https://doi.org/10.1016/j.neurobiolaging.2010.08.015.
11. Herholz K. Acetylcholine esterase activity in mild cognitive impairment and Alzheimer's disease. Eur J Nucl Med Mol Imaging. 2008;35:25–9. https://doi.org/10.1007/s00259-007-0699-4.
12. Iovino S, Burkart AM, Warren L, Patti ME, Kahn CR. Myotubes derived from human-induced pluripotent stem cells mirror in vivo insulin resistance. Proc Natl Acad Sci U S A. 2016;113:1889–94. https://doi.org/10.1073/pnas.1525665113.
13. Janson J, Laedtke T, Parisi JE, O'Brien P, Petersen RC, Butler PC. Increased risk of type 2 diabetes in Alzheimer disease. Diabetes. 2004;53:474–81.
14. Krstic D, Knuesel I. Deciphering the mechanism underlying late-onset Alzheimer disease. Nat Rev Neurol. 2012;9:25–34. https://doi.org/10.1038/nrneurol.2012.236.
15. Laws SM, Gaskin S, Woodfield A, Srikanth V, Bruce D, Fraser PE, Porter T, Newsholme P, Wijesekara N, Burnham S, Doré V, Li Q-X, Maruff P, Masters CL, Rainey-Smith S, Rowe CC, Salvado O, Villemagne VL, Martins RN, Verdile G. Insulin resistance is associated with reductions in specific cognitive domains and increases in CSF tau in cognitively normal adults. Sci Rep. 2017;7:9766. https://doi.org/10.1038/s41598-017-09577-4.
16. Mandelkow EM, Mandelkow E. Tau in Alzheimer's disease. Trends Cell Biol. 1998;8:425–7.
17. Masters CL, Simms G, Weinman NA, Multhaup G, McDonald BL, Beyreuther K. Amyloid plaque core protein in Alzheimer disease and Down syndrome. Proc Natl Acad Sci U S A. 1985;82:4245–9.
18. Moloney AM, Griffin RJ, Timmons S, O'Connor R, Ravid R, O'Neill C. Defects in IGF-1 receptor, insulin receptor and IRS-1/2 in Alzheimer's disease indicate possible resistance to IGF-1 and insulin signalling. Neurobiol Aging. 2010;31:224–43. https://doi.org/10.1016/j.neurobiolaging.2008.04.002.
19. Ortiz-Virumbrales M, Moreno CL, Kruglikov I, Marazuela P, Sproul A, Jacob S, Zimmer M, Paull D, Zhang B, Schadt EE, Ehrlich ME, Tanzi RE, Arancio O, Noggle S, Gandy S. CRISPR/Cas9-correctable mutation-related molecular and physiological phenotypes in iPSC-derived Alzheimer's PSEN2 N141I neurons. Acta Neuropathol Commun. 2017;5:77. https://doi.org/10.1186/s40478-017-0475-z.
20. Ott A, Stolk RP, Hofman A, van Harskamp F, Grobbee DE, Breteler MM. Association of diabetes mellitus and dementia: the Rotterdam study. Diabetologia. 1996;39:1392–7.
21. Paull D, Sevilla A, Zhou H, Hahn AK, Kim H, Napolitano C, Tsankov A, Shang L, Krumholz K, Jagadeesan P, Woodard CM, Sun B, Vilboux T, Zimmer M, Forero E, Moroziewicz DN, Martinez H, Malicdan MCV, Weiss KA, Vensand LB, Dusenberry CR, Polus H, Sy KTL, Kahler DJ, Gahl WA, Solomon SL, Chang S,

Meissner A, Eggan K, Noggle SA. Automated, high-throughput derivation, characterization and differentiation of induced pluripotent stem cells. Nat Methods. 2015;12:885–92. https://doi.org/10.1038/nmeth.3507.

22. Peila R, Rodriguez BL, Launer LJ, Honolulu-Asia Aging Study. Type 2 diabetes, APOE gene, and the risk for dementia and related pathologies: the Honolulu-Asia aging study. Diabetes. 2002;51:1256–62. https://doi.org/10.2337/DIABETES.51.4.1256.
23. Plum L, Belgardt BF, Brüning JC. Central insulin action in energy and glucose homeostasis. J Clin Invest. 2006;116:1761–6. https://doi.org/10.1172/JCI29063.
24. Ruiz HH, Chi T, Lindtner C, Hsieh W, Ehrlich M, Gandy S, Buettner C. Increased susceptibility to metabolic dysregulation in a mouse model of Alzheimer's disease is associated with impaired hypothalamic insulin signaling and elevated BCAA levels. Alzheimers Dement. 2016; https://doi.org/10.1016/j.jalz.2016.01.008.
25. Saber H, Himali JJ, Beiser AS, Shoamanesh A, Pikula A, Roubenoff R, Romero JR, Kase CS, Vasan RS, Seshadri S. Serum insulin-like growth factor 1 and the risk of ischemic stroke. Stroke. 2017;48:1760–5. https://doi.org/10.1161/STROKEAHA.116.016563.
26. Shekhar S, Wang S, Mims PN, Gonzalez-Fernandez E, Zhang C, He X, Liu CY, Lv W, Wang Y, Huang J, Fan F. Impaired cerebral autoregulation-a common neurovascular pathway in diabetes may play a critical role in diabetes-related Alzheimer's disease. Curr Res diabetes Obes J. 2017;2(3):555587.
27. Sparling DP, Yu J, Kim K, Zhu C, Brachs S, Birkenfeld AL, Pajvani UB. Adipocyte-specific blockade of gamma-secretase, but not inhibition of notch activity, reduces adipose insulin sensitivity. Mol Metab. 2016;5:113–21. https://doi.org/10.1016/j.molmet.2015.11.006.
28. Sproul AA, Jacob S, Pre D, Kim SH, Nestor MW, Navarro-Sobrino M, Santa-Maria I, Zimmer M, Aubry S, Steele JW, Kahler DJ, Dranovsky A, Arancio O, Crary JF, Gandy S, Noggle SA. Characterization and molecular profiling of PSEN1 familial Alzheimer's disease iPSC-derived neural progenitors. PLoS One. 2014;9:e84547. https://doi.org/10.1371/journal.pone.0084547.
29. Steen E, Terry BM, Rivera EJ, Cannon JL, Neely TR, Tavares R, Xu XJ, Wands JR, de la Monte SM. Impaired insulin and insulin-like growth factor expression and signaling mechanisms in Alzheimer's disease–is this type 3 diabetes? J Alzheimers Dis. 2005;7:63–80.
30. Stoeckel LE, Arvanitakis Z, Gandy S, Small D, Kahn CR, Pascual-Leone A, Pawlyk A, Sherwin R, Smith P. Complex mechanisms linking neurocognitive dysfunction to insulin resistance and other metabolic dysfunction. F1000Research. 2016;5:353. https://doi.org/10.12688/f1000research.8300.2.
31. Talboom JS, Velazquez R, Oddo S. The mammalian target of rapamycin at the crossroad between cognitive aging and Alzheimer's disease. npj Aging Mech Dis. 2015;1:15008. https://doi.org/10.1038/npjamd.2015.8.
32. Talbot K, Wang H-Y, Kazi H, Han L-Y, Bakshi KP, Stucky A, Fuino RL, Kawaguchi KR, Samoyedny AJ, Wilson RS, Arvanitakis Z, Schneider JA, Wolf BA, Bennett DA, Trojanowski JQ, Arnold SE. Demonstrated brain insulin resistance in Alzheimer's disease patients is associated with IGF-1 resistance, IRS-1 dysregulation, and cognitive decline. J Clin Invest. 2012;122:1316–38. https://doi.org/10.1172/JCI59903.
33. Vandal M, White PJ, Tremblay C, St-Amour I, Chevrier G, Emond V, Lefrançois D, Virgili J, Planel E, Giguere Y, Marette A, Calon F. Insulin reverses the high-fat diet–induced increase in brain Aβ and improves memory in an animal model of Alzheimer disease. Diabetes. 2014;63(12):4291–301.
34. Willette AA, Bendlin BB, Starks EJ, Birdsill AC, Johnson SC, Christian BT, Okonkwo OC, La Rue A, Hermann BP, Koscik RL, Jonaitis EM, Sager MA, Asthana S. Association of Insulin Resistance with Cerebral Glucose Uptake in late middle-aged adults at risk for Alzheimer disease. JAMA Neurol. 2015;72:1013–20. https://doi.org/10.1001/jamaneurol.2015.0613.
35. Xu WL, Qiu CX, Wahlin A, Winblad B, Fratiglioni L. Diabetes mellitus and risk of dementia in the Kungsholmen project: a 6-year follow-up study. Neurology. 2004;63:1181–6.
36. Zhao N, Liu C-C, Van Ingelgom AJ, Martens YA, Linares C, Knight JA, Painter MM, Sullivan PM, Bu G. Apolipoprotein E4 impairs neuronal insulin signaling by trapping insulin receptor in the endosomes. Neuron. 2017;96:115–129.e5. https://doi.org/10.1016/j.neuron.2017.09.003.
37. Zucker RS. Calcium- and activity-dependent synaptic plasticity. Curr Opin Neurobiol. 1999;9:305–13. https://doi.org/10.1016/S0959-4388(99)80045-2.

6

New insights into the role of TREM2 in Alzheimer's disease

Maud Gratuze[1,2,3], Cheryl E. G. Leyns[1,2,3] and David M. Holtzman[1,2,3*]

Abstract

Alzheimer's disease (AD) is the leading cause of dementia. The two histopathological markers of AD are amyloid plaques composed of the amyloid-β (Aβ) peptide, and neurofibrillary tangles of aggregated, abnormally hyperphosphorylated tau protein. The majority of AD cases are late-onset, after the age of 65, where a clear cause is still unknown. However, there are likely different multifactorial contributors including age, enviornment, biology and genetics which can increase risk for the disease. Genetic predisposition is considerable, with heritability estimates of 60–80%. Genetic factors such as rare variants of TREM2 (triggering receptor expressed on myeloid cells-2) strongly increase the risk of developing AD, confirming the role of microglia in AD pathogenesis. In the last 5 years, several studies have dissected the mechanisms by which TREM2, as well as its rare variants affect amyloid and tau pathologies and their consequences in both animal models and in human studies. In this review, we summarize increases in our understanding of the involvement of TREM2 and microglia in AD development that may open new therapeutic strategies targeting the immune system to influence AD pathogenesis.

Keywords: Alzheimer's disease, Neurodegeneration, TREM2, ApoE, Microglia, Gliosis

Background

Alzheimer's disease (AD) was first described more than a century ago by the German neuropsychiatrist, Dr. Alois Alzheimer ([1], English translation [2]), and today is the leading cause of dementia worldwide [3–5]. In the United States, deaths attributed to AD have increased by 71% between 2000 and 2013, ranking this disease as the 6th leading cause of death [6]. Although symptoms can vary greatly from one patient to another, AD results in progressive memory loss and irreversible cognitive decline. The two histopathological markers of AD are extracellular amyloid plaques composed of the amyloid-β peptide (Aβ), and neurofibrillary tangles (NFTs) within neurons derived from abnormally aggregated, hyperphosphorylated tau protein [3–5]. These defining protein aggregates are accompanied by synaptic and neuronal loss.

In addition to protein aggregation, neuroinflammatory changes are present in AD brains, including alterations in the morphology, activation and distribution of microglia and astrocytes (microgliosis and astrogliosis) as well as increased expression of inflammatory mediators [7–9]. However, the exact contributions of both microgliosis and astrogliosis in AD are not clear. While first hypothesized to contribute to AD neuropathology, gliosis and neuroinflammation seem to have more complex effects and could be either beneficial or damaging in those with AD (for review [10]). For example, reactive microglia and astrocytes can contribute to the clearance of Aβ [11–13]. Conversely, the production of pro-inflammatory cytokines like TNFα (Tumor necrosis factor α) or IL1-β (Interleukin 1β) resulting from glial activation are harmful and toxic to neurons (for review [14, 15]). Many studies also suggest that neuroinflammation exacerbates tau phosphorylation [16–18]. Altogether, these data suggest the possibility that gliosis and neuroinflammation have neuroprotective roles early in AD by controlling amyloid load, but later can become toxic to neurons and act as a catalyst for neurodegeneration.

Recent genomic studies have identified several novel genetic risk factors linking neuroinflammation and AD. Highly penetrant mutations in *APP*, *PSEN1*, and *PSEN2* are known to cause rare, autosomal dominant AD, where individuals develop the disease in mid-life [19]. However, the majority of AD cases are sporadic and late-onset, the causes of which are still unknown. Late-onset AD (LOAD)

* Correspondence: holtzman@wustl.edu
[1]Department of Neurology, St. Louis, USA
[2]Hope Center for Neurological Disorders, St. Louis, USA
Full list of author information is available at the end of the article

seems to be multifactorial, with age, environmental, and genetic factors contributing to disease risk, manifestation and progression. Interestingly, the genetic predisposition in LOAD patients is considerable, with a heritability estimate of 60–80% [20]. The most common genetic risk factor is the apolipoprotein E (ApoE) gene (for review [21]). *APOE* is encoded by three common alleles: ε2, ε3, and ε4. One copy of the ε4 allele of APOE increases LOAD risk approximately 3-4 fold while two ε4 copies increases LOAD risk by as much as 12-fold [22, 23]. Interestingly, the ε2 allele is associated with a decreased risk for LOAD and a later onset of disease. There are several mechanisms by which ApoE appears to play a role in AD pathogenesis. One important effect is that ApoE isoforms influence Aβ clearance, aggregation and metabolism [24–26]. In addition, recent studies suggest that ApoE modulates tau-mediated neurodegeneration in an isoform-specific manner [27].

For the last ten years, new whole-genome sequencing studies and genome wide association studies (GWAS) have made it possible to highlight several novel genetic factors linked with increased risk of LOAD. Several of these genetic risk factors encode proteins involved in microglial function and inflammation including TREM2, CD33, CR1, ABCA7 and SHIP1 (for reviews [28, 29]). In this review, we summarize the recent explosion of studies aiming to understand the role of microglia in LOAD. In particular, we focus on TREM2, a receptor of the innate immune system expressed in several types, as variants in the *TREM2* gene have been found to increase LOAD-risk by 2-4 fold, similarly to what has been observed in patients with one copy of APOE ε4. Many new models have been created to better understand the contributions of TREM2 in LOAD in light of this finding. Thus far, TREM2 studies further reiterate both the beneficial and detrimental effects of gliosis on neuronal health and degeneration, which are dependent on the context of the pathological insult and stage of disease. We further explore potential mechanisms by which TREM2 signaling may alter LOAD neuropathology. A better understanding of TREM2 and its impact in the disease is critical as TREM2 is currently being explored as a therapeutic target in LOAD.

1) TREM2 structure and expression

TREM2 belongs to a family of receptors referred to as the triggering receptors expressed on myeloid cells (TREM). Members of the TREM family are cell surface transmembrane glycoproteins with V-immunoglobulin extra-cellular domains and cytoplasmic tails [30]. The TREM2 gene is located on human chromosome 6p21 and encodes a 230-amino acid glycoprotein [31]. The TREM2 gene is expressed in a subgroup of myeloid cells including dendritic cells, granulocytes, and tissue-specific macrophages like osteoclasts, Kuppfer cells and alveolar macrophages [32–38]. In the brain, TREM2 is exclusively expressed by microglia [39–44]; however, there is some discordance regarding the level of its expression//translation [45–47] and whether or not TREM2 is present in all or only a subgroup of microglia [48] in mice and humans. Interestingly, the expression of TREM2 varies depending on the particular region of the central nervous system (CNS) [39, 49], with a higher expression in the hippocampus, the spinal cord and the white matter [41]. Its expression is modulated by inflammation, although inflammatory effects appear to be opposite *in vitro* and *in vivo*. Expression of anti-inflammatory molecules enhances TREM2 expression [50] while expression of pro-inflammatory molecules, such as TNFα, IL1β or lipopolysaccharide (LPS), decrease TREM2 expression *in vitro* [32, 51, 52]. TREM2 expression is up regulated in pathological conditions such as Parkinson's disease (PD) [53], Amyotrophic lateral sclerosis (ALS) [54], stroke [55], traumatic brain injury [56] and AD [47, 57–59]. In AD, increased expression of TREM2 has been confirmed in patients [47, 57–59] and in mouse models of amyloid and tau pathology [45, 60–63] and seems to be associated with the recruitment of microglia to amyloid plaques [59, 64]. Interestingly, aging is also a factor that increases TREM2 expression in both mice and humans [41, 60]. We could speculate that the acute inflammation mimicked by *in vitro* studies first induces a decrease of TREM2 expression while chronic inflammation observed in pathological conditions, such as AD, results in an increase of TREM2 expression.

2) TREM2 signaling and ligands

TREM2 acts principally through the intracellular adaptor DAP12 (DNAX-activation protein 12, also known as TYROBP) through its short cytoplasmic tail [32, 65, 66]. Indeed, ligand-bound TREM2 is incapable of initiating intracellular signaling without DAP12 [43]. The association of TREM2 with DAP12 is coordinated by an electrostatic interaction between a conserved positively-charged lysine in TREM2 (aa186) and a negatively- charged aspartic acid residue in DAP12 (Figure 1) [66, 67]. TREM2 ligation generates tyrosine phosphorylation of DAP12 within its immunoreceptor tyrosine-based activation motifs (ITAMS) by Src family kinases (Figure 1). This phosphorylation creates a docking site for the SH2 domains of several molecules, initiating a signaling cascade and subsequent immune response [66]. The principal kinase recruited by the ITAM region of DAP12 is Syk, which activates downstream signaling components including phosphatidylinositol 3-kinase (PI3K), Akt, mitogen-activated protein kinases (MAPK) and increases intracellular calcium levels [43, 68–70]. TREM2 can also act through the DAP-10 adaptor, a relative of DAP-12, allowing the recruitment of PI3K [71].

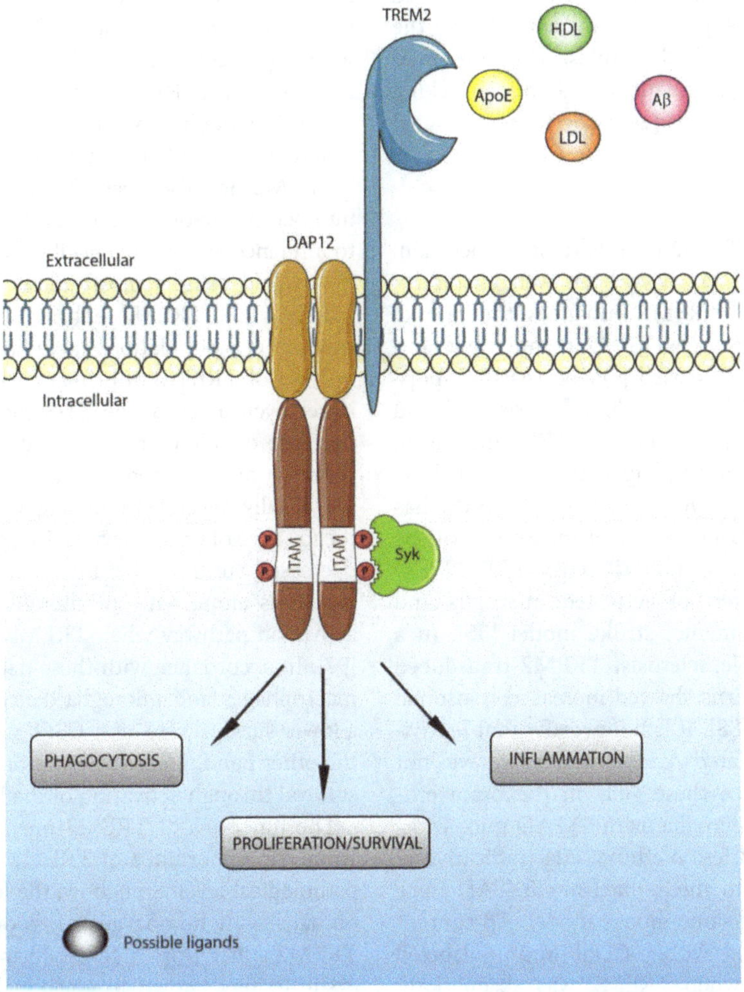

Fig. 1 TREM2 ligands, signaling and functions. Ligands binding to TREM2 induce the association of TREM2 to DAP12 through an electrostatic interaction between a conserved positively-charged lysine in TREM2 (aa186) and a negatively- charged aspartic acid residue in DAP12, generating tyrosine phosphorylation of DAP12 within its immunoreceptor tyrosine-based activation motifs (ITAMS) by Src family kinases

The exact identities of ligands that activate TREM2 remain uncertain. Early studies found that the TREM2 extracellular domain is able to bind microbial products such as LPS or lipoteichoic acids (LTA) [72]. Similarly to other TREM family members [73], lipids can bind and activate TREM2. Indeed, the putative structure of TREM2 contains a potential phospholipid binding site [73], which is confirmed by its crystal structure [74]. In addition, several studies demonstrated binding between TREM2 and lipids from cell membranes and lipoprotein complexes [73, 75, 76]. TREM2 has been reported to bind high-density lipoproteins (HDL), low-density lipoproteins (LDL) and several apolipoproteins such as ApoA1, ApoA2, ApoB and clusterin (ApoJ) [76–79]. However, one of the most well documented ligands of TREM2 is ApoE [76, 78, 79]. *In vitro* studies have demonstrated that lipidation of ApoE is not required for TREM2-ApoE binding [76, 78–80], although Yeh et al. suggested that ApoE lipidation enhanced this interaction [76].

It is interesting to note the interaction between TREM2, ApoE, and clusterin because all three are important genetic risk factors for LOAD, although binding between TREM2 and ApoE occurs with similar affinities between the three different AD-associated ApoE isoforms [64, 78, 79]. In addition, a recent paper characterized Aβ as a ligand of TREM2 [81]. The authors found that Aβ was able to directly bind to TREM2 and activate TREM2 signaling through DAP12 *in vitro*. Interestingly, an immunoprecipitation assay demonstrated a strong enhancement of TREM2-Aβ interaction with oligomeric forms of Aβ compared to monomers [81]. While most ligands of TREM2 have been identified *in vitro*, a recent *in vivo* study by Ulrich et al. strongly argues that ApoE and TREM2 are in the same pathway [82]. Given that a lack of TREM2 expression impairs plaque-associated microgliosis in amyloid models, Ulrich et al. tested whether a lack of ApoE expression similarly affected the microglial response to amyloid plaques. They observed that mice lacking ApoE phenocopied mice lacking TREM2 in regards to the plaque-associated microglial response.

3) TREM2 functions

While the identities of TREM2 ligands remain uncertain, several functions of TREM2 have been well characterized in the last decade. TREM2 enhances the rate of phagocytosis. *In vitro*, loss of TREM2 in microglia and macrophages results in decreased phagocytosis of apoptotic neurons [43, 55, 78, 83], cellular debris [43] and bacteria or bacterial products [84–87]; increasing TREM2 expression improved phagocytosis rate of these substrates [43, 63, 85, 87, 88]. Moreover, TREM2 has been associated with Aβ uptake *in vitro*, which will be discussed in a following section. *In vivo*, TREM2 KO mice had decreased levels of activated microglia and phagocytes in an experimental stroke model [55]. In a mouse model of multiple sclerosis, TREM2-transduced myeloid cells with lentivirus showed increased lysosomal and phagocytic activity [88]. It is noteworthy that lentiviruses and adeno-associated viruses (AAVs) have not been shown to transduce these cells in the brain efficiently. Regarding Aβ, microglia from 5XFAD mice without TREM2 internalized less methoxy-×04 (indicative of fibrillar Aβ) compared to microglia from 5XFAD mice with TREM2 [89]. In the same mouse model, Aβ content was significantly reduced within CD68-immunolabeled microglial phagosomes when TREM2 was absent [90]. These findings in TREM2 deficient mice from multiple pathological models corroborate *in vitro* studies regarding TREM2's role in phagocytosis.

TREM2 also modulates inflammatory signaling. Most studies agree on the anti-inflammatory properties of TREM2. Indeed, Toll-like receptor (TLR) stimulation induced a higher release of pro-inflammatory cytokines, including TNFα and IL6, by bone marrow-derived macrophages lacking TREM2 [50] or DAP12 [91]. Anti-inflammatory effects of TREM2 after TLR stimulation have been confirmed in several cell lines [88, 92, 93]. In microglia, the knockdown of TREM2 signaling increased TNFα and NO synthase-2 transcription (NOS2), while overexpression of TREM2 decreased gene transcription of TNFα, IL1β and NOS2 [43]. TREM2 also appears to signal through anti-inflammatory pathways in several pathological mouse models [55, 88, 94]. A recent study demonstrated that TREM2 mediates the switch from a homeostatic to a neurodegenerative microglia phenotype in APPPS1 and SOD1 (ALS mouse model) mice by inducing APOE signaling, a negative regulator of the homeostatic microglia transcription program [95]. Conversely, some studies reported that TREM2 promoted pro-inflammatory signaling [32, 96]. Inspection of genes with the highest connectivity to TREM2 revealed both anti- and pro-inflammatory gene clusters in the brain [41]. These last findings strongly suggest a more complex action of TREM2 on inflammatory processes.

TREM2 has also been shown to modulate myeloid cell number, proliferation and survival. The ability of TREM2 to influence and, more specifically, to increase the number of myeloid cells is mostly described in disease contexts [55, 56, 84]. TREM2 enhances proliferation of several myeloid cell populations including microglia. *In vitro*, reduction of TREM2 in primary microglia cultures resulted in cell cycle arrest at the G1/S checkpoint [97]. Similarly, a decrease of microglial proliferation has been observed in different disease models when deficient for TREM2 [89, 98]. Finally, several studies suggested TREM2 as a key factor for myeloid cell survival. Indeed, Zheng et al. reported decreased survival of primary microglia and BV2 microglial cells along with an alteration of the Wnt/β-catenin activation pathway when TREM2 expression was reduced [97]. In accordance with these data, bone marrow derived macrophages and microglia deficient for TREM2 showed a lower survival rate after CSF1 starvation [75, 77, 99]. On the other hand, TREM2 activation improved dendritic cell survival through activation of the ERK pathway [32].

The functions of TREM2 previously described demonstrate the importance of TREM2 at the physiological and pathological level. Somehow, the loss of these functions in humans with homozygous loss-of-function mutations in TREM2 suffer from a severe form of dementia with bone cystic lesions known as Nasu-Hakola disease [100, 101]. How and why this particular disease occurs due to loss of TREM2 function is not yet clear. Several TREM2 variants in the human population are able to impair but not block functional TREM2 signaling and impact the onset and progression of AD as will be described in an upcoming section of this review. It is noteworthy that studies have also associated some TREM2 variants with other neurodegenerative diseases such as ALS [54, 102], Parkinson's disease [102, 103] and frontotemporal dementia [104–106], although these observations are still somewhat controversial [102, 104, 107].

4) TREM2 variants and Alzheimer's disease

Thanks to the recent development of whole genome sequencing and genome-wide association studies (GWAS), several genetic variants have been identified that increase the risk of developing LOAD. Among them, several rare variants in TREM2 have emerged that significantly increase LOAD risk by 2- to 4- fold, comparable to the increased risk associated with having one copy of APOE ε4. The most common and most well studied TREM2 variant known to increase the risk of

AD is rs75932628, a single nucleotide polymorphism encoding an arginine-to-histidine missense substitution at amino acid 47 (R47H). The R47H variant was first identified as a risk factor for LOAD in 2013 by two independent studies on subjects of people of European or North American descent [108] and Icelandic subjects [109]. The association between the R47H variant and LOAD in populations of European descent was thereafter corroborated by several studies [104, 107, 110–118]. However, this risk variant has mostly present in European populations and the association of the R47H mutant with increased LOAD risk does not seem to exist in Chinese and African-American populations [119–123]. LOAD patients with the R47H variant display an earlier onset of symptoms [107, 109] and faster cognitive decline [124] compared to non-carriers, although these results are not always consistent between studies [107, 117, 125]. Interestingly, in a European cohort, the R47H variant of TREM2 increased the level of total tau protein in the CSF without affecting Aβ42 [102]. These data suggest a link between AD-associated pathologies and the R47H TREM2 variant. Other TREM2 variants have also been suggested as risk factors for developing LOAD, including R62H (rs143332484), D87N (rs142232675), T96K (rs2234353), L211P (rs2234256) and R136Q (rs149622783) [77, 108, 110, 112, 115, 126].

Identification of these new TREM2 variants as LOAD genetic risk factors has prompted many scientists to study their impact on TREM2 functions. Most of the studies have determined that AD-associated TREM2 variants do not affect folding, expression, stability or structure of TREM2 in AD brains [58, 77, 85]. However, Kober et al. do suggest that the R47H mutation induces a small, but measurable, conformational change in TREM2, and that the R47H and R62H TREM2 variants exhibited slightly decreased stability compared to the common variant [74]. AD-associated variants do appear to affect the affinity of TREM2 for its ligands. Indeed, binding assays revealed that R47H, R62H and D87N variants exhibit impaired interactions with lipoprotein ligands including ApoE, LDL and clusterin *in vitro* [74, 76, 78, 79]. Conversely, Kober et al. reported that the T96K variant increased TREM2 affinity to cell-surface ligands, while confirming reduced binding of cell-surface ligands by R47H [74]. AD-associated variants disturb TREM2 signaling in a pattern similar to that observed for affinity: R47H and R62H negatively affect TREM2 activity *in vitro*, while T96K activity was enhanced compared to the common variant of TREM2 [75, 77]. However, this correlation between affinity and signaling strength does not apply to the D87N variant, which induces a decrease in ligand binding but an increase in TREM2 signaling [77]. This highlights the need for better understanding of the complex action of TREM2. Finally, R47H and R62H variants have been shown to slightly alter phagocytic functions of TREM2 *in vitro* [76, 85]. Moreover, R47H missense mutation impairs TREM2 maturation and alters shedding by α-secretase [85]. Finally, Yeh et al. demonstrated a decrease of Aβ-lipoprotein complex uptake by blood monocyte-derived macrophages from patients heterozygous for the R62H variant [76].

Over the last 5 years, considerable efforts have been made to better understand how different TREM2 variants can affect the risk of AD *in vitro*. These studies have found that these variants result in a decrease of TREM2 functions. It is now essential to confirm and further explore these data *in vivo* using animal models of AD and in patients in order to elucidate the precise mechanisms linking the TREM2 variants to AD.

5) TREM2 and amyloid pathology in AD

TREM2 and amyloid burden

A large majority of *in vivo* studies aimed at understanding the link between TREM2 and AD have focused on amyloid pathology. Most of these studies used different mouse models of amyloid deposition with total or partial deletions of TREM2. Unfortunately, while *in vitro* studies suggested that TREM2 is strongly involved in Aβ40 and Aβ42 uptake by microglia [63, 85, 127], experiments performed *in vivo* found more inconsistent results regarding TREM2 function in Aβ uptake by microglia. The APPPS1-21 [128] and 5xFAD [129] mouse models have mainly been used to assess the effect of TREM2 deficiency or haplo-insufficiency on Aβ accumulation. In APPPS1-21 mice, TREM2 haplo-insufficiency did not affect Aβ accumulation in the cortex [130]. A total deletion of TREM2 in the APPPS1-21 mouse model resulted in a decreased Aβ burden in the cortex of 2-month-old mice but in a higher Aβ accumulation in the cortex of 8-month-old mice [131]. In 5xFAD mice, Wang et al. reported that TREM2 deletion increased Aβ pathology (insoluble Aβ42 and Aβ load) in the hippocampus but not in the cortex of 8.5-month-old mice, with an intermediate phenotype in TREM2-haplo-insufficient mice [75, 89]. These data suggest an age-dependent or Aβ burden-dependent effect of TREM2 on Aβ deposition. Therefore, TREM2 could result in greater Aβ deposition in the early stages of the disease and then result in less Aβ deposition in later stages. A time course analysis of Aβ burden in these two TREM2-deficient models will be necessary to confirm this hypothesis. Moreover, the use of a less aggressive model of Aβ deposition will be useful in order to finely dissect the effect of TREM2 on Aβ accumulation. [45, 75, 130] [132, 133]

TREM2 and microglial function

Whereas the effect of TREM2 on Aβ deposition remains unclear, studies have unanimously reported decreased microglial activation in APPPS1-21 and 5xFAD mice deficient or haplo-insufficient for TREM2, resulting in a subsequent reduction of plaque-associated microglia [45, 75, 130]. Importantly, microglia also failed to cluster around plaques in APPPS1-21 mice haplo-insufficient or deficient for DAP12 [90], confirming the need for TREM2 signaling to activate microglia and recruit them to the plaques. The inability of microglia to cluster around plaques without TREM2 was associated with defects in plaque compaction, microglia proliferation, and increased levels of dystrophic neurons [75, 89, 90]. Moreover, microglia that lacked TREM2 exhibited strong metabolic defects, including low ATP levels and elevated stress markers such as autophagic vesicles. This was caused by defective mammalian Target Of Rapamycin (mTOR) signaling [134]. These results suggest that TREM2 provides trophic support for microglia in stressful conditions. In cases of prolonged stress or activation, as seen in AD, a defective TREM2 could then alter microglial functions and survival through deficient mTOR signaling, resulting in exacerbation of AD neuropathologies.

Recently, Lee at al. used a BAC transgene to induce human TREM2 (hTREM2) expression in 5xFAD mice [135]. Compared to 5xFAD mice deficient or haplo-insufficient for TREM2 [75, 89, 136], 5xFAD mice expressing human TREM2 exhibited reduced insoluble and soluble Aβ42, diminished plaque area, more compact plaques and fewer dystrophic neurites in the cortex [135]. The authors demonstrated that expression of hTREM2 resulted in a reprogrammed microglial gene expression signature. Interestingly, human TREM2 expression was associated with the upregulation of some "disease-associated microglial genes" involved in microglial function, such as phagocytosis. Following this observation, the authors confirmed that phagocytic microglia markers such as CD68 and Lgasl3 in were increased in 5xFAD mice expressing hTREM2. This study confirmed several TREM2 functions previously described in TREM2-deletion mouse models and suggested that reprogrammed microglial gene expression is a key function of TREM2 in the Aβ-deposition models.

Recent findings by Zhao et al. revealed that TREM2 is an Aβ receptor that mediates microglial functions [81, 137]. As previously mentioned, the authors demonstrated TREM2-Aβ interactions using co-immunoprecipitation, cell-free, solid-phase and cell-based binding assay; this interaction was stronger with oligomeric forms of Aβ compared to monomers [81, 137]. Aβ/TREM2 binding activated TREM2 signaling and induced microglia depolarization and Aβ degradation. Moreover, microglia without TREM2 displayed defective clearance of Aβ, with longer internalization of Aβ and an impaired Aβ-induced pro-inflammatory response. *In vivo*, Zhao et al. described alterations in Aβ degradation as well as microglial proliferation and apoptosis in Aβ-injected TREM2 deficient mice [81]. Altogether, these data suggest that oligomeric forms of Aβ may activate TREM2 signaling through direct binding resulting in a pro-inflammatory response, Aβ degradation and microglial proliferation. Moreover, these results could explain why TREM2 is necessary for the recruitment of microglia to plaques.

Importantly, Zhao et al. also reported that the R47H and R62H hTREM2 variants compromised the interaction between oligomeric Aβ and TREM2-Fc [81]. We can therefore speculate that the mechanism by which TREM2 variants increase the risk of LOAD is by altering TREM2's Aβ-receptor functions. However, these *in vitro* data have not yet been confirmed by *in vivo* studies [82]. Indeed, Ulrich et al. demonstrated that a lack of ApoE expression affects microglial recruitment to amyloid plaques, which is phenotypically similar to what has been observed in mice lacking TREM2 expression. These *in vivo* observations suggest that if TREM2 is able to bind Aβ, as suggested by *in vitro* studies, it does not seem able to bind Aβ in plaques in the absence of ApoE to result in microglial recruitment and reduce neuritic dystrophy. Further studies characterizing AD-associated TREM2 variants in the context of amyloid pathology are thus needed to confirm this hypothesis and better understand how TREM2 variants promote LOAD.

The biologic impacts of hTREM2 variants

Two studies aimed at clarifying the impact of human TREM2 variants in LOAD have been published to date. In the first of these studies, Song et al. generated transgenic mice expressing the common variant or R47H variant of human TREM2 *via* BAC transgenes in a TREM2-deficient 5xFAD mouse background [132]. They reported that only the common variant of TREM2 was able to restore microgliosis and microglial activation induced by amyloid pathology in this model, while mice expressing the R47H variant displayed impaired microglial activation and recruitment to plaques. These results are similar to the observations made in TREM2-deficient 5xFAD mice [132]. Moreover, the authors found that soluble TREM2 released from microglia membranes is found in plaques and neurons of 5xFAD mice with the common variant of TREM2, but not in 5xFAD mice with the R47H variant of TREM2. Importantly, soluble TREM2 (corresponding to the TREM2 ectodomain previously described) was identified as a receptor for oligomeric Aβ [81, 137]. This suggests a possible direct binding between soluble TREM2 and plaques in the brains of 5xFAD mice expressing the common variant of TREM2 but not in the brains of mice expressing the R47H variant [81, 137]. However, the impact of this possible interaction between soluble TREM2 and oligomeric Aβ on AD remains to be further explored.

In a subsequent study, Cheng-Hathaway et al. used APPPS1-21 mice in which CRISPR/Cas9 was used to knock in the R47H TREM2 variant into the endogenous mouse TREM2 gene [133]. APPPS1-21 mice heterozygous for the R47H TREM2 variant exhibited reduced association of microglia to plaques, lowered Aβ-induced microglial activation and proliferation, more diffuse amyloid plaques and increased plaque-associated neuritic dystrophy. These results are comparable to observations made in both Aβ-deposition and APPPS1-21 mouse models that are haplo-insufficient or deficient for TREM2 [45, 75, 89, 130, 131]. Surprisingly, a strong reduction of TREM2 mRNA was observed in APPPS1-21 mice heterozygous for the R47H TREM2 variant, which differs from a human study that reported no change in TREM2 expression in the brain of AD patients heterozygous for the R47H variant [58]. Interestingly, a similar decrease of plaque-associated microglia, the presence of less compact plaques and higher neuritic dystrophy around plaques has also been observed in AD patients expressing the R47H variant of TREM2 compared to those patients expressing the common TREM2 variant, confirming the partial loss-of-function caused by the R47H variant [136]. Taken together, these *in vivo* studies confirmed the suspected partial TREM2 loss-of-function phenotype of the LOAD-associated R47H variant. Importantly, a new study by Xiang et al. has explored the cause of TREM2 RNA reduction in this CRISP/Cas9 model [138]. They reported that the R47H variant activated a cryptic splice site, which introduced a premature stop codon in mice but not in human TREM2, resulting in haplo insufficiency of the Cheng-Hathaway et al. model. These data strongly suggest that results obtained with this model should be interpreted carefully and may not be directly translatable to humans.

To conclude, these studies in mouse models of amyloid deposition indicate a critical function for TREM2 in the clustering of microglia around plaques, plaque compaction, and microglia proliferation and activation, which may be disturbed by some rare TREM2 variants. TREM2 signaling appears to both positively and negatively affect amyloid pathology depending on disease progression. AD-associated TREM2 variants may induce partial loss-of-function phenotypes, resulting in an inability of microglia to cluster around plaques. These findings advance our understanding of TREM2 involvement in the response of microglia to Aβ aggregation and its consequences and strongly encourage targeting and enhancing TREM2 expression and/or signaling early in AD pathogenesis to reduce Aβ-induced brain injury associated with TREM2 defects in AD. However, the Aβ deposition phase of AD occurs predominantly prior to symptom onset in humans. Questions still remain regarding the role of TREM2 and its different variants in later stages of AD, in particular in tau pathology and tau seeding.

6) TREM2 and tau pathology in AD

First clues linking TREM2 to tau pathology

Numerous findings in the literature suggest a link between tau pathology and TREM2 in LOAD. Indeed, in the cerebrospinal fluid (CSF) of AD patients, soluble TREM2 has been shown to correlate with total and phosphorylated tau (Thr181) levels, but not with levels of Aβ42 [139]. Moreover, AD patients harboring the R47H variant of TREM2 display higher levels of both total tau and phosphorylated tau (Thr181) in CSF compared to non-carriers, without any change in Aβ42 levels [102, 140]. Importantly, levels of phosphorylated tau in the CSF correlate with tau pathology burden in the brain (both in terms of neurofibrillary tangles and hyperphosphorylated tau loading) [141] and with neuronal loss and cognitive decline in AD patients [141–143]. Importantly, a study reported increased tau hyperphosphorylation and axonal dystrophy around amyloid plaques in humans harboring the R47H variant of TREM2 [90]. A study also found a positive correlation between TREM2 mRNA levels and tau burden in a cohort of 20 AD patients and 12 controls [57]. Additionally, microglia have been strongly characterized as key players in tau pathology and propagation [144–147]. Indeed, in a mouse model of tau propagation using an injection of AAV2/6-SYN1 promoter driving the expression of human P301L tau 1–441 mutant into the entorhinal cortex, Asai et al. report that depleting microglia dramatically suppressed the propagation of Tau [147]. Moreover, Luo et al. demonstrated that microglia degrade human tau species released from AD brains and eliminate NFTs from PS19 mice, a mouse model of tauopathy harboring the P301S human tau mutation [145]. In hTau mice, another tauopathy mouse model, microglial activation has been shown to correlate with a deficit in spatial memory and the spread of tau pathology [146]. While preliminary, these data suggest a role for microglia in tau pathology and tau propagation in AD, which can be affected by AD-associated TREM2 variants. However, only a few studies have investigated the link between tau and TREM2 compared to the extensive number of studies aimed at understanding the link between TREM2 and Aβ.

Some studies have assessed tau phosphorylation in Aβ-deposition mouse models deficient for TREM2. However, the results reported in these studies are inconsistent, and demonstrate either an increase [89] or decrease [45] of phosphorylated tau in mice deficient for TREM2. This may be because of differences in the mouse models used (5xFAD *vs.* APPPS1). A recent study also suggested that overexpression of TREM2 through

ICV injection of AAV encoding the murine TREM2 gene was able to decrease surgery-induced tau hyperphosphorylation in APPswe/PS1dE9 mice [148]. However, it is important to note that robust microglial transduction has not been reported *in vitro* using commonly used AAVs (1-9).

TREM2 functions in models of pure tau pathology

Although investigating the effects of TREM2 on tau pathology in the context of amyloid pathology is essential to better understand AD, studies of the direct link between TREM2 and tau pathology are very rare. Only 5 studies of TREM2 in pure tau pathology exist today in the literature. Two of these studies have been done by Jiang et al. in PS19 mice, a model of tauopathy harboring the P301S mutation [149, 150]. In the first study, the authors suggested that the silencing of brain TREM2 *via* injection of a lentivirus containing TREM2 shRNA was able to exacerbate tau phosphorylation through neuroinflammation-induced hyperactivation of tau kinases [150]. Moreover, data presented in this study suggests an exacerbation of neurodegeneration and higher spatial learning deficits in PS19 mice expressing TREM2 shRNA compared to mice not deficient in TREM2. In the second study, they induced TREM2 overexpression in microglia of PS19 mice with a lentivirus containing TREM2 cDNA. In agreement with their first study, the authors observed that overexpression of TREM2 in microglia reduced neurodegeneration, spatial cognitive impairments and tau hyperphosphorylation through the suppression of neuroinflammation-induced hyperactivation of tau kinases [149]. Although both articles have relevant hypotheses and provide encouraging results, a significant technical issue exists in these studies. Clear evidence that the lentiviruses utilized were able to infect and alter TREM2 levels in microglia is lacking. In the first study, the authors were able to confirm an increase in TREM2 mRNA levels specifically in microglia during disease progression in PS19 mice [150]. However, they did not use the same technique to assess the efficiency of their lentiviruses and only assessed TREM2 mRNA levels in whole cortex and hippocampus (not only in microglia) [149, 150]. To confirm that the lentiviruses altered TREM2 expression in microglia, they performed TREM2 immunofluorescence staining in mouse brains but the authors mention possible non-specific binding with the antibodies utilized [149, 150]. To summarize, due to the lack of important controls, results obtained in these studies are not sufficient to confidently understand how TREM2 affects tau pathology.

Three recent studies tackled this problem by crossing TREM2 knockout mice with two different murine models of tauopathies [151–153]. In the first study, Leyns et al. reported a decrease in neurodegeneration as well as attenuated microgliosis and astrogliosis in the brains of PS19 mice deficient for TREM2 [152]. Interestingly, no differences were observed for tau phosphorylation and insolubility in PS19 mice with or without TREM2. These unexpected results suggest that TREM2 promotes neuroinflammation and neurodegeneration in the context of tauopathy. In a second study, Sayed et al. [153] found that TREM2 haplo-insufficiency, but not complete loss of TREM2, increased tau pathology. Further, whereas complete TREM2 deficiency protected against tau-mediated microglial activation and atrophy as seen by Leyns et al. [152], TREM2 haplo-insufficiency elevated expression of proinflammatory markers and exacerbated atrophy at a late stage of disease. Taken together, these 2 studies suggest that partial or normal TREM2 function contributes to tauopathy as well as tau-mediated damage and that complete loss of function also decreases tau-mediated brain injury. In a third study, Bemiller et al. crossed TREM2 knockout mice with hTau mice [151], which is a mouse model of tauopathy expressing all human Tau isoforms in a murine tau knockout background [154]. Bemiller at al. confirmed the decrease of microgliosis in TREM2-deficient hTau mice, as previously seen in TREM2-deficient PS19 mice [151–153]. However, unlike studies on PS19 mice, complete deletion of TREM2 in hTau mice exacerbated tau phosphorylation and insolubility. The authors suggest that these changes are driven by the activation of stress-related tau protein kinases in TREM2-deficient hTau mice. Neurodegeneration was not evaluated in this study. These pure tauopathy mouse models suggest a complex relationship between TREM2 and Tau pathology, which requires further research. hTau and PS19 mice are independent mouse models and develop distinctive pathologies, which may explain differences between these models. Given the results of the current studies, it will be important to understand the effects of human TREM2 and human TREM2 variants in both pure tauopathy models that develop tau pathology and neurodegeneration as well as the effects of TREM2 in models that develop both Aβ and tau pathology.

Recently, an interesting study evaluated molecular and pathological interactions between Aβ42, tau, TREM2, and DAP12 in *Drosophila* models [155]. They created flies that expressed human tau in photoreceptor neurons and either WT or R47H TREM2/DAP12 complexes in glia cells simultaneously. Results obtained in this new model demonstrated that glial expression of both $TREM2^{WT}$/DAP12 and $TREM2^{R47H}$/TDAP12 complexes significantly exacerbated tau-mediated neurodegeneration without affecting tau phosphorylation and insolubility, in agreement with the Leyns et al. and Sayed et al. studies in TREM2 deficient PS19 mice [152, 153]. On the other hand, a recent *in vitro* study using a microglia/

neuron co-culture model, reported that depletion of TREM2 exacerbated tau phosphorylation *via* an increase in the microglial inflammatory response [156]. These results are in agreement with the findings reported by Bemiller et al.

Taken together, studies assessing the link between tau pathology and TREM2 suggest a biphasic effect of TREM2 loss-of-function, similar to what has been seen for amyloid pathology. In the early stages of the disease, dysfunctional TREM2 can promote tau pathology (both hyperphosphorylation and aggregation), while the complete loss of TREM2 function in advanced stages of the disease seems to protect from neurodegeneration.

7) TREM2 and ApoE: a close partnership in AD pathogenesis?

Beyond the direct contribution of TREM2 and its AD-related variants on the two histopathological markers of LOAD (i.e. amyloid plaques and NFTs), a new hypothesis has started to emerge suggesting a collaboration between ApoE and TREM2 in LOAD pathogenesis. This hypothesis is based on a combination of several observations. First, APOE and TREM2 are, to date, the two largest genetic risk factors that influence the development of LOAD [157]. Second, ApoE is now well-characterized as a TREM2 ligand *in vitro,* which may stimulate TREM2 functions [76, 78–80]. Interestingly, binding between TREM2 and ApoE occurs to a similar extent between the three different ApoE isoforms [64, 78–80]. Another study showed higher TREM2 expression in patient-derived mononuclear blood cells from ApoE ε4 carriers with mild cognitive impairment and AD compared to non-carriers [158]. Moreover, decrease of TREM2 in microglia has been reported in mice expressing ApoE ε4 [159]. Recently, Murray et al. suggested that ApoE ε4 is required in TREM2 R47H variant-carriers for AD to develop, although larger cohorts and statistical analyses are needed to support this hypothesis [160].

At the microglial level, quantification of ApoE transcripts isolated from both WT and TREM2-deleted mice using fluorescence-activated cell sorting and nanostring technology revealed a downregulation of ApoE expression in TREM2-deleted mice [161]. In PS19 mice, Leyns et al. reported the accumulation of ApoE-positive puncta specifically in microglia [152]. Deletion of TREM2 in this model strongly lowered the number of microglia containing ApoE puncta, and decreased the gene expression of ApoE in the cortex. Moreover, the same reduction in neurodegeneration induced by tau pathology in PS19 mice has been reported when mice lack TREM2 [152] or ApoE [27]. This suggests a strong contribution of TREM2 and ApoE in neurodegeneration in this model. Recent findings by Ulrich et al. also suggest that ApoE and TREM2 are in the same pathway [82]. Indeed, amyloid mice lacking ApoE phenocopied mice lacking TREM2 in regards to the plaque-associated microglial response. Taken together, these data suggest a possible relationship between TREM2 and ApoE in AD, although the exact nature of this alliance and its consequences in AD remained, until recently, poorly understood.

A new study has shed light on the function of the TREM2/ApoE connection in neurodegenerative diseases including AD [95]. In this study by Kraesmann et al., a specific molecular signature has was identified in microglia from several mouse models of neurodegenerative diseases, including AD [95]. This neurodegeneration-associated phenotype acquired by microglia (MGnD) is characterized by transcriptional changes, including decreased expression of 68 homeostatic genes, and increased expression of 28 inflammatory genes. Because the downregulation of ApoE observed in microglia during development is correlated with a homeostatic profile, the authors next aimed to assess the role of ApoE in the induction of MGnD in microglia [162]. To this end, they performed transcriptomic analysis in APOE-deleted microglia and observed that ApoE regulates the MGnD transcriptional program. Moreover, because TREM2 binds ApoE, the authors then evaluated if the ApoE-induced switch from a homeostatic profile to MGnD in microglia was TREM2-dependent. Deletion of TREM2 in APPPS1-21 mice suppressed the MGnD profile, locking microglia in the homeostatic phenotype. This suggests that the TREM2/ApoE pathway is able to drive the switch from homeostatic microglia to neurodegenerative microglia, MGnD being less effective at preventing neuronal loss. This novel study provides many answers regarding the relationship between TREM2 and ApoE in neurodegenerative diseases. However, it is still not clear whether ApoE or TREM2 are upstream or downstream of each other in this pathway.

Altogether, these data indicate a strong collaboration between TREM2 and ApoE in several neuropathological hallmarks of LOAD. However, these discoveries raise new questions regarding the exact mechanism underlying this collaboration and the origin of ApoE involved in this partnership, which require further investigation. Moreover, these data reveal that a more exhaustive study of ApoE specifically in microglia is now necessary to better understand the link between AD and microglia.

8) TREM2: a brain teaser for therapeutic strategy in AD

Despite more than a century of research on AD, there is currently no treatment to prevent or cure the disease. Current treatments aiming to slow the progression of the disease target neurotransmission pathways altered in AD. The U.S. Food and Drug Administration has approved two types of medications that aim to slow down

Table 1 Summary of the major findings on TREM2 in AD context

AD context	Major TREM2-AD related findings	Source	Citations
Risk factors	❖ Rare variants in TREM2 increase LOAD risk by 2- to 4- fold	AD patients	[104, 107–118]
Amyloid pathology	❖ Loss of functional TREM2 decreases microgliosis around plaques	5xFAD mice APPPS1-21 mice	[45, 75, 130, 132, 133]
	❖ Loss of functional TREM2 decreases plaque compaction	5xFAD mice APPPS1-21 mice	[75, 89, 90, 133]
Tau pathology	❖ TREM2 deletion decreases tau-mediated neurodegeneration	PS19 mice	[152, 153]
	❖ TREM2 deletion (1) or haploinsuficiency (2) increase tau pathology	hTau mice (1) PS19 mice (2)	[151] (1) [153] (2)
ApoE	❖ ApoE is a TREM2 ligand	*in vitro*	[76, 78, 79]
	❖ ApoE-induced switch from homeostatic to neurodegenerative microglia is TREM2-dependent	APPPS1-21 mice	[95]

AD: cholinesterase inhibitors (Aricept, Exelon, Razadyne) and the NMDA receptor antagonist memantine (Namenda). However, the efficiency of these drugs has often been questioned (for review [163]). Although a considerable effort has been made to find new treatments, none have been met with any success yet in clinical trials.

While a great interest in TREM2 as a therapeutic target in AD is emerging, many impediments make its use potentially challenging. First, TREM2 risk variants are found in less than one percent of the population. In comparison, ApoE ε4-carriers represent 20% of the population [113, 164]. Although several studies suggest that, in certain conditions, targeting TREM2 could decrease AD-related pathologies as previously described, it is still unknown whether a potential TREM2-targeting treatment will be effective in non-carrier AD patients, which represent the majority of cases. Moreover, it remains to be determined whether a therapeutic strategy targeting TREM2 should activate or inhibit it. Indeed, as

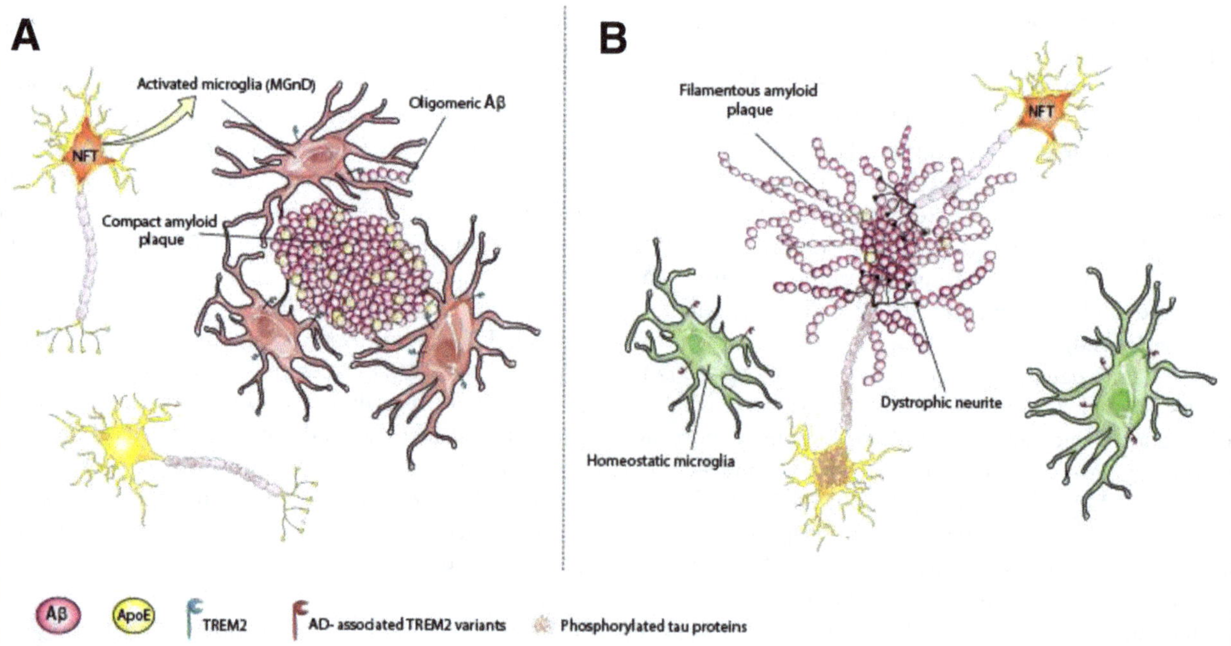

Fig. 2 Schematic summary of the role of TREM2 and its variants in AD. **a**. Functional TREM2 has been suggested to allow microglia activation (by amyloid and NFTs for example), promote microglia clustering around plaques, amyloid uptake (early stage of the disease) and plaque compaction through binding to plaque-associated ApoE or directly to oligomeric Aβ. **b**. AD-associated TREM2 variants resulting in TREM2 partial loss-of-function abolished microglia clustering around plaque and phagocytic activity. These changes could be caused by a blockage of microglia in homeostatic stages because of less plaque-associated ApoE or other reasons. The consequences are filamentous plaques associate with increased dystrophic neurites and a possible increase of tau pathology (in early stages)

previously discussed, TREM2 can be either beneficial or pathological in AD depending on the disease models used, the context of the pathological insult, and the stages of pathology. To date, the best strategy seems to involve stimulating TREM2 signaling in the early stages of the disease, when amyloid deposition starts and before tau pathology and neuronal loss occurs. However, because of the dual role of TREM2 in AD, this hypothesis must be carefully tested to avoid worsening disease pathology. A similar strategy would be to stimulate TREM2 even before amyloid deposits form in the brain. Indeed, TREM2 deficiency prevents the transition of microglia to the MGnD phenotype, which prevents the beneficial effects of microglia on amyloid pathology [165]. Stimulating the microglial transition from homeostatic states to MGnD prior to amyloid accumulation may therefore delay the evolution of AD. Conversely, the observation that deletion of TREM2 in APPPS1-21 mice decreased the Aβ burden in 2-months-old animals but resulted in higher Aβ accumulation in the cortex of 8-months-old animals [131] suggests that MGnD could be beneficial in the later stages of amyloid pathology. This example highlights the complexity of targeting TREM2.

While the timing of when to stimulate TREM2 in order to treat AD pathology needs to be resolved, the question of how to target TREM2 also remains unaddressed. Immunotherapy using antibodies to stimulate TREM2 signaling are being developed by a number of groups. TREM2-activating antibodies have been tested *in vitro* and have been shown to induce activation of calcium and ERK signaling in human dendritic cells [32]. Such a strategy requires particular thoughtfulness because antibodies could alter binding of TREM2 ligands [75]. Modulating TREM2 expression or protein levels is another strategy of interest. Indeed, overexpression of TREM2 *in vitro* decreases inflammation and promotes phagocytosis [43]. *In vivo*, lentiviral approaches aiming to increase TREM2 expression in the brains of mice attenuated both cognitive and neuropathologic alterations [63]. However, it is important to note that lentiviral strategies cannot be used in humans because of the high risk of inducing oncogenic transformation.

Regardless of the strategy chosen to modulate TREM2 in AD, it is important to remember that microglia are not the only cells that express TREM2. Targeting of this receptor outside the brain will need to be assessed to make sure there are not unwanted side effects. Further, even in the brain, microglial functions are not limited to inflammatory responses (for review [166]) and modulating TREM2 signaling could induce several deleterious side effects that will have to be assessed. It seems obvious that the targeting of TREM2 in AD is a promising avenue to explore. However, there are clearly several obstacles that will need to be addressed before moving forward with such a strategy. The growing interest in TREM2, especially in the context of AD, may hopefully provide a better characterization of its roles and thus help to find a way around the possible barriers to its therapeutic targeting.

Conclusion

Despite a continually growing number of cases, AD is still under-characterized. In addition to the role of amyloid pathology, it is now clear that the pathogenesis of AD involves many alterations in the brain that interact synergistically, ultimately resulting in neuronal death. Beyond tau and amyloid pathologies, growing evidence suggests that neuroinflammation plays a crucial role in AD. Recent genetic studies (GWAS and whole genome sequencing) have confirmed this by identifying numerous genetic risk factors for AD associated with the immune system. Within these new genetic risk factors, a special interest has been directed at TREM2 in the last 5 years. Together, the data presented in this review strongly suggest an important role of TREM2 in AD at the level of amyloid and tau pathologies and inflammation, alone or in collaboration with other molecules such as ApoE (Table 1). Figure 2 illustrates current thinking and hypotheses regarding the role of TREM2 and its rare AD-associated variants in AD pathogenesis. Studies on TREM2 in the context of AD highlight its complexity. Indeed, *in vivo* studies suggest that TREM2 is injurious in the early stages of the disease and then becomes beneficial in the later stages. Finally, both ApoE and oligomeric forms of Aβ are able to bind and activate TREM2 making the elucidating of the TREM2 mechanism of action in AD difficult.

Therefore, there are many outstanding questions that require further investigation. Most of the previously performed studies evaluated how TREM2 influences AD pathogenesis through partial or total deletion of TREM2. However, AD-related risk factors have also been associated with partial loss-of-function of TREM2. Consequently, further studies are needed to understand how these specific human risk variants affect AD. Furthermore, it is also necessary to understand the dual role of TREM2 in AD, which can reflect the often-reported dual role of neuroinflammation in this disease. In the same way, how TREM2 variants exactly alter AD remains unclear. Is it because of altered phagocytosis resulting in the accumulation of amyloid plaques and damaged neurons? Perhaps TREM2 variants increase the expression of pro-inflammatory molecules. Is TREM2 role in AD dependent of its interaction with ApoE? Is ApoE upstream or downstream of TREM2? It would be interesting to assess if similar TREM2 partial loss-of-function is observed in AD patients without AD-related TREM2 risk variants. This may occur through the interaction between TREM2 and APOE or oligomeric forms of Aβ, both of which are able to bind TREM2 and modulate its functions. Data obtained during the last 5 years has provided many answers regarding the role of TREM2 in AD, and has identified TREM2 as a therapeutic target. However, substantial questions regarding the potential targeting of TREM2 remain unclear. Is TREM2 beneficial or damaging at particular disease stages? The trigger of the disease? Or just a catalyst of an inevitable AD? The complexity of TREM2 in AD is beyond doubt and brings new questions with each new discovery. Addressing these questions first will be necessary to explain the role of TREM2 and microglia in AD and will help determine whether targeting it is a viable therapeutic strategy.

Abbreviations

AAV: Adeno-associated virus; AD: Alzheimer's disease; ApoE: Apolipoprotein E; Aβ: Amyloid-β peptide; ALS: Amyotrophic lateral sclerosis; CNS: Central nervous system; CSF: Cerebral spinal fluid; DAP: DNAX-activation protein; Fc: Fragment crystallizable; GSK-3β: Glycogen synthase kinase 3; GWAS: Genome wide association studies; HDL: High-density lipoproteins; ITAMs: Immunoreceptor tyrosine-based activation motifs; IL: Interleukin; IL-1β: Interleukin 1 beta; JNK: c-Jun N-terminal kinase; LDL: Low-density lipoproteins; LPS: Lipopolysaccharide; LOAD: Late-onset Alzheimer's disease; LTA: Lipoteichoic acids; MAPK: Mitogen activated protein kinase; mTOR: Mammalian target of rapamycin; NOS2: NO synthase-2 transcription; NFT: Neurofibrillary tangle; PD: Parkinson's disease; PI3K: Phosphatidylinositol 3-kinase; TLR: Toll-like receptor; TREM: Triggering receptors expressed on myeloid cells; TNF-α: Tumor necrosis factor alpha

Acknowledgments

The authors would like to thank InPrint, a scientific editing network, and Elise Alspach and Angela Schlegel for assisting in editing and correcting the structure/grammar of the manuscript. The author would like to thank Servier Medical Art that provides professionally designed biological elements for figures design.

Funding

This review was supported by grants from the Charles and Helen Schwab Foundation (DMH) and the Edward N. and Della L. Thome Memorial Foundation, Bank of America, N.A., Trustee (DMH).

Authors' contributions

MG reviewed the literature, drafted and revised the manuscript. MG constructed the figures. CEGL and DMH critically revised the manuscript. All authors read and approved the final manuscript.

Competing interests

DMH is listed as an inventor on a provisional patent from Washington University on TREM2 antibodies. CEGL and DMH are listed as inventors on a patent licensed by Washington University to C2N Diagnostics on the therapeutic use of anti-tau antibodies. DMH co-founded and is on the scientific advisory board of C2N Diagnostics, LLC. C2N Diagnostics, LLC has licensed certain anti-tau antibodies to AbbVie for therapeutic development. DMH is on the scientific advisory board of Proclara and Denali and consults for Genentech, AbbVie, and Idorsia.

Author details

[1]Department of Neurology, St. Louis, USA. [2]Hope Center for Neurological Disorders, St. Louis, USA. [3]Knight Alzheimer's Disease Research Center, Washington University School of Medicine, St. Louis, MO 63110, USA.

References

1. Alzheimer A. Über eine eigenartige Erkrankung der Hirnrinde. Allgemeine Zeitschrift fur Psychiatrie und Psychisch-gerichtliche Medizin. 1907;64:146–8.
2. Alzheimer A, Stelzmann RA, Schnitzlein HN, Murtagh FR. An English translation of Alzheimer's 1907 paper, "Uber eine eigenartige Erkankung der Hirnrinde". Clin Anat. 1995;8:429–31.
3. Castellani RJ, Rolston RK, Smith MA. Alzheimer disease. Dis Mon. 2010;56: 484–546.
4. Holtzman DM, Morris JC, Goate AM. Alzheimer's disease: the challenge of the second century. Sci Transl Med. 2011;3:77sr1.
5. Serrano-Pozo A, Frosch MP, Masliah E, Hyman BT. Neuropathological alterations in Alzheimer disease. Cold Spring Harb Perspect Med. 2011;1: a006189.
6. Alzheimer's A. Alzheimer's disease facts and figures. Alzheimers Dement. 2016;2016(12):459–509.
7. Beach TG, Walker R, McGeer EG. Patterns of gliosis in Alzheimer's disease and aging cerebrum. Glia. 1989;2:420–36.
8. Itagaki S, McGeer PL, Akiyama H, Zhu S, Selkoe D. Relationship of microglia and astrocytes to amyloid deposits of Alzheimer disease. J Neuroimmunol. 1989;24:173–82.
9. McGeer PL, Itagaki S, Tago H, McGeer EG. Reactive microglia in patients with senile dementia of the Alzheimer type are positive for the histocompatibility glycoprotein HLA-DR. Neurosci Lett. 1987;79:195–200.
10. Wyss-Coray T, Mucke L. Inflammation in neurodegenerative disease--a double-edged sword. Neuron. 2002;35:419–32.
11. Wyss-Coray T, Loike JD, Brionne TC, Lu E, Anankov R, Yan F, Silverstein SC, Husemann J. Adult mouse astrocytes degrade amyloid-beta in vitro and in situ. Nat Med. 2003;9:453–7.
12. Mandrekar S, Jiang Q, Lee CY, Koenigsknecht-Talboo J, Holtzman DM, Landreth GE. Microglia mediate the clearance of soluble Abeta through fluid phase macropinocytosis. J Neurosci. 2009;29:4252–62.
13. Paresce DM, Ghosh RN, Maxfield FR. Microglial cells internalize aggregates of the Alzheimer's disease amyloid beta-protein via a scavenger receptor. Neuron. 1996;17:553–65.
14. Akiyama H, Barger S, Barnum S, Bradt B, Bauer J, Cole GM, Cooper NR, Eikelenboom P, Emmerling M, Fiebich BL, et al. Inflammation and Alzheimer's disease. Neurobiol Aging. 2000;21:383–421.
15. Calsolaro V, Edison P. Neuroinflammation in Alzheimer's disease: Current evidence and future directions. Alzheimer's & dementia : the journal of the Alzheimer's Association. 2016;12:719–32.
16. Yoshiyama Y, Higuchi M, Zhang B, Huang SM, Iwata N, Saido TC, Maeda J, Suhara T, Trojanowski JQ, Lee VM. Synapse loss and microglial activation precede tangles in a P301S tauopathy mouse model. Neuron. 2007;53:337–51.
17. Roe AD, Staup MA, Serrats J, Sawchenko PE, Rissman RA. Lipopolysaccharide-induced tau phosphorylation and kinase activity--modulation, but not mediation, by corticotropin-releasing factor receptors. Eur J Neurosci. 2011;34:448–56.
18. Gorlovoy P, Larionov S, Pham TT, Neumann H. Accumulation of tau induced in neurites by microglial proinflammatory mediators. Faseb J. 2009;23:2502–13.
19. Harvey RJ, Skelton-Robinson M, Rossor MN. The prevalence and causes of dementia in people under the age of 65 years. J Neurol Neurosurg Psychiatry. 2003;74:1206–9.
20. Gatz M, Reynolds CA, Fratiglioni L, Johansson B, Mortimer JA, Berg S, Fiske A, Pedersen NL. Role of genes and environments for explaining Alzheimer disease. Arch Gen Psychiatry. 2006;63:168–74.
21. Karch CM, Goate AM. Alzheimer's disease risk genes and mechanisms of disease pathogenesis. Biol Psychiatry. 2015;77:43–51.
22. Corder EH, Saunders AM, Strittmatter WJ, Schmechel DE, Gaskell PC, Small GW, Roses AD, Haines JL, Pericak-Vance MA. Gene dose of apolipoprotein E type 4 allele and the risk of Alzheimer's disease in late onset families. Science. 1993;261:921–3.
23. Strittmatter WJ, Weisgraber KH, Huang DY, Dong LM, Salvesen GS, Pericak-Vance M, Schmechel D, Saunders AM, Goldgaber D, Roses AD. Binding of

human apolipoprotein E to synthetic amyloid beta peptide: isoform-specific effects and implications for late-onset Alzheimer disease. Proc Natl Acad Sci U S A. 1993;90:8098–102.

24. Castellano JM, Kim J, Stewart FR, Jiang H, DeMattos RB, Patterson BW, Fagan AM, Morris JC, Mawuenyega KG, Cruchaga C, et al. Human apoE isoforms differentially regulate brain amyloid-beta peptide clearance. Sci Transl Med. 2011;3:89ra57.
25. Kim J, Basak JM, Holtzman DM. The role of apolipoprotein E in Alzheimer's disease. Neuron. 2009;63:287–303.
26. Verghese PB, Castellano JM, Garai K, Wang Y, Jiang H, Shah A, Bu G, Frieden C, Holtzman DM. ApoE influences amyloid-beta (Abeta) clearance despite minimal apoE/Abeta association in physiological conditions. Proc Natl Acad Sci U S A. 2013;110:E1807–16.
27. Shi Y, Yamada K, Liddelow SA, Smith ST, Zhao L, Luo W, Tsai RM, Spina S, Grinberg LT, Rojas JC, et al. ApoE4 markedly exacerbates tau-mediated neurodegeneration in a mouse model of tauopathy. Nature. 2017;549:523–7.
28. Malik M, Parikh I, Vasquez JB, Smith C, Tai L, Bu G, LaDu MJ, Fardo DW, Rebeck GW, Estus S. Genetics ignite focus on microglial inflammation in Alzheimer's disease. Mol Neurodegener. 2015;10:52.
29. Zhang ZG, Li Y, Ng CT, Song YQ. Inflammation in Alzheimer's Disease and Molecular Genetics: Recent Update. Arch Immunol Ther Exp (Warsz). 2015; 63:333–44.
30. Bouchon A, Dietrich J, Colonna M. Cutting edge: inflammatory responses can be triggered by TREM-1, a novel receptor expressed on neutrophils and monocytes. J Immunol. 2000;164:4991–5.
31. Allcock RJ, Barrow AD, Forbes S, Beck S, Trowsdale J. The human TREM gene cluster at 6p21.1 encodes both activating and inhibitory single IgV domain receptors and includes NKp44. Eur J Immunol. 2003;33:567–77.
32. Bouchon A, Hernandez-Munain C, Cella M, Colonna M. A DAP12-mediated pathway regulates expression of CC chemokine receptor 7 and maturation of human dendritic cells. J Exp Med. 2001;194:1111–22.
33. Cella M, Buonsanti C, Strader C, Kondo T, Salmaggi A, Colonna M. Impaired differentiation of osteoclasts in TREM-2-deficient individuals. J Exp Med. 2003;198:645–51.
34. Goncalves LA, Rodrigues-Duarte L, Rodo J. Vieira de Moraes L, Marques I, Penha-Goncalves C: TREM2 governs Kupffer cell activation and explains belr1 genetic resistance to malaria liver stage infection. Proc Natl Acad Sci U S A. 2013;110:19531–6.
35. Hu N, Tan MS, Yu JT, Sun L, Tan L, Wang YL, Jiang T, Tan L. Increased expression of TREM2 in peripheral blood of Alzheimer's disease patients. J Alzheimers Dis. 2014;38:497–501.
36. Humphrey MB, Daws MR, Spusta SC, Niemi EC, Torchia JA, Lanier LL, Seaman WE, Nakamura MC. TREM2, a DAP12-associated receptor, regulates osteoclast differentiation and function. J Bone Miner Res. 2006;21:237–45.
37. Koth LL, Cambier CJ, Ellwanger A, Solon M, Hou L, Lanier LL, Abram CL, Hamerman JA, Woodruff PG. DAP12 is required for macrophage recruitment to the lung in response to cigarette smoke and chemotaxis toward CCL2. J Immunol. 2010;184:6522–8.
38. Paloneva J, Mandelin J, Kiialainen A, Bohling T, Prudlo J, Hakola P, Haltia M, Konttinen YT, Peltonen L. DAP12/TREM2 deficiency results in impaired osteoclast differentiation and osteoporotic features. J Exp Med. 2003;198: 669–75.
39. Sessa G, Podini P, Mariani M, Meroni A, Spreafico R, Sinigaglia F, Colonna M, Panina P, Meldolesi J. Distribution and signaling of TREM2/DAP12, the receptor system mutated in human polycystic lipomembraneous osteodysplasia with sclerosing leukoencephalopathy dementia. Eur J Neurosci. 2004;20:2617–28.
40. Garcia-Alloza M, Borrelli LA, Thyssen DH, Hickman SE, El Khoury J, Bacskai BJ. Four-dimensional microglia response to anti-Abeta treatment in APP/ PS1xCX3CR1/GFP mice. Intravital. 2013;2.
41. Forabosco P, Ramasamy A, Trabzuni D, Walker R, Smith C, Bras J, Levine AP, Hardy J, Pocock JM, Guerreiro R, et al. Insights into TREM2 biology by network analysis of human brain gene expression data. Neurobiol Aging. 2013;34:2699–714.
42. Kiialainen A, Hovanes K, Paloneva J, Kopra O, Peltonen L. Dap12 and Trem2, molecules involved in innate immunity and neurodegeneration, are co-expressed in the CNS. Neurobiol Dis. 2005;18:314–22.
43. Takahashi K, Rochford CD, Neumann H. Clearance of apoptotic neurons without inflammation by microglial triggering receptor expressed on myeloid cells-2. J Exp Med. 2005;201:647–57.
44. Neumann H, Takahashi K. Essential role of the microglial triggering receptor expressed on myeloid cells-2 (TREM2) for central nervous tissue immune homeostasis. J Neuroimmunol. 2007;184:92–9.
45. Jay TR, Miller CM, Cheng PJ, Graham LC, Bemiller S, Broihier ML, Xu G, Margevicius D, Karlo JC, Sousa GL, et al. TREM2 deficiency eliminates TREM2 + inflammatory macrophages and ameliorates pathology in Alzheimer's disease mouse models. J Exp Med. 2015;212:287–95.
46. Satoh J, Tabunoki H, Ishida T, Yagishita S, Jinnai K, Futamura N, Kobayashi M, Toyoshima I, Yoshioka T, Enomoto K, et al. Immunohistochemical characterization of microglia in Nasu-Hakola disease brains. Neuropathology. 2011;31:363–75.
47. Lue LF, Schmitz CT, Serrano G, Sue LI, Beach TG, Walker DG. TREM2 Protein Expression Changes Correlate with Alzheimer's Disease Neurodegenerative Pathologies in Post-Mortem Temporal Cortices. Brain Pathol. 2015;25:469–80.
48. Schmid CD, Sautkulis LN, Danielson PE, Cooper J, Hasel KW, Hilbush BS, Sutcliffe JG, Carson MJ. Heterogeneous expression of the triggering receptor expressed on myeloid cells-2 on adult murine microglia. J Neurochem. 2002;83:1309–20.
49. Chertoff M, Shrivastava K, Gonzalez B, Acarin L, Gimenez-Llort L. Differential modulation of TREM2 protein during postnatal brain development in mice. PLoS One. 2013;8:e72083.
50. Turnbull IR, Gilfillan S, Cella M, Aoshi T, Miller M, Piccio L, Hernandez M, Colonna M. Cutting edge: TREM-2 attenuates macrophage activation. J Immunol. 2006;177:3520–4.
51. Bhattacharjee S, Zhao Y, Dua P, Rogaev EI, Lukiw WJ. microRNA-34a-Mediated Down-Regulation of the Microglial-Enriched Triggering Receptor and Phagocytosis-Sensor TREM2 in Age-Related Macular Degeneration. PLoS One. 2016;11:e0150211.
52. Zheng H, Liu CC, Atagi Y, Chen XF, Jia L, Yang L, He W, Zhang X, Kang SS, Rosenberry TL, et al. Opposing roles of the triggering receptor expressed on myeloid cells 2 and triggering receptor expressed on myeloid cells-like transcript 2 in microglia activation. Neurobiol Aging. 2016;42:132–41.
53. Liu G, Liu Y, Jiang Q, Jiang Y, Feng R, Zhang L, Chen Z, Li K, Liu J. Convergent Genetic and Expression Datasets Highlight TREM2 in Parkinson's Disease Susceptibility. Mol Neurobiol. 2016;53:4931–8.
54. Cady J, Koval ED, Benitez BA, Zaidman C, Jockel-Balsarotti J, Allred P, Baloh RH, Ravits J, Simpson E, Appel SH, et al. TREM2 variant p.R47H as a risk factor for sporadic amyotrophic lateral sclerosis. JAMA Neurol. 2014;71:449–53.
55. Kawabori M, Kacimi R, Kauppinen T, Calosing C, Kim JY, Hsieh CL, Nakamura MC, Yenari MA. Triggering receptor expressed on myeloid cells 2 (TREM2) deficiency attenuates phagocytic activities of microglia and exacerbates ischemic damage in experimental stroke. J Neurosci. 2015;35:3384–96.
56. Saber M, Kokiko-Cochran O, Puntambekar SS, Lathia JD, Lamb BT. Triggering Receptor Expressed on Myeloid Cells 2 Deficiency Alters Acute Macrophage Distribution and Improves Recovery after Traumatic Brain Injury. J Neurotrauma. 2017;34:423–35.
57. Celarain N, Sanchez-Ruiz de Gordoa J, Zelaya MV, Roldan M, Larumbe R, Pulido L, Echavarri C, Mendioroz M. TREM2 upregulation correlates with 5-hydroxymethycytosine enrichment in Alzheimer's disease hippocampus. Clin Epigenetics. 2016;8:37.
58. Ma L, Allen M, Sakae N, Ertekin-Taner N, Graff-Radford NR, Dickson DW, Younkin SG, Sevlever D. Expression and processing analyses of wild type and p.R47H TREM2 variant in Alzheimer's disease brains. Mol Neurodegener. 2016;11:72.
59. Perez SE, Nadeem M, He B, Miguel JC, Malek-Ahmadi MH, Chen K, Mufson EJ. Neocortical and hippocampal TREM2 protein levels during the progression of Alzheimer's disease. Neurobiol Aging. 2017;54:133–43.
60. Raha AA, Henderson JW, Stott SR, Vuono R, Foscarin S, Friedland RP, Zaman SH, Raha-Chowdhury R. Neuroprotective Effect of TREM-2 in Aging and Alzheimer's Disease Model. J Alzheimers Dis. 2017;55:199–217.
61. Matarin M, Salih DA, Yasvoina M, Cummings DM, Guelfi S, Liu W, Nahaboo Solim MA, Moens TG, Paublete RM, Ali SS, et al. A genome-wide gene-expression analysis and database in transgenic mice during development of amyloid or tau pathology. Cell Rep. 2015;10:633–44.
62. Savage JC, Jay T, Goduni E, Quigley C, Mariani MM, Malm T, Ransohoff RM, Lamb BT, Landreth GE. Nuclear receptors license phagocytosis by trem2+ myeloid cells in mouse models of Alzheimer's disease. J Neurosci. 2015;35: 6532–43.
63. Jiang T, Tan L, Zhu XC, Zhang QQ, Cao L, Tan MS, Gu LZ, Wang HF, Ding ZZ, Zhang YD, Yu JT. Upregulation of TREM2 ameliorates neuropathology

and rescues spatial cognitive impairment in a transgenic mouse model of Alzheimer's disease. Neuropsychopharmacology. 2014;39:2949–62.
64. Yeh FL, Hansen DV, Sheng M. TREM2, Microglia, and Neurodegenerative Diseases. Trends Mol Med. 2017;23:512–33.
65. Daws MR, Lanier LL, Seaman WE, Ryan JC. Cloning and characterization of a novel mouse myeloid DAP12-associated receptor family. Eur J Immunol. 2001;31:783–91.
66. Lanier LL, Corliss BC, Wu J, Leong C, Phillips JH. Immunoreceptor DAP12 bearing a tyrosine-based activation motif is involved in activating NK cells. Nature. 1998;391:703–7.
67. Call ME, Wucherpfennig KW, Chou JJ. The structural basis for intramembrane assembly of an activating immunoreceptor complex. Nat Immunol. 2010;11:1023–9.
68. Mocsai A, Ruland J, Tybulewicz VL. The SYK tyrosine kinase: a crucial player in diverse biological functions. Nat Rev Immunol. 2010;10:387–402.
69. Sada K, Takano T, Yanagi S, Yamamura H. Structure and function of Syk protein-tyrosine kinase. J Biochem. 2001;130:177–86.
70. Sun M, Zhu M, Chen K, Nie X, Deng Q, Hazlett LD, Wu Y, Li M, Wu M, Huang X. TREM-2 promotes host resistance against Pseudomonas aeruginosa infection by suppressing corneal inflammation via a PI3K/Akt signaling pathway. Invest Ophthalmol Vis Sci. 2013;54:3451–62.
71. Peng Q, Malhotra S, Torchia JA, Kerr WG, Coggeshall KM, Humphrey MB. TREM2- and DAP12-dependent activation of PI3K requires DAP10 and is inhibited by SHIP1. Sci Signal. 2010;3:ra38.
72. Daws MR, Sullam PM, Niemi EC, Chen TT, Tchao NK, Seaman WE. Pattern recognition by TREM-2: binding of anionic ligands. J Immunol. 2003;171: 594–9.
73. Cannon JP, O'Driscoll M, Litman GW. Specific lipid recognition is a general feature of CD300 and TREM molecules. Immunogenetics. 2012;64:39–47.
74. Kober DL, Alexander-Brett JM, Karch CM, Cruchaga C, Colonna M, Holtzman MJ, Brett TJ. Neurodegenerative disease mutations in TREM2 reveal a functional surface and distinct loss-of-function mechanisms. Elife. 2016;5.
75. Wang Y, Cella M, Mallinson K, Ulrich JD, Young KL, Robinette ML, Gilfillan S, Krishnan GM, Sudhakar S, Zinselmeyer BH, et al. TREM2 lipid sensing sustains the microglial response in an Alzheimer's disease model. Cell. 2015; 160:1061–71.
76. Yeh FL, Wang Y, Tom I, Gonzalez LC, Sheng M. TREM2 Binds to Apolipoproteins, Including APOE and CLU/APOJ, and Thereby Facilitates Uptake of Amyloid-Beta by Microglia. Neuron. 2016;91:328–40.
77. Song W, Hooli B, Mullin K, Jin SC, Cella M, Ulland TK, Wang Y, Tanzi RE, Colonna M. Alzheimer's disease-associated TREM2 variants exhibit either decreased or increased ligand-dependent activation. Alzheimers Dement. 2017;13:381–7.
78. Atagi Y, Liu CC, Painter MM, Chen XF, Verbeeck C, Zheng H, Li X, Rademakers R, Kang SS, Xu H, et al. Apolipoprotein E Is a Ligand for Triggering Receptor Expressed on Myeloid Cells 2 (TREM2). J Biol Chem. 2015;290:26043–50.
79. Bailey CC, DeVaux LB, Farzan M. The Triggering Receptor Expressed on Myeloid Cells 2 Binds Apolipoprotein E. J Biol Chem. 2015;290:26033–42.
80. Jendresen C, Arskog V, Daws MR, Nilsson LN. The Alzheimer's disease risk factors apolipoprotein E and TREM2 are linked in a receptor signaling pathway. J Neuroinflammation. 2017;14:59.
81. Zhao Y, Wu X, Li X, Jiang LL, Gui X, Liu Y, Sun Y, Zhu B, Pina-Crespo JC, Zhang M, et al. TREM2 Is a Receptor for beta-Amyloid that Mediates Microglial Function. Neuron. 2018;97:1023–31 e1027.
82. Ulrich JD, Ulland TK, Mahan TE, Nystrom S, Nilsson KP, Song WM, Zhou Y, Reinartz M, Choi S, Jiang H, et al. ApoE facilitates the microglial response to amyloid plaque pathology. J Exp Med. 2018;215:1047–58.
83. Hsieh CL, Koike M, Spusta SC, Niemi EC, Yenari M, Nakamura MC, Seaman WE. A role for TREM2 ligands in the phagocytosis of apoptotic neuronal cells by microglia. J Neurochem. 2009;109:1144–56.
84. Gawish R, Martins R, Bohm B, Wimberger T, Sharif O, Lakovits K, Schmidt M, Knapp S. Triggering receptor expressed on myeloid cells-2 fine-tunes inflammatory responses in murine Gram-negative sepsis. FASEB J. 2015;29: 1247–57.
85. Kleinberger G, Yamanishi Y, Suarez-Calvet M, Czirr E, Lohmann E, Cuyvers E, Struyfs H, Pettkus N, Wenninger-Weinzierl A, Mazaheri F, et al. TREM2 mutations implicated in neurodegeneration impair cell surface transport and phagocytosis. Sci Transl Med. 2014;6:243ra286.
86. Stefano L, Racchetti G, Bianco F, Passini N, Gupta RS, Panina Bordignon P, Meldolesi J. The surface-exposed chaperone, Hsp60, is an agonist of the microglial TREM2 receptor. J Neurochem. 2009;110:284–94.
87. N'Diaye EN, Branda CS, Branda SS, Nevarez L, Colonna M, Lowell C, Hamerman JA, Seaman WE. TREM-2 (triggering receptor expressed on myeloid cells 2) is a phagocytic receptor for bacteria. J Cell Biol. 2009;184: 215–23.
88. Takahashi K, Prinz M, Stagi M, Chechneva O, Neumann H. TREM2-transduced myeloid precursors mediate nervous tissue debris clearance and facilitate recovery in an animal model of multiple sclerosis. PLoS Med. 2007;4:e124.
89. Wang Y, Ulland TK, Ulrich JD, Song W, Tzaferis JA, Hole JT, Yuan P, Mahan TE, Shi Y, Gilfillan S, et al. TREM2-mediated early microglial response limits diffusion and toxicity of amyloid plaques. J Exp Med. 2016;213:667–75.
90. Yuan P, Condello C, Keene CD, Wang Y, Bird TD, Paul SM, Luo W, Colonna M, Baddeley D, Grutzendler J. TREM2 Haplodeficiency in Mice and Humans Impairs the Microglia Barrier Function Leading to Decreased Amyloid Compaction and Severe Axonal Dystrophy. Neuron. 2016;90:724–39.
91. Hamerman JA, Tchao NK, Lowell CA, Lanier LL. Enhanced Toll-like receptor responses in the absence of signaling adaptor DAP12. Nat Immunol. 2005;6: 579–86.
92. Gao X, Dong Y, Liu Z, Niu B. Silencing of triggering receptor expressed on myeloid cells-2 enhances the inflammatory responses of alveolar macrophages to lipopolysaccharide. Mol Med Rep. 2013;7:921–6.
93. Zhong L, Chen XF, Zhang ZL, Wang Z, Shi XZ, Xu K, Zhang YW, Xu H, Bu G. DAP12 Stabilizes the C-terminal Fragment of the Triggering Receptor Expressed on Myeloid Cells-2 (TREM2) and Protects against LPS-induced Pro-inflammatory Response. J Biol Chem. 2015;290:15866–77.
94. Piccio L, Buonsanti C, Mariani M, Cella M, Gilfillan S, Cross AH, Colonna M, Panina-Bordignon P. Blockade of TREM-2 exacerbates experimental autoimmune encephalomyelitis. Eur J Immunol. 2007;37:1290–301.
95. Krasemann S, Madore C, Cialic R, Baufeld C, Calcagno N, El Fatimy R, Beckers L, O'Loughlin E, Xu Y, Fanek Z, et al. The TREM2-APOE Pathway Drives the Transcriptional Phenotype of Dysfunctional Microglia in Neurodegenerative Diseases. Immunity. 2017;47:566–81 e569.
96. Kobayashi M, Konishi H, Sayo A, Takai T, Kiyama H. TREM2/DAP12 Signal Elicits Proinflammatory Response in Microglia and Exacerbates Neuropathic Pain. J Neurosci. 2016;36:11138–50.
97. Zheng H, Jia L, Liu CC, Rong Z, Zhong L, Yang L, Chen XF, Fryer JD, Wang X, Zhang YW, et al. TREM2 Promotes Microglial Survival by Activating Wnt/beta-Catenin Pathway. J Neurosci. 2017;37:1772–84.
98. Seno H, Miyoshi H, Brown SL, Geske MJ, Colonna M, Stappenbeck TS. Efficient colonic mucosal wound repair requires Trem2 signaling. Proc Natl Acad Sci U S A. 2009;106:256–61.
99. Wu K, Byers DE, Jin X, Agapov E, Alexander-Brett J, Patel AC, Cella M, Gilfilan S, Colonna M, Kober DL, et al. TREM-2 promotes macrophage survival and lung disease after respiratory viral infection. J Exp Med. 2015;212:681–97.
100. Bianchin MM, Capella HM, Chaves DL, Steindel M, Grisard EC, Ganev GG, da Silva Junior JP, Neto Evaldo S, Poffo MA, Walz R, et al. Nasu-Hakola disease (polycystic lipomembranous osteodysplasia with sclerosing leukoencephalopathy--PLOSL): a dementia associated with bone cystic lesions. From clinical to genetic and molecular aspects. Cell Mol Neurobiol. 2004;24:1–24.
101. Paloneva J, Manninen T, Christman G, Hovanes K, Mandelin J, Adolfsson R, Bianchin M, Bird T, Miranda R, Salmaggi A, et al. Mutations in two genes encoding different subunits of a receptor signaling complex result in an identical disease phenotype. Am J Hum Genet. 2002;71:656–62.
102. Lill CM, Rengmark A, Pihlstrom L, Fogh I, Shatunov A, Sleiman PM, Wang LS, Liu T, Lassen CF, Meissner E, et al. The role of TREM2 R47H as a risk factor for Alzheimer's disease, frontotemporal lobar degeneration, amyotrophic lateral sclerosis, and Parkinson's disease. Alzheimers Dement. 2015;11:1407–16.
103. Rayaprolu S, Mullen B, Baker M, Lynch T, Finger E, Seeley WW, Hatanpaa KJ, Lomen-Hoerth C, Kertesz A, Bigio EH, et al. TREM2 in neurodegeneration: evidence for association of the p.R47H variant with frontotemporal dementia and Parkinson's disease. Mol Neurodegener. 2013;8:19.
104. Ruiz A, Dols-Icardo O, Bullido MJ, Pastor P, Rodriguez-Rodriguez E, Lopez de Munain A, de Pancorbo MM, Perez-Tur J, Alvarez V, Antonell A, et al. Assessing the role of the TREM2 p.R47H variant as a risk factor for Alzheimer's disease and frontotemporal dementia. Neurobiol Aging. 2014; 35(444):e441–4.
105. Cuyvers E, Bettens K, Philtjens S, Van Langenhove T, Gijselinck I, van der Zee J, Engelborghs S, Vandenbulcke M, Van Dongen J, Geerts N, et al.

Investigating the role of rare heterozygous TREM2 variants in Alzheimer's disease and frontotemporal dementia. Neurobiol Aging. 2014;35(726):e711–29.
106. Lattante S, Le Ber I, Camuzat A, Dayan S, Godard C, Van Bortel I, De Septenville A, Ciura S, Brice A, Kabashi E, et al. TREM2 mutations are rare in a French cohort of patients with frontotemporal dementia. Neurobiol Aging. 2013;34(2443):e2441–2.
107. Slattery CF, Beck JA, Harper L, Adamson G, Abdi Z, Uphill J, Campbell T, Druyeh R, Mahoney CJ, Rohrer JD, et al. R47H TREM2 variant increases risk of typical early-onset Alzheimer's disease but not of prion or frontotemporal dementia. Alzheimers Dement. 2014;10:602–8 e604.
108. Guerreiro R, Wojtas A, Bras J, Carrasquillo M, Rogaeva E, Majounie E, Cruchaga C, Sassi C, Kauwe JS, Younkin S, et al. TREM2 variants in Alzheimer's disease. N Engl J Med. 2013;368:117–27.
109. Jonsson T, Stefansson H, Steinberg S, Jonsdottir I, Jonsson PV, Snaedal J, Bjornsson S, Huttenlocher J, Levey AI, Lah JJ, et al. Variant of TREM2 associated with the risk of Alzheimer's disease. N Engl J Med. 2013;368:107–16.
110. Benitez BA, Cooper B, Pastor P, Jin SC, Lorenzo E, Cervantes S, Cruchaga C. TREM2 is associated with the risk of Alzheimer's disease in Spanish population. Neurobiol Aging. 2013;34(1711):e1715–7.
111. Finelli D, Rollinson S, Harris J, Jones M, Richardson A, Gerhard A, Snowden J, Mann D, Pickering-Brown S. TREM2 analysis and increased risk of Alzheimer's disease. Neurobiol Aging. 2015;36(546):e549–13.
112. Ghani M, Sato C, Kakhki EG, Gibbs JR, Traynor B, St George-Hyslop P, Rogaeva E. Mutation analysis of the MS4A and TREM gene clusters in a case-control Alzheimer's disease data set. Neurobiol Aging. 2016;42(217):e217–3.
113. Gonzalez Murcia JD, Schmutz C, Munger C, Perkes A, Gustin A, Peterson M, Ebbert MT, Norton MC, Tschanz JT, Munger RG, et al. Assessment of TREM2 rs75932628 association with Alzheimer's disease in a population-based sample: the Cache County Study. Neurobiol Aging. 2013;34(2889):e2811–83.
114. Hooli BV, Parrado AR, Mullin K, Yip WK, Liu T, Roehr JT, Qiao D, Jessen F, Peters O, Becker T, et al. The rare TREM2 R47H variant exerts only a modest effect on Alzheimer disease risk. Neurology. 2014;83:1353–8.
115. Jin SC, Benitez BA, Karch CM, Cooper B, Skorupa T, Carrell D, Norton JB, Hsu S, Harari O, Cai Y, et al. Coding variants in TREM2 increase risk for Alzheimer's disease. Hum Mol Genet. 2014;23:5838–46.
116. Pottier C, Wallon D, Rousseau S, Rovelet-Lecrux A, Richard AC, Rollin-Sillaire A, Frebourg T, Campion D, Hannequin D. TREM2 R47H variant as a risk factor for early-onset Alzheimer's disease. J Alzheimers Dis. 2013;35:45–9.
117. Rosenthal SL, Bamne MN, Wang X, Berman S, Snitz BE, Klunk WE, Sweet RA, Demirci FY, Lopez OL, Kamboh MI. More evidence for association of a rare TREM2 mutation (R47H) with Alzheimer's disease risk. Neurobiol Aging. 2015;36(2443):e2421–46.
118. Sims R, van der Lee SJ, Naj AC, Bellenguez C, Badarinarayan N, Jakobsdottir J, Kunkle BW, Boland A, Raybould R, Bis JC, et al. Rare coding variants in PLCG2, ABI3, and TREM2 implicate microglial-mediated innate immunity in Alzheimer's disease. Nat Genet. 2017;49:1373–84.
119. Yu JT, Jiang T, Wang YL, Wang HF, Zhang W, Hu N, Tan L, Sun L, Tan MS, Zhu XC, Tan L. Triggering receptor expressed on myeloid cells 2 variant is rare in late-onset Alzheimer's disease in Han Chinese individuals. Neurobiol Aging. 2014;35(937):e931–3.
120. Wang P, Guo Q, Zhou Y, Chen K, Xu Y, Ding D, Hong Z, Zhao Q. Lack of association between triggering receptor expressed on myeloid cells 2 polymorphism rs75932628 and late-onset Alzheimer's disease in a Chinese Han population. Psychiatr Genet. 2018;28:16–8.
121. Ma J, Zhou Y, Xu J, Liu X, Wang Y, Deng Y, Wang G, Xu W, Ren R, Liu X, et al. Association study of TREM2 polymorphism rs75932628 with late-onset Alzheimer's disease in Chinese Han population. Neurol Res. 2014;36:894–6.
122. Jiao B, Liu X, Tang B, Hou L, Zhou L, Zhang F, Zhou Y, Guo J, Yan X, Shen L. Investigation of TREM2, PLD3, and UNC5C variants in patients with Alzheimer's disease from mainland China. Neurobiol Aging. 2014;35(2422): e2429–2 e2411.
123. Jin SC, Carrasquillo MM, Benitez BA, Skorupa T, Carrell D, Patel D, Lincoln S, Krishnan S, Kachadoorian M, Reitz C, et al. TREM2 is associated with increased risk for Alzheimer's disease in African Americans. Mol Neurodegener. 2015;10:19.
124. Del-Aguila JL, Fernandez MV, Schindler S, Ibanez L, Deming Y, Ma S, Saef B, Black K, Budde J, Norton J, et al. Assessment of the Genetic Architecture of Alzheimer's Disease Risk in Rate of Memory Decline. J Alzheimers Dis. 2018; 62:745–56.
125. Korvatska O, Leverenz JB, Jayadev S, McMillan P, Kurtz I, Guo X, Rumbaugh M, Matsushita M, Girirajan S, Dorschner MO, et al. R47H Variant of TREM2 Associated With Alzheimer Disease in a Large Late-Onset Family: Clinical, Genetic, and Neuropathological Study. JAMA Neurol. 2015;72:920–7.
126. Roussos P, Katsel P, Fam P, Tan W, Purohit DP, Haroutunian V. The triggering receptor expressed on myeloid cells 2 (TREM2) is associated with enhanced inflammation, neuropathological lesions and increased risk for Alzheimer's dementia. Alzheimers Dement. 2015;11:1163–70.
127. Melchior B, Garcia AE, Hsiung BK, Lo KM, Doose JM, Thrash JC, Stalder AK, Staufenbiel M, Neumann H, Carson MJ. Dual induction of TREM2 and tolerance-related transcript, Tmem176b, in amyloid transgenic mice: implications for vaccine-based therapies for Alzheimer's disease. ASN Neuro. 2010;2:e00037.
128. Radde R, Bolmont T, Kaeser SA, Coomaraswamy J, Lindau D, Stoltze L, Calhoun ME, Jaggi F, Wolburg H, Gengler S, et al. Abeta42-driven cerebral amyloidosis in transgenic mice reveals early and robust pathology. EMBO Rep. 2006;7:940–6.
129. Oakley H, Cole SL, Logan S, Maus E, Shao P, Craft J, Guillozet-Bongaarts A, Ohno M, Disterhoft J, Van Eldik L, et al. Intraneuronal beta-amyloid aggregates, neurodegeneration, and neuron loss in transgenic mice with five familial Alzheimer's disease mutations: potential factors in amyloid plaque formation. J Neurosci. 2006;26:10129–40.
130. Ulrich JD, Finn MB, Wang Y, Shen A, Mahan TE, Jiang H, Stewart FR, Piccio L, Colonna M, Holtzman DM. Altered microglial response to Abeta plaques in APPPS1-21 mice heterozygous for TREM2. Mol Neurodegener. 2014;9:20.
131. Jay TR, Hirsch AM, Broihier ML, Miller CM, Neilson LE, Ransohoff RM, Lamb BT, Landreth GE. Disease Progression-Dependent Effects of TREM2 Deficiency in a Mouse Model of Alzheimer's Disease. J Neurosci. 2017;37: 637–47.
132. Song WM, Joshita S, Zhou Y, Ulland TK, Gilfillan S, Colonna M. Humanized TREM2 mice reveal microglia-intrinsic and -extrinsic effects of R47H polymorphism. J Exp Med. 2018;215:745–60.
133. Cheng-Hathaway PJ, Reed-Geaghan EG, Jay TR, Casali BT, Bemiller SM, Puntambekar SS, von Saucken VE, Williams RY, Karlo JC, Moutinho M, et al. The Trem2 R47H variant confers loss-of-function-like phenotypes in Alzheimer's disease. Mol Neurodegener. 2018;13:29.
134. Ulland TK, Song WM, Huang SC, Ulrich JD, Sergushichev A, Beatty WL, Loboda AA, Zhou Y, Cairns NJ, Kambal A, et al. TREM2 Maintains Microglial Metabolic Fitness in Alzheimer's Disease. Cell. 2017;170:649–63 e613.
135. Lee CYD, Daggett A, Gu X, Jiang LL, Langfelder P, Li X, Wang N, Zhao Y, Park CS, Cooper Y, et al. Elevated TREM2 Gene Dosage Reprograms Microglia Responsivity and Ameliorates Pathological Phenotypes in Alzheimer's Disease Models. Neuron. 2018;97:1032–48 e1035.
136. Yuan P, Condello C, Keene CD, Wang Y, Bird TD, Paul SM, Luo W, Colonna M, Baddeley D, Grutzendler J. TREM2 Haplodeficiency in Mice and Humans Impairs the Microglia Barrier Function Leading to Decreased Amyloid Compaction and Severe Axonal Dystrophy. Neuron. 2016;92:252–64.
137. Zhong L, Wang Z, Wang D, Wang Z, Martens YA, Wu L, Xu Y, Wang K, Li J, Huang R, et al. Amyloid-beta modulates microglial responses by binding to the triggering receptor expressed on myeloid cells 2 (TREM2). Mol Neurodegener. 2018;13:15.
138. Xiang X, Piers TM, Wefers B, Zhu K, Mallach A, Brunner B, Kleinberger G, Song W, Colonna M, Herms J, et al. The Trem2 R47H Alzheimer's risk variant impairs splicing and reduces Trem2 mRNA and protein in mice but not in humans. Mol Neurodegener. 2018;13:49.
139. Piccio L, Deming Y, Del-Aguila JL, Ghezzi L, Holtzman DM, Fagan AM, Fenoglio C, Galimberti D, Borroni B, Cruchaga C. Cerebrospinal fluid soluble TREM2 is higher in Alzheimer disease and associated with mutation status. Acta Neuropathol. 2016;131:925–33.
140. Cruchaga C, Kauwe JS, Harari O, Jin SC, Cai Y, Karch CM, Benitez BA, Jeng AT, Skorupa T, Carrell D, et al. GWAS of cerebrospinal fluid tau levels identifies risk variants for Alzheimer's disease. Neuron. 2013;78:256–68.
141. Buerger K, Ewers M, Pirttila T, Zinkowski R, Alafuzoff I, Teipel SJ, DeBernardis J, Kerkman D, McCulloch C, Soininen H, Hampel H. CSF phosphorylated tau protein correlates with neocortical neurofibrillary pathology in Alzheimer's disease. Brain. 2006;129:3035–41.
142. Andersson C, Blennow K, Almkvist O, Andreasen N, Engfeldt P, Johansson SE, Lindau M, Eriksdotter-Jonhagen M. Increasing CSF phospho-tau levels during cognitive decline and progression to dementia. Neurobiol Aging. 2008;29:1466–73.
143. de Leon MJ, DeSanti S, Zinkowski R, Mehta PD, Pratico D, Segal S, Clark C, Kerkman D, DeBernardis J, Li J, et al. MRI and CSF studies in the early diagnosis of Alzheimer's disease. J Intern Med. 2004;256:205–23.

144. Cherry JD, Tripodis Y, Alvarez VE, Huber B, Kiernan PT, Daneshvar DH, Mez J, Montenigro PH, Solomon TM, Alosco ML, et al. Microglial neuroinflammation contributes to tau accumulation in chronic traumatic encephalopathy. Acta Neuropathol Commun. 2016;4:112.
145. Luo W, Liu W, Hu X, Hanna M, Caravaca A, Paul SM. Microglial internalization and degradation of pathological tau is enhanced by an anti-tau monoclonal antibody. Sci Rep. 2015;5:11161.
146. Maphis N, Xu G, Kokiko-Cochran ON, Jiang S, Cardona A, Ransohoff RM, Lamb BT, Bhaskar K. Reactive microglia drive tau pathology and contribute to the spreading of pathological tau in the brain. Brain. 2015;138:1738–55.
147. Asai H, Ikezu S, Tsunoda S, Medalla M, Luebke J, Haydar T, Wolozin B, Butovsky O, Kugler S, Ikezu T. Depletion of microglia and inhibition of exosome synthesis halt tau propagation. Nat Neurosci. 2015;18:1584–93.
148. Jiang Y, Li Z, Ma H, Cao X, Liu F, Tian A, Sun X, Li X, Wang J. Upregulation of TREM2 Ameliorates Neuroinflammatory Responses and Improves Cognitive Deficits Triggered by Surgical Trauma in Appswe/PS1dE9 Mice. Cell Physiol Biochem. 2018;46:1398–411.
149. Jiang T, Zhang YD, Chen Q, Gao Q, Zhu XC, Zhou JS, Shi JQ, Lu H, Tan L, Yu JT. TREM2 modifies microglial phenotype and provides neuroprotection in P301S tau transgenic mice. Neuropharmacology. 2016;105:196–206.
150. Jiang T, Tan L, Zhu XC, Zhou JS, Cao L, Tan MS, Wang HF, Chen Q, Zhang YD, Yu JT. Silencing of TREM2 exacerbates tau pathology, neurodegenerative changes, and spatial learning deficits in P301S tau transgenic mice. Neurobiol Aging. 2015;36:3176–86.
151. Bemiller SM, McCray TJ, Allan K, Formica SV, Xu G, Wilson G, Kokiko-Cochran ON, Crish SD, Lasagna-Reeves CA, Ransohoff RM, et al. TREM2 deficiency exacerbates tau pathology through dysregulated kinase signaling in a mouse model of tauopathy. Mol Neurodegener. 2017;12:74.
152. Leyns CEG, Ulrich JD, Finn MB, Stewart FR, Koscal LJ, Remolina Serrano J, Robinson GO, Anderson E, Colonna M, Holtzman DM. TREM2 deficiency attenuates neuroinflammation and protects against neurodegeneration in a mouse model of tauopathy. Proc Natl Acad Sci U S A. 2017;114:11524–9.
153. Sayed FA, Telpoukhovskaia M, Kodama L, Li Y, Zhou Y, Le D, Hauduc A, Ludwig C, Gao F, Clelland C, et al. Differential effects of partial and complete loss of TREM2 on microglial injury response and tauopathy. Proc Natl Acad Sci U S A. 2018;115:10172–7.
154. Andorfer C, Kress Y, Espinoza M, de Silva R, Tucker KL, Barde YA, Duff K, Davies P. Hyperphosphorylation and aggregation of tau in mice expressing normal human tau isoforms. J Neurochem. 2003;86:582–90.
155. Sekiya M, Wang M, Fujisaki N, Sakakibara Y, Quan X, Ehrlich ME, De Jager PL, Bennett DA, Schadt EE, Gandy S, et al. Integrated biology approach reveals molecular and pathological interactions among Alzheimer's Abeta42, Tau, TREM2, and TYROBP in Drosophila models. Genome Med. 2018;10:26.
156. Jiang T, Zhang YD, Gao Q, Ou Z, Gong PY, Shi JQ, Wu L, Zhou JS. TREM2 Ameliorates Neuronal Tau Pathology Through Suppression of Microglial Inflammatory Response. Inflammation. 2018;41:811–23.
157. Guerreiro R, Bras J, Hardy J. SnapShot: genetics of Alzheimer's disease. Cell. 2013;155:968 e961.
158. Casati M, Ferri E, Gussago C, Mazzola P, Abbate C, Bellelli G, Mari D, Cesari M, Arosio B. Increased expression of TREM2 in peripheral cells from mild cognitive impairment patients who progress into Alzheimer's disease. Eur J Neurol. 2018;25:805–10.
159. Li X, Montine KS, Keene CD, Montine TJ. Different mechanisms of apolipoprotein E isoform-dependent modulation of prostaglandin E2 production and triggering receptor expressed on myeloid cells 2 (TREM2) expression after innate immune activation of microglia. FASEB J. 2015;29: 1754–62.
160. Murray CE, King A, Troakes C, Hodges A, Lashley T. APOE epsilon4 is also required in TREM2 R47H variant carriers for Alzheimer's disease to develop. Neuropathol Appl Neurobiol. 2018.
161. Mazaheri F, Snaidero N, Kleinberger G, Madore C, Daria A, Werner G, Krasemann S, Capell A, Trumbach D, Wurst W, et al. TREM2 deficiency impairs chemotaxis and microglial responses to neuronal injury. EMBO Rep. 2017;18:1186–98.
162. Butovsky O, Jedrychowski MP, Moore CS, Cialic R, Lanser AJ, Gabriely G, Koeglsperger T, Dake B, Wu PM, Doykan CE, et al. Identification of a unique TGF-beta-dependent molecular and functional signature in microglia. Nat Neurosci. 2014;17:131–43.
163. Zemek F, Drtinova L, Nepovimova E, Sepsova V, Korabecny J, Klimes J, Kuca K. Outcomes of Alzheimer's disease therapy with acetylcholinesterase inhibitors and memantine. Expert Opin Drug Saf. 2014;13:759–74.
164. Cuyvers E, Sleegers K. Genetic variations underlying Alzheimer's disease: evidence from genome-wide association studies and beyond. Lancet Neurol. 2016;15:857–68.
165. Xiang X, Werner G, Bohrmann B, Liesz A, Mazaheri F, Capell A, Feederle R, Knuesel I, Kleinberger G, Haass C. TREM2 deficiency reduces the efficacy of immunotherapeutic amyloid clearance. EMBO Mol Med. 2016;8:992–1004.
166. Tremblay ME, Stevens B, Sierra A, Wake H, Bessis A, Nimmerjahn A. The role of microglia in the healthy brain. J Neurosci. 2011;31:16064–9.

7

A multifunctional therapeutic approach to disease modification in multiple familial mouse models and a novel sporadic model of Alzheimer's disease

Jia Luo[1], Sue H. Lee[1], Lawren VandeVrede[1], Zhihui Qin[1], Manel Ben Aissa[1,5], John Larson[2], Andrew F. Teich[3], Ottavio Arancio[3], Yohan D'Souza[4], Ahmed Elharram[4], Kevin Koster[5], Leon M. Tai[5], Mary Jo LaDu[5], Brian M. Bennett[4] and Gregory R. J. Thatcher[1*]

Abstract

Background: Clinical failures singularly targeting amyloid-β pathology indicate a critical need for alternative Alzheimer's disease (AD) therapeutic strategies. The mixed pathology reported in a large population of AD patients demands a multifunctional drug approach. Since activation of cAMP response element binding protein (CREB) plays a crucial role in synaptic strengthening and memory formation, we retooled a clinical drug with known neuroprotective and anti-inflammatory activity to activate CREB, and validated this novel multifunctional drug, NMZ, in 4 different mouse models of AD.

Results: NMZ was tested in three mouse models of familial AD and one model of sporadic AD. In 3 × Tg hippocampal slices, NMZ restored LTP. In vivo, memory was improved with NMZ in all animal models with robust cognitive deficits. NMZ treatment lowered neurotoxic forms of Aβ in both APP/PS1 and 3 × Tg transgenic mice while also restoring neuronal plasticity biomarkers in the 3 × Tg mice. In EFAD mice, incorporation of the major genetic AD risk factor, h*APOE4*, did not mute the beneficial drug effects. In a novel sporadic mouse model that manifests AD-like pathology caused by accelerated oxidative stress in the absence of any familial AD mutation, oral administration of NMZ attenuated hallmark AD pathology and restored biomarkers of synaptic and neuronal function.

Conclusions: The multifunctional approach, embodied by NMZ, was successful in mouse models of AD incorporating Aβ pathology (APP/PS1), tau pathology (3xTg), and *APOE4*, the major human genetic risk factor for AD (EFAD). The efficacy observed in a novel model of sporadic AD (*Aldh2*$^{-/-}$) demonstrates that the therapeutic approach is not limited to rare, familial AD genetic mutations. The multifunctional drug, NMZ, was not designed directly to target Aβ and tau pathology; however, the attenuation of this hallmark pathology suggests the approach to be a highly promising, disease-modifying strategy for AD and mixed pathology dementia.

Keywords: CREB activation, NO/cGMP signaling, CMZ, NMZ, Neuroprotection, Alzheimer's disease modifying approach, Mixed pathology dementia, AD mouse models, *Aldh2*$^{-/-}$ mice

* Correspondence: thatcher@uic.edu
[1]Department of Medicinal Chemistry and Pharmacognosy, College of Pharmacy, University of Illinois at Chicago, Chicago, IL, USA
Full list of author information is available at the end of the article

Background

Alzheimer disease (AD), the most common form of dementia, has reached epidemic proportions, presenting a severe economic and social burden worldwide. Currently, no effective therapy exists. Early onset familial AD (FAD) which represents 1-4 % of cases [1], is linked to mutations in *APP*, *PS1*, and *PS2* which increase deposition of insoluble amyloid-β peptide (Aβ) [2]. According to the Amyloid Hypothesis, Aβ leads to neuronal death and the second hallmark neuropathology, tau-containing neurofibrillary tangles (NFT). Consequently, the search for AD therapeutics has been dominated by use of transgenic mouse models that overexpress mutant human genes linked to familial AD. Of AD cases, >96 % are multifactorial in origin, and importantly, hallmark AD pathology is often accompanied by other neuropathologic changes. Not unexpectedly, in this substantial population with AD neuropathology, the correlation of Aβ histopathology with cognitive decline is poor [3, 4]; providing one possible contributor to the failure of at least eight therapeutics in late stage clinical trials singularly targeting Aβ [5, 6]. While not dismissing a role for Aβ in AD pathogenesis, cogent arguments have been made that a new strategy is needed towards an effective pharmacotherapeutic response [7–10].

Expert opinion has recognized that AD treatment must target two or more factors in disease pathogenesis [8]. Drug repositioning is also attractive with particular promise shown by anticonvulsants [11]. Zendra (chlomethiazole, CMZ), an anticonvulsant with a history of clinical use, has been shown extensively to be neuroprotective against oxidative stress in animal models and targets inflammation, mitochondrial dysfunction, and excitotoxicity [12–14]; all of which are proposed to contribute to AD pathogenesis. CMZ is suggested as a potential component of future combination therapies for neuronal injury [14], and we have shown that CMZ protected primary neurons against oxygen glucose deprivation (OGD) and neurotoxic oligomeric Aβ (oAβ) insult [15]. Additional contributors to onset and progression of AD include early synaptic failure [16], cerebrovascular impairment [17], and depletion of neurotrophins [18]. We hypothesized that a small chemical modification to CMZ, as in the novel therapeutic agent, 4-methyl-5-(2-(nitrooxy) ethyl) thiazol-3-ium chloride (NMZ), would address these contributors (Fig. 1) [19, 20].

Our approach was inspired by the early work of Lipton [21] and that of Kandel linking nitric oxide (NO) and cyclic guanosine monophosphate (cGMP) to cAMP-response element binding protein (CREB) activation and long-term potentiation (LTP) [22]. Activation of CREB by phosphorylation has been shown to be necessary for memory formation and synaptic strengthening, therefore we hypothesized that the incorporation of a NO/cGMP signaling capability in NMZ would restore circuits dependent on CREB activation essential for learning and memory [23] (Fig. 1). Recent evidence links decreased CREB activity and dysregulated CREB-mediated gene regulation directly to the pathogenesis of AD [24–26]. Therefore NMZ, although not targeted at a specific component of Aβ accumulation, might reduce brain Aβ consequent to activation of NO/cGMP/CREB [27, 28]. We previously demonstrated that NMZ retained attributes of CMZ including potentiation of gamma-aminobutyric acid (GABA) signaling at the $GABA_A$ receptor [19, 20]. We also reported procognitive actions associated with NO/cGMP, including reversal of scopolamine-induced cognitive deficits, and demonstrated a high therapeutic index and efficacy at low nanomolar concentrations of NMZ in the brain [19].

Testing of NMZ was initiated in a variety of models demonstrating various subtypes of AD pathology, achieving a task set by expert opinion, in engagement of multiple targets in multiple AD transgenic models [8, 29]. First, NMZ was tested in the well-established young APP/PS1 and older 3 × Tg transgenic mouse models of FAD. LTP in hippocampal slices was restored by NMZ, in both APP/PS1 and 3 × Tg mice. Since human *apolipoprotein E4* (*APOE4*) [30] is the strongest genetic risk factor for sporadic AD, testing proceeded to the E4FAD AD mouse model that incorporates targeted replacement of mouse *APOE* with h*APOE4*. Oxidative stress is a primary driving force in AD pathogenesis [31, 32], linked to the lipid peroxidation product 4-hydroxynonenal (HNE) that accumulates in the brains of late-stage and presymptomatic AD patients, and is linked to apoE4 negative function [33, 34]. Loss of the enzyme aldehyde dehydrogenase 2 (ALDH2), which is important for 4-hydroxynonenal (4-HNE) detoxification, leads to HNE accumulation, neurodegeneration, and memory loss [35]. Therefore, NMZ was tested in the *Aldh2*$^{-/-}$ mouse that develops age-dependent cognitive deficits [36], providing validation of NMZ in a model of sporadic AD. NMZ, as a brain-bioavailable small molecule, was observed to protect against neuronal loss and synaptic dysfunction, improve memory, lower pro-inflammatory cytokines, and attenuate hallmark Alzheimer's pathology in these multiple mouse models.

Results

NMZ protects primary neurons from oAβ and oxygen glucose deprivation insult

NMZ retained the neuroprotective actions of CMZ [15], providing efficacy against OGD (Fig. 2a) and against exposure to oAβ (250nM or 5 μM). Cell viability was reduced by ~ 15 % and 60 % after vehicle treatment and exposure to oAβ, 250nM and 5 μM, respectively (Fig. 2b, c).

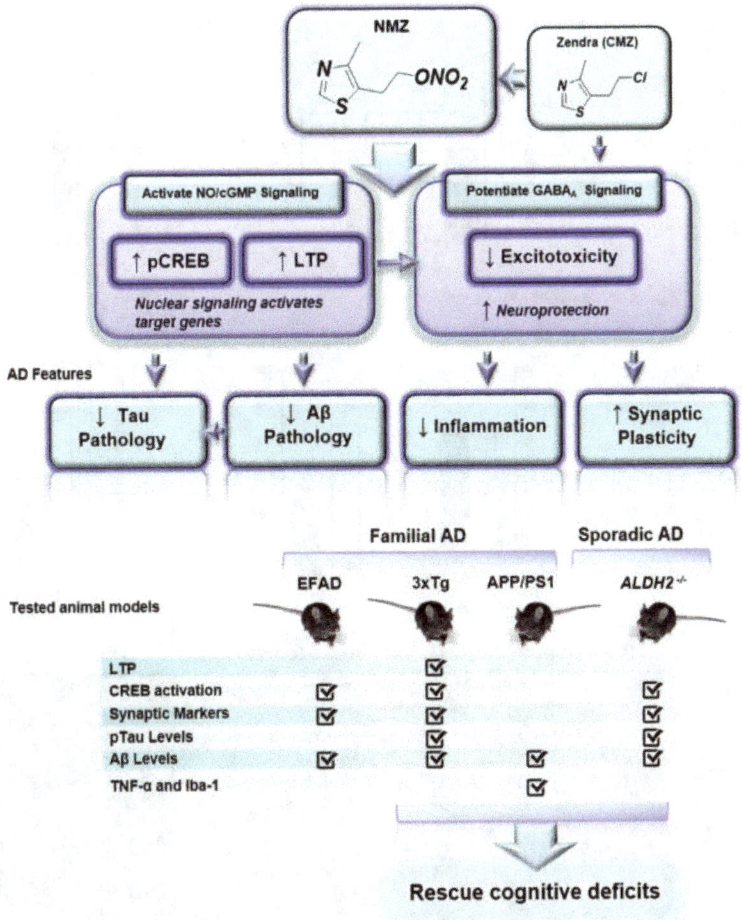

Fig. 1 Redesigning of the anticonvulsant Zendra for treatment of AD and dementia. The redesigned small molecule, NMZ, should retain the reported neuroprotective properties, while additionally targeting synaptic dysfunction, the case for which in AD is persuasive [16]. NMZ was designed to restore synaptic function via NO/cGMP/CREB signaling, and to retain the beneficial actions of CMZ. The desired activity profile was observed in multiple animal models on treatment with NMZ. Table indicates a summary of performed assays in used mouse models

NMZ demonstrated superior protection compared to CMZ in mitigating oxidative and low and high dose oAβ insults.

In APP/PS1 mice, NMZ restores cognition and lowers Aβ

NMZ was first tested in APP/PS1 double transgenic mice that manifest aberrant accumulation of human Aβ driven by FAD mutations in $APP_{695}{}^{K670N/M671L}$ and $PS1^{M146L}$. We have previously measured NMZ brain bioavailability and correlated brain levels with efficacy in cognition enhancement in scopolamine-induced amnestic mice, demonstrating that the brain concentration of NMZ required for memory consolidation after amnestic insult is approximately 0.5–1.0 nM [19]. Our previous PK/PD studies [19] guided dose selection herein, since NMZ was effective by both i.p. and p.o. drug administration at doses of 1 mg/kg and 20 mg/kg/day, respectively. Therefore, NMZ was administered at 1 mg/kg/day i.p. and 20 mg/kg/day in drinking water, treating randomized groups of both transgenic and age- and sex-matched wildtype (WT) littermates from 2.5 months of age for 12 weeks. In the last 2 weeks of treatment, animals were tested in the radial arm water maze (RAWM). NMZ treated transgenic animals performed significantly better than APP/PS1 control animals in trial blocks 2 and 4 ($p < 0.05$) (Fig. 2d).

In addition to improvement of cognition, whole brain homogenates were analyzed for various biomarkers. In whole brain homogenates, a significant reduction of oAβ was observed for NMZ treated animals for $A\beta_{1-42}$ species (Fig. 2e). Classic Aβ pathology was studied using quantitative Thioflavin S stereological analysis of serial coronal sections. NMZ treatment demonstrated almost a 3-fold reduction in Thioflavin S-positive Aβ deposit

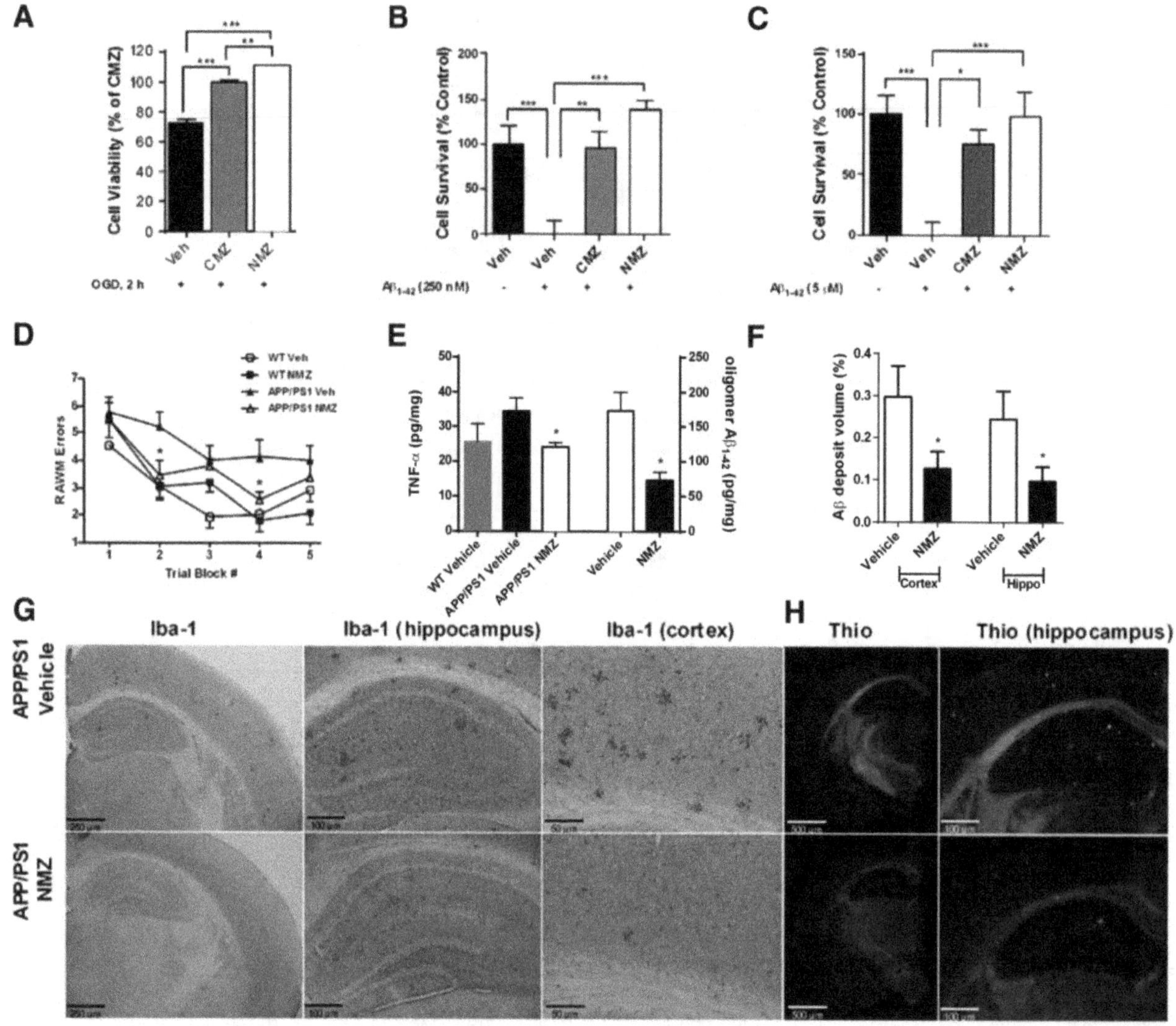

Fig. 2 Retention of neuroprotective activity (**a**-**c**) and the effects of NMZ treatment in APP/PS1 mice (**d**-**h**). Primary neuronal cultures treated with NMZ showed neuroprotection when exposed to 2 h OGD (**a**) and both low (**b**) and high (**c**) doses of Aβ oligomers. Data show mean ± S.E.M. normalized to insult and non-insult vehicle controls. Male APP/PS1 mice (n = 6–8) treated for 12 weeks with NMZ (1 mg/kg, i.p. plus 20 mg/kg/day in drinking water) demonstrated an improvement in the RAWM task (**d**) and reduction in levels of the pro-inflammatory marker, TNF-α, and in neurotoxic oAβ, in whole brain homogenates (**e**). Data show mean ± S.E.M compared to vehicle. NMZ also reduced total $A\beta_{1-42}$ deposit volumes compared to vehicle control in cortex and hippocampal homogenates (**f**). Data show mean ± S.E.M of total deposit volume determined by fluorescent staining and were analyzed by two-tailed student's *t*-test. All statistical significance is indicated by $^{*}p < 0.05$, $^{**}p < 0.01$, $^{***}p < 0.001$. Representative images of hippocampi and cortices with histochemical staining reveal significantly less activated microglia shown with Iba-1 (magnification: 4×, 10×, and 20× from left to right) (**g**) and reduced thioflavin-S staining of amyloid plaques in NMZ treatment compared to vehicle (magnification: 2× and 6×) (**h**)

volume in both the cortex and hippocampus (Fig. 2f and h). Lower levels of inflammatory markers in human blood and in rat models of hypoxia-ischemia in vivo and ex vivo, including the pro-inflammatory cytokine tumor necrosis factor alpha (TNF-α), have been reported previously for CMZ [12]. Total brain homogenates from APP/PS1 mice and WT littermates analyzed for TNF-α showed significant NMZ-induced reduction (Fig. 2e). This was mirrored by Iba-1 staining of coronal slices that showed reductions in activated microglia in the hippocampi and cortex of NMZ treated mice (Fig. 2g). Thus, in the one FAD model, in which WT mice are littermates, NMZ treatment significantly reduced elevation of TNF-α; a result compatible with the reported anti-inflammatory actions of CMZ.

In 3xTg mice, NMZ restores LTP via NO/cGMP, reverses cognitive deficits, and reduces Aβ and p-tau

The increased age of LaFerla's 3 × Tg ($APP_{695}^{K670N/M671L}$, $PS1^{M146L}$, tau^{P301L}) transgenic mouse model at treatment onset and the more complex pathology represents an increased therapeutic challenge. The effect of NMZ was first studied in LTP in the CA3-CA1 pathway in hippocampal slices from 16-month-old male mice [37]. Since the 3 × Tg is a homozygous line, the 129/SvJ x C57BL/6 background was used as an outbred line to provide control slices to give baseline performance. NMZ treatment resulted in a significant increase in fEPSP after LTP induction compared to untreated transgenics, to levels similar to WT control (Fig. 3a). To investigate the involvement of the

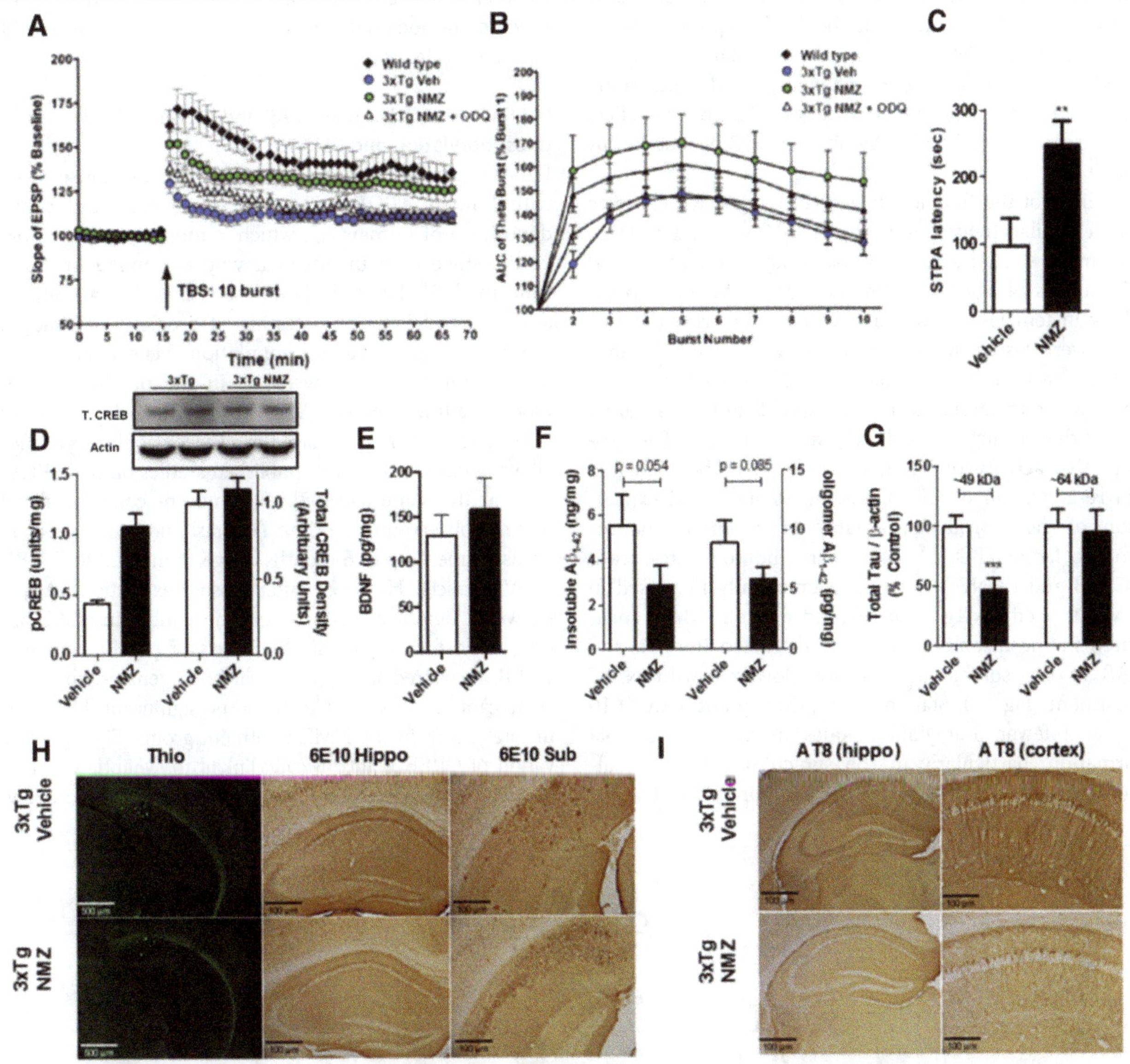

Fig. 3 NMZ treated 3xTg mice show improvements in LTP, behavior, synaptic biomarkers, and Aβ pathology. LTP was measured in the CA1 region of hippocampal sections from 16 month male 3 × Tg mice (n = 9-12) or in littermate controls treated with NMZ (50 μM) and ODQ (10 μM) 30 min prior to TBS and continued throughout. Fifty min after LTP induction, NMZ showed restoration of LTP deficits to WT levels, while ODQ completely blocked this activity (**a**). Analysis of theta bursts showed an increase by NMZ during induction of long-term potentiation (**b**). Data show mean ± S.E.M. normalized to baseline. Male and female 3xTg mice (n = 8–12) treated for 10 weeks with NMZ (1 mg/kg, i.p. + 20 mg/kg/day p.o) showed reversal of memory deficits to levels observed in WT mice in the STPA task 24 h after training (**c**). NMZ treatment resulted in an elevation of biomarkers associated with synaptic and neuronal plasticity (pCREB and BDNF) in whole brain homogenates measured by ELISA however not changing the total amount of total CREB measured by western blot (**d** and **e**). NMZ treatment attenuated insoluble and oligomeric Aβ (**f**) and total tau (**g**), both markers of AD hallmark pathology, in whole brain homogenates. Data show mean ± S.E.M. compared to vehicle control. Statistical significance is indicated by $^*p < 0.05$, $^{**}p < 0.01$, $^{***}p < 0.001$ and were analyzed by unpaired student's t-test. NMZ treatment showed a decrease in Aβ staining in the CA1 region of the hippocampus in treated animals but a negligible effect on the cortex. Representative images are shown with thioflavin-S (magnification 4×) staining and 6E10 antibody in the hippocampus (magnification 4×) and subiculum (magnification 10×) (**h**). AT8 immunohistochemistry in hippocampus and cortex (magnification 6× and 20×) showed a decrease in phosphorylated tau in the NMZ treated compared to the vehicle (**i**)

NO/cGMP pathway in the action of NMZ, ODQ (1H-[1, 2, 4] oxadiazolo-[4, 3-a] quinoxalin-1-one), a selective inhibitor of soluble guanylyl cyclase (sGC) was used to block cGMP production, and added 30 min prior to induction. LTP induced in the presence of both NMZ and ODQ was not significantly different to that obtained in untreated 3 × Tg slices. Examination of the field responses during theta-burst stimulation (TBS) indicated that NMZ facilitated LTP in 3 × Tg mice by enhancing the depolarization induced by the high frequency bursts (Fig. 3b); this effect was also attenuated by inhibition of cGMP production by ODQ.

In light of the findings in APP/PS1 mice, we chose to use a similar treatment protocol in 3 × Tg mice. Drug treatment started at 10 months of age for females and 12 months of age for males (to account for early pathology in females). In the last week of the trial, the animals were tested in the step through passive avoidance (STPA) task. The performance of NMZ treated 3 × Tg mice was comparable to untreated WT and significantly better than vehicle treated 3xTg mice (Fig. 3c). The pro-cognitive activity of NMZ is proposed to be mediated via re-activation of CREB, leading to increased expression of gene products, notably brain-derived neurotrophic factor (BDNF). In cerebral homogenates, both pCREB and BDNF levels were significantly increased in NMZ treated 3 × Tg mice (Fig. 3d and e). $A\beta_{1-42}$ measured in the insoluble guanidine extracted fraction and oAβ in the soluble fraction was lowered with NMZ treatment (Fig. 3f). Staining using the Aβ antibody 6E10 revealed fewer β-amyloid plaques in the hippocampal formation, particularly in the subiculum (Fig. 3h), although the cortex did not show a significant difference in plaque pathology. Immunohistochemical analysis using AT8 an antibody directed against phosphorylated tau showed a significant decrease in staining in the CA1 region of NMZ treated mouse brains (Fig. 3i). In contrast, total tau was unchanged, measured by western blot of total brain extract using antibody HT7 (a human-specific monoclonal antibody recognizing amino acids 159–163) (Fig. 3g).

In EFAD mice, NMZ lowers Aβ and elevates CREB phosphorylation and PSD-95

E4FAD mice carry targeted replacement of mouse *APOE* with human *APOE4*. The 5 × FAD background causes deposition of human Aβ, which is more severe in apoE4 carrier mice than in mice carrying the apoE2 or apoE3 isoforms [30]. The E4FAD mouse is therefore an important AD model for drug testing of predictive efficacy in the human apoE4 carrier population. Male E4FAD mice at 3.5 months of age were, as in the previous mouse models, administered NMZ i.p. (1 mg/kg/day) and p.o. in hydrogel (20 mg/kg/day) for 12 weeks before sacrifice, allowing comparison with published studies on male EFAD mice at the same age [38]. A significant cognitive deficit was not observed using the STPA task, nor nesting behavior assessment up to 6 months of age, compared to C57BL/6 WT mice. However, after tissue extraction, $A\beta_{1-42}$ showed a significant reduction in the soluble, insoluble and oligomeric forms (Fig. 4a, b). Levels of pCREB and total CREB, measured in hippocampal homogenates, showed a significant increase in pCREB and no significant differences in total CREB in the NMZ treatment group (Fig. 4c). Activation of CREB is intrinsically linked to synaptic function; and the scaffold protein, postsynaptic density protein 95

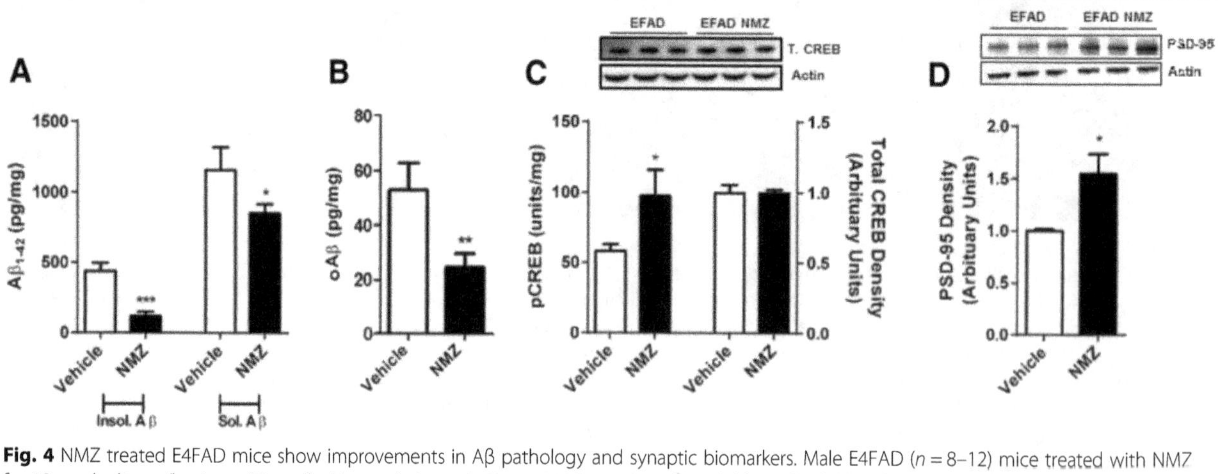

Fig. 4 NMZ treated E4FAD mice show improvements in Aβ pathology and synaptic biomarkers. Male E4FAD ($n = 8$–12) mice treated with NMZ for 12 weeks (1 mg/kg, i.p. + 20 mg/kg/day p.o.) showed attenuated formation of insoluble and soluble $A\beta_{1-42}$ (**a**) and oligomeric Aβ (**b**) in hippocampal homogenates measured by ELISA. NMZ treatment led to elevated pCREB in the hippocampal fraction (**c**) without a change in total CREB determined by western blot. NMZ treated mice restored levels of the synaptic marker PSD-95 determined by western blot (**d**). Data show mean ± S.E.M. compared to the vehicle control. Statistical significance is indicated by $^{*}p < 0.05$, $^{**}p < 0.01$, $^{***}p < 0.001$ and were analyzed by unpaired student's *t*-test

(PSD-95), plays a critical role in synaptic plasticity and synaptic dysfunction in AD [39, 40]. Immunoassay of homogenates from E4FAD mice showed a significant increase of PSD-95 in the hippocampus of E4FAD mic3 after treatment with NMZ (Fig. 4d).

In Aldh2 $^{-/-}$ mice, NMZ restores synaptic plasticity and attenuates AD hallmark pathology

Aldh2$^{-/-}$ mice, compared to age and sex-matched littermates, show a progressive decrease in performance, beginning at 2.5–3 months of age, in both the novel object recognition (NOR) and Y-maze tasks, measures of non-spatial and spatial working memory [36]. Given the positive outcomes of NMZ treatment in the three familial AD transgenic mouse models, we decided to forego i.p. delivery in *Aldh2*$^{-/-}$ mice, administering drug solely by the oral route (20 mg/kg/day) for 12 weeks from 3 months of age. The *Aldh2*$^{-/-}$ mouse represents a model for accelerated aging manifested by accumulation of lipid peroxidation products that fail to be cleared by Aldh2 enzyme action and pathology reflected by significantly increased levels of HNE-adducted proteins. We hypothesized that NMZ would counteract the downstream effects of this pathology on neuronal and synaptic function without impacting upstream HNE-adduct formation. Marked increases in HNE adduct formation occur early in *Aldh2*$^{-/-}$ mouse brains, characterized by increases in both the density and number of immunoreactive bands in immunoblots, which was not significantly perturbed by administration of NMZ (Fig. 5a). *Aldh2*$^{-/-}$ mice demonstrated age-related increases in soluble Aβ and phospho-tau that were significant at 6 months of age [36] and attenuated by NMZ treatment (Fig. 5b, c), without change in total tau. Age-related changes in synaptic and neuronal markers were also significantly attenuated by NMZ treatment (Fig. 5d), as were age-related increases in activated caspases 3 and 6 (Fig. 5e). These progressive biochemical changes linked to synaptic and neuronal dysfunction are intrinsically linked with AD in humans.

Aldh2$^{-/-}$ and WT mice were tested in the Y-maze and NOR before randomization into treatment groups. In both tasks, untreated *Aldh2*$^{-/-}$ mice showed a significant cognitive deficit that was more distinct with age; NMZ treatment having no effect on WT mice. A significant deficit was seen in *Aldh2*$^{-/-}$ mice prior to randomization; whereas, NMZ treated mice up to 6 months of age showed no cognitive deficit in the Y-maze and NOR (Fig. 6a, b).

A final ex vivo experiment was carried out using the acetylcholine receptor agonist, carbachol, applied to hippocampal slices from NMZ-treated *Aldh2*$^{-/-}$ mice, WT littermates, and their vehicle controls. Carbachol stimulation of hippocampal slices from 6 month old WT mice that had been administered NMZ or vehicle control for 12 weeks caused significant and similar elevation of pCREB (Fig. 6c). Slices from vehicle treated *Aldh2*$^{-/-}$ mice showed significantly attenuated basal pCREB response relative to WT and no significant effect of carbachol stimulation, whereas hippocampi from *Aldh2*$^{-/-}$ mice that had undergone NMZ treatment showed basal response and stimulation in response to carbachol comparable to WT littermates. NMZ treatment of *Aldh2*$^{-/-}$ mice was able to restore normal basal and stimulated pCREB signaling.

Discussion

The collected data presented herein profile an orally bioavailable small molecule, NMZ, that yields beneficial biochemical and functional outcomes in four diverse mouse models of Alzheimer's disease, building on animal data showing the ability of NMZ to restore memory consolidation in response to a variety of acute amnestic insults and in response to saporin-induced cholinergic lesions [19, 41]. Lowering brain Aβ levels has remained the primary and often exclusive target for therapeutic intervention in AD; however, the failure of such therapeutic agents to reach primary endpoints in phase 3 clinical trials, emphasizes the urgent need for new approaches. Nevertheless, any new therapeutic approach to AD should also positively impact hallmark neuropathology. NMZ targets multiple contributing mechanisms in AD and dementia. Beginning with the APP/PS1 mouse that manifests Aβ pathology and cognitive deficits, the efficacy of this approach was demonstrated. Adding tau pathology in older 3 × Tg mice and h*APOE4* in E4FAD mice did not blunt the efficacy of NMZ, which was also demonstrated in a novel mouse model of sporadic AD.

AD accounts for up to 80 % of dementia and half of those diagnosed with dementia have more than one pathology; for example vascular dementia, and dementia with Lewy bodies. However, in the population with AD pathology, Aβ histopathology with cognitive deficits have shown to be poorly correlated [3, 4], and Aβ-specific therapeutics might be expected to fail in this clinical population. AD is a multifactorial disease linked to other aging-associated maladies and to factors common to other neurodegenerative diseases, for example, glutamate excitotoxicity, oxidative stress, and inflammation [42]. Neuroprotective agents have been targeted to these and other contributors to neurodegeneration. For example, the clinical anticonvulsant Zendra/CMZ, was repurposed in Phase 3 clinical trials as a neuroprotective drug for use in spinal cord injury and ischemic stroke. CMZ, clinically prescribed for anxiety and agitation in the elderly, continues to be recommended as a component of combination therapy for stroke and neuronal injury [14]. GABA-potentiation [43] and TNF-α antagonism [44, 45] have been targeted for AD therapy and

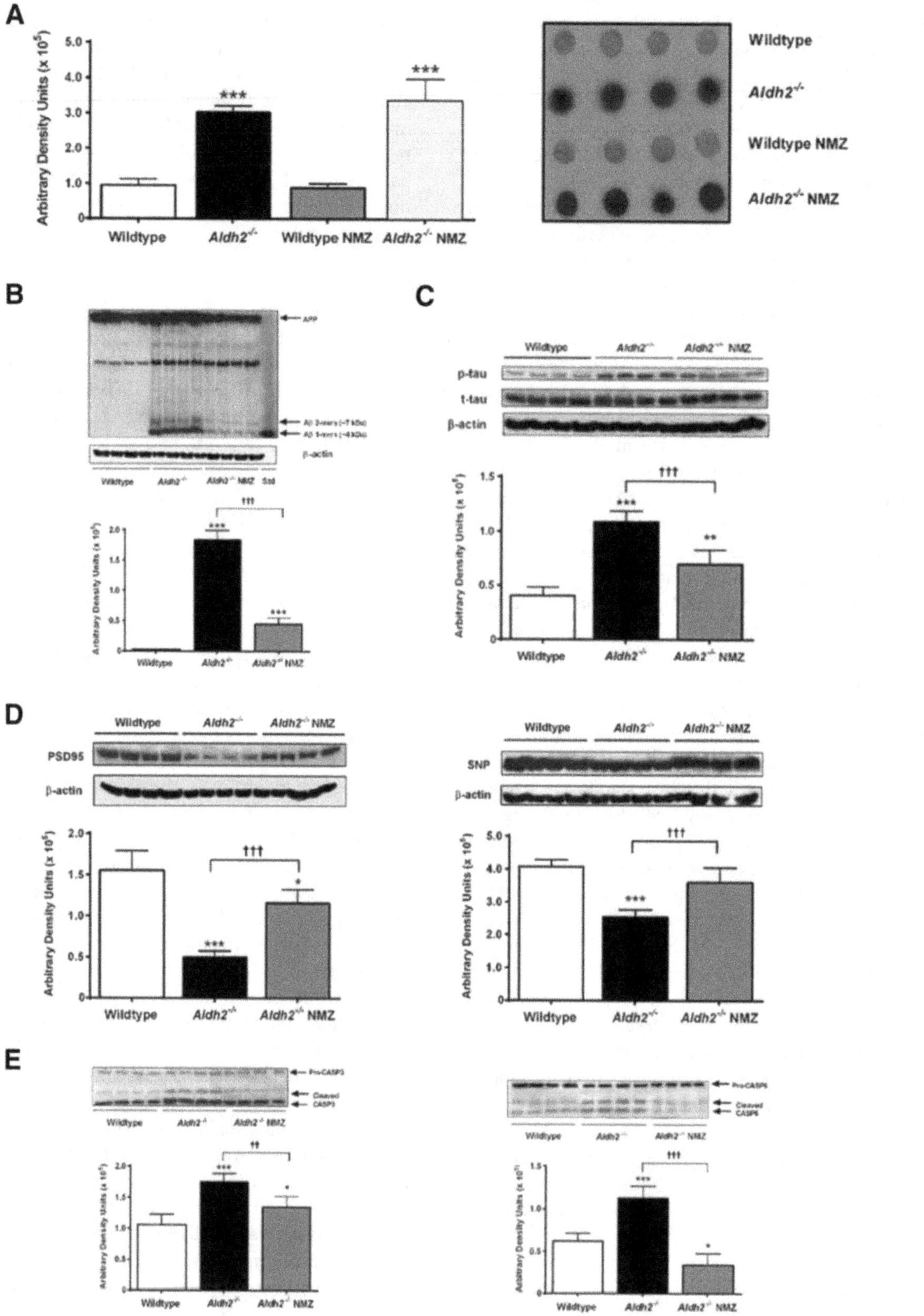

Fig. 5 (See legend on next page.)

(See figure on previous page.)
Fig. 5 NMZ treated Aldh2$^{-/-}$ mice show improvements in AD-like pathology, synaptic biomarkers and neuronal function. Hippocampal homogenates (30 µg protein) from *Aldh2$^{-/-}$* mice, treated with NMZ or vehicle for 12 weeks, showed no effect of NMZ on HNE adduct formation by dot-blot immunoassay of HNE protein adducts; whereas HNE adducts were significantly elevated relative to treated and untreated WT mice mice (**a**). Immunoblot analysis of hippocampal homogenates of WT and drug or vehicle treated *Aldh2$^{-/-}$* mice quantitated by densitometry with representative blots shown: monomeric Aβ (**b**) and p-tau (**c**); synaptic biomarkers PSD-95 and synaptophysin (**d**); and activated caspases (**e**). Data are presented as the mean ± S.D. and were analyzed by one-way ANOVA with Bonferroni post-hoc tests. Statistical significance is indicated by *$p < 0.05$, **$p < 0.01$, ***$p < 0.001$ compared with wildtype; †, significant difference from *Aldh2$^{-/-}$* (†† $p < 0.01$, ††† $p < 0.001$)

there is evidence that CMZ provides these attributes in addition to attenuation of mitochondrial and neuronal damage [12]. The early loss of synaptic function in both AD and mild cognitive impairment (MCI), which correlates with cognitive dysfunction and memory loss [46, 47], must be addressed; therefore CMZ, was chemically modified in the form of NMZ, to treat Alzheimer's and dementia [20] (Fig. 1). Importantly, NMZ was shown to retain the beneficial properties of CMZ [19].

Studies suggest that restoration of synaptic failure in AD can be achieved through CREB activation [48], and since CREB activation is coupled to NO/cGMP signaling in the hippocampus [22, 23], we hypothesized that incorporation of a CREB activating moiety would reactivate circuits associated with CREB which are vital to learning and memory [49]. NMZ was designed to activate CREB through the NO/cGMP signaling pathway [19], regulating the strength of synaptic transmission in an activity-dependent manner in the hippocampus [50] (Fig. 1). NMZ was effective in 3 × Tg mice, wherein LTP restoration was shown to be cGMP dependent (Fig. 3).

NMZ significantly restored cognitive function in different memory tasks in 6 month old APP/PS1 and 12–15 month old 3 × Tg mice (Figs. 2 and 3). Given this positive response in FAD mice to NMZ administered using daily i.p. delivery supplemented by oral delivery over 12 weeks, administration of NMZ to *Aldh2$^{-/-}$* mice was reduced to oral delivery alone. Working memory was measured in two further memory tasks (Fig. 6), showing a progressive decline in performance in *Aldh2$^{-/-}$* mice compared to the WT littermate control group. Before randomization for drug treatment at 2.5–3 months, *Aldh2$^{-/-}$* mice showed a deficit in both tasks. After 4 weeks treatment with NMZ, spontaneous alternation in the Y-maze was not different from that of WT controls; and after 8 weeks treatment, NOR performance recovered to that of WT controls. Thus, in 4 different behavioral assays of working and spatial memory and 3 different animal models, NMZ administration rescued the age-related decline in learning and memory.

Molecular network analysis and other clinical evidence converges on aberrant CREB-mediated gene regulation in the AD hippocampus [25, 26], compatible with the role of CREB phosphorylation in mediating synaptic plasticity through structural changes at synapses. In NMZ-treated 3×Tg, E4FAD, and *Aldh2$^{-/-}$* mice, levels of pCREB in either whole brain homogenates or hippocampi were significantly increased over vehicle control (Figs. 2, 3, 4 and 5). CREB acts upon downstream genes involved in synaptic and neuronal plasticity and neurogenesis, including BDNF. NMZ caused elevation of BDNF and of the protein biomarker of synaptic function, PSD-95 (Figs. 3, 4 and 5). The inability of CREB, in hippocampal slices from *Aldh2$^{-/-}$* mice, to respond to cholinergic stimulation further mirrors the loss of function of CREB in AD (Fig. 6). Given the evidence for direct dysregulation of CREB by oAβ and reciprocal regulation of amyloidogenesis by CREB [27, 28, 51], an agent that elevates pCREB and biomarkers of synaptic function in the AD brain may have a reciprocal and beneficial effect on production and/or clearance of Aβ. More direct links between NO/cGMP signaling and APP processing via beta-secretase-1 (BACE1) have been reported: the anti-amyloidogenic activity of an NO-donor was reported to be BACE1 and cGMP-dependent [52, 53], and intact endothelial NO synthase (eNOS) activity in the cerebral microvasculature [54] and brain tissues is linked with downregulation of BACE1 activity [52, 55, 56]. In three models of FAD, treatment with NMZ resulted in attenuated levels of Aβ (Figs. 2, 3, 4, 5 and 6).

Contemporary disease-modifying approaches to AD remain targeted at lowering brain Aβ aggregates, including immune-based approaches. Most recently the gantenerumab Aβ antibody was shown preferentially to bind aggregated brain Aβ and in APP/PS-1 mice, to reduce or halt Aβ plaque formation [57]; however, the Phase 3 clinical trial, in early stage symptomatic patients with evidence of amyloid, was halted in December 2014. Since AD is defined by the hallmark neuropathologies of aberrant Aβ and tau protein aggregates, any new disease-modifying therapy should attenuate these pathologies. The data presented herein for NMZ in 4 preclinical animal models suggest that therapeutic strategies targeting synaptic and neuronal dysfunction are also able to ameliorate hallmark pathology. NMZ treatment was shown to lower p-tau in the 3 × Tg mouse using antibodies that selectively recognize neurofibrillary filaments made up of hyperphosphorylated human tau and also to attenuate native p-tau formation in the *Aldh2$^{-/-}$* mouse (Figs. 3 and 5).

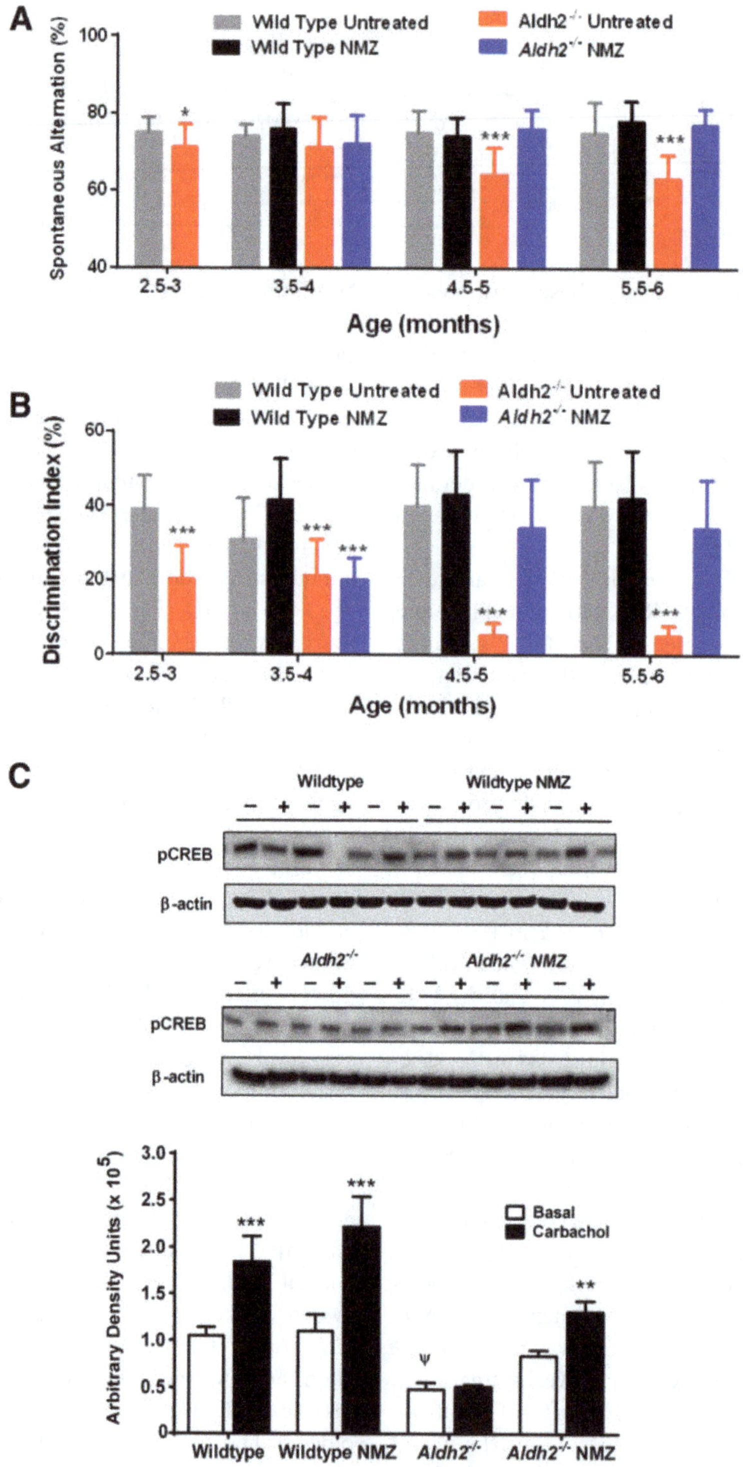

Fig. 6 (See legend on next page.)

(See figure on previous page.)
Fig. 6 NMZ-treated Aldh2$^{-/-}$ mice show rescued learning, memory and CREB responsiveness in carbachol treated hippocampal slices. Reversal of the age-dependent decline in the spontaneous alternation rate and discrimination index in the Y-maze task (**a**) and NOR task (**b**), respectively, was observed in male and female *Aldh2*$^{-/-}$ mice: after obtaining baseline measurements at 2.5–3 months, mice were randomized to drug or vehicle control groups ($n = 8$–11) and treated with NMZ (20/mg/kg/day p.o.) or vehicle at 3 months of age for a period of 12 weeks. Pre-randomization data were compared by an unpaired *t*-test and post-randomization groups by a one-way ANOVA with a Bonferroni post-hoc test. Hippocampal slices from 6 month old wild type and *Aldh2*$^{-/-}$ mice that had been treated with NMZ or vehicle control for 12 weeks, were incubated with 50 μM carbachol or vehicle (Basal) for 30 mins and snap frozen. Immunoblot analysis for pCREB was performed using 30 μg protein of hippocampal homogenate, and immunoreactive bands were quantitated by densitometry (**c**). Data are presented as the mean ± S.D. ($n = 3$) and were analyzed by a one-way ANOVA with a Bonferroni post-hoc test: * significant differences from basal (** $p < 0.01$, ***$p < 0.001$); ψ significant difference compared to basal in all other groups ($p < 0.05$)

Conclusions

Disease-modifying approaches to AD remain predominantly targeted at lowering Aβ aggregates in the brain. The development of effective therapies for AD and mixed pathology dementia has been limited by the lack of suitable animal models adequately reflecting the complexity of human AD. We successfully modified a neuroprotective, anti-inflammatory drug to retain these functions and to address synaptic dysfunction in AD: the new orally bioavailable small molecule was effective in three FAD models of increasing therapeutic challenge and in a new animal model of AD not linked to rare genetic mutations. The multifunctional approach incorporates NO/cGMP signaling which regulates the strength of synaptic transmission in an activity-dependent manner in the hippocampus [50]. Importantly, NMZ reactivated CREB signaling, effectively restored LTP, improved learning and memory, and attenuated TNFα and pathological hallmarks of AD. These observations should encourage alternate, parallel strategies to the singular targeting of Aβ. The increasing recognition that AD and age-related dementia may have underlying mixed pathology further supports a small molecule multifunctional approach to neurodegeneration and dementia.

Methods

Animals

All animal care and procedures were conducted with approved institutional animal care protocols at UIC (OACIB), Columbia University (IACUC) and Queen's University (UACC), in accordance with the NIH Guide for the Care and use of Laboratory Animals.

Mice were randomly grouped into NMZ or vehicle treatment groups and mice were treated with drug or vehicle for 10–12 weeks; where applicable littermates were sex and age-matched. APP/PS1 mice (6–8 weeks) were administered drug (1 mg/kg qd) or saline i.p. supplemented with drug (20 mg/kg qd in drinking water). 3 × Tg mice (males 12 months; females 10 months) and E4FAD mice (male 4 months) were administered drug using the same protocol, with the exception that drug in hydrogel replaced drinking water [38]. *Aldh2*$^{-/-}$ mice (3 months) were treated with drug (20 mg/kg qd) in hydrogel. Primary cultures of cortical neurons were prepared from DIV 16 days old rat embryos and subjected to transient OGD or oAβ insults as described [15].

Electrophysiology

LTP measurements were made on 400 μm 3 × Tg mouse slices from 16-month-old male mice using ten theta bursts. Slices were perfused with ODQ (10 μM) and/or NMZ (50 μM) in aCSF perfusate for 30 min before inducing LTP as measured by fEPSP slope measured for 50 min.

Behavior

The RAWM task has proven informative in the analysis of short-term spatial working memory in AD models and was performed as previously described [58]. NOR and Y-maze were performed as described: preliminary data, tested using a three-way analysis of variance, showed no sex differences in either task for *Aldh2*$^{-/-}$ mice, therefore NOR and Y-maze data from male and female mice were combined for analysis [36]. In the NOR, on the test day, animals were allowed to explore the objects until they accumulated a total of 30 s of exploration time, and the discrimination index (difference in time exploring the novel and familiar object, divided by total exploration time) determined. In the Y-maze, spontaneous alternation rate was calculated as the total triads containing entries into each of the three arms without repeated entry into a previously visited arm, divided by the total number of arm entries. STPA has been widely used to test long-term working memory and was performed as previously described [20].

Biomarkers and immunohistochemistry

Brains were separated by hemisphere for immunohistochemistry or ELISA/immunoblot studies. Frozen hemibrains were homogenized and serially extracted for biomarker measurement. For EFAD mice, proteins were extracted from the hippocampus using a three step serial extraction as described [38]. Levels of oAβ (Biosensis) Aβ42 (Invitrogen), TNF-α (Invitrogen), pCREB (Biosource), and BDNF (Promega) were determined for soluble and insoluble fractions using sandwich ELISA kits and reported as weight/unit per milligram of soluble protein. Samples for immunoblot analysis of Aβ were incubated in Laemmli buffer containing 6 M urea for 30 min prior to electrophoresis. The following antibodies were used: mouse monoclonal to Aβ (W0-2, Millipore, recognizes residues 4–10 of Aβ), rabbit polyclonal antibody to 4-hydroxynonenal (HNE11-S antibody, Alpha Diagnostics International), mouse monoclonal antibody to PHF-tau (AT8 antibody, Pierce Thermo Scientific), rabbit polyclonal antibody to caspase-3 (ab90437, Abcam), rabbit polyclonal antibody to caspase-6 (ab52295, Abcam), mouse monoclonal antibody to PSD-95 (Pierce Thermo Scientific), mouse monoclonal antibody to total tau (ab64193, Abcam), rabbit polyclonal antibody to phospho-CREB (Ser 133, 06–519, Upstate Biotechnology), rabbit polyclonal antibody to total CREB (06–863, Millipore), mouse monoclonal antibody to β-actin (Sigma). Serial coronal brain sections (30 μm) of paraformaldehyde-fixed hemi-brains were cut frozen using a Leica cryostat in six adjacent series and immunohistochemically processed using antibodies directed against Aβ/APP, a phospho-specific (Ser202/Thr205) tau antibody, and microglia marker Iba1 (primary, 6E10, Covance, 1:2000; AT8, ThermoFisher, 1:1000; anti-Iba-1, Wako, 1:1000; secondary goat anti-mouse IgG for 6E10/AT8, 1:200; goat anti-mouse IgM for anti-Iba-1, 1:200). Quantitative Thioflavine-S staining was performed on frozen hemi-brain 20 μm serial slides. Aβ deposition stereology in cortex and hippocampus were analyzed using quantitative Metamorph software. Brain slices, were incubated with carbachol or vehicle (Basal) for 30 mins and snap frozen. Immunoblot analysis for pCREB was performed using 30 μg protein of hippocampal homogenate, and immunoreactive bands were quantitated by densitometry. Hippocampal slices from WT and *Aldh2*$^{-/-}$ mice that had been treated with NMZ or vehicle control for 12 weeks, were incubated with carbachol (50 μM) or vehicle for 30 min and snap frozen, before immunoblot analysis of pCREB in homogenates.

Statistical analysis

Unless otherwise stated, all data are expressed as mean ± SD or SEM and were analyzed by one-, two- or three-way analysis of variance with either Bonferroni's or Tukey's post-hoc test, and/or a Student's *t* test for unpaired data. A *p*-value of 0.05 or less was considered statistically significant. All statistical analysis was done of GraphPad Prism.

Ethical committees

The Office of Animal Care and Institutional Biosafety (OACIB) UIC; The Institutional animal care and use committee (IACUC) Colombia University; The University Animal Care Committee (UACC) Queen's University.

Abbreviations

AD: Alzheimer's disease; ALDH2: aldehyde dehydrogenase 2; APOE: apolipoprotein; Aβ: amyloid-beta; BDNF: brain-derived neurotrophic factor; cGMP: cyclic guanosine monophosphate; CMZ: chlormethiazole (also clomethiazole); CREB: cAMP response element-binding protein; DIV: days in vitro; fEPSP: field excitatory postsynaptic potential; GABA: gamma-aminobutyric acid; HNE: 4-hydroxynonenal; LTP: long-term potentiation; MCI: mild cognitive impairment; NFT: neurofibrillary tangles; NMZ: 4-methyl-5-(2-(nitrooxy)ethyl)thiazol-3-ium chloride; NO: nitric oxide; NOR: novel object recognition; oAβ: oligomeric amyloid-β; ODQ: 1H-[1,2,4]oxadiazolo[4, 3-a]quinoxalin-1-one; OGD: oxygen-glucose deprivation; pCREB: phosphorylated cAMP response element-binding protein; PSD-95: postsynaptic density protein 95; RAWM: radial arm water maze; sGC: soluble guanylyl cyclase; STPA: step-through passive avoidance; TBS: theta burst stimulation; TNF-α: tumor necrosis factor alpha.

Competing interests

GRJT and BMB are inventors on patents associated with NMZ.

Authors' contributions

JL designed and directed experiments in primary cultures, immunoassays in APP/PS1 mice and behavioral and other studies in 3xTg and E4FAD mice and helped in drafting and revising the manuscript. SHL carried out experiments in E4FAD mice and drafted and revised the manuscript. LV conducted and interpreted LTP studies in 3xTg mice, assisted with studies in 3xTg and APP/PS1 mice and contributed to drafting the manuscript. ZQ prepared and characterized drugs and contributed to the manuscript draft. MBA generated Fig. 1, assisted with data interpretation and drafted and revised the manuscript. JL assisted with design and interpretation of 3xTg LTP experiments and helped draft the manuscript. OA and AFT designed, directed, and interpreted APP/PS1 mouse behavioral studies and helped draft the manuscript. BMB designed and directed all studies on *Aldh2*$^{-/-}$ mice and drafted and revised the manuscript. YD and AE equally participated in conducting experiments on *Aldh2*$^{-/-}$ mice and contributing to drafting the manuscript. MJL designed experiments on E4FAD mice and drafted and revised the manuscript. LMT and KK assisted with experiments on E4FAD mice and helped in drafting the manuscript. GRJT designed NMZ and conceived and coordinated the overall project, manuscript preparation and revision. All authors have read and approved the final manuscript.

Acknowledgements

Agnieszka Staniszewski and Hong Zhang are thanked for technical assistance. For funding: NIH U01 AG031294 (GRJT); Alzheimer's Drug Discovery Foundation and ISOA grants (New York, NY) (GRJT; MJL); NIH P01AG030128 (MJL); UIC Center for Clinical and Translational Science Grant UL1RR029879 (MJL; GRJT); Harry Botterell Foundation (BMB).

Author details

[1]Department of Medicinal Chemistry and Pharmacognosy, College of Pharmacy, University of Illinois at Chicago, Chicago, IL, USA. [2]Department of Psychiatry, Neuropsychiatric Institute, University of Illinois at Chicago, Chicago, IL, USA. [3]Department of Pathology, The Taub Institute for Research on Alzheimer's Disease and the Aging Brain, Columbia University, New York, NY, USA. [4]Department of Biomedical & Molecular Sciences, Faculty of Health Sciences, Queen's University, Kingston, ON, Canada. [5]Department of Anatomy and Cell Biology, College of Medicine, University of Illinois at Chicago, Chicago, IL, USA.

References

1. Tanzi RE, Kovacs DM, Kim TW, Moir RD, Guenette SY, Wasco W. The gene defects responsible for familial Alzheimer's disease. Neurobiol Dis. 1996;3:159–68.
2. McLean CACR, Fraser FW, Fuller SJ, Smith MJ, Beyreuther K, Bush AI, Masters CL. Soluble pool of Abeta amyloid as a determinant of severity of neurodegeneration in Alzheimer's disease. Ann Neurol. 1999;46:860–6.

3. Schneider JA, Arvanitakis Z, Yu L, Boyle PA, Leurgans SE, Bennett DA. Cognitive impairment, decline and fluctuations in older community-dwelling subjects with Lewy bodies. Brain. 2012;135:3005–14.
4. Negash S, Wilson RS, Leurgans SE, Wolk DA, Schneider JA, Buchman AS, Bennett DA, Arnold SE. Resilient brain aging: characterization of discordance between Alzheimer's disease pathology and cognition. Curr Alzheimer Res. 2013;10:844–51.
5. Extance A. Alzheimer's failure raises questions about disease-modifying strategies. Nat Rev Drug Discov. 2010;9:749–51.
6. Mikulca JA, Nguyen V, Gajdosik DA, Teklu SG, Giunta EA, Lessa EA, Tran CH, Terak EC, Raffa RB. Potential novel targets for Alzheimer pharmacotherapy: II. Update on secretase inhibitors and related approaches. J Clin Pharm Ther. 2014;39:25–37.
7. Drachman DA. The amyloid hypothesis, time to move on: Amyloid is the downstream result, not cause, of Alzheimer's disease. Alzheimers Dement. 2014;10:372–80.
8. Herrup K, Carrillo MC, Schenk D, Cacace A, Desanti S, Fremeau R, Bhat R, Glicksman M, May P, Swerdlow R, et al. Beyond amyloid: getting real about nonamyloid targets in Alzheimer's disease. Alzheimers Dement. 2013;9:452–8.
9. Teich AF, Arancio O. Is the amyloid hypothesis of Alzheimer's disease therapeutically relevant? Biochem J. 2012;446:165–77.
10. Querfurth HW, LaFerla FM. Alzheimer's disease. N Engl J Med. 2010;362:329–44.
11. Suzuki H, Gen K. Clinical efficacy of lamotrigine and changes in the dosages of concomitantly used psychotropic drugs in Alzheimer's disease with behavioural and psychological symptoms of dementia: a preliminary open-label trial. Psychogeriatrics. 2015;15:32–7.
12. Clarkson AN, Clarkson J, Jackson DM, Sammut IA. Mitochondrial involvement in transhemispheric diaschisis following hypoxia-ischemia: Clomethiazole-mediated amelioration. Neuroscience. 2007;144:547–61.
13. Gilby KL, Kelly ME, McIntyre DC, Robertson HA. Neuro-overprotection? A functional evaluation of clomethiazole-induced neuroprotection following hypoxic-ischemic injury. Neuroscience. 2005;131:785–92.
14. Wilby MJ, Hutchinson PJ. The pharmacology of chlormethiazole: a potential neuroprotective agent? CNS Drug Rev. 2004;10:281–94.
15. Vandevrede L, Tavassoli E, Luo J, Qin Z, Yue L, Pepperberg DR, Thatcher GR. Novel analogues of chlormethiazole are neuroprotective in four cellular models of neurodegeneration by a mechanism with variable dependence on GABAA receptor potentiation. Br J Pharmacol. 2014;171:389–402.
16. Selkoe DJ. Alzheimer's disease is a synaptic failure. Science. 2002;298:789–91.
17. Bangen KJ, Nation DA, Delano-Wood L, Weissberger GH, Hansen LA, Galasko DR, Salmon DP, Bondi MW. Aggregate effects of vascular risk factors on cerebrovascular changes in autopsy-confirmed Alzheimer's disease. Alzheimers Dement. 2014;11(4):394–403.
18. Connor B, Young D, Yan Q, Faull RL, Synek B, Dragunow M. Brain-derived neurotrophic factor is reduced in Alzheimer's disease. Brain Res Mol Brain Res. 1997;49:71–81.
19. Luo J, Lee SH, VandeVrede L, Qin Z, Piyankarage S, Tavassoli E, Asghodom RT, Aissa MB, Fa M, Arancio O, et al. Re-engineering a neuroprotective, clinical drug as a procognitive agent with high in vivo potency and with GABAA potentiating activity for use in dementia. BMC Neurosci. 2015;16:67.
20. Qin Z, Luo J, VandeVrede L, Tavassoli E, Fa M, Teich AF, Arancio O, Thatcher GR. Design and synthesis of neuroprotective methylthiazoles and modification as NO-chimeras for neurodegenerative therapy. J Med Chem. 2012;55:6784–801.
21. Lipton SA, Choi YB, Pan ZH, Lei SZ, Chen HS, Sucher NJ, Loscalzo J, Singel DJ, Stamler JS. A redox-based mechanism for the neuroprotective and neurodestructive effects of nitric oxide and related nitroso-compounds. Nature. 1993;364:626–32.
22. Arancio O, Kandel ER, Hawkins RD. Activity-dependent long-term enhancement of transmitter release by presynaptic 3',5'-cyclic GMP in cultured hippocampal neurons. Nature. 1995;376:74–80.
23. Lu YF, Kandel ER, Hawkins RD. Nitric oxide signaling contributes to late-phase LTP and CREB phosphorylation in the hippocampus. J Neurosci. 1999; 19:10250–61.
24. Saura CA, Valero J. The role of CREB signaling in Alzheimer's disease and other cognitive disorders. Rev Neurosci. 2011;22:153–69.
25. Pugazhenthi S, Wang M, Pham S, Sze CI, Eckman CB. Downregulation of CREB expression in Alzheimer's brain and in Abeta-treated rat hippocampal neurons. Mol Neurodegener. 2011;6:60.
26. Satoh J, Tabunoki H, Arima K. Molecular network analysis suggests aberrant CREB-mediated gene regulation in the Alzheimer disease hippocampus. Dis Markers. 2009;27:239–52.
27. Lazarov O, Robinson J, Tang YP, Hairston IS, Korade-Mirnics Z, Lee VM, Hersh LB, Sapolsky RM, Mirnics K, Sisodia SS. Environmental enrichment reduces Abeta levels and amyloid deposition in transgenic mice. Cell. 2005;120:701–13.
28. Zheng Z, Sabirzhanov B, Keifer J. Oligomeric amyloid-{beta} inhibits the proteolytic conversion of brain-derived neurotrophic factor (BDNF), AMPA receptor trafficking, and classical conditioning. J Biol Chem. 2010;285:34708–17.
29. Shineman DW, Basi GS, Bizon JL, Colton CA, Greenberg BD, Hollister BA, Lincecum J, Leblanc GG, Lee LB, Luo F, et al. Accelerating drug discovery for Alzheimer's disease: best practices for preclinical animal studies. Alzheimers Res Ther. 2011;3:28.
30. Youmans KL, Tai LM, Nwabuisi-Heath E, Jungbauer L, Kanekiyo T, Gan M, Kim J, Eimer WA, Estus S, Rebeck GW, et al. APOE4-specific changes in Abeta accumulation in a new transgenic mouse model of Alzheimer disease. J Biol Chem. 2012;287:41774–86.
31. Nunomura A, Perry G, Aliev G, Hirai K, Takeda A, Balraj EK, Jones PK, Ghanbari H, Wataya T, Shimohama S, et al. Oxidative damage is the earliest event in Alzheimer disease. J Neuropathol Exp Neurol. 2001;60:759–67.
32. Pratico D, Uryu K, Leight S, Trojanoswki JQ, Lee VM. Increased lipid peroxidation precedes amyloid plaque formation in an animal model of Alzheimer amyloidosis. J Neurosci. 2001;21:4183–7.
33. Montine KS, Olson SJ, Amarnath V, Whetsell Jr WO, Graham DG, Montine TJ. Immunohistochemical detection of 4-hydroxy-2-nonenal adducts in Alzheimer's disease is associated with inheritance of APOE4. Am J Pathol. 1997;150:437–43.
34. Butterfield DA, Reed T, Perluigi M, De Marco C, Coccia R, Cini C, Sultana R. Elevated protein-bound levels of the lipid peroxidation product, 4-hydroxy-2-nonenal, in brain from persons with mild cognitive impairment. Neurosci Lett. 2006;397:170–3.
35. Ohsawa I, Nishimaki K, Murakami Y, Suzuki Y, Ishikawa M, Ohta S. Age-dependent neurodegeneration accompanying memory loss in transgenic mice defective in mitochondrial aldehyde dehydrogenase 2 activity. J Neurosci. 2008;28:6239–49.
36. D'Souza Y, Elharram A, Soon-Shiong R, Andrew RD, Bennett BM. Characterization of Aldh2 (−/−) mice as an age-related model of cognitive impairment and Alzheimer's disease. Mol Brain. 2015;8:27.
37. Morrissette DA, Parachikova A, Green KN, LaFerla FM. Relevance of transgenic mouse models to human Alzheimer disease. J Biol Chem. 2009;284:6033–7.
38. Tai LM, Koster KP, Luo J, Lee SH, Wang YT, Collins NC, Ben Aissa M, Thatcher GR, LaDu MJ. Amyloid-beta Pathology and APOE Genotype Modulate Retinoid X Receptor Agonist Activity in vivo. J Biol Chem. 2014;289(44):30538–55.
39. Sultana R, Banks WA, Butterfield DA. Decreased levels of PSD95 and two associated proteins and increased levels of BCl2 and caspase 3 in hippocampus from subjects with amnestic mild cognitive impairment: Insights into their potential roles for loss of synapses and memory, accumulation of Abeta, and neurodegeneration in a prodromal stage of Alzheimer's disease. J Neurosci Res. 2010;88:469–77.
40. Almeida CG, Tampellini D, Takahashi RH, Greengard P, Lin MT, Snyder EM, Gouras GK. Beta-amyloid accumulation in APP mutant neurons reduces PSD-95 and GluR1 in synapses. Neurobiol Dis. 2005;20:187–98.
41. Bennett BM, Reynolds JN, Prusky GT, Douglas RM, Sutherland RJ, Thatcher GRJ. Cognitive deficits in rats after forebrain cholinergic depletion are reversed by a novel NO mimetic nitrate ester. Neuropsychopharmacology. 2007;32:505–13.
42. Li J, Wang YJ, Zhang M, Xu ZQ, Gao CY, Fang CQ, Yan JC, Zhou HD. Vascular risk factors promote conversion from mild cognitive impairment to Alzheimer disease. Neurology. 2011;76:1485–91.
43. Marcade M, Bourdin J, Loiseau N, Peillon H, Rayer A, Drouin D, Schweighoffer F, Desire L. Etazolate, a neuroprotective drug linking GABA(A) receptor pharmacology to amyloid precursor protein processing. J Neurochem. 2008;106:392–404.
44. Tweedie D, Sambamurti K, Greig NH. TNF-alpha inhibition as a treatment strategy for neurodegenerative disorders: new drug candidates and targets. Curr Alzheimer Res. 2007;4:378–85.

45. McAlpine FE, Lee JK, Harms AS, Ruhn KA, Blurton-Jones M, Hong J, Das P, Golde TE, LaFerla FM, Oddo S, et al. Inhibition of soluble TNF signaling in a mouse model of Alzheimer's disease prevents pre-plaque amyloid-associated neuropathology. Neurobiol Dis. 2009;34:163–77.
46. Masliah E, Mallory M, Alford M, DeTeresa R, Hansen LA, McKeel Jr DW, Morris JC. Altered expression of synaptic proteins occurs early during progression of Alzheimer's disease. Neurology. 2001;56:127–9.
47. Terry RD, Masliah E, Salmon DP, Butters N, DeTeresa R, Hill R, Hansen LA, Katzman R. Physical basis of cognitive alterations in Alzheimer's disease: synapse loss is the major correlate of cognitive impairment. Ann Neurol. 1991;30:572–80.
48. Phillips HS, Hains JM, Armanini M, Laramee GR, Johnson SA, Winslow JW. BDNF mRNA is decreased in the hippocampus of individuals with Alzheimer's disease. Neuron. 1991;7:695–702.
49. Barco A, Alarcon JM, Kandel ER. Expression of constitutively active CREB protein facilitates the late phase of long-term potentiation by enhancing synaptic capture. Cell. 2002;108:689–703.
50. Neitz A, Mergia E, Imbrosci B, Petrasch-Parwez E, Eysel UT, Koesling D, Mittmann T. Postsynaptic NO/cGMP increases NMDA receptor currents via hyperpolarization-activated cyclic nucleotide-gated channels in the hippocampus. Cereb Cortex. 2014;24:1923–36.
51. Espana J, Valero J, Minano-Molina AJ, Masgrau R, Martin E, Guardia-Laguarta C, Lleo A, Gimenez-Llort L, Rodriguez-Alvarez J, Saura CA. beta-Amyloid disrupts activity-dependent gene transcription required for memory through the CREB coactivator CRTC1. J Neurosci. 2010;30:9402–10.
52. Austin SA, Santhanam AV, Katusic ZS. Endothelial nitric oxide modulates expression and processing of amyloid precursor protein. Circ Res. 2010;107:1498–502.
53. Cai ZX, Guo HS, Wang C, Wei M, Cheng C, Yang ZF, Chen YW, Le WD, Li S. Double-Edged Roles of Nitric Oxide Signaling on APP Processing and Amyloid-beta Production In Vitro: Preliminary Evidence from Sodium Nitroprusside. Neurotox Res. 2016;29:21–34.
54. Santhanam AV, d'Uscio LV, He T, Das P, Younkin SG, Katusic ZS. Uncoupling of endothelial nitric oxide synthase in cerebral vasculature of Tg2576 mice. J Neurochem. 2015;134:1129–38.
55. Austin SA, Santhanam AV, Hinton DJ, Choi DS, Katusic ZS. Endothelial nitric oxide deficiency promotes Alzheimer's disease pathology. J Neurochem. 2013;127:691–700.
56. Katusic ZS, Austin SA. Endothelial nitric oxide: protector of a healthy mind. Eur Heart J. 2014;35:888–94.
57. Bohrmann B, Baumann K, Benz J, Gerber F, Huber W, Knoflach F, Messer J, Oroszlan K, Rauchenberger R, Richter WF, et al. Gantenerumab: a novel human anti-Abeta antibody demonstrates sustained cerebral amyloid-beta binding and elicits cell-mediated removal of human amyloid-beta. J Alzheimers Dis. 2012;28:49–69.
58. Puzzo D, Staniszewski A, Deng SX, Privitera L, Leznik E, Liu S, Zhang H, Feng Y, Palmeri A, Landry DW, Arancio O. Phosphodiesterase 5 inhibition improves synaptic function, memory, and amyloid-beta load in an Alzheimer's disease mouse model. J Neurosci. 2009;29:8075–86.

8

No diurnal variation of classical and candidate biomarkers of Alzheimer's disease in CSF

Claudia Cicognola[1,2], Davide Chiasserini[3], Paolo Eusebi[3], Ulf Andreasson[1,2], Hugo Vanderstichele[4], Henrik Zetterberg[1,2,5], Lucilla Parnetti[3*†] and Kaj Blennow[1,2†]

Abstract

Background: Cerebrospinal fluid (CSF) biomarkers have gained increasing importance in the diagnostic work-up of Alzheimer's disease (AD). The core CSF biomarkers related to AD pathology (Aβ42, t-tau and p-tau) are currently used in CSF diagnostics, while candidate markers of amyloid metabolism (Aβ38, Aβ40, sAPPα, sAPPβ), synaptic loss (neurogranin), neuroinflammation (YKL-40), neuronal damage (VILIP-1) and genetic risk (apolipoprotein E) are undergoing evaluation. Diurnal fluctuation in the concentration of CSF biomarkers has been reported and may represent a preanalytical confounding factor in the laboratory diagnosis of AD. The aim of the present study was to investigate the diurnal variability of classical and candidate CSF biomarkers in a cohort of neurosurgical patients carrying a CSF drainage.

Method: Samples were collected from a cohort of 13 neurosurgical patients from either ventricular ($n = 6$) or lumbar ($n = 7$) CSF drainage at six time points during the day, 1–7 days following the neurosurgical intervention. Concentrations of the core biomarkers were determined by immunoassays.

Results: Although absolute values largely varied among subjects, none of the biomarkers showed significant diurnal variation. Site of drainage (lumbar vs. ventricular) did not influence this result. The different immunoassays used for tau and Aβ markers provided similar results.

Conclusion: Time of day at CSF collection does not ultimately affect the concentration levels of classical and candidate AD biomarkers. Similar trends were found when using different immunoassays, thus corroborating the consistency of the data.

Background

Alzheimer's disease (AD) represents the most common neurodegenerative disease leading to dementia, and its prevalence is increasing and becoming a major health and socioeconomic issue [1]. AD pathology affects the brain several years before the clinical onset, which is characterized by a long asymptomatic phase followed by a prodromal phase with disturbances in episodic memory, ultimately leading to overt dementia [2]. To enable early initiation of treatment, especially the day disease-modifying drugs reach the clinic, early diagnosis is recommended, which is based on combining clinical symptoms and neuropsychological testing with biomarkers (CSF, imaging) reflecting AD pathology [3]. With respect to classical CSF biomarkers (Aβ42, total tau, phosphorylated tau), large evidence has been collected about their reliability in supporting the diagnosis of AD [4–6].

In order to introduce the use of biomarkers as part of the routine diagnostic assessment, standardization of the procedures is mandatory. Preanalytical factors are reported to be the cause of at least 40–60 % of the total variability in biomarker measurements [7]. Some key issues were identified for sample collection and analysis, such as presence of a CSF gradient, blood contamination of the sample, fasting state of the patient, and other laboratory procedures regarding collection and storage of

* Correspondence: lucilla.parnetti@unipg.it
†Equal contributors
[3]Section of Neurology, Department of Medicine, Center for Memory Disturbances, University of Perugia, Sant' Andrea delle Fratte, 06132 Perugia, Italy
Full list of author information is available at the end of the article

the samples (collection tubes, aliquot volume, centrifugation, length and temperature of storage, number of freeze/thaw cycles).

The major focus of our study is the influence of time of day at CSF collection which, in a clinical routine schedule, may influence the results obtained. If proved significant, the diurnal fluctuations would affect the reliability of the CSF analysis depending on time at withdrawal. Only few studies have addressed this issue, giving inconsistent results: Bateman et al. first observed a significant decreasing trend of Aβ during the 24 h in young individuals [8], an observation disproved in subsequent studies in older populations [9–11], the ones more likely to undergo CSF analysis to assess the risk of memory impairment and AD. There is also no consensus on the time intervals between the CSF withdrawals or the volume to be taken.

Regarding analytical factors, different methods and assays may also represent another source of variability [12], but no study has been done on the performance and reliability of different assays when considering diurnal variation as a confounding factor.

Candidate biomarkers

Along with core biomarkers of AD, other proteins are currently studied as candidate biomarkers, with significant results in their role in CSF diagnostics.

Biomarkers of the amyloidogenic pathway are being taken into account in AD diagnosis, since Aβ42 is produced from cleavage of amyloid precursor protein (APP). APP can be cleaved either by α- or β-secretase, releasing sAPPα or sAPPβ, respectively. After β-secretase cleavage, the remaining C-terminal fragment is further processed by γ-secretase which releases Aβ42 along with Aβ38 and Aβ40 fragments, whereas no amyloidogenic fragments are produced after α-secretase cleavage followed by γ-secretase. Since sAPPα was found decreased and sAPPβ increased in AD subjects, α- and β- pathway were considered mutually exclusive [13–16]; however, subsequent studies showed positively correlated concentrations of sAPPα and β [17–19], challenging the hypothesis of an imbalance between the two isoforms. The several critical steps of amyloid metabolism can also cause Aβ fluctuations during the day: Dobrowolska et al. found diurnal fluctuations in sAPPα, sAPPβ, Aβ40, and Aβ42, diminishing with increased age [20].

Regarding genetic risk factors for AD, ApoE is probably the most important and acknowledged. The three different isoforms exert a different effect on AD predisposition: ApoE4 increases the risk of AD, whereas ApoE2 is a protective factor, compared to the most common variant ApoE3. Quantifying ApoE isoforms, especially ApoE4, could be a useful biological correlate in the study of AD pathology, but CNS and peripheral ApoE isoform turnover rates differ substantially, probably because the ApoE metabolism pathways are different in the central nervous system (CNS) and the periphery, as observed in a study by Wildsmith et al. [21]. Time-dependent fluctuations were also observed [21, 22].

Also neurogranin (a calmodulin-binding postsynaptic protein, involved in synaptic signaling, plasticity, long-term potentiation and memory consolidation) is currently studied as a potential biomarker. Synaptic loss has been reported to occur very early in the natural history of AD, therefore neurogranin can be a valuable biomarker of early, possible preclinical, stage of the disease [23]. Neurogranin concentrations are significantly increased in mild cognitive impairment (MCI) [24, 25] and can be a predictive factor of conversion to dementia.

Among inflammatory markers we find YKL-40 (also known as chitinase-3-like protein 1), a protein mainly expressed by astrocytes. Even if its physiological function remains unclear [26], it was found to be upregulated in the AD brain from the preclinical stages of the disease and may have a role in Aβ deposition [27]. Besides, as a biomarker, it could also give additional information on the inflammatory status of the AD brain. However, studies on its diagnostic and prognostic value still give conflicting results [26, 28].

Neuronal damage markers include VILIP-1 (visinin-like protein 1), a neuronal calcium sensor protein involved in calcium-mediated neurotoxicity. Not only VILIP-1 is significantly increased in AD and could help differentiate AD from other dementia, but it may also have an influence on tau metabolism [29, 30]. Moreover, when combined with Aβ42, it is also a good predictor of cognitive decline [31, 32].

The diurnal variability of the aforementioned biomarkers has been poorly investigated and no studies are available on neurogranin, YKL-40 and VILIP-1. Also, most studies only use one immunoassay type and do not provide a comparison between different methods.

Aim

In this study we wanted to measure classical (Aβ42, t-tau, p-tau) and candidate (Aβ38, Aβ40, sAPPα, sAPPβ, apolipoprotein E, neurogranin, YKL-40 and VILIP-1) AD biomarkers in CSF collected at six time points (08:00; 12:00; 16:00; 20:00, 00:00, 08:00) during 24 h to assess these markers for diurnal variation.

Methods

Participants

We enrolled a total of 13 patients, 8 males (61.5 %) and 5 females (38.5 %), with an age span between 26 and 82 years (Tables 1 and 2). All patients carried a CSF drainage after neurosurgical intervention for tumors, traumas or hemorrhages ($n = 9$) or for monitoring CSF pressure ($n = 4$). 7 patients had a lumbar drainage (53.8 %) and 6 patients had a ventricular drainage (46.2 %), with no

Table 1 Age, clinical features of the patients and type of drainage

Patient	Age	Case of drainage placement	Type of drainage
1	48	Third ventricle tumor	ventricular
2	73	Left middle cerebral artery infarct	ventricular
3	81	Subarachnoid hemorrhage	ventricular
4	72	Intracranial hemorrhage	lumbar
5	67	Cerebellar hemorrhage	ventricular
6	69	Cerebellopontine angle tumor	lumbar
7	74	Normal pressure hydrocephalus	lumbar
8	36	Head trauma	ventricular
9	63	Intracranial hemorrhage	ventricular
10	58	Tetraventricular hydrocephalus	lumbar
11	77	Normal pressure hydrocephalus	lumbar
12	82	Normal pressure hydrocephalus	lumbar
13	26	Pseudotumor cerebri	lumbar

filter (Codman&Shurtleff, Inc, Raynham, MA, USA). CSF was collected according to a standard protocol following international guidelines [33]. The study was approved by the local Ethical Committee and informed written consent was signed by all patients enrolled. The work was carried out according to the Declaration of Helsinki.

CSF collection

According to our protocol, 4 mL CSF were collected at six time points: 8.00, 12.00, 16.00, 20.00, 00.00 and 8.00. Haemorrhagic CSF samples were excluded; if the drainage was put after a trauma, haemorrhage or tumor surgery CSF samples collected had to be either clear or slightly and stably xantochromic (<1000 rbc/μL). CSF was collected in polypropylene (PP) tubes (Sarsted, code: 62.610.201) and all samples were centrifuged (2000 g × 10 min, room temperature) no longer than 15 min after collection, aliquoted in 0.5 ml aliquots (Sarsted, code: 72.730.007) and frozen at −80 °C pending analysis (Table 3).

Table 2 Demographics (mean ± standard deviation or count with percentages)

Age	63.5 ± 17.3
Sex	Male: 8 (61.5 %)
	Female: 5 (38.5 %)
Type of drainage	Lumbar: 7 (53.8 %)
	Ventricular: 6 (46.2 %)
Cause of drainage placement	Cerebellar hemorrhage: 1 (7.7 %)
	Cerebellopontine angle tumor: 1 (7.7 %)
	Head trauma: 1 (7.7 %)
	Intracranial hemorrhage: 2 (15.4 %)
	Left middle cerebral artery infarct: 1 (7.7 %)
	Normal pressure hydrocephalus: 3 (23.1 %)
	Pseudotumor cerebri: 1 (7.7 %)
	Subarachnoid hemorrhage: 1 (7.7 %)
	Tetraventricular hydrocephalus: 1 (7.7 %)
	Third ventricle tumor: 1 (7.7 %)

Assays

Aβ42, t-tau and p-tau were determined with ELISA kit (Fujirebio) in the Clinical Neurochemistry Laboratory of the University of Perugia (Perugia, Italy), according to the manufacturer's protocol.

Aβ38, Aβ 40, Aβ 42, sAPPα, sAPPβ, neurogranin, VILIP-1 and YKL-40 were analyzed in the Clinical Neurochemistry Laboratory of The Sahlgrenska Academy, University of Gothenburg (Mölndal, Sweden).

MSD V-PLEX Plus kits were used for Aβ38, Aβ40, Aβ42, sAPPα and sAPPβ, according to the manufacturer's protocol. ELISA kits from R&D and Biovendor were used for YKL-40 and VILIP-1, respectively, according to the manufacturer's protocol.

An in-house developed assay was used for neurogranin, according to previous reports [24]. Briefly, in-house antibody Ng7 diluted in PBS was used as coating, a rabbit anti-neurogranin antibody (ab23570, cat. no. 07-425, Upstate, Lake Placid, NY, USA) as primary and a goat anti-rabbit sulfo-tag antibody (MSD) for detection. Full-length Ng 1–78 protein (ADx) was used as calibrator for the standard curve.

Aβ38, Aβ40, Aβ42, t-tau, and ApoE were also measured with Euroimmun kits at ADx NeuroSciences (Gent, Belgium).

Table 3 CSF collection procedures and sample processing

Subjects:	13 neurosurgical patients carrying a CSF drainage
	8 M, 5 F; 26 to 82 y
	Admitted for tumor, trauma, hemorrhage ($n = 9$), CSF pressure monitoring ($n = 4$)
CSF collection:	From lumbar ($n = 7$) or ventricular ($n = 6$) drainage
	Volume: 4 mL in PP Sarsted tubes, code: 62.610.201
	Time of day: 8.00, 12.00, 16.00, 20.00, 00.00, 8.00
CSF processing:	Centrifugation within 15 min, 2000 g × 10 min at RT
	0.5 mL aliquots in PP Sarsted tubes, code: 72.730.007
CSF storage:	−80 °C freezer, with controlled temperature, alarm and CO2 backup system
Thawing:	RT with gentle shaking
Biomarker measurement:	Immunoassay (Fujirebio): Aβ1-42, t-tau, p-tau181
	Immunoassay (Biovendor): VILIP-1
	Immunoassay (R&D): YKL-40
	Immunoassay (Euroimmun): Aβ1-38, Aβ1-40, Aβ1-42, t-tau, ApoE
	Immunoassay (in-house): neurogranin
	Immunoassay (MSD): Aβx-38, Aβx-40, Aβx-42, sAPPα, sAPPβ

Together with the quality control (QC) samples included in the kits, CSF pools were run in each plate as further internal controls to check for variability, as previously described [34]. Performance data (inter- and intra assay variability, recovery and linearity) can be found at the following references [34, 35].

Statistical analysis

Statistical analysis was performed using R v 13.1 and Graph Pad v 6.0. Continuous variables were reported as means, standard deviations and ranges. Categorical variables were shown as counts and percentages. Continuous variables were tested for normality with Shapiro–Wilk test. Differences in biomarkers levels across time points were tested by means of non-parametric version of repeated measurement ANOVA based on aligned ranks, due to the non-normality of the majority of parameters. Spearman's r correlation coefficients of biomarkers concentrations were calculated pooling all the time points. Drainage type was tested as potential confounder in the fluctuations of biomarkers across time points. Bland-Altman plots were drawn to investigate the agreement of different assays for some of the investigated biomarkers (Aβ38, Aβ40, Aβ42, t-tau). $P < 0.05$ was chosen as the minimum level of statistical significance.

Results

Circadian trends in the individual classical and candidate biomarkers

Aβ38, Aβ40, Aβ42 and t-tau measured with different methods, i.e. immunoassay by Euroimmun, Fujirebio, and MSD, showed significant positive correlations (Fig. 1). Results from Euroimmun vs. MSD highly correlated for both Aβ38 ($r = 0.89$, $p < 0.01$, 95 % confidence interval (CI) = 0.82 to 0.94) and Aβ40 ($r = 0.87$, $p < 0.01$, 95 % CI = 0.74 to 0.9). Similar results were found for Aβ42 when comparing Euroimmun vs. MSD ($r = 0.92$, $p < 0.01$, 95 % CI = 0.82 to 0.93), Euroimmun vs. Fujirebio ($r = 0.81$, $p < 0.01$, 95 % CI = 0.74 to 0.9) and MSD vs. Fujirebio ($r = 0.86$, $p < 0.01$, 95 % CI = 0.74 to 0.89) (Fig. 1).

There was also a positive correlation for tau when measured with Fujirebio and Euroimmun ($r = 0.67$, $p < 0.01$, 95 % CI = 0.48 to 0.8). Bland-Altman analysis was used to assess the agreement among the

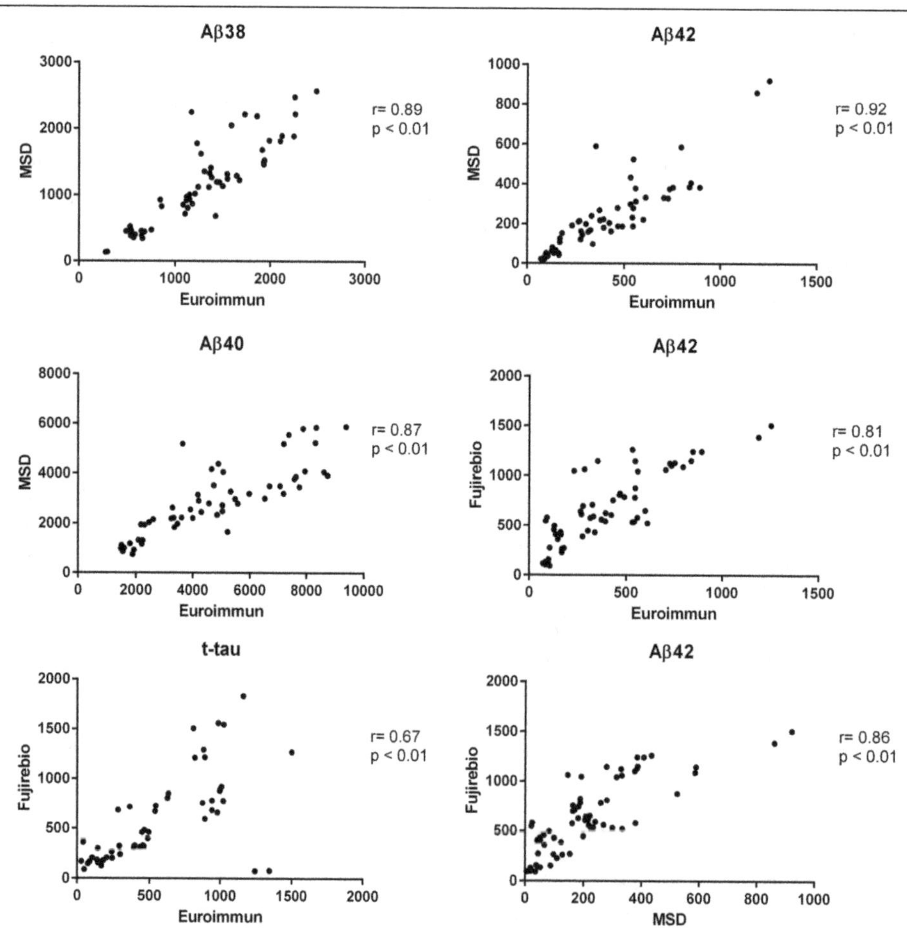

Fig. 1 Correlation of the levels of biomarkers measured with different assays (Euroimmun, MSD, Fujirebio)

different assays for measuring absolute concentrations of the biomarkers (Additional file 1).

Notably, MSD assays overall showed differences either when compared to Euroimmun or Fujirebio assays. This was especially evident for Aβ42 and Aβ40 which showed the largest variation in the difference between the two assays across the whole range of concentrations (Additional file 1).

As expected from the different admittance diagnosis, sex and age of the population (Tables 1 and 2), absolute concentrations of the biomarkers were very different among patients (Table 4). For what concerns classical biomarkers, in the whole population Aβ42 ranged from 71 to 1253.4 pg/mL, t-tau from 29 to 1501 pg/mL and p-tau from 15 to 113 pg/mL.

Possibly due to their common metabolism pathway, amyloid metabolism markers (Aβ38, Aβ40, Aβ42, sAPPα, sAPPβ) showed similar trends over time in the whole population (Figs. 2 and 3). However, none of them had significant variation across time points ($p > 0.05$). sAPPα, sAPPβ and β-amyloid fragments correlated positively with each other, with r values ranging from to 0.54 to 0.97 ($p > 0.01$) (Additional file 2). When measured with Euroimmun kits, Aβ42/β40 and Aβ38/40 ratio showed no significant oscillations ($p > 0.05$). No significant intraindividual fluctuations over time were found for any of the Aβ markers when measured with the different assays (for Aβ42, see Additional file 3).

Neither T-tau nor P-tau did show a significant diurnal variation (Figs. 2 and 3). No significant oscillations were observed for Neurogranin, ApoE, YKL-40 and VILIP-1 ($p > 0.05$) (Fig. 3). Single patients showed some variations for specific proteins but globally no significant fluctuations over time were observed.

Table 4 Concentration range of the biomarkers (with median)

Biomarker	Median (IQR)	Min - Max
$Aβ_{38}$ MSD (pg/mL)	990.9 (440.1–1396.0)	33.3–2573.0
$Aβ_{40}$ MSD (pg/mL)	2514.9 (1154.8–3356.5)	79.3–5880.5
$Aβ_{42}$ MSD (pg/mL)	182.1 (54.1–266.6)	5.5–921.2
$Aβ_{38}$ Euroimmun (pg/mL)	1247.7 (1120.9–1462.0)	277.5–2492.5
$Aβ_{40}$ Euroimmun (pg/mL)	4669.0 (3605.0–5305.0)	1487.0–9382.2
$Aβ_{42}$ Euroimmun (pg/mL)	337.9 (191.9–521.8)	70.6–1253.4
t-tau Euroimmun (pg/mL)	464.7 (223.0–917.6)	29.3–1501.0
$Aβ_{42}$ Fujirebio (pg/mL)	568.0 (294.5–786.0)	91.0–1507.0
t-tau Fujirebio (pg/mL)	319.0 (180.2–742.2)	72.0–1832.0
p-tau (pg/mL)	43.0 (30.3–52.8)	15.0–113.0
sAPPα (ng/mL)	60.4 (32.5–178.8)	4.3–429.6
sAPPβ (ng/mL)	66.4 (25.5–175.0)	1.4–313.6
YKL-40 (ng/mL)	264.6 (151.9–348.4)	65.4–1020.0
VILIP-1 (pg/mL)	113.5 (99.0–135.0)	72.0–781.0
Neurogranin (pg/mL)	354.5 (275.9–435.4)	46.3–1291.1
ApoE (ng/mL)	24.5 (18.8–44.4)	3.4–104.2

Site of drainage

When site of drainage was considered as a covariate in non-parametric repeated measurements ANOVA based on aligned ranks, variability in some of the proteins (Aβ38, Aβ40, YKL40, t-tau) was found to be significantly explained by the site of drainage ($p < 0.05$), with generally higher concentration in CSF from ventricular catheter. Anyway, subgroup analyses restricted to lumbar or ventricular catheter showed no significant changes across the time points analysed ($p > 0.05$) (Fig. 4). Similar results were obtained when the analysis was repeated considering only patients with normal pressure hydrocephalus ($n = 3$, $p > 0.05$).

Discussion

In our study we assessed the possible circadian oscillation of classical (Aβ42, t-tau, p-tau) and candidate (Aβ38, Aβ40, sAPPα, sAPPβ, apolipoprotein E, neurogranin, YKL-40, VILIP-1) CSF AD biomarkers. Previous studies addressed the issue of diurnal fluctuations of Aβ and tau in CSF (for review see [36]), however, a significant circadian oscillation of Aβ was detected only in the study by Bateman and colleagues [8]. Moreover, the study included subjects significantly younger than the ones who usually undergo lumbar puncture as a diagnostic procedure (23 to 78 years old).

Subsequent studies did not observe the same trend [9–11]. Bjerke et al. led a study in healthy subjects undergoing knee surgery and observed a slight decrease in Aβ42 levels, which tended to return to baseline after 24 h [10]. Slats et al. compared the trends of Aβ in healthy and mild AD subjects, noticing no significant diurnal variation and also a less pronounced circadian pattern compared with the one in younger subjects (59 to 85 years old) [11]. Only Moghekar et al. examined also tau along with Aβ, in a cohort of normal pressure hydrocephalus subjects, but no diurnal fluctuation of the biomarkers was reported [9].

Our study is in line with the majority of the results from previous ones, but we also investigated the possible oscillations of the latest candidate AD biomarkers (neurogranin, YKL-40, VILIP-1). We collected a smaller volume of CSF (4 mL) than in previous studies (from 6 to 40 mL) to avoid possible fluctuations due to tapping large volumes of CSF, and we compared results from ventricular CSF and lumbar CSF to detect a possible gradient effect.

Although CSF protein concentrations were significantly different from one patient to another, none of the biomarkers showed a significant diurnal variation. The ranges of the biomarkers were very different from the ones available from the literature on optimal cut-offs for

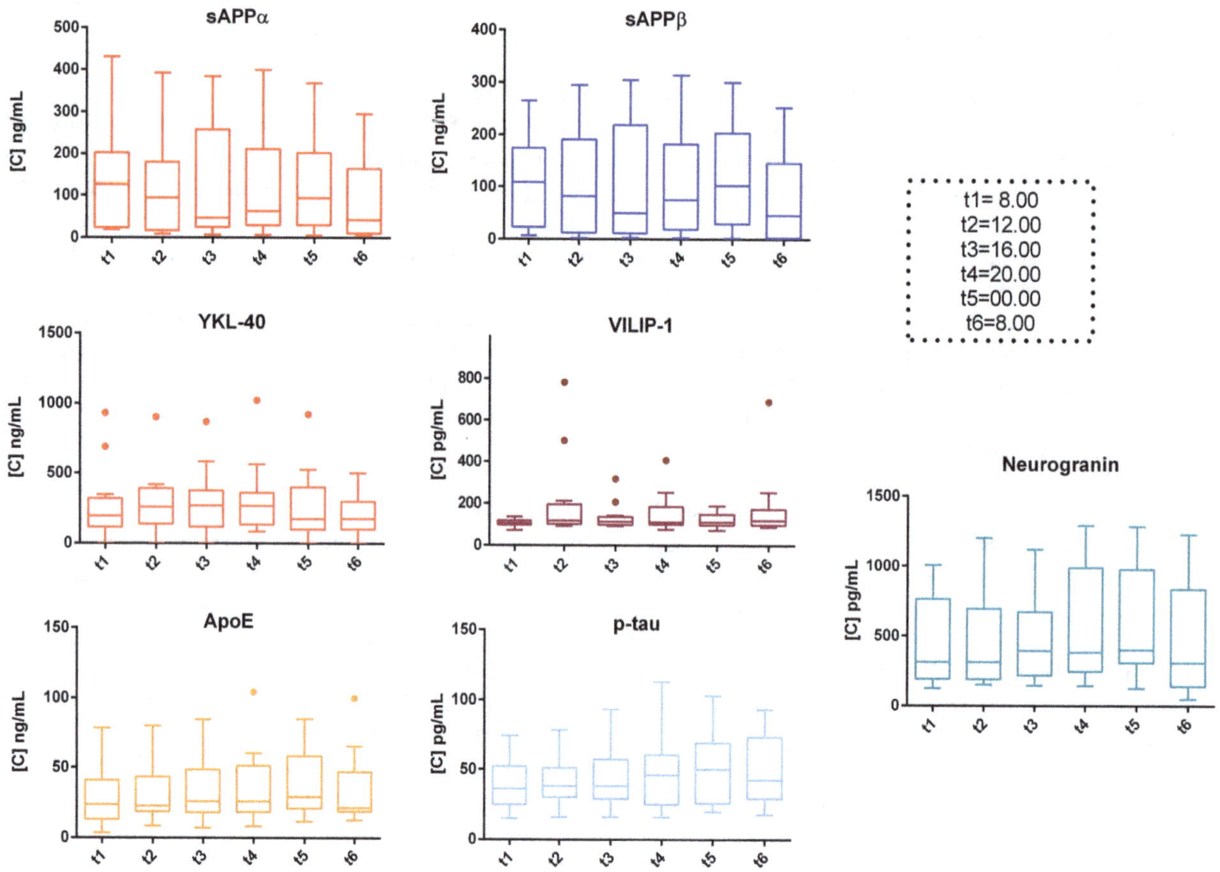

Fig. 2 Concentration levels of the biomarkers across time points (horizontal lines representing the median, box representing the 25th and 75th percentiles, whiskers representing the 5th and 95th percentiles, and outliers represented by dots)

AD biomarkers [37]. This is mostly due to the heterogeneity of the population, different for sex, age and diagnosis at admission (Tables 1 and 2). The subjects did all undergo an invasive procedure for catheter insertion, which might have affected the levels of the biomarkers in CSF. Moreover, 9 out of 13 subjects underwent brain surgery for tumours, haemorrhage or head trauma prior to drainage placement, which is most likely the reason for the generally upregulated values of inflammatory and brain injury markers (tau, YKL-40) in the population. Not to be excluded is also the presence of a possible underlying AD pathology in the older subjects. It is remarkable, however, that even if set on different ranges between subjects, the overall levels of the individual biomarkers are very stable over time and do not seem to be affected by external factors.

Site of drainage significantly influenced the variability of some of the biomarkers (Aβ38, Aβ40, YKL40, t-tau), as previously described [38], with generally higher concentration in CSF from ventricular catheter, most likely due to the increased concentrations of injury markers in the site of the surgical intervention or brain damage in patients carrying a ventricular drainage.

Some of the analytes tested in this work were measured with different immunoassays (Fujirebio, MSD, and Euroimmun). Absolute concentrations of the biomarkers using different immunoassays varied widely, possibly due to the different sources for the calibrators used by the manufacturers, as well as to the different antibodies used for coating and detection. No previous studies on circadian rhythms of CSF biomarkers have been performed comparing these three different techniques, which nevertheless showed good inter-assay correlations, proving the reliability of the methods in use and supporting the lack of circadian oscillations independently from the technique.

The main limitation of this study was the population, mostly admitted to hospital for traumatic intervention, limited in number and very different for age and disease. However, patients with normal pressure hydrocephalus, which were admitted to hospital only for diagnostic purposes and represented a more selected population, did not show significant diurnal variability as well. Obviously, to find ventricular CSF samples suitable for biomarker analysis is not easily manageable, due to the severe underlying conditions that lead to the insertion of a ventricular

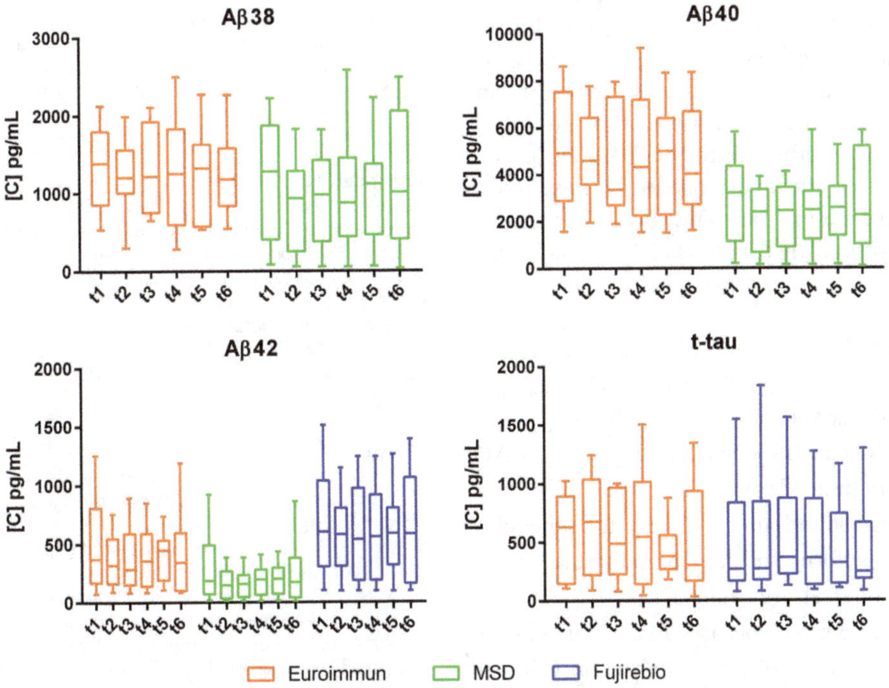

Fig. 3 Concentration levels of several biomarkers measured with different assays (Euroimmun, MSD, Fujirebio) across time points (horizontal lines representing the median, box representing the 25th and 75th percentiles, whiskers representing the 5th and 95th percentiles)

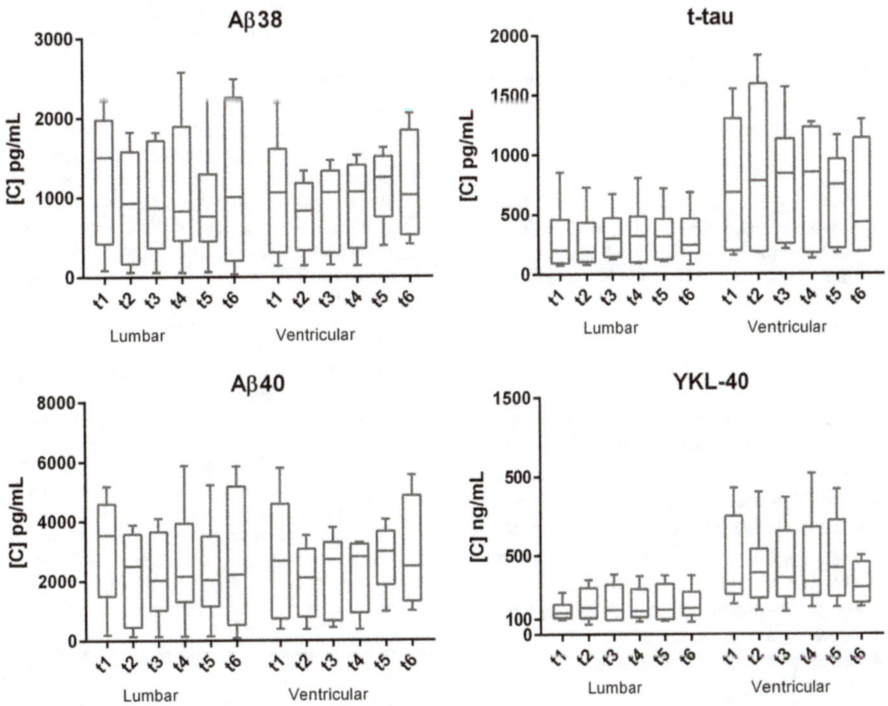

Fig. 4 Concentration levels of several biomarkers with different type of drainage (lumbar or ventricular) across time points (horizontal lines representing the median, box representing the 25th and 75th percentiles, whiskers representing the 5th and 95th percentiles). Pictures not showed for non-significant comparisons

catheter. Same is for lumbar CSF: not being possible to perform multiple lumbar punctures during the day, repeated measurements at different time points can only be done after insertion of a drainage, which is seen as a dangerous procedure by most of the population, making it problematic to enrol healthy controls and AD subjects in larger studies. Further efforts are needed to raise public awareness about the minor risks of this kind of procedure, especially in view of an early diagnosis of AD pathology.

Conclusions

In view of standardizing CSF collection and analysis procedures, the absence of an influence on classical and candidate CSF biomarker of time at sampling make them a valuable asset in the diagnostic work-up of AD. Independence from time of day is also crucial for clinical practitioners: being bound to fixed hospital schedules, the possibility to perform the lumbar puncture at any time of the day is of great importance.

An increasing number of tools are already being developed for the measurement of these analytes in CSF and preliminary results show robustness and significant overlap between different methods, proving their reliability and reproducibility for biomarker analysis. However, larger and selected populations are needed to increase the power of these findings.

Acknowledgments
The authors would like to thank Cristiano Spaccatini, Ulrika Törnqvist and Leentje Demeyer for their technical assistance and Professor Paolo Lunardi for allowing access to the Section of Neurosurgery (Santa Maria della Misericordia Hospital, University of Perugia, Italy).

Funding
Blennow received funding from Research Council, Sweden; the Swedish Brain Foundation; the Swedish Alzheimer Foundation; and Torsten Söderberg Foundation, Sweden. Parnetti received funding from Michael J. Fox Foundation for Parkinson's Disease.

Authors' contributions
CC collected the samples, performed the experiments, analyzed the data and wrote the manuscript. DC performed the experiments, designed and supervised the analysis and participated in the drafting of the manuscript. PE performed the statistical analysis and participated in the drafting of the manuscript. UA coordinated the analysis at the Clinical Neurochemistry Laboratory of The Sahlgrenska Academy, University of Gothenburg (Mölndal, Sweden) and reviewed the manuscript. HV run the analysis at ADx NeuroSciences (Gent, Belgium) and reviewed the manuscript. HZ participated in the design of the study and reviewed the manuscript. LP and KB designed the study, gave financial support and reviewed the manuscript. All authors read and approved the final manuscript.

Authors' information
Not applicable.

Competing interests
Blennow has served at advisory boards and as a consultant for IBL International, Fujirebio Europe, and Roche Diagnostics. Parnetti obtained research reagents from Fujirebio and Euroimmun AG. Vanderstichele is co-founder of ADx NeuroSciences and founder of Biomarkable bvba. The other authors report no disclosures for this paper.

Author details
[1]Institute of Neuroscience and Physiology, Department of Psychiatry and Neurochemistry, The Sahlgrenska Academy at University of Gothenburg, House V3, SU / Mölndal hospital, Göteborgsvägen 31, SE-431 80 Mölndal, Sweden. [2]Clinical Neurochemistry Laboratory, Sahlgrenska University Hospital, SE-431 80 Mölndal, Sweden. [3]Section of Neurology, Department of Medicine, Center for Memory Disturbances, University of Perugia, Sant' Andrea delle Fratte, 06132 Perugia, Italy. [4]ADx NeuroSciences, Gent, Belgium. [5]UCL Institute of Neurology, Queen Square, London, UK.

References

1. Prince M, Bryce R, Albanese E, Wimo A, Ribeiro W, Ferri CP. The global prevalence of dementia: a systematic review and metaanalysis. Alzheimers Dement. 2013;9(1):63–75. e62.
2. Sperling RA, Aisen PS, Beckett LA, Bennett DA, Craft S, Fagan AM, Iwatsubo T, Jack Jr CR, Kaye J, Montine TJ, et al. Toward defining the preclinical stages of Alzheimer's disease: recommendations from the National Institute on Aging-Alzheimer's Association workgroups on diagnostic guidelines for Alzheimer's disease. Alzheimers Dement. 2011;7(3):280–92.
3. Dubois B, Feldman HH, Jacova C, Hampel H, Molinuevo JL, Blennow K, DeKosky ST, Gauthier S, Selkoe D, Bateman R, et al. Advancing research diagnostic criteria for Alzheimer's disease: the IWG-2 criteria. The Lancet Neurology. 2014;13(6):614–29.
4. Blennow K, Zetterberg H. The past and the future of Alzheimer's disease CSF biomarkers-a journey toward validated biochemical tests covering the whole spectrum of molecular events. Frontiers in neuroscience. 2015;9:345.
5. Rosen C, Hansson O, Blennow K, Zetterberg H. Fluid biomarkers in Alzheimer's disease - current concepts. Mol Neurodegener. 2013;8:20.
6. Molinuevo JL, Blennow K, Dubois B, Engelborghs S, Lewczuk P, Perret-Liaudet A, Teunissen CE, Parnetti L. The clinical use of cerebrospinal fluid biomarker testing for Alzheimer's disease diagnosis: a consensus paper from the Alzheimer's Biomarkers Standardization Initiative. Alzheimers Dement. 2014;10(6):808–17.
7. Vanderstichele H, Bibl M, Engelborghs S, Le Bastard N, Lewczuk P, Molinuevo JL, Parnetti L, Perret-Liaudet A, Shaw LM, Teunissen C, et al. Standardization of preanalytical aspects of cerebrospinal fluid biomarker testing for Alzheimer's disease diagnosis: a consensus paper from the Alzheimer's Biomarkers Standardization Initiative. Alzheimers Dement. 2012;8(1):65–73.
8. Bateman RJ, Wen G, Morris JC, Holtzman DM. Fluctuations of CSF amyloid-beta levels: implications for a diagnostic and therapeutic biomarker. Neurology. 2007;68(9):666–9.
9. Moghekar A, Goh J, Li M, Albert M, O'Brien RJ. Cerebrospinal fluid Abeta and tau level fluctuation in an older clinical cohort. Arch Neurol. 2012;69(2):246–50.
10. Bjerke M, Portelius E, Minthon L, Wallin A, Anckarsater H, Anckarsater R, Andreasen N, Zetterberg H, Andreasson U, Blennow K: Confounding factors influencing amyloid Beta concentration in cerebrospinal fluid. Int J Alzheimers Dis. 2010;2010. doi: 10.4061/2010/986310
11. Slats D, Claassen JA, Spies PE, Borm G, Besse KT, van Aalst W, Tseng J, Sjogren MJ, Olde Rikkert MG, Verbeek MM. Hourly variability of cerebrospinal fluid biomarkers in Alzheimer's disease subjects and healthy older volunteers. Neurobiol Aging. 2012;33(4):831. e831-839.
12. Mattsson N, Andreasson U, Persson S, Carrillo MC, Collins S, Chalbot S, Cutler N, Dufour-Rainfray D, Fagan AM, Heegaard NH, et al. CSF biomarker variability in the Alzheimer's Association quality control program. Alzheimers Dement. 2013;9(3):251–61.
13. Olsson A, Hoglund K, Sjogren M, Andreasen N, Minthon L, Lannfelt L, Buerger K, Moller HJ, Hampel H, Davidsson P, et al. Measurement of alpha- and beta-secretase cleaved amyloid precursor protein in cerebrospinal fluid from Alzheimer patients. Exp Neurol. 2003;183(1):74–80.
14. Sennvik K, Fastbom J, Blomberg M, Wahlund LO, Winblad B, Benedikz E. Levels of alpha- and beta-secretase cleaved amyloid precursor protein in the cerebrospinal fluid of Alzheimer's disease patients. Neurosci Lett. 2000;278(3):169–72.

15. Lannfelt L, Basun H, Wahlund LO, Rowe BA, Wagner SL. Decreased alpha-secretase-cleaved amyloid precursor protein as a diagnostic marker for Alzheimer's disease. Nature medicine. 1995;1(8):829–32.
16. Vassar R. beta-Secretase, APP and Abeta in Alzheimer's disease. Sub-cellular biochemistry. 2005;38:79–103.
17. Alexopoulos P, Tsolakidou A, Roselli F, Arnold A, Grimmer T, Westerteicher C, Leante MR, Forstl H, Livrea P, Kurz A, et al. Clinical and neurobiological correlates of soluble amyloid precursor proteins in the cerebrospinal fluid. Alzheimers Dement. 2012;8(4):304–11.
18. Gabelle A, Roche S, Geny C, Bennys K, Labauge P, Tholance Y, Quadrio I, Tiers L, Gor B, Chaulet C, et al. Correlations between soluble alpha/beta forms of amyloid precursor protein and Abeta38, 40, and 42 in human cerebrospinal fluid. Brain Res. 2010;1357:175–83.
19. Lewczuk P, Kamrowski-Kruck H, Peters O, Heuser I, Jessen F, Popp J, Burger K, Hampel H, Frolich L, Wolf S, et al. Soluble amyloid precursor proteins in the cerebrospinal fluid as novel potential biomarkers of Alzheimer's disease: a multicenter study. Mol Psychiatry. 2010;15(2):138–45.
20. Dobrowolska JA, Kasten T, Huang Y, Benzinger TL, Sigurdson W, Ovod V, Morris JC, Bateman RJ. Diurnal patterns of soluble amyloid precursor protein metabolites in the human central nervous system. PLoS One. 2014;9(3):e89998.
21. Wildsmith KR, Basak JM, Patterson BW, Pyatkivskyy Y, Kim J, Yarasheski KE, Wang JX, Mawuenyega KG, Jiang H, Parsadanian M, et al. In vivo human apolipoprotein E isoform fractional turnover rates in the CNS. PLoS One. 2012;7(6):e38013.
22. Yamauchi K, Tozuka M, Nakabayashi T, Sugano M, Hidaka H, Kondo Y, Katsuyama T. Apolipoprotein E in cerebrospinal fluid: relation to phenotype and plasma apolipoprotein E concentrations. Clin Chem. 1999;45(4):497–504.
23. Thorsell A, Bjerke M, Gobom J, Brunhage E, Vanmechelen E, Andreasen N, Hansson O, Minthon L, Zetterberg H, Blennow K. Neurogranin in cerebrospinal fluid as a marker of synaptic degeneration in Alzheimer's disease. Brain Res. 2010;1362:13–22.
24. Kvartsberg H, Duits FH, Ingelsson M, Andreasen N, Ohrfelt A, Andersson K, Brinkmalm G, Lannfelt L, Minthon L, Hansson O, et al. Cerebrospinal fluid levels of the synaptic protein neurogranin correlates with cognitive decline in prodromal Alzheimer's disease. Alzheimers Dement. 2015;11(10):1180–90.
25. De Vos A, Jacobs D, Struyfs H, Fransen E, Andersson K, Portelius E, Andreasson U, De Surgeloose D, Hernalsteen D, Sleegers K, et al. C-terminal neurogranin is increased in cerebrospinal fluid but unchanged in plasma in Alzheimer's disease. Alzheimers Dement. 2015;11:1461.
26. Craig-Schapiro R, Perrin RJ, Roe CM, Xiong C, Carter D, Cairns NJ, Mintun MA, Peskind ER, Li G, Galasko DR, et al. YKL-40: a novel prognostic fluid biomarker for preclinical Alzheimer's disease. Biol Psychiatry. 2010;68(10):903–12.
27. Rosen C, Andersson CH, Andreasson U, Molinuevo JL, Bjerke M, Rami L, Llado A, Blennow K, Zetterberg H. Increased levels of chitotriosidase and YKL-40 in cerebrospinal fluid from patients with Alzheimer's disease. Dement Geriatr Cogn Dis Extra. 2014;4(2):297–304.
28. Mattsson N, Tabatabaei S, Johansson P, Hansson O, Andreasson U, Mansson JE, Johansson JO, Olsson B, Wallin A, Svensson J, et al. Cerebrospinal fluid microglial markers in Alzheimer's disease: elevated chitotriosidase activity but lack of diagnostic utility. Neuromolecular Med. 2011;13(2):151–9.
29. Luo X, Hou L, Shi H, Zhong X, Zhang Y, Zheng D, Tan Y, Hu G, Mu N, Chan J, et al. CSF levels of the neuronal injury biomarker visinin-like protein-1 in Alzheimer's disease and dementia with Lewy bodies. J Neurochem. 2013;127(5):681–90.
30. Schnurra I, Bernstein HG, Riederer P, Braunewell KH. The neuronal calcium sensor protein VILIP-1 is associated with amyloid plaques and extracellular tangles in Alzheimer's disease and promotes cell death and tau phosphorylation in vitro: a link between calcium sensors and Alzheimer's disease? Neurobiol Dis. 2001;8(5):900–9.
31. Tarawneh R, D'Angelo G, Macy E, Xiong C, Carter D, Cairns NJ, Fagan AM, Head D, Mintun MA, Ladenson JH, et al. Visinin-like protein-1: diagnostic and prognostic biomarker in Alzheimer disease. Ann Neurol. 2011;70(2):274–85.
32. Tarawneh R, Lee JM, Ladenson JH, Morris JC, Holtzman DM. CSF VILIP-1 predicts rates of cognitive decline in early Alzheimer disease. Neurology. 2012;78(10):709–19.
33. Teunissen CE, Petzold A, Bennett JL, Berven FS, Brundin L, Comabella M, Franciotta D, Frederiksen JL, Fleming JO, Furlan R, et al. A consensus protocol for the standardization of cerebrospinal fluid collection and biobanking. Neurology. 2009;73(22):1914–22.
34. Chiasserini D, Biscetti L, Farotti L, Eusebi P, Salvadori N, Lisetti V, Baschieri F, Chipi E, Frattini G, Stoops E, et al. Performance Evaluation of an Automated ELISA System for Alzheimer's Disease Detection in Clinical Routine. J Alzheimers Dis. 2016;54(1):55–67.
35. Sutphen CL, Jasielec MS, Shah AR, Macy EM, Xiong C, Vlassenko AG, Benzinger TL, Stoops EE, Vanderstichele HM, Brix B, et al. Longitudinal cerebrospinal fluid biomarker changes in preclinical Alzheimer disease during middle age. JAMA Neurol. 2015;72(9):1029–42.
36. Cicognola C, Chiasserini D, Parnetti L. Preanalytical confounding factors in the analysis of cerebrospinal fluid biomarkers for Alzheimer's disease: the issue of diurnal variation. Front Neurol. 2015;6:143.
37. Fourier A, Portelius E, Zetterberg H, Blennow K, Quadrio I, Perret-Liaudet A. Pre-analytical and analytical factors influencing Alzheimer's disease cerebrospinal fluid biomarker variability. Clin Chim Acta. 2015;449:9–15.
38. Brandner S, Thaler C, Lelental N, Buchfelder M, Kleindienst A, Maler JM, Kornhuber J, Lewczuk P. Ventricular and lumbar cerebrospinal fluid concentrations of Alzheimer's disease biomarkers in patients with normal pressure hydrocephalus and posttraumatic hydrocephalus. J Alzheimers Dis. 2014;41(4):1057–62.

9

High-density lipoproteins suppress Aβ-induced PBMC adhesion to human endothelial cells in bioengineered vessels and in monoculture

Jérôme Robert[1,2†], Emily B. Button[1,2†], Sophie Stukas[1,2], Guilaine K. Boyce[1,2], Ebrima Gibbs[2,3], Catherine M. Cowan[4], Megan Gilmour[1,2], Wai Hang Cheng[1,2], Sonja K. Soo[1,2], Brian Yuen[1,2], Arvin Bahrabadi[1,2], Kevin Kang[1,2], Iva Kulic[1,2], Gordon Francis[5], Neil Cashman[2,3] and Cheryl L. Wellington[1,2*]

Abstract

Background: Alzheimer's Disease (AD), characterized by accumulation of beta-amyloid (Aβ) plaques in the brain, can be caused by age-related failures to clear Aβ from the brain through pathways that involve the cerebrovasculature. Vascular risk factors are known to increase AD risk, but less is known about potential protective factors. We hypothesize that high-density lipoproteins (HDL) may protect against AD, as HDL have vasoprotective properties that are well described for peripheral vessels. Epidemiological studies suggest that HDL is associated with reduced AD risk, and animal model studies support a beneficial role for HDL in selectively reducing cerebrovascular amyloid deposition and neuroinflammation. However, the mechanism by which HDL may protect the cerebrovascular endothelium in the context of AD is not understood.

Methods: We used peripheral blood mononuclear cell adhesion assays in both a highly novel three dimensional (3D) biomimetic model of the human vasculature composed of primary human endothelial cells (EC) and smooth muscle cells cultured under flow conditions, as well as in monolayer cultures of ECs, to study how HDL protects ECs from the detrimental effects of Aβ.

Results: Following Aβ addition to the abluminal (brain) side of the vessel, we demonstrate that HDL circulated within the lumen attenuates monocyte adhesion to ECs in this biofidelic vascular model. The mechanism by which HDL suppresses Aβ-mediated monocyte adhesion to ECs was investigated using monotypic EC cultures. We show that HDL reduces Aβ-induced PBMC adhesion to ECs independent of nitric oxide (NO) production, miR-233 and changes in adhesion molecule expression. Rather, HDL acts through scavenger receptor (SR)-BI to block Aβ uptake into ECs and, in cell-free assays, can maintain Aβ in a soluble state. We confirm the role of SR-BI in our bioengineered human vessel.

Conclusion: Our results define a novel activity of HDL that suppresses Aβ-mediated monocyte adhesion to the cerebrovascular endothelium.

Keywords: Alzheimer's disease, Beta-amyloid, High-density lipoprotein, Engineered vessel, Endothelial cells

* Correspondence: wcheryl@mail.ubc.ca
†Equal contributors
[1]Department of Pathology and Laboratory Medicine, University of British Columbia, Vancouver, BC V6T 1Z3, Canada
[2]Djavad Mowafaghian Centre for Brain Health, University of British Columbia, 2215 Wesbrook Mall, Vancouver, BC V6T 1Z3, Canada
Full list of author information is available at the end of the article

Background

Alzheimer's disease (AD) is the leading cause of dementia with over 44 million affected persons worldwide and has no effective treatment [1]. AD is believed to arise from the toxic effects of amyloidogenic beta-amyloid peptides (Aβ), which form higher order structures including oligomers and fibrils that accumulate as amyloid plaques in the brain parenchyma and cerebral vessels [2]. The role of the cerebrovasculature in AD has gained increased recognition in the last decade, as AD risk is increased by vascular risk factors, including hypertension, type 2 diabetes mellitus (T2DM), and hypercholesterolemia [3–5]. Most AD autopsy cases have evidence of cerebral small vessel disease, including cerebral amyloid angiopathy (CAA) and microvascular degeneration, with micro- and macro-infarcts reported in over 80% of very old AD subjects [6]. The cerebrovasculature plays a pivotal role in clearing Aβ from the brain [7], and activation of cerebrovascular endothelial cells (ECs) has been reported in AD brain [8].

High-density lipoproteins (HDL) are a heterogeneous mixture of circulating lipoprotein particles that are composed of, in addition to apoA-I, cholesterol and phospholipids, over 200 lipid species and at least 95 proteins in normolipidemic plasma [9, 10]. Intriguingly, the elevated concentration of plasma high-density lipoprotein cholesterol (HDL-C), which is associated with reduced cardiovascular disease risk [11], is also negatively correlated with cognitive decline [12]. Preclinical studies also support a beneficial role of HDL on the cerebrovasculature. Specifically, transgenic overexpression of human apoA-I, the major protein component on HDL, from its endogenous promoter in the liver and intestine, reduces neuroinflammation, improves cognitive function and selectively reduces cerebrovascular amyloid in the APP/PS1 model of amyloidosis, whereas deletion of apoA-I, the major protein component of HDL, has the opposite effects [13, 14]. We recently reported that a single intravenous injection of reconstituted HDL reduces soluble brain Aβ40 and Aβ42 levels after 24 h in symptomatic APP/PS1 mice [15].

Systemically circulating HDL may therefore benefit the brain, however, the mechanisms by which it may do so are unknown. HDL is well established to possess several potent vasoprotective functions in peripheral vascular endothelial cells (ECs) including reducing inflammation, increasing vascular tone through promoting endothelial nitric oxide (NO) synthase activity, and suppressing vascular adhesion molecule expression [16]. Using peripheral blood mononuclear cell (PBMC) adherence assays, here we show that Aβ induces PMBC adhesion, a classical measure of EC activation, in cerebral microvascular ECs through a mechanism distinct from classical inflammatory stimulation by tumor necrosis factor-alpha (TNF-α). We also demonstrate that HDL robustly suppresses Aβ-induced monocyte adhesion to ECs both in monolayer cultures as well as in a novel 3 dimensional (3D) tissue engineered human vessel.

Methods

Fabrication of tissue engineered vessels

Scaffold-directed human engineered vessels were generated under flow bioreactor conditions as described [17]. Briefly, non-woven polyglycolic-acid meshes (PGA; BMS) were coated with polycoprolactone (PCL, Purac) and polyglycolic acid (PLA, Purac) by dipping into a 1.75% (*w*/w/w) solution of PCL/PLA/tetrahydrofuran (Sigma Aldrich). A tubular shape (length 10 mm and inner diameter 2 mm) was obtained by heat welding before external coating with a 10% (*w*/w) PCL/tetrahydrofuran solution. After sterilization with 70% ethanol for 30 min followed by 3 washes with PBS, scaffolds were pre-incubated in advanced DMEM overnight before cell seeding. Human umbilical cord smooth muscle cells were isolated as described [17] and 2 × 10^6 cells/cm^2 were seeded in the inner surface of the vascular scaffold using fibrinogen (10 mg/mL clottable protein, Sigma Aldrich) and thrombin (10 mU) as cell carriers [18]. After a short static incubation period of 3 days, vascular constructs were exposed to dynamic conditioning in a flow bioreactor, where the flow of nutrient medium (Advanced DMEM (Invitrogen) with 10% FBS; 0.05% Penicillin/Streptomycin, 1% L-glutamine and 1.5 mM L-ascorbic acid) was directed through the inner lumen of the bioreactor circulation loop at 6 mL/min. After 14 days of flow conditioning, vascular grafts were endothelialzed with HUVECs (1.5 × 10^6 cells/cm^2) seeded into the lumen followed by cultivation under static conditions for 5 days in complete endothelial growth medium (EBM-2; Lonza) supplemented with 10% foetal bovine serum (FBS) and growth supplements to form EGM complete media FBS. After the static phase, vascular grafts were placed back in the bioreactor for 14 additional days with increasing medium flow (4 to 6 mL/min) in complete EGM-2 with 10% FBS.

Characterization of engineered vascular tissue

For histological characterization, engineered vessels were fixed in formalin (Fisher), dehydrated through a graded ethanol series using a Sakura Tissue Processor (Sakura), embedded in paraffin and sectioned at 7 μm thickness. Sections were deparaffinised, rehydrated through a graded ethanol series and stained using haematoxylin & eosin (SigmaAldrich) following the manufacture's instructions. For immunofluorescence analyses, tissues were cryopreserved in Cryomatrix (ThermoFisher) and sectioned at 20 μm thickness using a cryotome (Leica). Immunostaining was performed as described [17] using antibodies specific for the EC marker CD31 (clone JC/70A Biolegend, 1:50) and α-smooth muscle actin (clone 1A4 SigmaAldrich, 1:200). Sections were counter-stained with DAPI and imaged with an inverted microscope (Carl Zeiss). Endothelium barrier integrity was analyzed by injecting Evans blue (Sigma Aldrich) at a final concentration of 0.5% in the circulation loop of the bioreactor for 10 min followed by continuous PBS washing for 20 min. Vessels were cut open longitudinally and *en face* preparations were analysed macroscopically with photo documentation.

Preparation of HDL and PBMCs

All experiments were conducted under an approved clinical protocol (UBC Clinical Ethics Research Board H14–03357). Upon receipt of written informed consent, 100 mL of fasted blood was collected from normolipidemic healthy donors into vacutainer tubes. Plasma HDL (1.063–1.21 g/mL) was isolated by sequential potassium bromide gradient ultracentrifugation as described [19]. The purity of the HDL preparations was verified by sodium dodecyl sulphate-polyacrylamide gel electrophoresis (SDS-PAGE) followed by Coomassie blue staining to ensure no low-density lipoprotein (LDL) or albumin contamination. Eight independent donors were used across the experiments, 6 isolated in-house and 2 commercially obtained (Leebioscience). Human-derived, lipid free apoA-I was a kind gift from CSL-Behring. Immortalized human THP1 monocytes (ATCC) were cultured in RPMI containing 10% FBS, 1% Pen/Strep, 2 mM L-glutamine and 0.1% β-mercaptoethanol. Primary human PBMC were isolated from healthy donors by centrifugation on a continuous density gradient (Lymphoprep™, Stemcell) following the manufacturer's instructions. Freshly isolated PBMC were fluorescently labeled with 10 μM of Cell-Tracker Red for 30 min (Invitrogen) following the manufacturer's recommendations.

Monocyte adhesion in engineered vessels

Vascular grafts were perfused with complete EGM-2 with 2% FBS. 1 μM Aβ42 or Aβ40 monomers were injected directly into the graft chamber to mimic Aβ originating from the brain (antelumen) side of the vessel. At time points ranging from 2 to 72 h, THP1 cells were fluorescently labeled with Cell-Tracker Red as described above, injected in the graft circulation at a concentration of 1×10^6 cells/mL and maintained under flow conditions for 3 h. For HDL experiments, vascular grafts were perfused with luminal HDL (200 μg/mL) for 2 h before injecting Aβ in the antelumen side for 8 h. Tissues were longitudinally cut open, washed extensively with PBS and fixed with 4% PFA. After 20 min, tissues were washed 3 times with PBS and mounted in Prolong Gold antifade reagent with DAPI. For each independently seeded tissue, adherent monocytes and monocytes undergoing diapedesis were counted in 3 random squares of 1.23 mm^2 using a z-stack covering the whole tissue thickness with a SP8 confocal microscope (Leica), averaged and expressed as percent of vehicle normalized to 100% for Fig. 1d and f or percent of Aβ normalized to 100% for Fig. 1 h and j, and Fig. 8a and b.

Static monotypic cell culture

hCMEC/D3 (Fisher; passage 27–35), and HUVEC (passage 4–7, isolated as described [17]) cells were cultured using complete EGM-2 with 2% FBS, ECs were cultured in a humidified incubator at 37 °C at 5% carbon dioxide. For mechanistic experiments, ECs were treated with SR-BI blocking antibody (NB440–113 Novus, 1:500), the SR-BI inhibitor block lipid transport-1 (BLT-1, SigmaAldrich, 10 μM), the eNOS inhibitor L–NG-nitroarginne methyl ester (L-NAME, SigmaAldrich, 1 mM), the receptor associated protein (RAP, Oxford biome, 1 μM), the RAGE blocking antibody (176,902, R&D Systems, 1:50), heparin (10 mU), heparinase (SigmaAldrich, 0.2 mM) or the CD36 blocking antibody (JC63.1, ABCAM, 1:500) for 1 h before HDL priming. For miRNA experiments, cells were transiently transfected using Lipofectamine 2000 (Life Technology) 2 h before Aβ stimulation with the miR-223 mimetic (Life Technology, 4,464,066 (MC12301), 100 nM) or miR-223 inhibitor (Life Technology, 4,464,084 (MH12301), 100 nM) in EBM-2 containing 0.2% BSA.

Monolayer PBMC adhesion assay

ECs were seeded at 1×10^5 cells/well in 24-well plates and cultured until confluent for 2 to 3 days. On the day of the assay, ECs were primed for 2 h with 100 μg/mL bovine serum albumin as vehicle control or 100 μg/mL HDL before stimulation with 1 ng/mL of TNF-α (Preprotech) or various concentrations of monomeric Aβ40 and Aβ42 (0.001–1 μM, California Peptide), prepared as described below. After 3 h, 5×10^5 Cell-Tracker Red-labeled PBMC per well were added to ECs for 3 additional hours before washing 3 times with PBS to remove non-adherent PBMC. Cells were then fixed with 4% PFA for 15 min before 3 additional PBS washes and 4′,6-diamidino-2-phenylindole (DAPI) counterstaining. For each independent experiment, adherent monocytes were counted in 5 random squares of 7.84 mm^2 using a fluorescent inverted microscope (Zeiss), averaged and expressed as percent of vehicle normalized to 100%. DAPI counterstaining was used to ensure endothelial cell coverage.

Aβ oligomerization/fibrilization and electron microscopy confirmation

Recombinant Aβ40 and Aβ42 peptides (California Peptide) were dissolved in ice-cold hexafluoroisopropanol (HFIP).

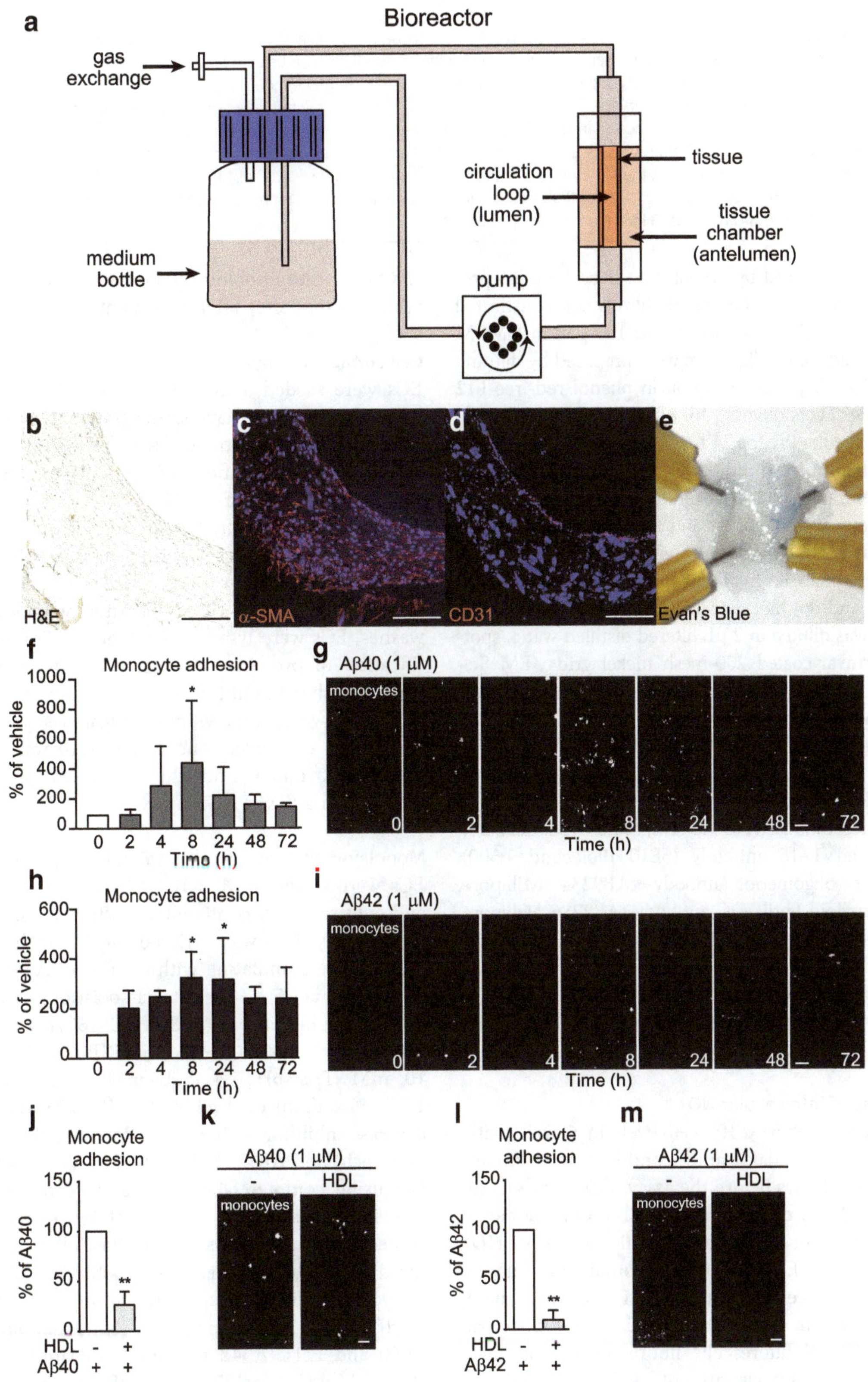

Fig. 1 (See legend on next page.)

(See figure on previous page.)
Fig. 1 Aβ induces monocyte adhesion in engineered vessels, which is suppressed by HDL. **a** Schematic representation of bioengineered tissue. **b** Histological structure of engineered tissue using hematoxalin-eosin staining to reveal a dense tissue formation composed of cells and extracellular matrix in engineered vessels. **c** α-smooth muscle actin (α-SMA) confirmed the smooth muscle phenotype of cells in the inner layers and **d** CD31 confirmed an endothelial monolayer. Scale bar represents 200 μm. **e** Evans blue staining confirmed a tight endothelium. **f-g** 1 μM of Aβ40 or **h-i** Aβ42 monomers were injected within the tissue chamber (abluminal). Fluorescently labeled human monocytes (THP1, *white*) were circulated in the lumen of the engineered vessels. Tissues were counterstained with DAPI (*blue*) and analyzed using confocal microscopy over time. **j-m** 200 μg/mL of HDL were circulated through the lumen of the grafts for 2 h prior injection of 1 μM of **j-k** Aβ40 or **l-m** Aβ42 monomers within the tissue chamber (abluminal) for 8 h prior to circulating fluorescent THP1 in the lumen. Graphs represent means ± SD of adhered monocytes relative to Aβ treated tissues from at least 3 individual grafts. $^*p < 0.05$, $^{**}p < 0.01$

The HFIP was removed by evaporation overnight. To prepare soluble monomers, the peptide film was reconstituted in DMSO to 5 mM, diluted further to 100 μM in DMEM and used immediately. Oligomers were prepared by diluting the 5 mM DMSO peptide solution in phenol red-free F12 medium (Life Technologies) to a final concentration of 100 μM and incubating for 24 h 4 °C. Fibrils were prepared by diluting the 5 mM peptide solution in 0.1 uM of HCl to a final concentration of 100 μM and incubating for 24 h at 37 °C. Aβ monomer, oligomer and fibril preparations were then either used to stimulate hCMEC/D3 monolayers, as given, or were analysed by Transmission Electron Microscopy (TEM) and dot blot. For TEM, 0.5 μL of 100 μM Aβ preparation was diluted in 2 μL filtered distilled water, spotted onto formvar-coated 200-mesh nickel grids (EM Sciences) and allowed to dry. Grids were then negatively stained with 0.5% aqueous uranyl acetate for 30 s, and viewed on a FEI Tecnai G2 Spirit Transmission Electron Microscope. For dot blot, aliquots of Aβ(0.1 μM) were added to PVDF membrane, which were dried and blocked in 3% skimmed milk PBST. After 1 h, blots were incubated with β-amyloid 1–16 antibody (6E10 Biolegend 1:500), amyloid A11 oligomeric antibody (AB9234 Millipore, 1:1000) or amyloid fibrils OC antibody (AB2286 Millipore, 1:1000) in blocking buffer for 16 h, washed extensively in PBST and incubated with anti-mouse or anti-rabbit (1:1000) secondary antibody in blocking buffer. After 1 h, blots were washed as above and developed using enhanced ECL and a ChemiDoc MP imager.

Measurement of intracellular NO

ECs were seeded at 5 × 10^5 cells/well in 6-well plates and cultured for 2 days until confluent in complete EBM-2. Sixteen hours before the assay, ECs were serum-depleted in EBM-2 containing 0.2% FBS. On the day of the assay, ECs were incubated with 100 μg/mL of HDL in serum-depleted EBM-2 medium containing 1 μM of 4,5-diaminofluorescein diacetate (DAF2, Caymanchem) at 37 °C. After 6 h, ECs were washed with PBS, trypsinized, and triazolofluorescein fluorescence was measured (excitation wavelength of 485 nm, emission 538 nm), using an Infinite M200Pro plate reader (Tecan). In addition to DAF2 measurement, the phosphorylation of eNOS at Ser1177 was compared to total eNOS by immunoblotting (below) in cell lysates harvested 15 min after HDL treatment.

Cell surface biotinylation

ECs were seeded at 5 × 10^5 cells/well in 6-well plates and cultured for 2 days until confluent. On the day of the assay, ECs were treated with HDL, Aβ or TNF-α as above. After stimulation, EC monolayers were washed twice with ice cold PBS (pH 8), cooled on ice for 15 min and biotinylated with 250 μg/mL EZ-link™-sulfo-NHS-biotin (ThermoFisher Scientific) in PBS (pH 8) at 4 °C. After 1 h the reaction was stopped with a 5 min incubation in DMEM with 10% FBS. After two additional PBS washes, ECs were lysed in RIPA buffer. Following quantification of protein concentration using a BCA assay (Thermofisher Scientific), at least 100 μg of protein were incubated with streptavidin-conjugated sepharose beads (Pierce) at 4 °C overnight. Beads were washed 3 times with RIPA buffer and the recovered proteins were resolved on a SDS-PAGE.

Monolayer aβ association, binding and uptake

ECs were seeded at 3 × 10^5 cells/well in 12-well plates and cultured until confluent for 2 to 3 days. On the day of the assay, ECs were primed for 2 h with 100 μg/mL HDL before stimulating with 0.1 μM of Aβ40 and Aβ42 monomers at 37 °C for total association, or at 4 °C for cell surface binding. After 3 h, hCMEC/D3 were washed 3 times with PBC and lysed in RIPA buffer containing 10 mM Tris pH 7.4, 150 mM NaCl, 1.0% NP-40, 1.0````% sodium deoxycholate, 0.1% SDS and cOmplete protease inhibitor with EDTA (Roche). Aβ40 (KHB3442, Life Tech) and Aβ42 (KHB3482, Life Tech) were quantified using commercial ELISAs and normalized to total protein concentration. For Aβ uptake, hCMEC/D3 were seeded at 1 × 10^5 cells/well in 24-well plates and cultured to confluence for 2 to 3 days. On the day of the assay endothelial, ECs were primed for 2 h with 1 mg/mL of HDL before stimulating with 1 μM monomeric FITC-Aβ40 and FITC-Aβ42 (Bachem) prepared as described above. After 3 h at 37 °C, hCMEC/D3 were washed 3 times with PBS and fixed in 4% PFA for 20 min. After one Tris-HCl and two PBS washes, hCMEC/D3 were mounted in Prolong antifade reagent.

Molecular biology

For mRNA, cells were lysed in Trizol (Invitrogen) and RNA was extracted and treated with DNase I (Invitrogen) according to the manufacturer's protocol. cDNA was generated using oligo-dT primers and Taqman reverse transcription reagents (Applied Biosystems). Real-time quantitative PCR was done using FastStart Universal SYBR Green Master reagent (Roche) on a Light Cycler 96 system (Roche) to quantify gene expression relative to vehicle using specific primer against ICAM-1 (fwd: ATGGCAACGAC TCCTTCTCG; rev: CGCCGGAAAGCTGTAGATGG) and VCAM-1 (fwd: TGTTTGCAGCTTCTCAAGCTTTT; rev: GATGTGGTCCCCTCATTCGT) and normalized to GAPDH (fwd: CCTGCACCACCAACTGCTTA; rev: CATGAGTCCTTCCACGATACCA). MiRNA was isolated using an miRNeasy mini kit (Qiagen) following the manufacturer's instructions, respectively. Reverse transcription was performed using 2 μg of total RNA with specific miRNA primers (Life Technology). MiR223 and U6 were quantified using specific TaqMan probes (Life Technology).

Immunoblot

ECs were lysed in RIPA buffer containing either cOmplete protease inhibitor or Phosphostop (Roche) and quantified using a BCA assay. Equal amounts of total protein were separated by SDS-PAGE followed by electrophoretic transfer to polyvinylidene fluoride (PVDF) membranes (Millipore). After blocking membranes for 1 h with 5% skim milk powder in PBST, or 5% BSA in TBST for phosphoproteins, ICAM-1, (EP1442Y Abcam, 1:1000), VCAM 1 (EPR5047 Novus, 1:1000), peNOS (ser1177 Cellsignalling, 1:1000), eNOS (M221 ABCAM, 1:1000), AnxA1 (D5V2T, Cellsignalling, 1:1000), p-Akt (Ser473 D9E, Cellsignalling, 1:2000), Akt (9272, Cellsignalling, 1:1000), p-NF-κB p65 (Ser536 93H1, Cellsignalling, 1:1000), NF-κB p65 (D14E12, Cellsignalling, 1:1000), p-SAPK/JNK (Thr183/Tyr185 G9, Cellsignalling, 1:1000), JNK (2C6, Cellsignalling, 1:1000), p-p42/44 MAPK (Erk1/2) (Thr202/Tyr204 D13.14.4E, Cellsignalling, 1:1000), p42/44 MAPK (Erk1/2) (137F5, Cellsignalling, 1:1000), p-Stat3 (Tyr705, Cellsignalling 1:1000), Stat3 (124H6, Cellsignalling, 1:1000) and GAPDH (MAB374 1:10,000, Millipore) were immunodetected by incubating for 16 h in primary antibody in blocking buffers. Membranes were washed extensively with PBST or TBST, and incubated with anti-mouse or anti-rabbit (1:1000–10′000, Jackson ImmunoResearch) secondary antibody in blocking buffer. After 1 h, membranes were washed as above and developed using enhanced chemiluminescence (ECL, Amersham) and a ChemiDoc MP imager (Biorad). Densitometric images were captured with ImageJ and band intensity normalized to GAPDH as a loading control.

Beta-sheet formation assay

Cell-free Thioflavin-T fibrillization assays were performed on an Infinite M2000 Pro plate reader (Tecan) as described (Truran 2015). Briefly, 10 μM monomeric Aβ40 or Aβ42 were incubated in a buffer consisting of 20 mM of Thioflavin-T in 150 mM NaCl and 5 μM of HEPES at pH 7.4, with and without 1 mg/mL of HDL, at 37 °C with 20 s of orbital shaking (3 mm amplitude) every 5 min in a black 96-well plate. Formation of fibrillar β-amyloid pleated sheets over time was monitored by excitation at 440 nm and measuring emission intensity at 490 nm every 5 min up to 12 h in total.

Human brain protein extraction and ELISA

Frozen brain tissues (cortex Brodmann area 9 and cerebellum) were provided by the Harvard Brain Tissue Resource Center under an approved UBC protocol (C04–0595) and extracted with 8 volumes of ice-cold carbonate buffer (100 mM Na_2CO_3, 50 mM NaCl, pH 11.5) containing cOmplete protease inhibitor (Roche Applied Science) by manual homogenization with a tissue probe. After incubating on ice for 10 min, lysates were clarified by centrifugation at 16,600 rcf for 45 min at 4 °C. The supernatant was removed and neutralized by adding 1.5-volumes of 1 M Tris-HCl pH 6.8 to give a final pH of approximately 7.4. Brain tissues from all samples were extracted in an identical manner, and fractions were aliquoted and immediately frozen at −80 °C until analysis. Protein concentrations were determined using the Lowry Protein Assay (Biorad). ICAM-1 (ab174445, ABCAM), VCAM-1 (ab187393, ABCAM), Aβ40 (KHB3442, Life Tech) and Aβ42 (KHB3482, Life Tech) in carbonate extracts were quantified using commercial ELISAs. ELISA data were normalized to total protein concentration of the extract. For immunofluorescent staining, brains were sectioned at 20 μm, rehydrated in PBS and blocked in 4% paraformaldehyde (PFA). After 20 min, sections were washed once with Tris-HCl (0.5 mM, pH 8), twice with PBS, and blocked in blocking buffer (5% goat serum and 1% BSA). After 60 min, section were incubated at 4 °C with antibodies against CD31 (WM59 Biolegend, 1:50), ICAM-1 (EP1442Y ABCAM 1:200), and VCAM-1 (EPR5047 ABCAM 1:200) in blocking buffer overnight. Sections were washed 3 times in PBS and incubated at RT with Alexa-488 anti-mouse and Alexa-594 anti-rabbit fluorescently labeled secondary antibodies (LifeTechnologies, 1:600). After 45 min and 3 additional PBS washes, sections were mounted in Prolong Gold antifade reagent with DAPI (LifeTechnologies) and imaged on an inverted fluorescent microscope (Zeiss)

Statistical analysis

All statistical analyses were performed using SPSS and p-values <0.05 were considered significant. Data were obtained from at least 3 independent experiments and are presented as mean ± SD if not indicated otherwise. Data were first log transformed and analyzed by two-way ANOVA with a blocking factor (experiment) with direct comparison when comparing two treatments or Dunnett's or Bonferonni multi-comparison tests. After statistical calculations, vehicle data were normalized to 100% and represented as a dashed line in the graph, and tested conditions were expressed and graphed as percentage of vehicle if not otherwise stated.

Results

HDL suppresses aβ-mediated monocyte adhesion to ECs in three-dimensional dynamic engineered human vessels

To mimic the complexity of native cell-cell and/or cell-matrix interactions observed in native human vessels, we used innovative tissue engineering technology to generate in vitro 3D human vessels composed of primary human umbilical vein ECs (HUVEC) and primary human smooth muscle cells (SMC) to maximize translational relevance of our studies relative to in vitro studies that solely use traditional static cell culture models. Our system uses a scaffold-directed dynamic, semi-pulsatile flow bioreactor system, on which primary human cells are sequentially seeded into 2 mm diameter biodegradable polyglycolic-acid (PGA)/polycaprolactone (PCL) composite matrices. After a short static incubation, vascular constructs are exposed to dynamic flow in a bioreactor, where nutrient medium is directed through the lumen of the bioreactor circulation loop to mimic native blood flow. We previously demonstrated that these scaffold-directed engineered vessels are useful for studies of endothelial activation in 3D culture [17]. A schematic of the bioreactor system is presented in Fig. 1a. Under our flow bioreactor conditions, haematoxylin and eosin staining confirmed a dense tissue formation composed of cells with extracellular matrix on the luminal side of the scaffold (Fig. 1b-d). Immunofluorescent staining confirmed a SMC phenotype of cells in the inner layers and an EC monolayer on the luminal side (Fig. 1c,d). Integrity of the endothelial barrier was functionally assessed by injecting Evans blue dye into the bioreactor circulation loop, which was excluded after EC seeding, demonstrating a functionally tight endothelial barrier (Fig. 1e).

Having established a 3D human vascular model, we injected 1 μM Aβ40 or Aβ42 directly into the graft chamber to mimic Aβ coming from the brain anteluminal side, followed by injection of human THP-1 monocytes into the lumen chamber to mimic circulating monocytes. Both Aβ40 and Aβ42 led to THP1 adhesion to endothelium in the engineered vessels, with the most robust response appearing 8 h after Aβ injection (Fig. 1f-h). We then tested the ability of HDL, isolated from healthy human donors using KBr density gradient ultracentrifugation, to suppress Aβ-induced monocyte adhesion to ECs in engineered vessels by circulating either media alone or 200 μg/mL of HDL for 2 h prior to injecting 1 μM Aβ into the graft chamber. In this engineered vascular model, HDL robustly suppressed monocyte adhesion to endothelium by both Aβ40 (5 fold, p = 0.0286) and Aβ42 (10 fold, p = 0.0016) (Fig. 1i-l).

HDL attenuates aβ-induced peripheral blood mononuclear cell (PBMC) adhesion in monotypic ECs

To define the mechanisms by which HDL attenuates Aβ-induced monocyte binding to ECs, we used static monolayer EC cultures and peripheral blood mononuclear cells (PBMC) isolated by continuous density gradient ultracentrifugation from healthy human donors. We first confirmed that Aβ induces PBMC adhesion in monotypic HUVEC cultures and that HDL attenuates this activity (Fig. 2a,b). As Aβ originates within the brain and the primary pathways by which Aβ is cleared from the brain involve cerebral vessels [7], we also showed that the human brain microvascular endothelial cell line hCMEC/D3, a commonly used cell line for in vitro studies of the blood brain barrier (BBB) [20], also exhibit increased PBMC adhesion upon Aβ treatment and that this too is attenuated by HDL (Fig. 2c,d). As HUVEC and hCMEC/D3 give nearly identical results, we focused on hCMEC/D3 cells for all subsequent mechanistic experiments.

Our first question was to determine if lipid-free apoA-I was functionally equivalent to mature HDL in its ability to suppress Aβ-mediated PBMC binding to hCMEC/D3. Our results clearly showed that pre-incubation of hCMEC/D3 with lipid-free apoA-I (50 and 100 μg/mL) did not alter Aβ-induced PBMC adhesion (Fig. 2e,f), demonstrating that mature HDL particles are required to attenuate Aβ-induced PBMC adhesion to brain-derived ECs.

To establish the experimental conditions to investigate how HDL suppresses Aβ-mediated PBMC adhesion to hCMEC/D3, we performed PMBC adhesion assays in hCMEC/D3 after a 3 h exposure to increasing concentrations human Aβ40 and Aβ42 monomers. Compared to baseline, Aβ40 concentrations of 0.01, 0.1 and 1.0 μM led to significant 175%, 169% and 179% increases in PMBC adhesion (p = 0.033, 0.002 and 0.019 respectively, Additional file 1a), The same concentrations of Aβ42 also led to significant 184%, 161% and 223% increases in PMBC adhesion (p = 0.019, 0.0406 and 0.0421, respectively) relative to baseline (Additional file 1b). Having demonstrated that 0.1 μM of monomeric Aβ40 or Aβ42 is sufficient to induce PMBC adhesion in hCMEC/D3, we then tested whether pre-treating hCMEC/D3 for 2 h with 0 to 400 μg/mL HDL could attenuate Aβ-induced PBMC adhesion. Significant suppression of PBMC adhesion was observed at concentrations of HDL from 100 μg/mL and above. At 100 μg/mL HDL there was an

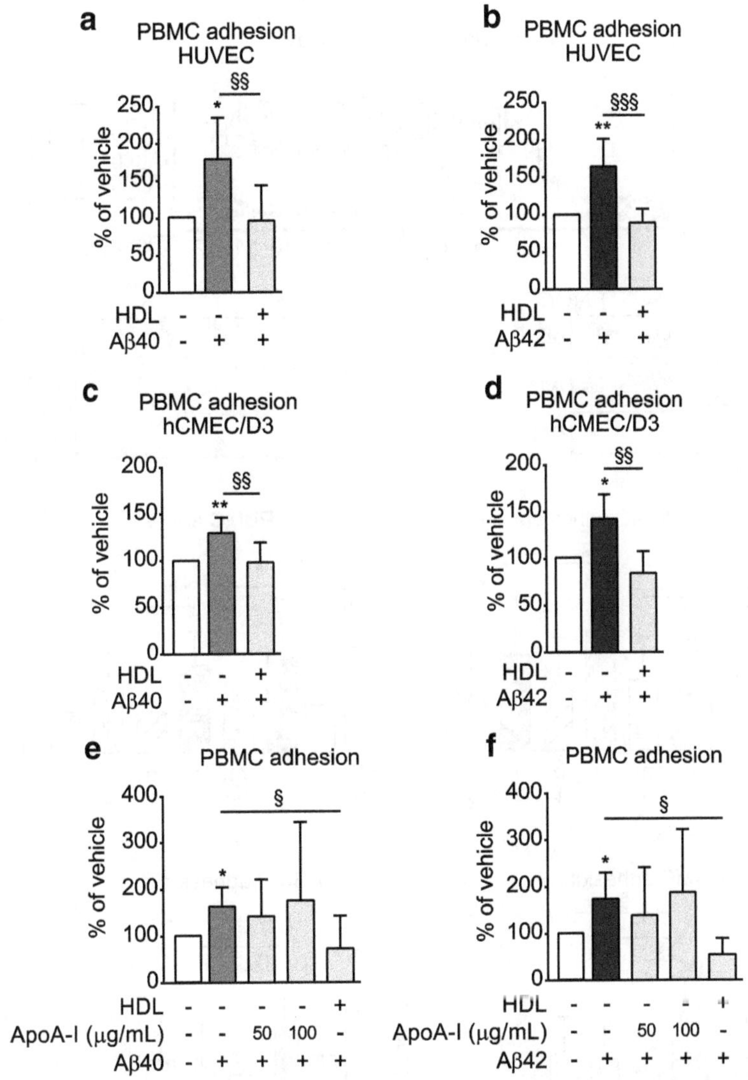

Fig. 2 Aβ40 and Aβ42 induce PBMC adhesion to ECs, which is suppressed by HDL. HUVEC (**a-b**) or hCMEC/D3 (**c-d**) were primed with 100 μg/mL of HDL and stimulated with 0.1 μM **a, c** Aβ40 (*light grey*) or **b, d**Aβ42 (*dark grey*) monomers for 3 h. Fluorescently labelled PBMC were allowed to adhere to stimulated cells for 3 h followed by washing, fixation, imaging, and counting. hCMEC/D3 were primed with either 100 μg/mL of HDL or 50 μg/mL or 100 μg/mL lipid-free human apoA-I for 2 h followed by stimulation with 0.1 μM **e** Aβ40 (*light grey*) or **f** Aβ42 (*dark grey*) monomers for 3 h. Cells were washed, imaged and counted as above. Graphs represent mean ± SD of adhered PBMC relative to vehicle control from at least 3 independent trials where * $p < 0.05$, ** $p < 0.01$, *** $p < 0.001$ versus vehicle, § $p < 0.05$, §§ $p < 0.01$ versus Aβ

80% and 60% reduction of adhered PBMCs in cells induced by 0.1 μM Aβ40 ($p = 0.017$) or 0.1 μM Aβ42 ($p = 0.018$) respectively (Additional file 1c,d).

HDL reduces the fibrillization rate of aβ42 and aβ40 in cell-free conditions

As Aβ has been reported to bind HDL-like particles in both cerebrospinal fluid (CSF) and blood [21], and apoA-I has been reported to affect Aβ aggregation [13, 22], we reasoned that one mechanism by which HDL may attenuate PBMC adhesion to hCMEC/D3 could be by affecting Aβ structure to prevent the formation of toxic higher order species [23]. A cell-free Thioflavin-T reporter assay was used to determine whether HDL affects the fibrillization kinetics of Aβ40 or Aβ42 over a 12 h period, using 10 μM Aβ and 10 mg/mL HDL (ratio: 1:1), which is the same Aβ:HDL ratio used for our cellular PBMC adhesion assays and allows detection of fluorescence signal using a plate reader (Fig. 2c,d). Under these conditions, in the absence of HDL, the onset of Aβ fibrillization requires at least 3 h for Aβ42 and at least 10 h for Aβ40. Notably, in the presence of HDL, we observed delayed onset of fibrillization for both Aβ42 and Aβ40, and a slower rate of Aβ42 fibrillization (Fig. 3a). As HDL can suppress PBMC

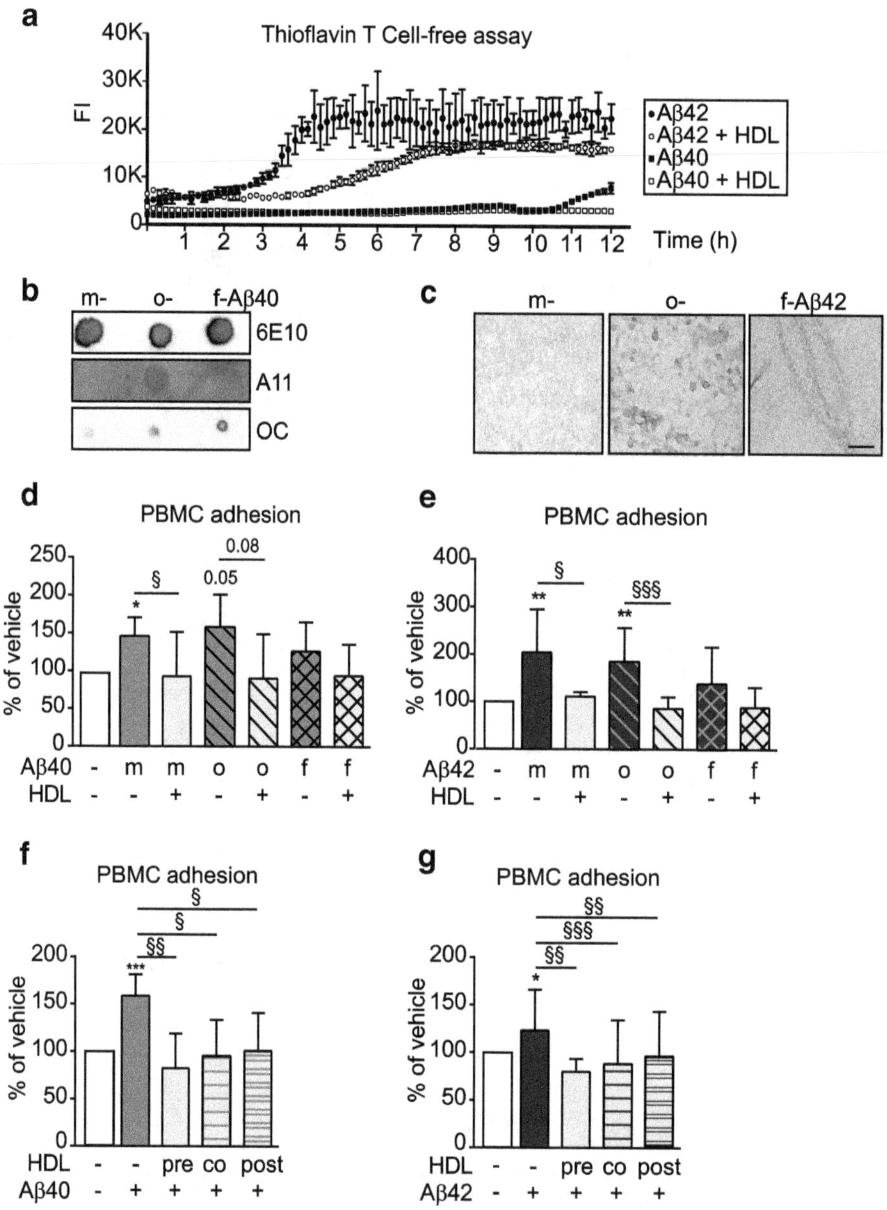

Fig. 3 HDL delays beta-sheet formation and attenuates Aβ-induced PBMC adherence independent of Aβ structure. **a** Representative graph ± SD of technical triplicates of 3 individual experiments where 10 μM Aβ40 or Aβ42 with or without 10 mg/mLl HDL were incubated with 20 μM of Thio-T in 150 mM NaCl and 5 μM of HEPES (pH 7.4) for 12 h at 37 °C. Formation of β-amyloid pleated sheets was monitored every 5 min at excitation 440 nm and emission 490 nm. **b-c** Aβ structures were confirmed using dot blot with antibodies against oligomers (A11) or fibrils (OC) and electron microscopy (EM). **d-e** hCMEC/D3 were stimulated for 3 h with 0.1 μM monomeric (m-Aβ, *solid bar*), oligomeric (o-Aβ, *striped bar*) or fibrillar-aggregated (f-A Aβ, *cross-hatched bar*) **d** Aβ40 or **e** Aβ42 in the presence or absence of HDL. **f-g** hCMEC/D3 were pre-incubated for 2 h with 100 μg/mL HDL prior to Aβ addition (pre, *solid bar*), co-incubated with 100 μg/mL HDL and Aβ (co, *striped bar*), or post-incubated by adding 100 μg/mL HDL 1 h following Aβ stimulation (post, *double striped bar*). Graphs represent means ± SD of adhered PBMC relative to vehicle treated cells from at least 5 independent trials where. *$p < 0.05$, **$p < 0.01$, ***$p < 0.001$ * $p < 0.05$, **$p < 0.01$, ***$p < 0.001$ versus vehicle, § $p < 0.05$, §§ $p < 0.01$, §§§$p < 0.001$ versus Aβ

adhesion to hCMEC/D3 induced by both Aβ40 and Aβ42 within 3 h of Aβ addition, we conclude that suppression of Aβ fibrillization cannot be the only mechanism by which HDL functions to protect ECs from the detrimental effects of Aβ.

Aβ structure does not affect HDL's ability to reduce PBMC adhesion to hCMEC/D3

Several experiments were then performed to further test whether Aβ structure affects HDL's anti-inflammatory activity on hCMEC/D3. We varied the structural species of the Aβ preparation added to hCMEC/D3, reasoning that if HDL acts primarily through maintaining Aβ in a soluble monomeric state, the protective effect of HDL should be diminished if ECs are stimulated with pre-formed Aβ oligomers or fibrils. Soluble monomeric and oligomeric, and insoluble fibrillar Aβ were prepared as described [24] and structures were confirmed using a dot blot assay as well as electron microscopy (Fig. 3b,c). Interestingly, monomeric and oligomeric Aβ40 and Aβ42 preparations induced comparably robust PBMC adherence, whereas the insoluble fibrillary form failed to significantly increase PBMC adhesion. Importantly, the ability of HDL to suppress PMBC adhesion was unaffected by input of either Aβ monomers or oligomers (Fig. 3d-e). These results suggest that delayed Aβ fibrillization may not be the major pathway by which HDL suppresses PBMC adhesion to ECs under our experimental conditions as HDL maintained its protective effect when ECs are treated with pre-formed oligomers. To confirm this, we also varied the timing of HDL and Aβ addition to hCMEC/D3 such that, in addition to a 2 h HDL pre-incubation as above, HDL was added at the same time as Aβ (co-incubation) or 1 h after Aβ addition (post-incubation). We reasoned that if HDL acts primarily through maintaining Aβ solubility, pre-incubation and co-incubation designs should give equivalent and maximal suppression of Aβ-induced PBMC adhesion as, in both scenarios, Aβ is always in the presence of HDL and aggregation could be delayed. In contrast, as the post-incubation scenario would allow Aβ aggregation to begin prior to addition of HDL, the protective effect of HDL should be reduced if added after the Aβ stimulus if Aβ structure is the key driver of PBMC adhesion to ECs. We observed that PMBC adhesion was significantly and similarly reduced regardless of when HDL was added to hCMEC/D3 relative to Aβ40 or Aβ42 providing additional support that HDL's ability to attenuate Aβ-mediated PBMC adhesion to hCMEC/D3 is independent of whether Aβ input is monomeric or oligomeric (Fig. 3f,g).

These two lines of evidence suggest that, although HDL can affect Aβ structure in cell-free conditions, these effects are neither rapid nor robust enough to fully explain how HDL suppresses Aβ mediated PBMC adhesion to hCMEC/D3. We next evaluated signalling pathways implicated in HDL's anti-inflammatory effects on ECs.

The ability of HDL to suppresses aβ-induced PBMC adhesion to hCMEC/D3 is independent of nitric oxide (NO) production and Annexin A1 (Anx1)

Stimulation of NO synthesis by HDL is reported to reduce arterial EC activation [25]. We therefore tested whether HDL induces NO production in hCMEC/D3 using the cell permeable indicator 4,5-Diaminofluorescein diacetate (DAF2), which reacts with NO to produce highly fluorescent trizaolo-fluorescein. Compared to baseline conditions, HDL-treated hCMEC/D3 showed a significant 130% increase ($p = 0.01$) in NO production (Fig. 4a), as well as significantly elevated phosphorylated endothelial NO synthase (eNOS) on serine 1177 (161%, $p = 0.047$) (Fig. 4b,c). These results confirm that HDL can induce NO production in hCMEC/D3, as observed in ECs derived from other origins.

To test whether NO generation is required for HDL to suppress Aβ-mediated PBMC adhesion to hCMEC/D3, we treated cells with the eNOS inhibitor L-NAME, followed by the addition of HDL, and finally stimulation with either Aβ40, Aβ42 or TNF-α. We observed that blocking eNOS with L-NAME had no effect on the ability of HDL to suppress either Aβ- or TNF-α-mediated PBMC adhesion to hCMEC/D3 (Fig. 4d-f). Additional experiments confirmed the potency of L-NAME to block eNOS in HDL-stimulated HUVEC (Additional file 2a), yet this also had no effect on the ability of HDL to suppress either Aβ- or TNF-α- mediated PBMC binding in HUVEC (Additional file 2b–d). We further ruled out a role for the NO pathway in hCMEC/D3 by measuring the effect of HDL in the presence of VPC23019, an antagonist of sphingosine-1 phosphate receptor 1 (S1P1) and S1P3, receptors that are required for eNOS activity [26], and again found no effect on the ability of HDL to suppress either Aβ- or TNF-α-mediated PBMC adhesion to hCMEC/D3 (Fig. 4g-i) or HUVEC (Additional file 2e–h). Taken together, these results provide strong support that the eNOS pathway is not involved in the ability of HDL to suppress PBMC adhesion to Aβ- or TNF-α-activated hCMEC/D3 and HUVEC.

In contrast to a recent report suggesting that HDL upregulates Anx1, which affects HDL's ability to suppress ECs activation [27], we observed no significant change in Anx1 protein levels in hCMEC/D3 after either HDL or Aβ treatment (Additional file 2i).

HDL-mediated suppression of aβ-induced PBMC adhesion to hCMEC/D3 is independent of miR-233

In addition to numerous proteins and lipid species, HDL particles carry microRNAs (miRNAs) that can correlate with vascular disease risk [28]. One of the most abundant miRNAs in HDL is miR-233, which has recently been shown to affect gene expression in human coronary artery ECs including suppressing ICAM-1 expression [29]. Three lines of evidence suggest that HDL-mediated suppression of Aβ-mediated PBMC binding to hCMEC/D3 is independent of miR-233. First, direct transfection of a miR-223 mimetic did not prevent Aβ40 or TNF-α-mediated PBMC adhesion to hCMEC/D3, although a statistically significant reduction with Aβ42 was observed (Additional file 3a–c). Second, priming hCMEC/D3 with HDL in the presence of

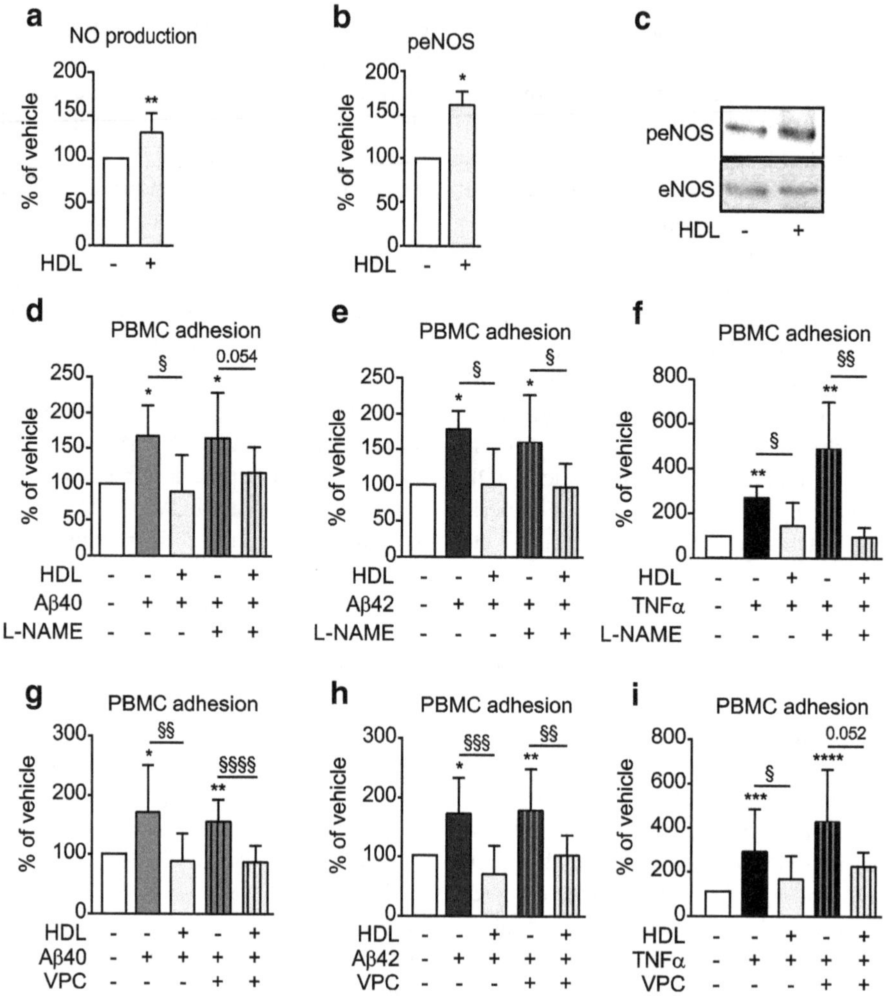

Fig. 4 HDL suppression of Aβ-induced inflammation is independent of eNOS and S1P. **a** Intracellular NO production was measured by treating hCMEC/D3 with 100 μg/mL HDL in the presence of 1 μM DAF-2 for 6 h. Fluorescence was measured at 485 nm. **b** Phosphorylation of eNOS was measured by treating hCMEC/D3 with 100 μg/mL HDL for 15 min before immunoblotting for phosphorylated eNOS (p-eNOS) or total eNOS. Representative immunoblots are shown in (**c**). hCMEC/D3 were pretreated for 1 h with the eNOS inhibitor L-NAME (**d-f**) or the S1P1 and S1P3 inhibitor VPC23019 (**g-i**) followed by 100 μg/mL HDL for 2 h. Cells were then stimulated with 0.1 μM Aβ40 (**d,g**) Aβ42 monomers, (**e,h**) or 1 ng/mL of TNF-α (**f,i**) for 3 h before testing PBMC adherence. Graphs represent means ± SD of adhered PBMC relative to vehicle treated cells for at least 5 independent trials. *$p < 0.05$, **$p < 0.01$, ***$p < 0.001$ * $p < 0.05$, **$p < 0.01$, ***$p < 0.001$ versus vehicle, § $p < 0.05$, §§ $p < 0.01$, §§§$p < 0.001$ versus Aβ or TNF-α

a specific miR-223 inhibitor did not diminish the ability of HDL to suppress PMBC adhesion by Aβ40 , Aβ42 or TNF-α (Additional file 3d–f). Third, in the 5 h period where hCMEC/D3 were exposed to HDL (2 h pre-treatment then 3 h with Aβ), no significant transfer of miR-223 was detected (see Additional file 3g), consistent with a previous report that after 6 h, miR-223 was not transferred from HDL to several types of ECs including HUVEC [30]. These results suggest that, although the miR-233 mimetic can suppress Aβ42-mediated PBMC binding to hCMEC/D3 when added directly, miR-233 is unlikely to underlie the ability of HDL to suppress PBMC adhesion to hCMEC/D3 triggered by Aβ40, Aβ42 or TNF-α.

HDL-mediated suppression of aβ-induced PBMC adhesion to hCMEC/D3 is independent of ICAM-1 and VCAM-1. ICAM-1 and VCAM-1 are canonical markers of EC activation that mediate PBMC adhesion by classical inflammatory stimuli [31]. Several studies have reported elevated microvascular inflammatory markers in the AD brain [32, 33]. Using ELISA, we confirmed that protein levels of intercellular adhesion molecule 1 (ICAM-1) but not vascular cell adhesion molecule 1 (VCAM-1) are increased in the cortex of AD patients compared to either cerebellum from the same individual or the cortex from non-cognitively impaired (NCI) control subjects (Additional file 4). Increased ICAM-1 levels were further confirmed using immunofluorescence revealing both vascular and glial ICAM-1 reactivity whereas VCAM-1 remained unchanged (Additional file 5a–b). As expected, soluble Aβ40 and Aβ42 levels were elevated in the cortex of AD patients compared to their corresponding cerebellum or to the cortex of NCI subjects (Additional file 4). Because ICAM-1 is a classical marker of EC activation and HDL can attenuate PBMC adherence by reducing ICAM-1 levels in aortic derived ECs [34], we also evaluated the roles of ICAM-1 and VCAM-1 in hCMEC/D3 activation. Using Western blotting, we observed that pretreatment of monotypic hCMEC/D3 cultures with HDL significantly suppressed TNF-α-mediated induction of ICAM-1 (from 1343% to 920%, $p = 0.041$) and VCAM-1 (from 2838% to 1928% $p = 0.012$), relative to untreated cells (Additional file 6a–c), results that are consistent with HDL's anti-inflammatory effects on peripherally derived ECs. By contrast, Aβ treatment did not affect either mRNA levels or total protein levels of VCAM-1 and ICAM-1 in hCMEC/D3 (Additional file 6d–m). Although total ICAM-1 levels showed no significant change in response to either Aβ40 or Aβ42 treatment, biotinylation assays revealed significantly increased cell surface ICAM-1 levels, but not VCAM-1 levels, in response to 0.1 μM of Aβ40 ($p = 0.009$) and a strong trend in response to Aβ42 ($p = 0.06$) (Additional file 6 h–j). Unexpectedly, however, we observed that cell surface ICAM-1 levels were not reduced by a 2 h exposure to HDL (Additional file 6 k–m), showing that cell surface ICAM-1 levels do not correlate with PMBC adhesion in Aβ-activated hCMEC/D3. We next analysed the effects of Aβ on the phosphorylation of multifunctional serine/threonine protein kinases that are involved in EC activation, survival, apoptosis, proliferation and migration. TNF-α activated NFκB p-P65 ($p = 0.002$), SAPK/JNK ($p = 0.005$), MAPK/ERK ($p = 0.01$), but not Akt or STAT2 pathways, whereas Aβ did not alter any of these pathways in hCMEC/D3 (Additional file 7). Taken together, these results suggest that Aβ does not activate any of classical inflammatory pathways known to increase PBMC adhesion through ICAM-1 or VCAM-1.

Suppressing aβ uptake into hCMEC/D3 blocks PBMC adherence

As our results show that Aβ activates hCMEC/D3 through a mechanism that is independent of canonical EC activation intracellular signalling pathways, we hypothesised that binding or uptake of Aβ to ECs might influence PBMC adhesion. To test this hypothesis, we first used temperature modulation experiments to investigate how HDL affects the interactions of Aβ with hCMEC/D3 and observed that HDL pre-treatment significantly reduced total association measured at 37 °C (Fig. 5a,b), cell surface binding measured at 4 °C measured by ELISA (Fig. 5c,d) and intracellular uptake of fluorescently labeled Aβ40 and Aβ42 (Fig. 5e). Second, we tested whether blocking RAGE and LRP1, known receptors that modulate Aβ binding and uptake in ECs [35], might reduce PBMC adhesion. Blocking RAGE with a specific antibody abrogated PBMC adhesion to both Aβ40 and Aβ42 but not TNF-α stimulated hCMEC/D3(Fig. 5f-h). Similarly, blocking LRP1 with receptor associated protein (RAP) abolished Aβ40 and Aβ42 but not TNF-α effects (Fig. 5i-k). Finally, as heparin sulphate proteoglycans (HSPG) are also involved in binding and uptake of Aβ in neuron [36], we then saturated or removed HSPG by treating hCMEC/D3 with heparin or heparinase III, respectively. Both treatments abolished the ability of Aβ40 and Aβ42 to induce PBMC binding whereas TNF-α induced-PBMC adhesion remained significant (Fig. 5l-n). Together, these observations show that, unlike TNF-α, Aβ induces PBMC adhesion to ECs through a pathway that requires interactions with or internalization through Aβ receptors on the EC surface. We also observed that HDL does not decrease the expression of RAGE or LRP1 (Additional file 8), suggesting that down-regulation of these receptors cannot explain the protective effect of HDL on Aβ-induced PBMC binding to hCMEC/D3.

Scavenger receptor-BI (SR-BI) is necessary for HDL to suppress aβ-induced PBMC adhesion to ECs

Scavenger receptor BI (SR-BI) is the principal HDL receptor on ECs and activates several HDL signalling pathways in addition to mediating selective cholesterol uptake upon HDL docking [37]. We observed that inhibiting SR-BI binding with a specific blocking antibody abolished the ability of HDL to suppress both Aβ- and TNF-α-mediated PBMC adhesion to hCMEC/D3 (Fig. 6a-c). Selectivity to SR-BI was confirmed by demonstrating that blocking scavenger receptor CD36 with a specific antibody had no effect on the ability of HDL to suppress either Aβ- or TNF-α-mediated PBMC adhesion to hCMEC/D3 (Fig. 6d-f). Intriguingly, inhibiting SR-BI-mediated selective cholesterol uptake with block lipid transfer 1 (BLT1) did not affect the ability of HDL to suppress either Aβ- or TNF-α-mediated PBMC adhesion to hCMEC/D3 (Fig. 6g-i). We further observed that inhibiting SR-BI with a specific blocking antibody abolished the ability of HDL to suppress Aβ uptake in hCMEC/D3 (Fig. 6j). These results demonstrate that HDL requires SR-BI-mediated signalling to inhibit Aβ uptake and subsequently suppress PBMC adhesion to hCMEC/D3 in response to Aβ- or TNF-α in a manner independent of lipid uptake.

Having used monotypic static cell cultures to demonstrate that HDL suppresses Aβ-induced PBMC adhesion to endothelial cells through a mechanism that requires SR-BI and is independent of ICAM-1 expression, we confirmed that this mechanism also explains the results in our 3D bioengineered vessels. We observed that inhibiting SR-BI

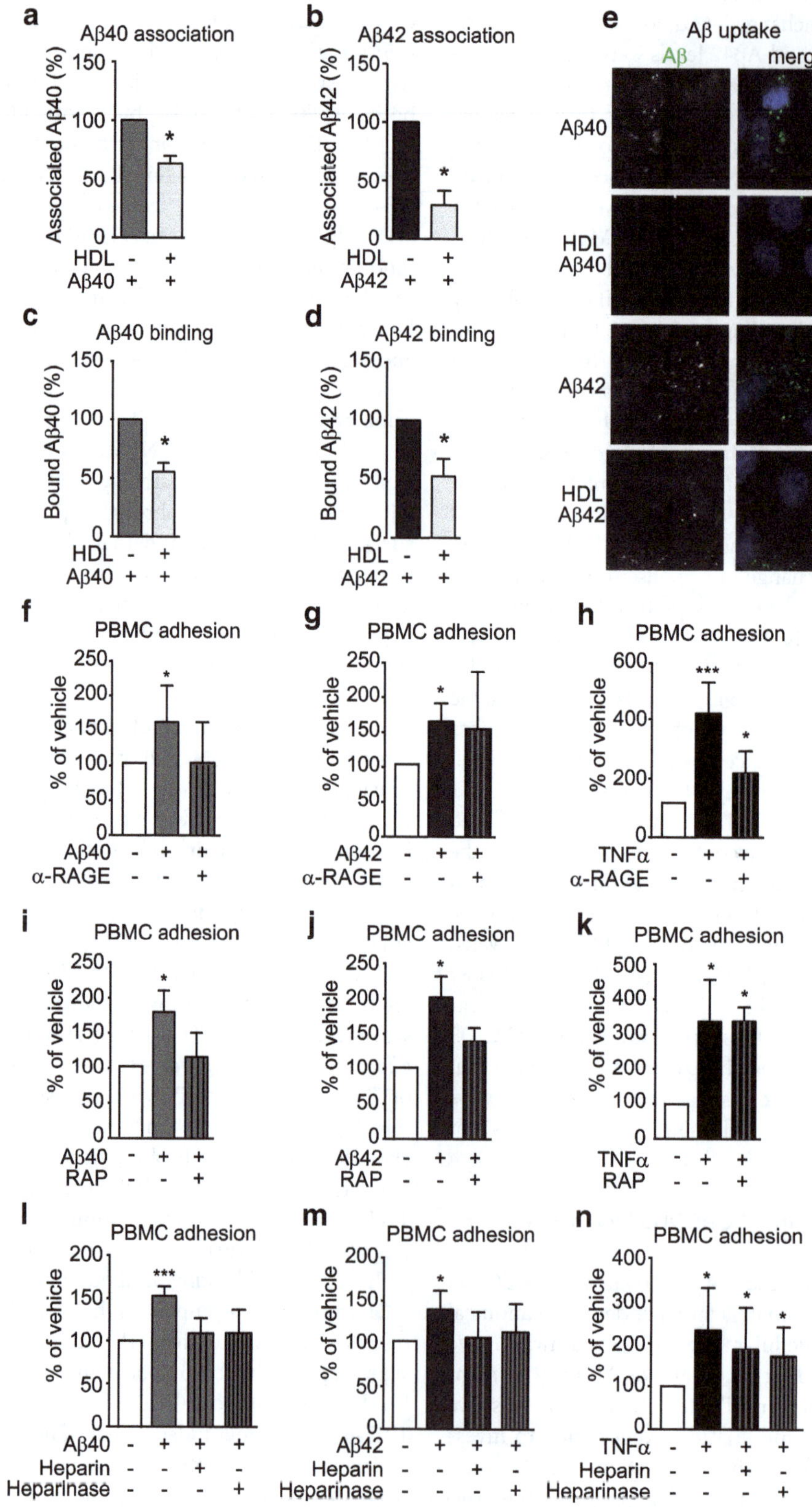

Fig. 5 (See legend on next page.)

(See figure on previous page.)
Fig. 5 HDL reduces Aβ association, binding and uptake to hCMEC/D3 whereas blocking Aβ binding or uptake reduces PBMC adhesion to hCMEC/D3. **a-d** hCMEC/D3 were pre-treated with 100 μg/mL of HDL and 0.1 μM **a,c** Aβ40 or **b,d** Aβ42 monomers as described in Fig. 2 at either 37 °C (association **a,b**) or at 4 °C (binding **c,d**). Cells were lysed in RIPA buffer and Aβ were measured using commercial ELISA. **e** hCMEC/D3 were pre-treated with HDL (1 mg/mL) for 2 h before stimulating with 1 mM of fluorescently labelled Aβ40 or Aβ42 monomers. Scale bar represents 10 μm. **f-n** hCMEC/D3 were pre-treated with (**f-h**) RAGE blocking antibody, **i-k** RAP or **l-n** heparin or heparinase III 60 min before stimulation with Aβ40 or Aβ42 monomers or TNF-α for 3 h. PBMC adhesion assays were conducted as described in Fig. 2. Graphs represent means ± SD relative to vehicle treated cells for at least 3 independent trials. *$p < 0.05$, **$p < 0.01$ versus vehicle

with a specific antibody circulated through the vessel lumen abolished the ability of HDL to suppress Aβ-mediated monocyte adhesion to the vascular endothelium (Fig. 7a-b) without reducing ICAM-1 expression (Fig. 7c-d).

Discussion

Far from being an inert vascular lining, ECs form a metabolically active and specialized interface between blood and underlying tissues. In response to an inflammatory stimulus, ECs undergo activation, which is classically defined by increased interaction with blood leukocytes. EC dysfunction plays a central role in peripheral vascular disease, stroke, heart disease, diabetes, insulin resistance, chronic kidney failure, tumor growth, metastasis, venous thrombosis, and severe viral infectious diseases [38]. The richly vascularized human brain contains ECs that form the nearly impenetrable BBB, which regulates the flux of substances in and out of the CNS. The contribution of cerebrovascular dysfunction in dementia and cognitive decline is well acknowledged [39, 40], yet pathways that mediate cerebrovascular EC dysfunction and protection are not well understood.

Using classical PMBC adhesion assays, we demonstrate that Aβ can act as an inflammatory stimulus to increase PBMC adhesion to brain microvascular ECs that can be suppressed by HDL. Our results show that the ability of HDL to attenuate Aβ-induced PBMC adhesion to ECs is independent of Aβ structure, NO production, miR-223 and, unexpectedly, of ICAM-1 and VCAM-1 expression. Rather, HDL requires SR-BI to suppress Aβ-mediated PBMC adhesion to ECs, which can also be attenuated by inhibiting internalization of Aβ by blocking RAGE or LRP1, or by inhibiting Aβ-HSPG interactions. We also show that HDL can also prevent Aβ fibrillization, suggesting that HDL may also help to maintain Aβ solubility as it transits across the BBB. However, as this function of HDL is relatively slow, it is unlikely to account for HDL's ability to suppress Aβ-mediated PBMC adhesion to ECs. Our observations are consistent with a previous study that demonstrated that deficiency of SR-BI increases cerebrovascular amyloid deposition in the J20 mouse model of AD [41].

As ICAM-1 levels are clearly elevated in AD cortex, and previous studies have reported induced adhesion molecule expression after Aβ stimulation [42], we were surprised to observe that Aβ had negligible effects on adhesion molecule expression and kinase activation under our experimental conditions, whereas TNF-α robustly induces ICAM-1 and VCAM-1 expression as well as NFκB, MAPK/ERK, and SAPK/JNK signalling. The cellular processes triggered by internalized Aβ that promote PBMC adhesion remain to be determined.

In cultured aortic ECs, HDL reduces adhesion molecule expression and subsequent monocyte binding via a mechanism involving SR-BI signalling through eNOS, which requires the S1P receptor [25]. Our observations that HDL's ability to suppress Aβ- and TNF-α-mediated PBMC adhesion to hCMEC/D3 is independent of NO production and S1P activity suggests that brain ECs may have pathways distinct from ECs derived from arterial sources, at least under the culture conditions used here. Reduced eNOS expression in the AD brain has been hypothesized to increase Aβ deposition and promote production of reactive oxygen species production, which reduces vasomotor regulation of penetrating arterioles [43, 44]. HDL clearly induces NO production in hCMEC/D3 and HUVEC, and although NO production is not required to protect hCMEC/D3 from Aβ- or TNF-α mediated PBMC adhesion per se, HDL-stimulated NO production may provide beneficial effects on other cerebrovascular EC functions.

A wealth of studies have explored in vitro associations of Aβ with lipoprotein components, primarily focussing on apoE as genetic variants of apoE have established effects on Aβ metabolism in AD [45]. As Aβ is a hydrophobic peptide, it is not surprising that it associates with lipoprotein particles, and also to amphipathic apolipoproteins. Elucidating the structure-function relationships of Aβ with lipoproteins remains an active area of research. While Aβ might associate with plasma lipoproteins [46], the effect of HDL on Aβ structure remains poorly understood. Interestingly, HDL constituents on their own have been reported to both interact with Aβ and diminish its toxic effects. Specifically, small liposomes (<50 μm) accelerate Aβ40 fibrillization and the amounts of amorphous aggregates become larger as liposome increase (>50 μm) [47]. By contrast, nanoliposomes (100 nm) prevent Aβ42 fibrillization and reduces Aβ42-induced EC dysfunctions [48]. In addition, lipid-free apoA-I induces Aβ aggregation and generation of

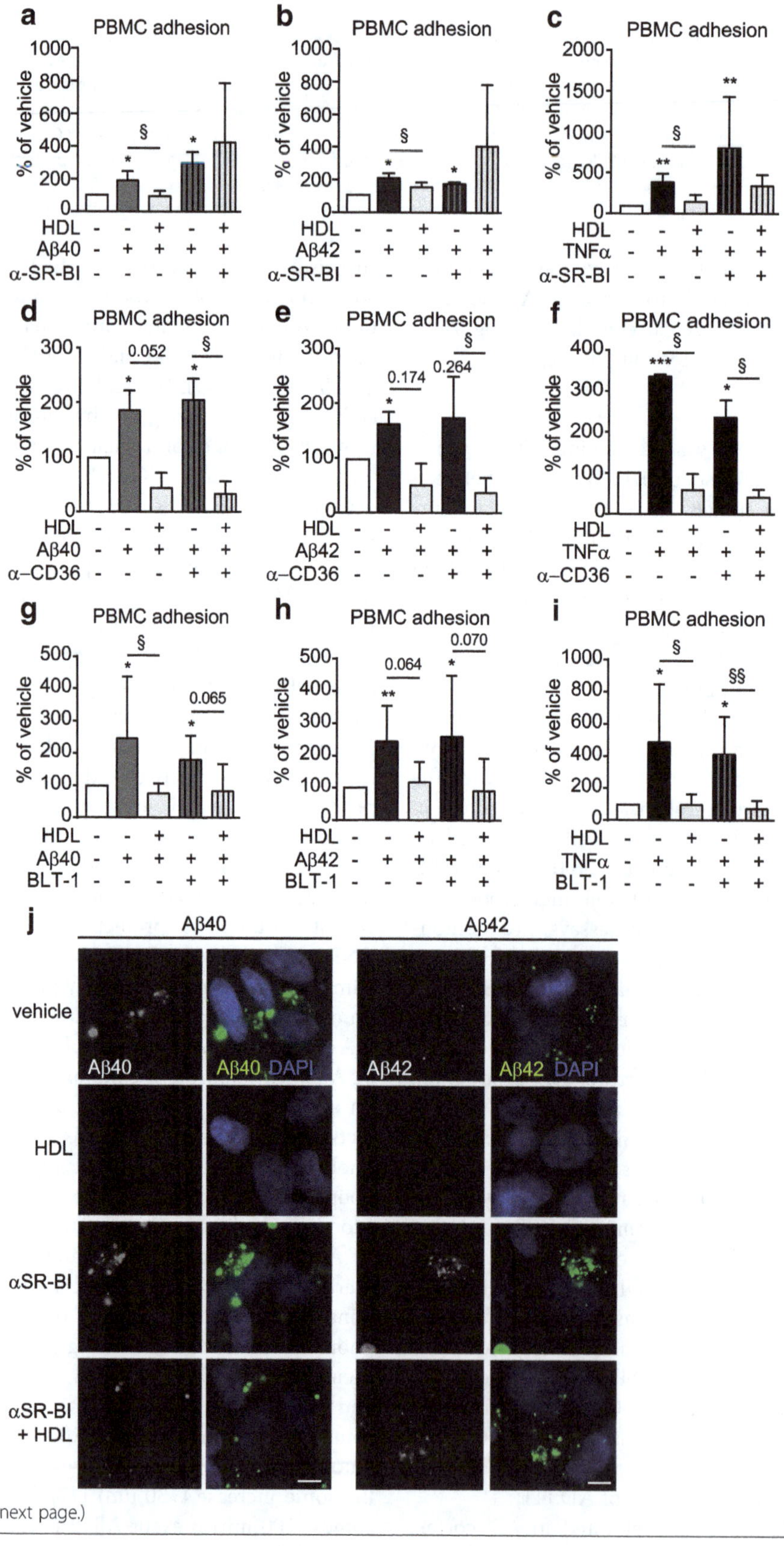

Fig. 6 (See legend on next page.)

(See figure on previous page.)
Fig. 6 HDL suppression of Aβ-induced inflammation requires SR-BI. hCMEC/D3 were pre-treated for 1 h with **a-c** SR-BI or **d-f** CD36 blocking antibodies or **g-i** BLT1 followed by 100 μg/mL HDL for 2 h. Cells were then stimulated with 0.1 μM monomeric **a,d,g** Aβ40 or **b,e,h** Aβ42 or (**c,f,i**) 1 ng/mL of TNF-α for 3 h before evaluating PBMC adherence. **j** hCMEC/D3 were pre-treated for 1 h with SR-BI blocking antibody followed by HDL (1 mg/mL) for 2 h before stimulating with 1 mM of fluorescently labelled Aβ40 or Aβ42 monomers. Scale bar represents 10 μm. Graphs represent means ± SD of adhered PBMC relative to vehicle treated cells from at least 4 independent trials. *$p < 0.05$, **$p < 0.01$, ***$p < 0.001$ * $p < 0.05$, **$p < 0.01$, ***$p < 0.001$ versus vehicle, § $p < 0.05$ versus Aβ or TNF-α.

amorphous complexes, both of which reducing amyloid toxicity [22]. Our results clearly show that mature HDL delays Aβ fibrillization in a cell-independent assay with substantially slower kinetics than HDL's ability to attenuate Aβ-induced PBMC adhesion to ECs. As HDL also reduces Aβ-induced PBMC adhesion to ECs independent of monomeric vs. oligomeric input structures, we believe that HDL's ability to delay Aβ fibrillization is a distinct function compared to reduce Aβ-inflammation, which relies exclusively to a cellular process involving SR-BI.

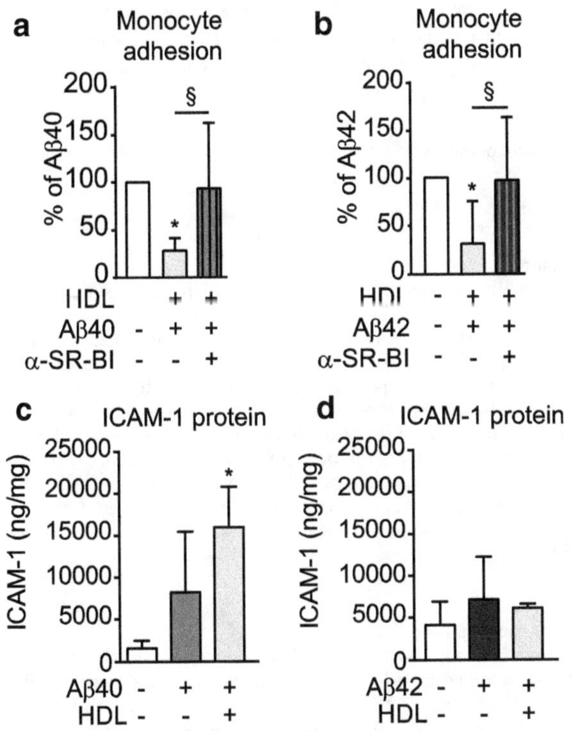

Fig. 7 HDL suppresses Aβ-induced monocyte adhesion in engineered vessels via SR-BI. SR-BI blocking antibody was circulated through the lumen of engineered vessels prepared using HUVEC for 1 h prior treatment with 200 μg/mL of HDL for 2 h followed by injection of 1 μM of monomeric **a** Aβ40 or **b** Aβ42 within the tissue chamber (abluminal) for 8 h prior to injecting circulating fluorescent THP1 into the lumen. **c-d** ICAM-1 protein was measured in tissue lysates prepared in RIPA buffer by commercial ELISA. Graphs represent means ± SD of adhered monocytes relative to Aβ treated tissues from at least 4 individual grafts. * and # $p < 0.05$

As traditional static monotypic cell cultures do not reproduce the physiological complexity of the native vascular bed, we also used a 3D model of the human vasculature in our studies. These engineered vessels mimic a native vessel with a luminal monolayer of human ECs surrounded by several layers of human SMCs, through which human mononuclear cells can be circulated under flow conditions. This model has been previously used to study atherosclerosis in peripheral arteries [17]. Here, we injected Aβ on the anteluminal side to mimic brain-produced Aβ and circulated HDL and monocytes through the lumen. We confirmed that Aβ induces monocyte adhesion to ECs under native-like flow conditions in engineered human vessels, which can be suppressed by HDL through a mechanism that requires SR-BI and that is independent of changes in ICAM-1 levels.

Conclusion

Numerous studies show that HDL has several properties that are associated with improved vascular function [49]. While some lines of evidence also suggest a beneficial role for HDL in protecting from cognitive decline, the nature of this association remains largely unknown. Whereas lipid-free apoA-I can be transported into the CNS [50], there is thus far no evidence that mature HDL might cross the BBB, supporting the view that HDL might act predominately from the blood compartment and would therefore primarily affect ECs. Our data suggest at least three mechanisms by which HDL could have beneficial effects on cerebral vessels. First, HDL prevents Aβ-induced PBMC adhesion to brain microvascular ECs through a mechanism that requires SR-BI and suppresses Aβ uptake. The cellular pathways by which internalized Aβ promotes PBMC adhesion to ECs remains to be defined, and appears to be distinct from those induced by classical inflammatory stimuli. Second, similar to its effects in peripheral EC, HDL induces NO secretion in hCMEC/D3. Although we ruled out a role for eNOS in Aβ-induced PBMC adhesion, HDL-stimulated NO production may still help to attenuate vasomotor dysfunction as observed in the aging brain [44]. Third, although HDL can protect hCMEC/D3 from PBMC adhesion independent of Aβ structure, the ability of HDL to maintain Aβ in a soluble state may facilitate efficient Aβ clearance out of the brain.

Additional files

Additional file 1: Aβ induced dose dependent PBMC adhesion and HDL attenuate dose dependent Aβ-induced PBMC adhesion to hCMEC/D3. In all conditions, hCMEC/D3 were stimulated with 0–1 μM Aβ40 (light grey) or Aβ42 (dark grey) monomers for 3 h. Fluorescently labelled PBMC were allowed to adhere to (**a**) Aβ40- or (**b**) Aβ42- stimulated cells for 3 additional hours. Cells were washed, fixed, and imaged to count adhered PBMC. hCMEC/D3 were primed with increasing doses (25–400 μg/mL) of HDL for 2 h and stimulated with 0.1 μM (**c**) Aβ40 (light grey) or (**d**) Aβ42 (dark grey) for 3 h. Fluorescently labelled PBMC were allowed to adhere to stimulated cells for 3 h followed by washing, fixation, imaging, and counting. Graphs represent mean ± SD of adhered PBMC relative to vehicle control from at least 3 independent trials where * $p < 0.05$, ** $p < 0.01$, *** $p < 0.001$ versus vehicle, § $p < 0.05$, §§ $p < 0.01$ versus Aβ (PDF 422 kb)

Additional file 2 HDL suppression of Aβ-induced inflammation is independent of eNOS and S1P in HUVEC. (**a**) L-NAME and (**e**) VPC23019 potency was tested by measuring intracellular NO production in HUVEC after incubating with 100 μg/mL HDL and 1 μM DAF-2 for 6 h. Fluorescence was measured at 485 nm. (**b-d, f-h**) In all conditions, HUVEC or hCMEC/D3 were stimulated with 0.1 μM **monomeric** Aβ40 or Aβ42 or 1 ng/mL of TNF-α for 3 h prior to measuring PBMC adherence. HUVEC were pre-treated for 1 h with (**b-d**) the eNOS inhibitor L-NAME or (**f-h**) the S1P1 and S1P3 inhibitor VPC23019 followed by 100 μg/mL HDL for 2 h. (**i**) hCMEC/D3 were pre-treated with 100 μg/mL of HDL for 2 h before simulating with Aβ40 or Aβ42. Total cellular expression of Annexin-1 (Anx1) was analysed by immunoblotting and compared to GAPDH. Graphs represent means ± SD from at least 3 independent trials. * $p < 0.05$, ** $p < 0.01$, *** $p < 0.001$, **** $p < 0.0001$ versus vehicle, § $p < 0.05$, §§ $p < 0.01$, §§§ $p < 0.001$, §§§§ $p < 0.0001$ versus Aβ or TNF-α (PDF 1059 kb)

Additional file 3: HDL does not signal through miR-223 to reduce Aβ-induced inflammation in hCMEC/D3. (**a-c**) hCMEC/D3 were pre-treated with 100 μg/mL of HDL as described in Fig. 2 with or without 10 nM of miR-223 mimetic nucleotides or (**d-f**) in the absence or presence of a specific miR223 inhibitor for 2 h before stimulation with (**a,d**) Aβ40, (**b,e**) Aβ42 or (**c, f**) TNF-α before testing PBMC adherence to ECs. (**g**) Intracellular levels of mature miR-223 in hCMEC/D3 were quantified by real-time PCR and normalized to U6 after a 5 h treatment with 100 μg/mL of HDL. Graphs represent means ± SD of adhered PBMC relative to vehicle treated cells for at least 5 independent trials. * $p < 0.05$, ** $p < 0.01$, *** $p < 0.001$ * $p < 0.05$, ** $p < 0.01$, *** $p < 0.001$ versus vehicle, § $p < 0.05$, §§ $p < 0.01$, §§§ $p < 0.001$ versus Aβ or TNF-α (PDF 464 kb)

Additional file 4: Demographic data, Aβ40 and Aβ42, and adhesion molecule quantification in Alzheimer's disease patients and non-cognitive impaired controls (PDF 431 kb)

Additional file 5: Cortical ICAM-1 expression is increased in AD. Cryopreserved cortex and cerebellum of AD or NCI patients were cut at 20 μm. After PFA fixation sections were washed with PBS and stained against (**a**) ICAM-I or (**b**) VCAM-1 and CD31 as a vascular marker and imaged using an inverted fluorescent microscope. Arrow demonstrates colocalization of ICAM-1 and CD31. Bar represents 50 μm (PDF 62676 kb)

Additional file 6: Adhesion molecules are enhanced by TNF-α but not Aβ.(**a-c**) hCMEC/D3 were primed with 100 μg/mL HDL for 2 h followed by stimulation with 1 ng/mL TNF-α for 3 h. Cell lysates were prepared in RIPA and protein levels of (**a**) ICAM-1 and (**b**) VCAM-1 were measured by denaturing immunoblotting (**c**). (**d-g**) hCMEC/D3 were stimulated with monomeric (**d,f**) Aβ40 or (**e,g**) Aβ42 at the indicated concentrations and (**d,e**) *ICAM-1* and (**f,g**) *VCAM-1* mRNA levels were measured by real-time PCR. (**h-j**) Following Aβ stimulation, cell surface proteins were biotinylated and isolated by immunoprecipitation. Protein levels of cell surface and total (**h**) ICAM-1 and (**i**) VCAM-1 were measured by denaturing immunoblotting (**j**). (**k-m**) hCMEC/D3 were pre-treated with 100 μg/mL of HDL for 2 h followed by stimulation with Aβ. After 3 h total and cell surface ICAM-1 expression were measured as above. Graphs represent means ± SD from at least 3 independent trials. *** $p < 0.001$ versus vehicle, § $p < 0.05$, versus Aβ or TNF-α (PDF 2282 kb)

Additional file 7: Aβ does not activate phosphorylation of multifunctional serine/threonine protein kinases. hCMEC/D3 were stimulated with 0.1 mM of monomeric Aβ or 1 ng/mL of TNF-αfor 15 min before lysing cells in RIPA containing phosphostop. Phosphorylation of (**a-b**) p65, (**c**) STAT3, (**d**) Akt, (**e**) SAPK/JNK and (**f**) p42/44 MAPK were analysed by immunoblotting and compared to respective total p65, STAT3, Akt, SAPK/JNK and p42/44 MAPK respectively. (**b**) Nuclear translocation of p65 was analysed by immunofluorescence 15 min after Aβ stimulation. Graphs represent means ± SD relative to vehicle treated cells in 4 trials. * $p < 0.05$, ** $p < 0.01$ (PDF 9645 kb)

Additional file 8: HDL treatment does not alter LRP1 or RAGE protein levels in hCMEC/D3. (**a-c**) hCMEC/D3 were treated with HDL (0–400 μg/mL) for 5 h before lysing in RIPA. (**a**) LRP1 and (**b**) RAGE protein levels were quantified by immunoblotting (**c**). Graphs represent means ± SD relative to vehicle treated cells in 3 trials (PDF 1114 kb)

Abbreviations

AD: Alzheimer Disease; Aβ: Beta-amyloid peptide; BLT-1: Block lipid transport 1; CAA: Cerebral amyloid angiopathy; CNS: Central nervous system; EBM-2: Endothelial growth basal medium; EC: Endothelial cell; eNOS: Endothelial nitric oxide synthase; FBS: Fetal bovine serum; FITC: Fluorescein isothiocyanate; hBMEC: Human brain microvascular endothelial cell; hCMEC/D3: Human cortical microvascular endothelial cell line D3; HDL: High density lipoprotein; hSMC: Human smooth muscle cell; HSPG: Heparan sulphate proteoglycan; ICAM-1: Inducible cellular adhesion molecule-1; L-NAME: L NG-nitroarginne methyl ester; LRP1: Low density lipoprotein receptor related protein-1; NO: Nitric oxide; PBMC: Peripheral blood mononuclear cell; RAGE: Receptor of advanced glycation endproducts; SR-BI: Scavenger receptor BI; VCAM-1: Vascular cell adhesion molecule –1

Acknowledgements

Not applicable

Funding

This work was supported by operating grants from the Canadian Institutes of Health Research (CIHR), a Canadian Consortium of Neurodegeneration and Aging (CCNA), a Djavad Mowafaghian Centre for Brain Health Catalyst grant, philanthropic funding from the Jack Brown and Family Alzheimer's Research Foundation, the Y.P. Heung Foundation, and a private BC-based foundation to CLW, and a Weston Brain Institute Rapid Response grant to JR. JR was supported by a BrightFocus postdoctoral fellowship and a Swiss National Science Foundation Early.postdoctoral fellowship. EB was supported by a CIHR Doctoral Scholarship. GKB was supported by a UBC four years doctoral Fellowship. IK was supported in part by a Weston Brain Institute Rapid Response grant. NC was supported by CIHR and Brain Canada and GF was supported by a CIHR Project Grant 148,883 (GAF).

Author contributions

JR, EB and CLW conceived the project. JR and EB made equivalent contributions to this study and performed most of the experiments with assistance from SS, GKB, EG, CC, WHC, SKS, BY, MG, AB, KK and IK. Data analysis was primarily performed by JR. EB, and CLW, who together wrote the manuscript with assistance from EG, GF and NC. The authors declare no competing financial interests. All authors read and approved the final manuscript.

Authors' information

Not applicable

Competing interests:

The authors declare that they have no competing interests.

BC V6T 1Z3, Canada. [3]Department of Neurology, University of British Columbia, Vancouver, BC V6T 2B5, Canada. [4]Department of Zoology, University of British Columbia, Vancouver, BC V6T 2B5, Canada. [5]Department of Medicine, University of British Columbia, Vancouver, BC V6Z 1Y6, Canada.

Author details

[1]Department of Pathology and Laboratory Medicine, University of British Columbia, Vancouver, BC V6T 1Z3, Canada. Djavad Mowafaghian Centre for Brain Health, University of British Columbia, 2215 Wesbrook Mall, Vancouver,

References

1. Alzheimer's Association. 2015 Alzheimer's disease facts and figures. Alzheimer's & dementia : the journal of the Alzheimer's Association. 2015;11(3):332–84.
2. Perl DP. Neuropathology of Alzheimer's disease. The Mount Sinai journal of medicine, New York [Internet]. 2010;77(1):32–42.
3. Debette S. Vascular risk factors and cognitive disorders. Rev Neurol. 2013; 169(10):757–64.
4. Justin BN, Turek M, Hakim AM. Heart disease as a risk factor for dementia. Clin Epidemiol. 2013;5:135–45.
5. Craft S. The role of metabolic disorders in Alzheimer disease and vascular dementia: two roads converged. Arch Neurol. 2009;66(3):300–5.
6. Schneider JA, Arvanitakis Z, Bang W, Bennett DA. Mixed brain pathologies account for most dementia cases in community-dwelling older persons. Neurology. 2007;69(24):2197–204.
7. Tarasoff-Conway JM, Carare RO, Osorio RS, Glodzik L, Butler T, Fieremans E, Axel L, Rusinek H, Nicholson C, Zlokovic BV, Frangione B, Blennow K, Ménard J, Zetterberg H, Wisniewski T, de Leon MJ. Clearance systems in the brain-implications for Alzheimer disease. Nat Rev Neurol. 2015;11(8):457–70.
8. Grammas P. Neurovascular dysfunction, inflammation and endothelial activation: implications for the pathogenesis of Alzheimer's disease. J Neuroinflammation. 2011;8:26.
9. Kontush A, Lhomme M, Chapman MJ. Unraveling the complexities of the HDL lipidome. J Lipid Res. 2013;54(11):2950–63.
10. Shah AS, Tan L, Lu Long J, Davidson WS. The proteomic diversity of high density lipoproteins: our emerging understanding of its importance in lipid transport and beyond. J Lipid Res. 2013 Feb;24
11. Mahdy Ali K, Wonnerth A, Huber K, Wojta J. Cardiovascular disease risk reduction by raising HDL cholesterol–current therapies and future opportunities. Br J Pharmacol. 2012;167(6):1177–94.
12. Zuliani G, Cavalieri M, Galvani M, Volpato S, Cherubini A, Bandinelli S, Corsi AM, Lauretani F, Guralnik JM, Fellin R, Ferrucci L. Relationship between low levels of high-density lipoprotein cholesterol and dementia in the elderly. The InChianti study. J Gerontol A Biol Sci Med Sci. 2010;65(5):559–64.
13. Lefterov I, Fitz NF, A CA, Fogg A, Lefterov P, Kodali R, Wetzel R, Koldamova R. Apolipoprotein A-I deficiency increases cerebral amyloid angiopathy and cognitive deficits in APP/PS1DeltaE9 mice. J Biol Chem. 2010;285(47):36945–57.
14. Lewis TL, Cao D, Lu H, Mans RA, Su YR, Jungbauer L, Linton MF, Fazio S, Mj LD, Li L. Overexpression of human apolipoprotein A-I preserves cognitive function and attenuates neuroinflammation and cerebral amyloid angiopathy in a mouse model of Alzheimer disease. J Biol Chem. 2010; 285(47):36958–68.
15. Robert J, Stukas S, Button E, Cheng WH, Lee M, Fan J, Wilkinson A, Kulic I, Wright SD, Wellington CL. Reconstituted high-density lipoproteins acutely reduce soluble brain Aβ levels in symptomatic APP/PS1 mice. Biochim Biophys Acta. 2015;1862(5):1027–36.
16. Riwanto M, Landmesser U. High-density lipoproteins and endothelial functions: mechanistic insights and alterations in cardiovascular disease. J Lipid Res. 2013;54(12):3227–43.
17. Robert J, Weber B, Frese L, Emmert MY, Schmidt D, von Eckardstein A, Rohrer L, Hoerstrup SP. A three-dimensional engineered artery model for in vitro atherosclerosis research. PLoS One. 2013;8(11):e79821.
18. Hoerstrup SP, Cummings Mrcs I, Lachat M, Schoen FJ, Jenni R, Leschka S, Neuenschwander S, Schmidt D, Mol A, Günter C, Gössl M, Genoni M, Zund G. Functional growth in tissue-engineered living, vascular grafts: follow-up at 100 weeks in a large animal model. Circulation. 2006;114:I159–66.
19. Robert J, Lehner M, Frank S, Perisa D, von Eckardstein A, Rohrer L. Interleukin 6 stimulates endothelial binding and transport of high-density lipoprotein through induction of endothelial lipase. Arterioscler Thromb Vasc Biol. 2013;33(12):2699–706.
20. Czupalla CJ, Liebner S, Devraj K. In vitro models of the blood-brain barrier. Methods in molecular biology (Clifton, NJ). 2014;1135:415–37.
21. Koudinov AR, Berezov TT, Koudinova NV. The levels of soluble amyloid beta in different high density lipoprotein subfractions distinguish Alzheimer's and normal aging cerebrospinal fluid: implication for brain cholesterol pathology. Neurosci Lett. 2001;314(3):115–8.
22. Paula-Lima AC, Tricerri MA, Brito-Moreira J, Bomfim TR, Oliveira FF, Magdesian MH, Grinberg LT, Panizzutti R, Ferreira ST. Human apolipoprotein A-I binds amyloid-beta and prevents Abeta-induced neurotoxicity. Int J Biochem Cell Biol. 2009;41(6):1361–70.
23. Lee SJC, Nam E, Lee HJ, Savelieff MG, Lim MH. Towards an understanding of amyloid-β oligomers: characterization, toxicity mechanisms, and inhibitors. Chem Soc Rev. 2016;46(2):310–23.
24. Stine WB, Jungbauer L, Yu C, LaDu MJ. Preparing synthetic Aβ in different aggregation states. Methods in molecular biology (Clifton, NJ). 2011;670:13–32.
25. Besler C, Heinrich K, Rohrer L, Doerries C, Riwanto M, Shih DM, Chroni A, Yonekawa K, Stein S, Schaefer N, Mueller M, Akhmedov A, Daniil G, Manes C, Templin C, Wyss C, Maier W, Tanner FC, Matter CM, Corti R, Furlong C, Lusis AJ, von Eckardstein A, Fogelman AM, Luscher TF, Landmesser U. Mechanisms underlying adverse effects of HDL on eNOS-activating pathways in patients with coronary artery disease. J Clin Invest. 2011;121(7):2693–708.
26. Tölle M, Klöckl L, Wiedon A, Zidek W, van der Giet M, Schuchardt M. Regulation of endothelial nitric oxide synthase activation in endothelial cells by S1P1 and S1P3. Biochem Biophys Res Commun. 2016;476(4):627–34.
27. Pan B, Kong J, Jin J, Kong J, He Y, Dong S, Ji L, Liu D, He D, Kong L, Jin DK, Willard B, Pennathur S, Zheng L. A novel anti-inflammatory mechanism of high density lipoprotein through up-regulating annexin A1 in vascular endothelial cells. Biochim Biophys Acta. 2016;1861(6):501–12.
28. Vickers KC, Palmisano BT, Shoucri BM, Shamburek RD, Remaley AT. MicroRNAs are transported in plasma and delivered to recipient cells by high-density lipoproteins. Nat Cell Biol. 2011;13(4):423–33.
29. Tabet F, Vickers KC, Cuesta Torres LF, Wiese CB, Shoucri BM, Lambert G, Catherinet C, Prado-Lourenco L, Levin MG, Thacker S, Sethupathy P, Barter PJ, Remaley AT, Rye K-A. HDL-transferred microRNA-223 regulates ICAM-1 expression in endothelial cells. Nat Commun. 2014;5:3292.
30. Wagner J, Riwanto M, Besler C, Knau A, Fichtlscherer S, Röxe T, Zeiher AM, Landmesser U, Dimmeler S. Characterization of levels and cellular transfer of circulating lipoprotein-bound microRNAs. Arterioscler Thromb Vasc Biol. 2013;33(6):1392–400.
31. Lawson C, Wolf S. ICAM-1 signaling in endothelial cells. Pharmacol Rep. 2009;61(1):22–32.
32. Canobbio I, Abubaker AA, Visconte C, Torti M, Pula G. Role of amyloid peptides in vascular dysfunction and platelet dysregulation in Alzheimer's disease. Front Cell Neurosci. 2015;9:65.
33. Tchalla AE, Wellenius GA, Sorond FA, Gagnon M, Iloputaife I, Travison TG, Dantoine T, Lipsitz LA. Elevated soluble vascular cell adhesion molecule-1 is associated with cerebrovascular resistance and cognitive function. J Gerontol A Biol Sci Med Sci. 2016;72(4):560–6.
34. Calabresi L, Gomaraschi M, Villa B, Omoboni L, Dmitrieff C, Franceschini G. Elevated soluble cellular adhesion molecules in subjects with low HDL-cholesterol. Arterioscler Thromb Vasc Biol. 2002;22(4):656–61.
35. Qosa H, Abuasal BS, Romero IA, Weksler B, Couraud P-O, Keller JN, Kaddoumi A. Differences in amyloid-β clearance across mouse and human blood-brain barrier models: kinetic analysis and mechanistic modeling. Neuropharmacology. 2014;79:668–78.
36. Liu C-C, Zhao N, Yamaguchi Y, Cirrito JR, Kanekiyo T, Holtzman DM, Bu G. Neuronal heparan sulfates promote amyloid pathology by modulating brain amyloid-β clearance and aggregation in Alzheimer's disease. Sci Transl Med. 2016;8(332):332ra44.
37. Rohrer L, Ohnsorg PM, Lehner M, Landolt F, Rinninger F, von Eckardstein A. High-density lipoprotein transport through aortic endothelial cells involves scavenger receptor BI and ATP-binding cassette transporter G1. Circ Res. 2009;104(10):1142–50.
38. Rajendran P, Rengarajan T, Thangavel J, Nishigaki Y, Sakthisekaran D, Sethi G, Nishigaki I. The vascular endothelium and human diseases. Int J Biol Sci. 2013;9(10):1057–69.
39. Snyder HM, Corriveau RA, Craft S, Faber JE, Greenberg SM, Knopman D, Lamb BT, Montine TJ, Nedergaard M, Schaffer CB, Schneider JA, Wellington C, Wilcock DM, Zipfel GJ, Zlokovic B, Bain LJ, Bosetti F, Galis ZS, Koroshetz W, Carrillo MC. Vascular contributions to cognitive impairment and dementia including Alzheimer's disease. Alzheimers Dement. 2015;11(6):710–7.

40. Raz L, Knoefel J, Bhaskar K. The neuropathology and cerebrovascular mechanisms of dementia. J Cereb Blood Flow Metab. 2016;36(1):172–86.
41. Thanopoulou K, Fragkouli A, Stylianopoulou F, Georgopoulos S. Scavenger receptor class B type I (SR-BI) regulates perivascular macrophages and modifies amyloid pathology in an Alzheimer mouse model. Proc Natl Acad Sci U S A. 2010;107(48):20816–21.
42. Giri R, Selvaraj S, Miller CA, Hofman F, Yan SD, Stern D, Zlokovic BV, Kalra VK. Effect of endothelial cell polarity on beta-amyloid-induced migration of monocytes across normal and AD endothelium. Am J Physiol Cell Physiol. 2002;283(3):C895–904.
43. Lamoke F, Mazzone V, Persichini T, Maraschi A, Harris MB, Venema RC, Colasanti M, Gliozzi M, Muscoli C, Bartoli M, Mollace V. Amyloid β peptide-induced inhibition of endothelial nitric oxide production involves oxidative stress-mediated constitutive eNOS/HSP90 interaction and disruption of agonist-mediated Akt activation. J Neuroinflammation. 2015;12:84.
44. Katusic ZS, Austin SA. Endothelial nitric oxide: protector of a healthy mind. Eur Heart J. 2014;35(14):888–94.
45. Kanekiyo T, Xu H, Bu G. ApoE and Abeta in Alzheimer's disease: accidental encounters or partners. Neuron. 2014;81(4):740–54.
46. Wilson LM, Pham CLL, Jenkins AJ, Wade JD, Hill AF, Perugini MA, Howlett GJ. High density lipoproteins bind Abeta and apolipoprotein C-II amyloid fibrils. J Lipid Res. 2006;47(4):755–60.
47. Terakawa MS, Yagi H, Adachi M, Lee Y-H, Goto Y. Small liposomes accelerate the fibrillation of amyloid β (1-40). J Biol Chem. 2015;290(2):815–26.
48. Truran S, Weissig V, Madine J, Davies HA, Guzman-Villanueva D, Franco DA, Karamanova N, Burciu C, Serrano G, Beach TG, Migrino RQ. Nanoliposomes protect against human arteriole endothelial dysfunction induced by β-amyloid peptide. J Cereb Blood Flow Metab. 2015;36(2):405–12.
49. Di Angelantonio E, Sarwar N, Perry P, Kaptoge S, Ray KK, Thompson A, Wood AM, Lewington S, Sattar N, Packard CJ, Collins R, Thompson SG, Danesh *J. major* Lipids, apolipoproteins, and risk of vascular disease. JAMA. 2009;302(18):1993–2000.
50. Stukas S, Robert J, Lee M, Kulic I, Carr M, Tourigny K, Fan J, Namjoshi D, Lemke K, DeValle N, Chan J, Wilson T, Wilkinson A, Chapanian R, Kizhakkedathu JN, Cirrito JR, Oda MN, Wellington CL. Intravenously injected human apolipoprotein A-I rapidly enters the central nervous system via the choroid plexus. J Am Heart Assoc. 2014;3(6):e001156.

10

Network-driven plasma proteomics expose molecular changes in the Alzheimer's brain

Philipp A. Jaeger[1,2,3*], Kurt M. Lucin[1,17], Markus Britschgi[1,18], Badri Vardarajan[4], Ruo-Pan Huang[5,6], Elizabeth D. Kirby[1], Rachelle Abbey[1], Bradley F. Boeve[7], Adam L. Boxer[8], Lindsay A. Farrer[4,9], NiCole Finch[10], Neill R. Graff-Radford[11], Elizabeth Head[12], Matan Hofree[13], Ruochun Huang[5,6], Hudson Johns[1], Anna Karydas[8], David S. Knopman[7], Andrey Loboda[14], Eliezer Masliah[15], Ramya Narasimhan[1], Ronald C. Petersen[7], Alexei Podtelezhnikov[14], Suraj Pradhan[1], Rosa Rademakers[10], Chung-Huan Sun[1], Steven G. Younkin[10], Bruce L. Miller[8], Trey Ideker[3] and Tony Wyss-Coray[1,16*]

Abstract

Background: Biological pathways that significantly contribute to sporadic Alzheimer's disease are largely unknown and cannot be observed directly. Cognitive symptoms appear only decades after the molecular disease onset, further complicating analyses. As a consequence, molecular research is often restricted to late-stage post-mortem studies of brain tissue. However, the disease process is expected to trigger numerous cellular signaling pathways and modulate the local and systemic environment, and resulting changes in secreted signaling molecules carry information about otherwise inaccessible pathological processes.

Results: To access this information we probed relative levels of close to 600 secreted signaling proteins from patients' blood samples using antibody microarrays and mapped disease-specific molecular networks. Using these networks as seeds we then employed independent genome and transcriptome data sets to corroborate potential pathogenic pathways.

Conclusions: We identified Growth-Differentiation Factor (GDF) signaling as a novel Alzheimer's disease-relevant pathway supported by in vivo and in vitro follow-up experiments, demonstrating the existence of a highly informative link between cellular pathology and changes in circulatory signaling proteins.

Background

Plasma proteins provide a sampling of biological processes throughout the organism and have been applied to diagnose or monitor human disease. However, in neurodegenerative disorders it has so far been more difficult to use unbiased large-scale proteomic approaches to discover blood-based biomarkers for diagnostics [1–3]. While individual patient samples might be insufficient for reliable classification tasks based on plasma proteins alone, patient populations could instead be used to smoothen variability and identify underlying common changes linked to disease mechanisms. To achieve this, we propose a medium-scale proteomic strategy that concentrates on secreted signaling proteins involved in cellular communication. Changes in these signaling proteins may result from pathogenic processes or indicate cellular responses to disease. A screen focused on these proteins may not only reduce the proteome test space dramatically but also provide mechanistic insight [4]. Here, we examined whether this approach can robustly identify proteins and biological pathways linked to sporadic late-onset Alzheimer's disease dementia (AD).

* Correspondence: pjaeger@ucsd.edu; twc@stanford.edu
[1]Department of Neurology and Neurological Sciences, Stanford University School of Medicine, Stanford, CA, USA
[16]Center for Tissue Regeneration, Repair and Restoration, VA Palo Alto Health Care System, Palo Alto, CA, USA
Full list of author information is available at the end of the article

Results

To monitor the secreted signaling proteome in plasma, we manufactured glass-based microarrays with commercially available antibodies to measure the relative levels of close to 600 distinct secreted signaling proteins. Using these arrays, we obtained quantifiable results for 582 signaling proteins (Additional file 1: Figure S1A to D and Additional file 2) in archived blood plasma from 47 sporadic, cognitively impaired AD patients and 52 non-demented, closely age- and sex-matched controls obtained from two clinical centers (Additional file 1: Table S1). While these proteins do not encompass all secreted signaling proteins, they do provide a strong representation of all major signaling pathways and represent the largest dataset of this kind available today (Additional file 1: Figure S1A). Raw data were processed, normalized (Additional file 1: Figure S2), and then subjected to three parallel analyses, aimed at integrating both molecular and clinical data, followed by external and internal validation steps (Fig. 1a).

To identify signaling proteins with significantly changed plasma levels in AD we calculated corrected p-values for the quality controlled, centered, and normalized array data. Principal component analysis showed that our data were relatively free of obvious batch effects or confounding factors (Additional file 1: Figure S3). Clustering of the top 50 most different proteins illustrated clear differences between AD and control samples (Fig. 1b and c). Using the most significant proteins (FDR < 0.05, corresponding to $p_{corr} < 0.015$) as a starting point, we then queried known pathway or physical interaction databases to test the hypothesis that the signaling proteome could be mined to identify pathologically disturbed pathways (i.e., deregulated pathways should reveal themselves through changes in multiple receptors and/or ligands). This approach greatly reduces the chance of false-positive discoveries in contrast to following individually significant but unconnected leads. Using this methodology we identified highly interconnected clusters of receptors and ligands with growth factor activity ("TGFβ/GDF/BMP signaling" and "Angiogenesis") or with activity linked to apoptosis (Fig. 1d). Reassuringly, the direction of changes was often coherent within each cluster/sub-cluster (Fig. 1d). Individual proteins can show highly significant differences between cohorts and, at the same time, exhibit large overlaps in the observed protein level ranges, highlighting the need for sufficient sample sizes and cohort stratification (Fig. 1e and Additional file 1: Figure S4).

To determine to what extent the observed changes in the AD signaling proteome are AD specific or the result of general neurodegeneration or other unrelated processes, we collected plasma samples from an additional 92 patients (Additional file 1: Table S2) suffering from semantic-variant primary progressive aphasia (svPPA), a sub-type of frontotemporal lobar degeneration (FTLD). SvPPA is almost always associated with Trans-activation response element (TAR) DNA-binding protein 43 (TDP-43)-aggregate pathology and appears to have weak genetic linkage [5–7]. This makes svPPA an ideal candidate to compare distinct neurological pathologies between two unrelated, sporadic, progressive dementias (svPPA *vs.* AD) *via* signaling proteome analysis [8]. The svPPA samples were prepared, handled, and analyzed in parallel to the AD samples to minimize experimental variations.

We found 39 proteins with significant changes in both AD and svPPA (Fig. 2a, inset; $p = 7.3 \times 10^{-5}$ by hypergeometric test). Intriguingly, when we compared significance and direction of protein changes between the two pathologies, we found a perfect correlative trend of up/up or down/down amongst the 39 overlapping proteins ($p < 1.8 \times 10^{-12}$ by binominal test), indicating that a more general disease-profile does exist (Fig. 2a, red boxes). Additionally, we were able to identify proteins with svPPA-specific (Fig. 2a, purple box) and AD-specific proteome signatures (Fig. 2a and b, yellow box), respectively. A more detailed analysis of the svPPA findings is published elsewhere [9]. Manual literature curation of the AD-specific hits yielded numerous proteins involved in TGFβ/GDF/BMP signaling, complement activation, apoptosis, or with otherwise strong AD literature, suggesting that those pathways could play a role in AD (Fig. 2b). These findings indicate that a mixture of both disease-specific and nonspecific signaling profiles can be obtained from blood and that comparative proteomics can be applied to identify disease-specific changes.

Changes in protein levels provide a binary view on AD (significantly changed or not). However, disease is a gradual process with patient's cognition becoming increasingly more impaired. To explore the relationship between cognitive performance and relative plasma protein levels, we correlated the levels of 582 proteins with the Mini-mental state [10] examination (MMSE) scores of the respective patient (Fig. 3a and b, and Additional file 2; Spearman rank correlation and p-value [p_{rho}] as well as explicit p-values through 1000-fold sample permutations [p_{perm}]). Applying the same network exploration method as before, we identified again many proteins involved in TGFβ/GDF/BMP signaling and apoptosis to be positively or negatively correlated with cognitive performance (Fig. 3c), lending further support to our AD-specific findings above. While proteins involved in "Complement" activation were detected by the MMSE correlation analysis, they did not meet the cutoff criteria in the differential analysis, indicating that the complement driven effects are more subtle and gradual in nature (Fig. 3c). This finding highlights the fact that analyzing a continuous functional parameter such as MMSE can retrieve additional non-binary pathways of interest.

Testing for mean differences in plasma protein levels allows us to identify proteins with significantly different levels of expression between AD and controls. However, we hypothesized that additional insight could be gained

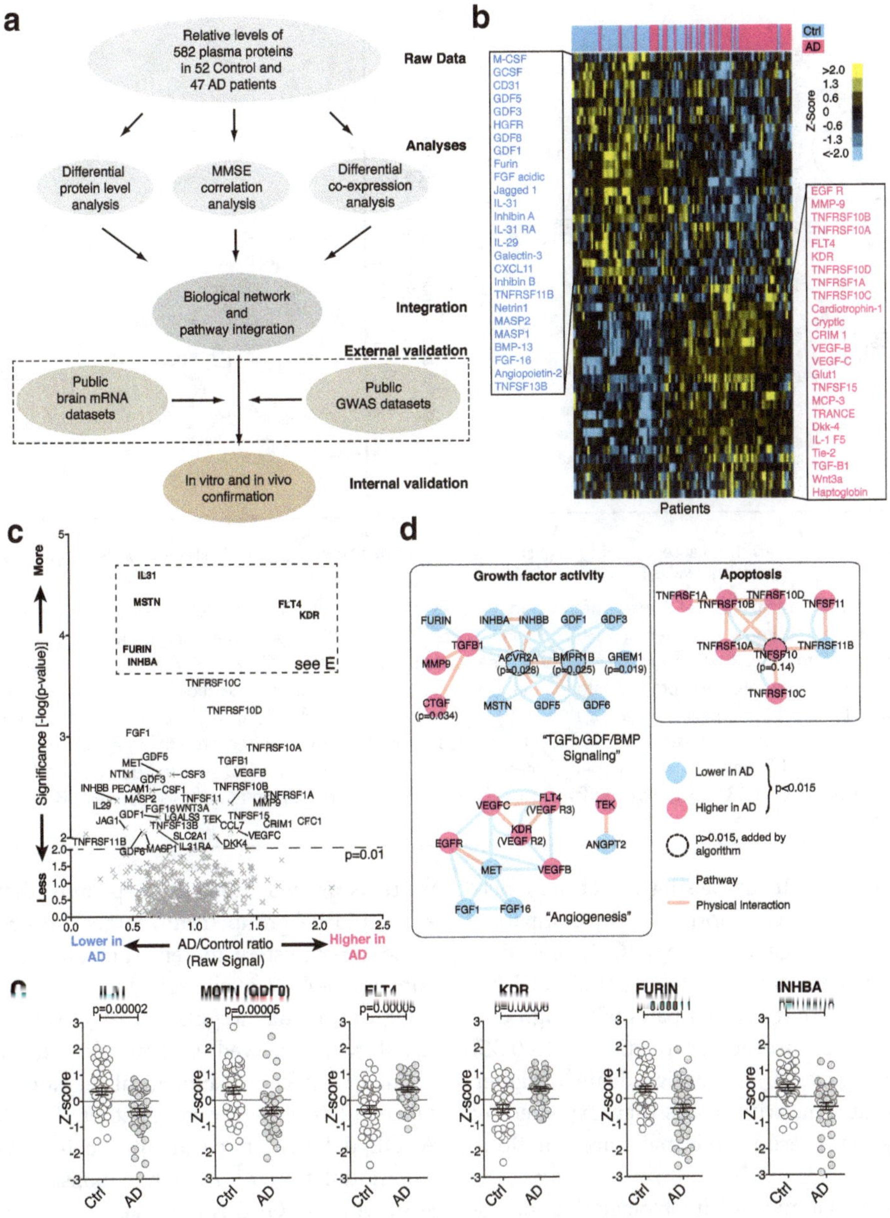

Fig. 1 The circulatory AD signaling proteome reveals changes in cellular communication. **a** Overview of the experimental and analysis workflow. Plasma samples were collected at clinical centers, relative protein abundance was determined by antibody microarray and three types of analyses were performed: Protein level, MMSE correlation (cognitive performance), and protein co-secretion analysis. The analyses results were then integrated in a network and pathway enrichment framework and finally subjected to internal and external validation. **b** Heat map representation of the protein level analysis showing the top 50 most different proteins after unsupervised clustering ($q < 0.05$), separating samples into AD (pink, right) and controls (blue, left) and proteins into higher in control (blue, top) and higher in AD (pink, bottom). **c** Volcano-plot showing the distribution of all proteins and naming those significantly different between AD and control subjects ($p_{corr} < 0.01$). **d** A network representation of the most significantly changed proteins ($p_{corr} < 0.015$; un-connected proteins omitted) after integration with known pathway and physical interaction data reveals many densely connected hits in pathways related to TGFβ/GDF/BMP, angiogenesis, and apoptosis signaling. **e** Example scatter plots of the six top changed proteins (see dashed box in e, mean ± s.e.m; all p-values are corrected for multiple hypothesis testing)

from comparing changes in co-expression of signaling molecules as this might carry information on the pairwise relationship between the underlying signaling proteins and regulatory pathways, and on how this relationship is affected in disease [11].

To assess changes in co-expression, we calculated the Spearman correlation between each protein pair under healthy control and under AD conditions and then subtracted these correlations from each other, creating co-expression and differential co-expression networks

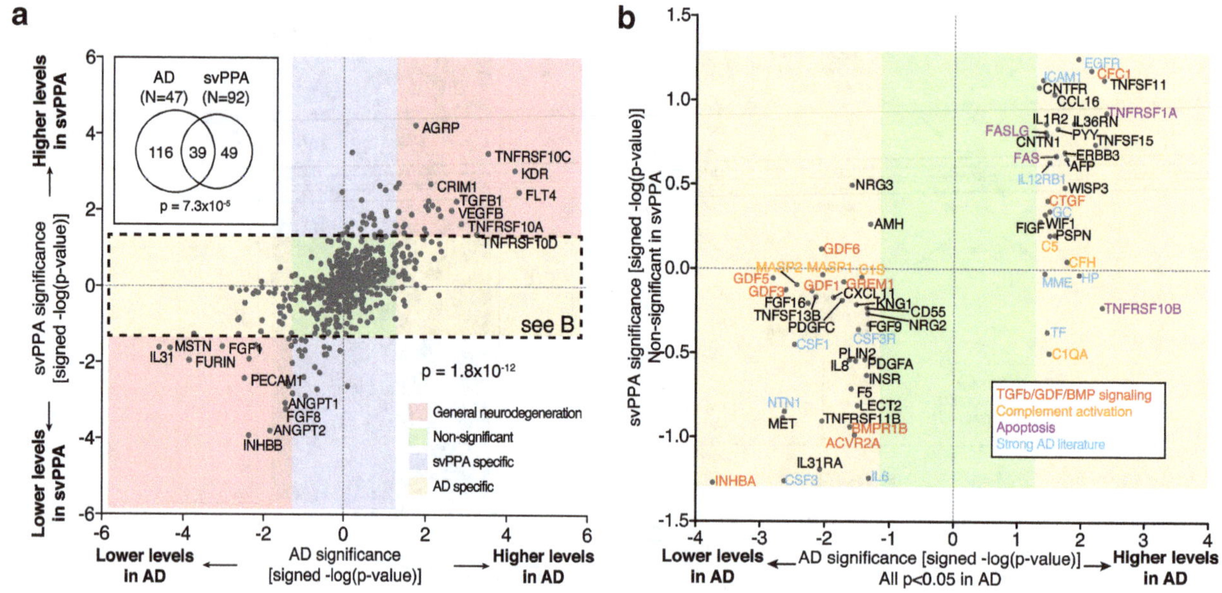

Fig. 2 The plasma proteome contains disease specific information. To assess the specificity of the proteins identified in the expression level analysis, AD samples were compared to another, unrelated progressive dementia (svPPA = semantic-variant primary progressive aphasia). **a** Plotting signed, log-transformed p_{corr}-values (more extreme = greater significance) of the AD *vs.* svPPA analysis show preserved directionality (binominal test) and can be used to categorize proteins into four distinct groups: "General neurodegeneration" (p_{AD} & $p_{svPPA} < 0.05$, same direction of changes in both diseases; red box); "Non-significant" (p_{AD} & $p_{svPPA} > 0.05$; green box), "svPPA specific" ($p_{AD} > 0.05$, $p_{svPPA} < 0.05$; purple box); "AD specific" ($p_{AD} < 0.05$, $p_{svPPA} > 0.05$; yellow box). Venn diagram showing the overlap of significantly changed proteins in AD or svPPA samples (top-left inset; threshold $p_{corr} < 0.05$; overlap significance by hypergeometric test). **b** Zooming into the "AD specific" box (see dashed box in a), many proteins can be identified as part of TGFβ/GDF/BMP, complement, or apoptosis signaling in addition to numerous proteins with strong supporting AD literature (manual curation)

respectively (Fig. 4a and b). It can be shown that these networks carry valuable biological information by comparing co-expression profiles and gene ontology (GO) biological process similarity between genes/proteins (Additional file 1: Figure S5). We found that protein pairs with high differential co-expression profile correlation ($R > 0.35$; Additional file 1: Figure S5) have significantly higher median GO semantic similarity scores than expected by chance, indicating that these protein pairs are functionally related.

Having established that meaningful biological information is contained within the co-expression profiles, we used hierarchical clustering [12] to arrange signaling proteins based on their co-expression profile correlations (Fig. 4c). Using DAVID [13, 14], we identified several clusters of proteins that were significantly enriched for a number of ontology terms (Fig. 4c). These protein clusters represent signaling molecules whose co-expression profiles change in a highly parallel fashion in AD, which in turn could indicate that the underlying regulatory pathways participate in AD pathogenesis. The most significantly enriched clusters were "Complement" ($p = 9.7 \times 10^{-10}$), "Regulation of growth" ($p = 0.00018$) and "Apoptosis" ($p = 0.0037$; all EASE score p-value based on 562 unique gene background). In this approach, the size (and number) of clusters identifiable is limited by the overall number of proteins probed: While it is apparent that cluster a-d and e-g could be grouped into larger "superclusters", probing these superclusters for enrichment is not useful as they contain 25–45 % of all probed proteins (Fig. 4c).

Exploring the "Regulation of growth" cluster in more detail, we observed several sub-clusters that partially aligned with known biological relationships, often bridging regulatory pathways together (Fig. 4d). For example APOE deficient mice are prone to atherosclerosis, but C3 modulation of lipid metabolism can protect them [15], while VEGFC is a marker for advanced atherosclerosis and hypercholesterolemia in the same animals [16]. TGFβ and interferons (IFN) have antagonizing relationships in the control of inflammation [17], while interferons reduce ghrelin (GHRL) expression [18], and Follistatin-like 1 (FSTL1) is controlled by TGFβ [19]. We also noticed that numerous proteins were directly or indirectly associated with or regulated by TGFβ/GDF/BMP signaling (e.g., TGFBR1, FSTL1, THBS1, MMP11, GREM1, GDF3, GDF5, GDF9), making that pathway a lead candidate to test for its involvement in AD. These data suggest that co-expression analysis can be used to identify clusters of proteins and regulatory pathways that are linked through similar co-expression profiles, potentially indicating pathways that are affected by or affecting AD pathology simultaneously.

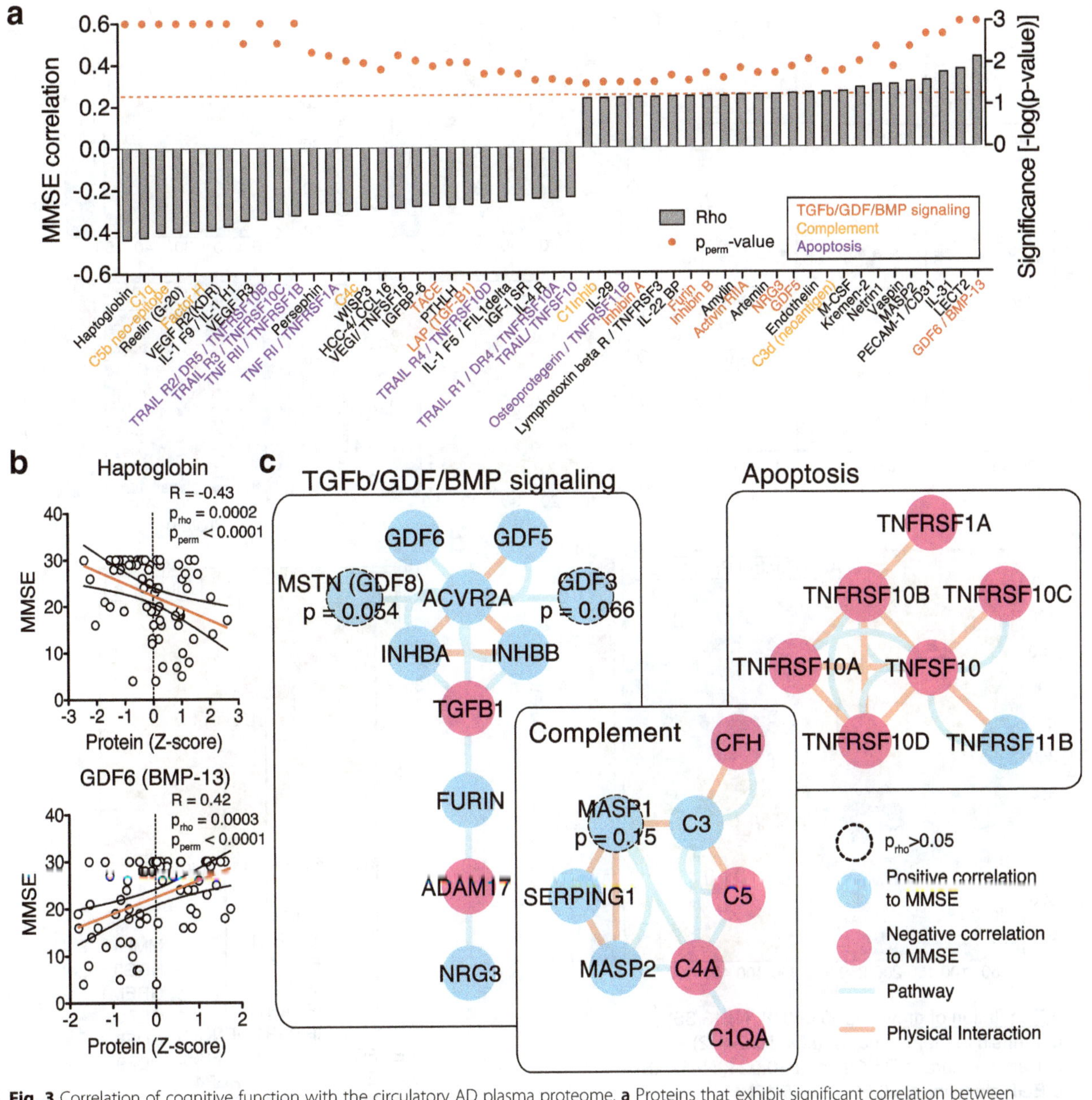

Fig. 3 Correlation of cognitive function with the circulatory AD plasma proteome. **a** Proteins that exhibit significant correlation between cognitive function (evaluated by MMSE = Mini-mental state examination score) and protein levels ranked by correlation (cutoff $p_{rho} < 0.05$, Spearman rank correlation; p_{perm} based on 1000 MMSE-score permutations; dashed red line indicates $p_{perm} = 0.05$ threshold). Many proteins are part of TGFβ/GDF/BMP, complement, or apoptosis signaling. **b** Example scattergrams of the top positive and negative MMSE-correlated proteins (red line indicates regression with 95 % confidence intervals). **c** Network representation of significantly correlated proteins after integration with known pathway and physical interaction data reveals many densely connected hits in pathways related to TGFβ/GDF/BMP, complement, and apoptosis signaling

Because protein quantification is notoriously difficult [1, 2, 20, 21] we examined the existing published literature for suitable non-proteomics data that could be used to validate our experimental approach. Recently, a large post-mortem study examined the mRNA expression levels in tissue from late-onset AD and control patients (cerebellum, pre-frontal cortex, and visual cortex) and provided data on the correlation between transcript levels and brain atrophy and Braak staging, which provides a measure of tangle pathology [22]. Using this dataset, we asked whether proteins that we found to be significantly correlated to cognitive performance (MMSE) also show a significant correlation between pre-frontal cortex transcript level and brain pathology (Braak stage and

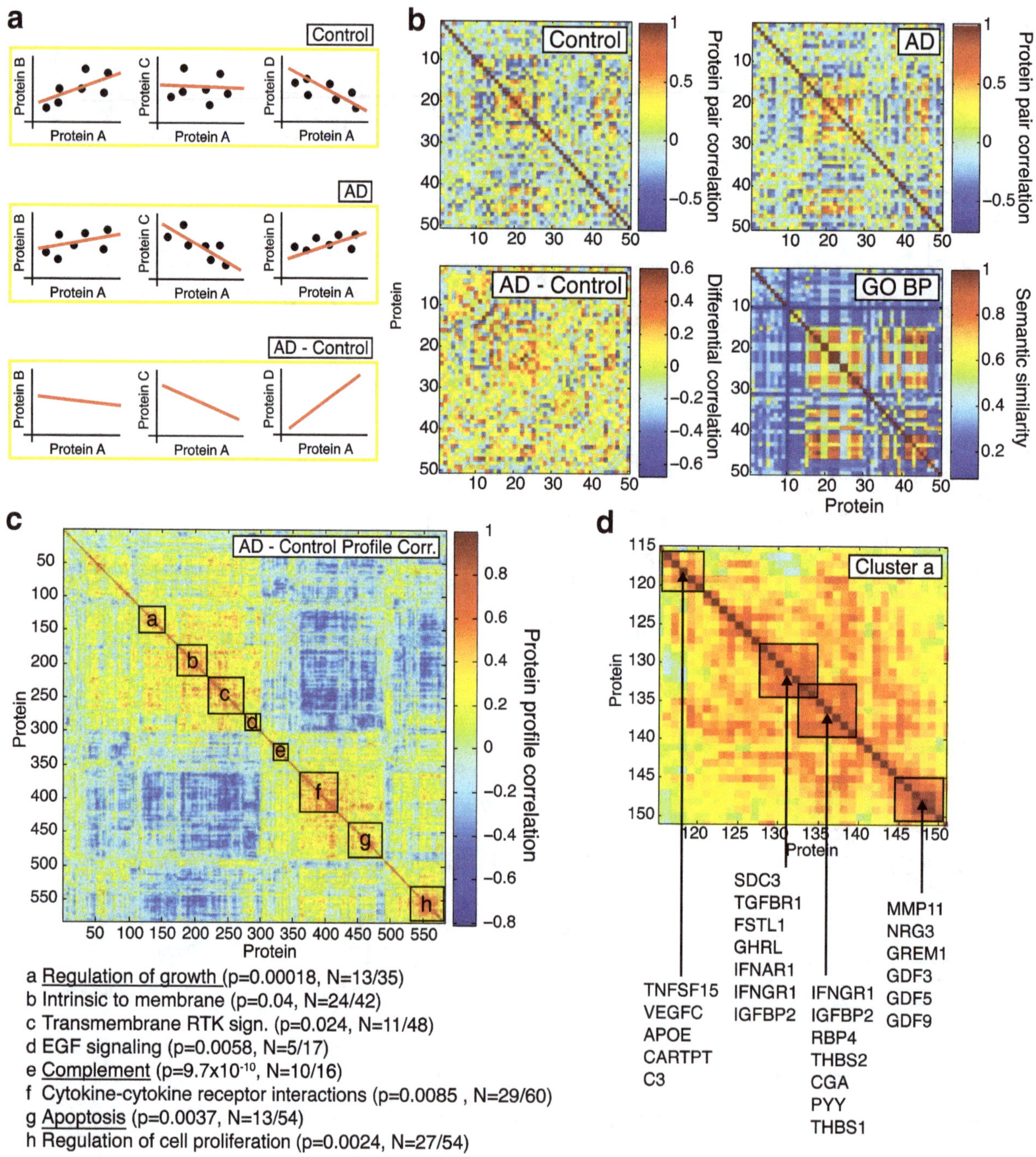

Fig. 4 Protein co-expression analysis. **a** Schematic, hypothetical example of differential protein correlation: Proteins A to D exhibit a certain correlation pattern in control samples (top row) and a different pattern in AD samples (middle row). Subtracting the control correlations from the AD correlations yields the differential correlation "AD-Control" that captures the direction and magnitude of the correlation changes in disease (bottom row). **b** Zoomed-in correlation matrices for 50 proteins out of 582: Pairwise protein correlation in control samples (top left), AD samples (top right) and calculated differential correlation (bottom left; random subset of proteins in alphabetical order, Spearman rank correlation). "GO BP" represents the pairwise semantic similarity score of the protein pairs from ~0.1 (very different) to ~0.9 (very similar) in the "biological process" gene ontology as a measure for distance in the ontology tree and shared membership in biological processes. **c** Heat map of the differential profile correlations of all 582 proteins after unsupervised clustering with optimal leaf ordering. Positive correlations between two proteins indicate that these proteins change their correlations to many other proteins in a highly parallel fashion. Different clusters of proteins with similar profiles can be identified and are each significantly enriched for biological processes (boxes a-h, annotation below heat map; *p*-value based on a modified Fisher exact *p*-value; *N* = members with annotation/cluster size; three most significantly enriched clusters are underlined). **d** Cluster "a Regulation of growth" zoomed in with detailed sub-structure (same color scale as c)

atrophy). And indeed, 29.4 % of the proteins (15/51) we had identified using MMSE as trait also have significant transcript-Braak stage correlations ($p = 0.0017$, Chi^2-test, Fig. 5a), while 33.3 % (17/51) exhibited transcript-atrophy correlations ($p = 0.0195$, Chi^2-test, Fig. 5a). This supports the notion that our experimental approach focusing on circulatory signaling proteins is able to enrich for proteins linked to AD brain pathology.

The results thus far from the differential protein level analysis, the correlations with cognitive function, and the co-expression network analysis consistently implicate the complement pathway, apoptosis, and a signaling network around the TGFβ superfamily in AD. We were particularly intrigued by this latter network, and its GDF family members, many of which had not been linked to AD. To further validate the significance of this finding we asked whether any of the proteins in this pathway – including intra- or extracellular ones not measured with the array – were additionally linked to AD at the genomic or transcript level. We used the Gene Ontology to identify a list of 114 genes linked to the TGFβ/GDF/BMP signaling pathway (Additional file 2) and queried two large AD data sets consisting of meta-data from 10 genome-wide association studies with a total of 8,309 AD cases and 7,366 cognitively normal elders [23] and AD brain transcriptome data from 181 AD and 125 controls [24] for significant SNPs or mRNA changes within the TGFβ/GDF/BMP pathway associated with AD.

We found significantly more SNPs in genes associated with TGFβ/GDF/BMP signaling than what would be expected by chance ($p = 8.0\times10^{-17}$, Kolmogorov-Smirnov test, Fig. 5b). Specifically, several genes that are involved in GDF3/Activin-receptor signaling had significant associations (GDF3, ACVR1B, SMAD3; see Additional file 2). Similarly, we found significantly more mRNAs with altered expression in AD brains associated with TGFβ/GDF/BMP signaling than what would be expected by chance ($p = 1.3\times10^{-20}$, Kolmogorov-Smirnov test, Fig. 5c and Additional file 2), including CFC1 (Cripto, a co-factor of GDF3), and Activin-receptor subunits 2B and 1C (ACVR2B/ACVR1C, GDF3 receptors). Taken together, multiple layers of experimental evidence suggest that changes at the genome, the transcriptome, and the proteome level in TGFβ/GDF/BMP signaling are associated with AD (Fig. 5d-f).

Activin receptors and its ligands Inhibin A and B, GDF1, GDF3, GDF5, and the ligand binding proteins CFC1/cripto and gremlin were most prominently altered in AD throughout our study (Figs. 1d, 3c, 4d, 5f). While TGFβ and TGFβ-receptor signaling has been studied extensively in the context of AD and neuroinflammation [25, 26], and BMP9/GDF2 has been identified as a regulator of cholinergic neuronal development [27], Activin receptor signaling and GDFs have not been studied in AD. GDF3 represents a particularly intriguing candidate: it is highly expressed in the human brain [28] and mouse dentate gyrus (Fig. 6a), is part of the co-expression cluster a (Fig. 4c and d), exhibits significant SNP enrichment (Additional file 2), is positively correlated with cognitive performance ($p_{perm} = 0.038$), yet its effects on neurons or the brain are unknown.

Given that we observed reduced GDF3 plasma levels, we first investigated whether these changes may be reflective of GDF3 levels in human AD brains. To do this, we measured the processed, active form of GDF3 in tissue extracts of AD and age matched control patients and found a significant reduction in the cortex ($n = 16$–18 subjects per group, $p = 0.02$, Fig. 6b), but not in the cerebellum, an area unaffected by AD ($n = 8$ subjects per group, $p = 0.15$, Additional file 1: Figure S6A and B). To evaluate our svPPA *vs* AD comparison, which predicted that GDF3 reduction is AD-specific, we measured activated GDF3 in cortical extracts from svPPA patients and controls and found no difference in GDF3 levels ($n = 5$ subjects per group, $p = 0.08$, opposite trend to AD, Additional file 1: Figure S6 C and D). While these studies support our plasma proteomic findings, the source and functional significance of GDF3 within the brain remain unclear.

Because GDF3 is highly expressed in the mouse dentate gyrus (a neurogenic area; Fig. 6c) and previous studies show a role for GDF3 in regulating embryonic and cancer stem cell fate and differentiation [29–31] we asked whether GDF3 regulates adult neurogenesis. We first cultured primary adult mouse neural progenitor cells (NPCs) under non-differentiating and differentiating conditions and measured GDF3 mRNA. Inducing NPC differentiation into neurons and astrocytes caused a marked upregulation of GDF3 (Fig. 6d), suggesting that, unlike in embryonic stem cells [32], adult NPCs are not the main source of secreted GDF3 and adult hippocampal GDF3 likely derives from mature cell types [28]. To assess whether GDF3 affects NPC function, we exposed primary adult NPCs to increasing concentrations of recombinant mouse GDF3 and measured proliferation. Indeed, GDF3 increased NPC proliferation as measured by BrdU incorporation (Fig. 6e) and changes in neurosphere number (Fig. 6f). Given that GDF3 has been implicated in embryonic stem cell fate [29, 30] and is capable of differentiating PC12 cells [33], we next investigated whether GDF3 promotes neuronal differentiation. To evaluate neuronal differentiation we utilized NTERA cells stably transfected with Doublecortin (Dcx) promoter-controlled eGFP, as previously described [34]. NTERA cells cultured with GDF3 showed a prominent increase in Dcx expression compared to control cells (Fig. 6g and h), which was also confirmed by western blot (Additional file 1: Figure S6E and F). Furthermore, a recent study demonstrated the potential importance of developmental factors

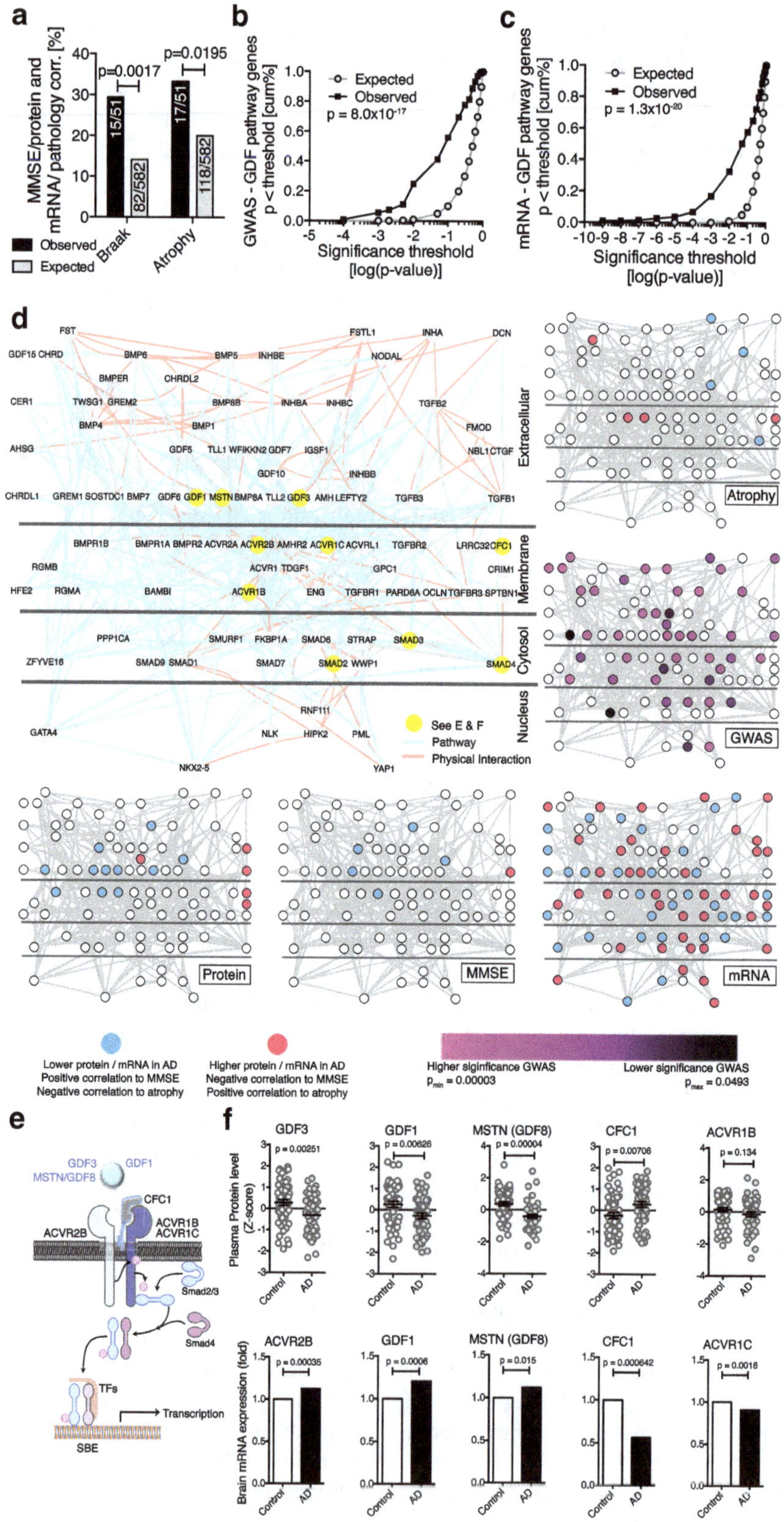

Fig. 5 (See legend on next page.)

(See figure on previous page.)

Fig. 5 External Validation. To assess the biological validity of our findings top proteins were cross-referenced at the transcript or genomic level to external datasets containing AD brain mRNA transcriptome data or AD genome-wide association data, respectively. **a** Pre-frontal cortex transcripts in AD brain corresponding to proteins that correlated with MMSE in our study (see Fig. 3a) correlate strongly with Braak stage or brain atrophy (pre-frontal cortex) beyond what is expected by chance (chi^2-test). **b** Based on meta-data from AD GWAS studies 114 genes which are part of "TGFβ/GDF/BMP signaling" exhibit higher than expected enrichment for significant SNPs (gene-wide *p*-value using VEGAS; cumulative curve comparison by Kolmogorov–Smirnov test). **c** Pre-fontal cortex transcripts for 120 genes of the TGFβ/GDF/BMP signaling pathway show many more significant transcript changes in AD than expected by chance (explicit p-value through sample permutation; cumulative curve comparison by Kolmogorov–Smirnov test). **d** Graphical representation of 92 proteins of TGFβ/GDF/BMP signaling pathway and integration with the findings from the various studies as indicated (only nodes with hits ≥ 1 are shown). Proteins are positioned relative to their location in the cells (extracellular, membrane bound, intracellular) and edges indicate physical or functional interactions (small border diagrams highlight proteins with associated significant changes). **e** Detailed pathway diagram for GDF-Activin receptor signaling. **f** Examples of protein (top row) and mRNA changes (bottom row) among the members of the GDF-Activin receptor signaling cascade (all corrected *p*-values)

such as the Repressor element 1-silencing transcription factor (REST) in AD pathology [35]. Intriguingly, GDF3 and REST appear to be controlled by shared transcription factor binding [36], potentially hinting at common upstream disturbances. Taken together these findings suggest that GDF3 plays an important role in NPC proliferation and neuronal differentiation and that it's levels are altered in AD.

Discussion

This study uses a new approach to discover biological pathways associated with AD dementia by measuring hundreds of circulatory proteins involved in cellular communication. Combined with multiple levels of statistical and bioinformatics analyses and leveraging current pathway knowledge, we were able to build networks of proteins deregulated in AD. We provide evidence that this approach has considerable robustness for the discovery of proteins and pathways linked to AD and successfully validate it against existing datasets. We show that genomic and transcriptomic data can be used to corroborate suspected disease-specific pathways and identify GDF3 as a new regulator of adult neurogenesis. Given the important function adult hippocampal neurogenesis has in rodent behavior related to memory and learning, the recent discovery of significant hippocampal neurogenesis in the adult human brain even with advanced age [37], and previous implications of disturbed neurogenesis in AD [38, 39], changes in neurogenesis caused by abnormal GDF3 signaling might well have a role in the development or progression of AD.

Currently, our approach is limited only by the availability of high-quality, verified antibodies able to reliably bind signaling molecules in plasma. Future developments in the production of antibodies or antibody alternatives such as aptamteres [40, 41] will likely enable researchers to probe even broader sets of circulating antigens. However, with increasingly large numbers of analytes ever-closer attention has to be paid to the statistical methods involved in identifying interesting candidates. Independent sample cohorts that are probed using different experimental approaches should always be considered, similar to the approach we are taking in this study. Nevertheless, there are certain limitations to consider when pursuing the biological interpretation of high-throughput proteomic studies [42]: (1) Protein coexpression data is currently still fairly noisy, resulting in networks with noisy edges making cluster definition challenging. To deal with this problem we based most of our analysis on much more vetted pathway or protein-protein interaction data. (2) Most proteins act in transient and changing complexes and how to define these overlapping clusters is not trivial. (3) Similarly difficult is to avoid arbitrarily breaking large clusters into random smaller ones and to identify the "correct" number of clusters from *a priori* knowledge. (4) If possible, running replicates will reduce clustering error and using learning through training and test sets can similarly improve the validity of the results [43]. However, availability of precious sample material and cohort sizes often limits the ability to perform these steps. Encouragingly, these limitations are subject to very active ongoing research efforts and novel methodologies will likely enable us to avoid many of these pitfalls in the future.

Motivated by the idea to specifically monitor the cellular communication factors secreted into the bloodstream, we naturally had a strong representation of inflammatory and growth factor related proteins in our screen. In the complete human proteome, additional proteins and protein fragments have the potential to being secreted into the bloodstream and could provide mechanistic insight into further pathological processes active in AD, which we likely missed in our current screening format. Additional pathways or protein sets could easily be added to future versions of the screening platform as antibodies become available. Conversely, there may be other inflammatory and signaling-related pathologies that were left undiscovered due to limited sample numbers and increasing cohort sizes could ameliorate this limitation, although we estimate to have recovered 50–75 % of the true positive hits (Additional file 1: Figure S4). Finally, using gene ontology enrichment to identify classes of interesting genes inherently carries over the annotation and research bias present

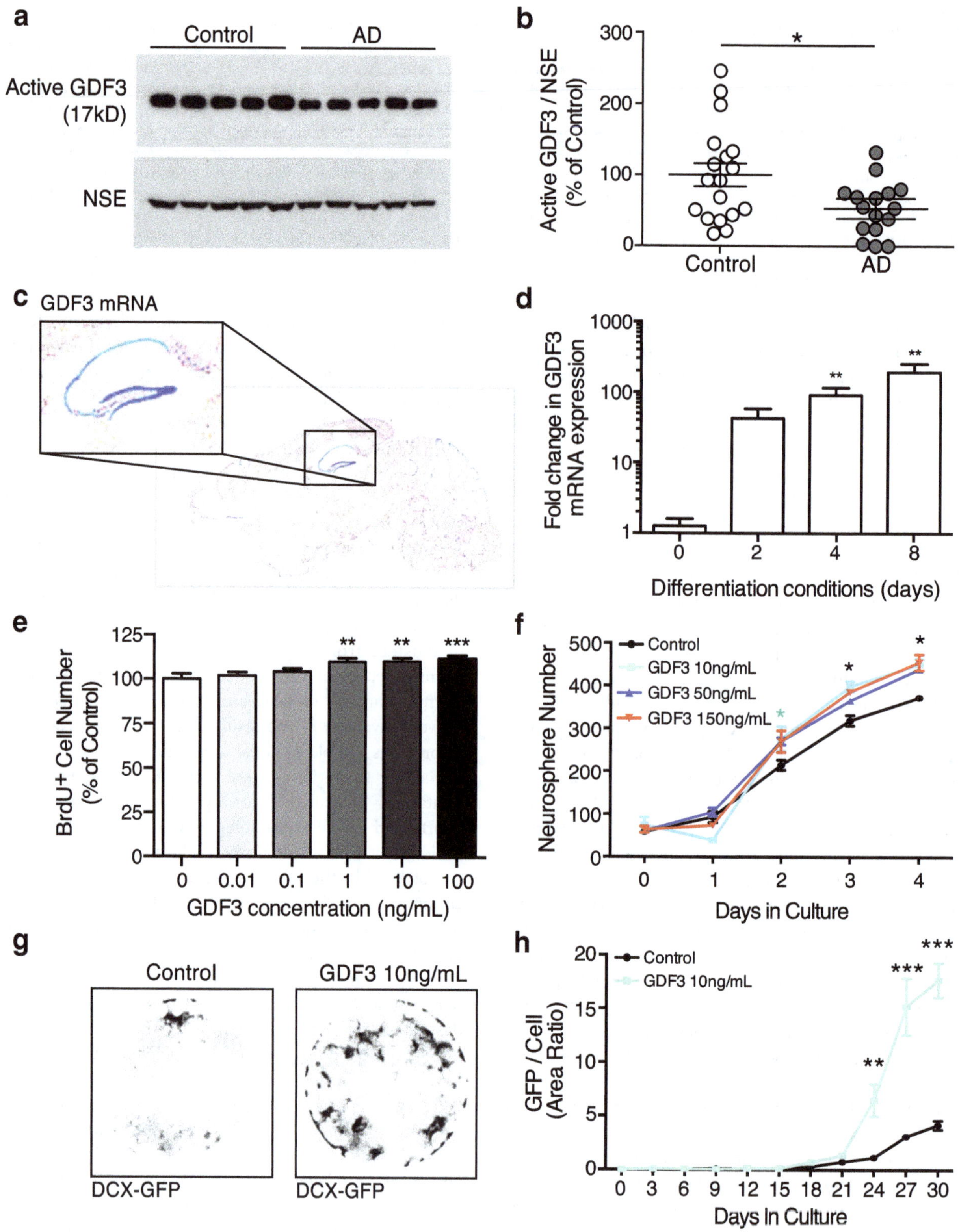

Fig. 6 (See legend on next page.)

(See figure on previous page.)

Fig. 6 GDF3 regulates neurogenesis and is reduced in AD brains. **a** To test whether GDF3 levels are also reduced in AD brains, Human AD and control cortical grey matter regions were lysed and the detergent soluble protein fraction was probed by western blot. Levels of active GDF3 (**b**) were quantified relative to neuron-specific enolase (NSE). **c** To identify areas in the brain where GDF3 may have a functional role, we referred to The Allen Brain Atlas, which showed strong RNA expression in the mouse hippocampus (blue = high expression). **d** Using qPCR, GDF3 mRNA expression was detected in non-differentiated adult mouse NPCs and NPCs cultured in differentiating conditions. **e** To determine whether GDF3 affects stem cell function, adult mouse NPCs were provided recombinant mouse GDF3 and NPC proliferation was assessed using BrdU. **f** Recombinant mouse GDF3 was also provided to dissociated adult mouse neurospheres and the number of newly formed neurospheres was subsequently quantified. **g** To investigate whether GDF3 promotes neurogenesis, human-derived NTERA cells stably transfected with Dcx promoter-controlled eGFP were provided recombinant human GDF3. Shown are representative images of DCX-GFP fluorescence expression from an entire well of NTERA cells treated with GDF3 or control for 30 days. **h** DCX-GFP fluorescence area was quantified relative to the cellular area detected by brightfield microscopy. Results were compared by a one-way ANOVA with a Dunnett's post-test (**b**,**e**), an unpaired Student's *t* test (**d**), or a two-way ANOVA with a Bonferroni post-test (**f**,**h**) and are representative of at least 2 independent experiments (b $n = 16-18$ per group, d,e,f,h; $n = 3$ per group). Values are mean ± s.e.m.. $^*p < 0.05$, $^{**}p < 0.01$, $^{***}p < 0.001$ compared to respective control groups

from GO [44]. This can be mediated somewhat by using more data-driven ontology approaches such as NeXO and CliXO [45, 46], although research bias cannot be overcome that way. We thus encourage the reader to not purely rely on the enrichment terms that we provide for the identified protein clusters, but to interpret the proteins of interest in the broader framework of biological knowledge.

Over the past decade, numerous studies [20, 21, 47–59] have been performed to identify biomarker sets in AD plasma samples (Additional file 1: Figure S1A), leading to the recognition of a number of biological pathways and proteins potentially affected in the disease [60]. Analyzing pathway enrichment in combined cohorts from multiple studies, Kiddle and colleagues [3] found the most significant enrichment in proteins linked to "Complement and coagulation cascades" ($p = 9.78 \times 10^{-25}$) and "Cytokine-cytokine receptor interaction" ($p = 2.07 \times 10^{-18}$), which is in good agreement with the pathways implicated in our screen (Figs. 3 and 4). Using a similar meta-analysis approach to identify individual proteins related to AD pathology, Chiam et al. report multi-cohort support for the involvement of Complement C3, Complement Factor H, and Plasma protease C1 inhibitor [60], all of which were identified in our screen as well (Fig. 3). For many of the other proteins and pathways implicated in this study (for example GDF), little comparable data exist, as they are not covered by the most widely used Rules Based Medicine (RBM) 190 analyte panel.

The approach presented here could be extended to study abnormal cellular processes in other CNS diseases or conditions where affected tissues are similarly difficult to access. Collectively, our data support the presence of an accessible and informative link between molecular (mRNA), cellular (Braak stages), structural (atrophy), and functional (MMSE) changes in the brain and circulatory signaling proteins. Exploiting this link, may aid in the design of novel therapeutic and early diagnostic strategies for sporadic AD.

Conclusion

Neurodegenerative disorders are widespread, devastating, poorly understood, and largely untreatable with current knowledge. One difficulty lies in the fact that the brain is extraordinarily sensitive and cannot easily be examined on the cellular or molecular level in the diseased patient. Here, we instead created and analyzed a large set of blood protein data from Alzheimer's disease and healthy control patients for changes in cellular communication factors, leading to the discovery and validation of altered GDF signaling in sporadic Alzheimer's disease brain tissue. We achieve this by integrating multiple levels of 'omics data, linking blood to brain tissue changes, thus opening up potentially new avenues for treatment and diagnosis.

Methods

Nomenclature

This is a proteomics study. To highlight this fact, we labeled hits in the first analyses (Figs. 1b and 2a) with protein names. Due to space restrictions in figure design, we labeled hits in all other figures with the HUPO *gene names* of the corresponding protein or mRNA products.

Human plasma samples

All participants underwent thorough and standardized history and physical exams. For the antibody arrays, we used a total of 99 archived human plasma samples with ethylenediaminetetraacetate (EDTA) as anticoagulant collected at the University of California San Francisco (San Francisco, CA) and the Mayo Clinic (Rochester, MN and Jacksonville, FL; Additional file 1: Table S1). Plasma was produced by standard blood processing, then aliquots were frozen and stored in aliquots at −80 °C, avoiding freeze thaw cycles. Informed consent was obtained from human subjects according to the ethics committee guidelines at the respective clinical centers. All patients were clinically diagnosed with AD based on the 1984 NINCDS-ADRDA Alzheimer's criteria with additional attention to the 2011 revisions [61] and (if possible) post-mortem tissue analysis (27 of the 47 AD cases). Details on the svPPA plasma samples are provided in Additional file 1: Table S2. A total of 92 svPPA patients from the University of California San Francisco or Mayo Clinic Jacksonville were identified whose clinical features conformed to revised consensus diagnostic criteria for svPPA [62]. Patient consent had been administered at the respective sample collection centers and research has been conducted according to the principles expressed in the Declaration of Helsinki. Analysis of de-identified samples was performed with research approval by the Stanford University institutional review board.

Antibody-microarray production

Plasma protein levels were measured using antibody-based protein microarrays. We used a custom-expanded, commercially available microarray with modified antibody content (custom L-Series, RayBiotech Inc., Norcross, GA) containing 474 antibodies against chemokines and cytokines printed in triplicates by the company, plus 17 control antibodies. Additionally, we produced a custom-made in-house array that contained a separate set of 119 antibodies against secreted signaling factors printed in quadruplicates, plus 7 control antibodies. A total of 617 antibodies were measured. Subsequent quality control steps removed 11 antibodies with extremely low or no signal and control antibodies (see *Antibody-Microarray Data Preparation* below) yielding a total of 582 analyzed antibodies (Additional file 2 and Additional file 1: Figure S1 and S2C). Some antibodies target the same protein multiple times (such as precursor/full-length/truncated forms, 14 proteins and 32 antibodies total; see Additional file 2). The microarray production protocol was the following: antibodies of interest were selected based on their biological role as secreted signaling factors and the availability of ELISA-grade quality batches to ensure likely detection of the epitope in liquid solution. The arrays were printed onto SuperEpoxy glass slides (Arrayit, Sunnyvale, CA) using a custom-built robotic microarrayer fitted with sixteen SMP4B pins (Arrayit). After drying the slides overnight they were vacuum-sealed and stored at −20 °C until use.

Plasma sample preparation and antibody-microarray incubation

The human plasma samples were thawed at room temperature and diluted 5-times in PBS without Ca^{2+}/Mg^{2+} (pH 6.5) followed by 10,000 g centrifugation in a swing bucket centrifuge for 10 min at Room temperature. The lipid layer on top was carefully removed with the house vacuum. Without disturbing the platelet pellet 300 μl was carefully removed for dialysis (96 well Dispodialyzer/5 kDa, Harvard Apparatus, Holliston, MA) into PBS (pH 6.5) at 4 °C in multiple steps including a last over-night step to yield a maximally pure plasma protein fraction in an appropriate buffer for the biotinylation reaction. The dialyzed plasma was diluted again 6-times in PBS and recombinant Green fluorescent protein (GFP) was spiked into the samples as positive control at a final concentration of 1 μg/ml. The plasma proteins were N-terminally biotinylated (NHS-SulfoBiotin, Thermo Scientific, Rockford, IL), reaction was stopped with 0.1 M glycin final concentration and unbound biotin removed by multiple dialysis against PBS (pH 6.5 and last at pH 8). Then samples were diluted in 3 % casein in PBS (pH 7.4) and the individual samples were incubated on blocked antibody arrays overnight at 4 °C. Blocking was performed by incubating dried arrays in 4 °C precooled 3 % casein in PBS (pH 7.4) overnight on a shaker (30 rpm) at 4 °C. After multiple washing steps antibody-bound protein was detected using 0.5 μg/ml Alexa Fluor 555 conjugated streptavidin (Invitrogen) on a GenePix Pro 4000B scanner (Molecular Devices, Sunnyvale, CA, Additional file 1: Figure S1D). Samples for both AD and svPPA studies were processed in parallel in randomized order in one batch.

Data processing and figure generation

Raw data from the array scanner were provided as images (.tif files) and spot intensities (Excel.xls files; Microsoft, Seattle, WA). Excel files were condensed into one file (tab-delimited.txt file) and non-analyzed data rows/ columns were removed using RDBmerge (Ron de Bruin, www.rondebruin.nl). Unless otherwise stated, data processing and statistical testing were performed in Matlab R2012a (MathWorks, Natick, MT). Figures were generated directly in Matlab or data were transferred and plotted in Prism 5.0f (GraphPad Software, La Jolla, CA). Figures were then arranged for publishing using Illustrator CS5 and Photoshop CS5 (both Adobe, San Diego, CA).

Antibody-microarray data preparation

To determine spot intensities, we calculated the mean pixel intensity per spot. To determine background intensities we calculated the median pixel intensity per background "doughnut" (Additional file 1: Figure S1D). Individual array spots were background subtracted locally (by subtracting the median background across spot replicates in each sample). Spots with a residual intensity less than 10 % above background were set to 'ND' (non-detectable). Antibodies with more than 55 % 'ND' values were excluded from the analysis ($N = 11$), yielding a total of 582 quantifiable antibodies (Additional file 2, for 'ND'-count distribution see Additional file 1: Figure S2C). 'ND' values were then replaced with the greater of the half the minimum non-'ND' value per sample replicates, the half the minimum non-'ND' value of that antibody across all samples (if the sample replicates were all 'ND'), or 1. The spot data were Log2 transformed, replicate averaged, and iteratively ($i = 50$) row- and column-wise median centered (subtract the column-wise median from the values in each column/row of data, so that the mean or median value of each column/row is 0) and normalized (multiply all values in each column/row of data by a scale factor S so that the sum of the squares of the values in each column/row is constant across columns/rows) following a procedure described in the Cluster 3.0 manual [63]. Finally the data were Z-scored, leaving approximately normally distributed data for analysis with a mean of 0 and a standard deviation of 1 (Additional file 1: Figure S2D to F, 86 % of all antibodies have normal distributions based on one-sample Kolmogorov-Smirnov test).

Principle component analysis

To assess the influence of potentially confounding factors such as plasma source, patient age, or patient gender, we performed a Principle Component Analysis in Matlab using the Z-scored data and the built-in *princomp* function.

Differential protein level analysis

To identify proteins with significant changes in plasma levels (based on Z-score values) we calculated permutation-corrected p-values (p_{corr}) for Control *vs.* AD for every protein (unpaired two-tailed t-test, 10,000 class label permutations) using the *mattest* Matlab function. To compute false-discovery rates, we adopted a direct approach to estimate q-values [64] using the *mafdr* Matlab function. Proteins with a significant difference between AD and Control samples and a $q < 0.05$ were considered having different plasma levels (a total of 50 proteins). An identical approach was used for the svPPA data.

Network representation

To link the proteins with changed plasma levels to biological pathways, we mapped these proteins onto known protein networks using the Genemania-app [65] in Cytoscape 3.0.1 [www.cytoscape.org, [66]]. Pathway data came from NCI-Nature [67], Reactome [68–70], and [71]. Physical interaction data came from Biogrid Small Scale [72], IREF Interact, and IREF Small Scale [73]. We allowed for some nodes above the significance threshold to be added by the algorithm to connect cliques (dashed nodes, p-value indicted in figure). To test for enrichment in biological function, we queried Gene Ontology [74, 75], KEGG [76], and Panther [77] databases using DAVID [13] with the 564 unique genes representing the 582 proteins tested as background.

Mini-mental State Exam (MMSE) correlation

MMSE scores were recorded at the time of plasma acquisition at the respective clinical centers. Scores were available for 44/47 AD patients and 26/52 Control patients (Additional file 2 and Additional file 1: Table S1). MMSE scores were correlated to Z-scored protein levels using Spearman's rank correlation. Correlation significance was assessed using Spearman's p-value (p_{Rho}: significance that slope is not 0) and by computing an empirical p-value by permuting protein scores over MMSE scores 1,000-times (p_{Perm}: Number of times that random MMSE-Protein data yields correlation greater than observed/1,000). Network representation was performed as described above.

Differential co-expression analysis

Co-expression analysis was performed to identify proteins involved in AD pathogenesis that would inform us on more specific pathways than the broad ones implicated in the differential analysis above. Besides the mere difference in expression levels, proteins may differ in how they correlate with each other between disease and controls. We sought to discover protein networks that are changed between AD and Control by evaluating differential correlation matrices in an approach analogous to methods developed for analyzing genetic interaction profiles [78]. We thus created separate correlation matrices (Spearman's rank correlation) in Matlab of all of the proteins measured for AD and Control signaling proteomes, respectively. Since cohort sizes were almost equal for AD and Controls we then calculated differential correlation profiles from these correlation matrices and used unsupervised clustering to identify 8 distinct clusters of proteins with highly similar differential correlation profiles (Fig. 4c, boxes). To demonstrate that differential co-expression data contains valuable biological information, we created semantic similarity scores for each protein pair [79]. Protein pairs with high differential co-expression profile correlation exhibited high semantic-similarity profile correlations as well (Additional file 1: Figure S5).

Braak staging and atrophy correlation

Braak staging and atrophy data were downloaded from the supplemental data file of [22]. We then filtered the data for mRNAs that had been reported to exhibit significant correlation to either Braak staging or atrophy data in the pre-frontal cortex. Expected values were calculated by determining the total number of *proteins tested* that were reported to have significant correlations. Observed values were calculated by determining the total number of proteins *within our MMSE correlation hit list* that were reported to have significant correlations. Significance testing was performed using the chi^2-test.

Single Nucleotide Polymorphism (SNP) analysis

Datasets and SNP association testing. Summarized information from tests of genetic association of AD with SNPs located in the candidate gene regions was culled from a recent large genome-wide association study (GWAS) conducted by the Alzheimer Disease Genetics Consortium

(ADGC) [23]. Naj et al. computed results for SNPs throughout the genome in their discovery sample composed of 8,309 AD cases and 7,366 cognitively normal elders from ten independent Caucasian data sets. Details of the procedures for quality control, genotype imputation, and population substructure adjustment are published elsewhere [23]. Genotyped and imputed SNPs were tested for association with AD in each dataset separately using a logistic generalized linear model (GLM) in case–control datasets and a logistic generalized estimating equation (GEE) in family-based datasets, controlling for intra-study population substructure. Genotyped SNPs were coded as 0, 1, or 2 according to the number of minor alleles under the additive genetic model. For imputed SNPs, a quantitative estimate between 0 and 2 for the dose of the minor allele were used to incorporate the uncertainty of the imputation estimates. All analyses were performed using the GEE [80] and GWAF [81] programs in the R statistical software package. SNP association results obtained from individual datasets were combined by meta-analysis using the inverse variance method implemented in the software package METAL [82] (http://www.sph.umich.edu/csg/abecasis/Metal/index.html).

Gene-based multiple testing corrections

We corrected for testing multiple SNPs in a gene after accounting for correlation between SNP genotypes due to linkage disequilibrium. Each gene tested was treated as an independent hypothesis and the effective number of tests per gene was obtained by a previously described method [83]. The Versatile Gene-based Association Study (VEGAS) approach [84] was used to summarize the strength of association of a gene with AD based on the number of SNPs tested in the gene and size of the gene. This method computes a gene-based test statistic based on the SNP p-values within the gene, and then uses simulation to calculate an empirical gene-based p-value. The distribution of empirical p-values was then plotted and tested against an expected distribution of p-values using the Kolmogorov-Smirnov test.

mRNA expression analysis

The dataset comprises gene expression data from brain tissues that were posthumously collected from more than 600 individuals with AD diagnosis, HD diagnosis, or with normal non-demented brains. We used a subset of dorsolateral prefrontal cortex (PFC, Brodmann area 9) samples from 181 AD case and 125 controls. Only neuropathologically confirmed AD subjects with Braak stage > III were included in this profiling experiment; Braak stage and atrophy were assessed by pathologists at McLean Hospital (Belmont, MA). The samples were flash frozen in liquid nitrogen vapor with an average postmortem interval (PMI) of about 18 h.

A total of 1 μg of mRNA extracted from each tissue sample was amplified to fluorescently labeled cRNA, and profiled by the Rosetta Gene Expression Laboratory in two phases using the Rosetta/Merck 44 k 1.1 microarray (GPL4372) (Agilent Technologies, Santa Clara, CA). The average RNA integrity number of 6.81 was sufficiently high for the microarray experiment monitoring 40,638 transcripts representing more than 31,000 unique genes. The expression levels were processed and normalized to the average of all samples in the batch from the same region using Rosetta Resolver (Rosetta Biosoftware, Seattle, WA).

All microarray data generated in this study are available through the National Brain Databank at the Harvard Brain Tissue Resource Center (http://www.brainbank.mclean.org/). This microarray dataset is MIAME compliant. The raw and final processed data for each hybridization are available upon request. The essential sample annotation including experimental factors and their values (e.g., gender, age, PMI, pH) is available and summarized in [24].

The differential gene expression was assessed using the standard t-test. The distribution of p-values was then plotted and tested against an expected distribution of p-values using the Kolmogorov-Smirnov test.

Western blot

Active GDF3 levels were determined in fresh tissue samples not part of the plasma screen (Additional file 1: Table S3). Hippocampal samples were a random subset picked blindly from the same donors as the cortical samples. All tissues or cells were lysed in RIPA buffer and total protein concentrations were determined with a BCA Protein Assay Kit (Thermo Scientific, Waltham, MA). 10–20 μg of total protein was loaded for each sample into pre-cast 4–12 % bis-tris gels and run with MOPS buffer (Invitrogen, Carlsbad, CA). Gels were transferred onto PVDF membranes (Millipore, Billerica, MA). Antigen specific primary antibodies were incubated overnight at 4 °C and detected with species-specific horseradish-peroxidase labeled secondary antibodies. An ECL Western Blotting Detection kit (GE Healthcare, Cleveland, OH) was used to obtain a chemiluminescence signal, which was detected using Amersham Hyperfilm ECL (GE Healthcare). Band quantification was performed using ImageJ software (version 1.46; NIH, Bethesda, MD). Bands of interest were normalized to actin or neuron specific enolase for a loading control. For active GDF3 we used anti-GDF3 antibodies from Novus Biologicals (Littleton, CO; NBP1-96508).

Cell culture assays

Human NTERA cells expressing eGFP under the DCX promoter were maintained in DMEM media containing 10 % FBS. To induce differentiation, cells were plated in 96 well plates. One day after seeding, 10 μM of retinoic acid and designated concentrations of recombinant carrier-free human GDF3 (R&D Systems, Minneapolis, MN; at 0, 10, 50, or 150 ng/mL) were added to the culture media of each corresponding NTERA treatment well. Cells were maintained under these conditions for 2 weeks, during which media was replaced every 3 days. Cells were then cultured for an additional 2 weeks with continued GDF3 treatment, in the absence of retinoic acid.

Cellavista

Adult neurosphere number, eGFP expression (relative to cell confluence), and number of proliferating NPCs were quantified after GDF3 treatment using an Innovatis Cellavista Imager (Dynamic Devices, Wilmington, DE). To quantify NPC proliferation, 10x images were collected by Cellavista and BrdU+ nuclei were detected and quantified by Cellavista software using the cell nuclei count function.

Adult hippocampal NPC isolation

Hippocampal NPCs were isolated from 6 week old male and female mice [85]. NPCs were maintained on poly-D-lysine (Sigma, St. Lous, MO) and laminin (Invitrogen) coated 10 cm plastic plates in neurobasal A media (Invitrogen) with 1× B27 supplement without vitamin A (Invitrogen) and 1× GlutaMAX-I supplement (Invitrogen) and 20 ng/ml each of recombinant human FGF-basic (Peprotech, Rocky Hill, NJ) and recombinant human EGF (Peprotech) at 37 °C and 5 % CO2. All experiments used NPCs below passage 20 and were repeated at least once with male NPCs and once with female NPCs.

GDF3 treatment of proliferating NPCs

5000 cells were plated per well in a 96 well poly-D-lysine/laminin-coated plate with 0, 0.01, 0.1, 1, 10 or 100 ng/ml recombinant mouse GDF3 (R&D Systems) in normal growth media. Cells were allowed to grow for 4 days, with a ½ media change on day 2 (which replaced full growth factors [85] and ½ of GDF3 treatment). After 4 days in treatment, 20 μM bromodeoxyuridine (BrdU, Sigma) in sterile PBS was added to all wells and cells were fixed with 4 % paraformaldehyde 2 h later for 10 min.

Immunocytochemistry

Fixed cells were rinsed with 0.1 M phosphate buffered saline (PBS) 3 times then blocked with 10 % normal donkey serum (NDS, Jackson ImmunoResearch, West Grove, PA) and 0.3 % Triton-X 100 (Sigma) in PBS for 30 min. Cells were incubated overnight in primary antibody, rat anti-BrdU (1:500, AbD Serotech, Raleigh NC) in 10 % NDS in PBS at 4 °C. Cells were then rinsed and incubated in secondary antibody, Alexa488 anti-rat (1:200, Invitrogen) in 10 % NDS in PBS. After rinsing, total BrdU+ cells were imaged and quantified using an automated Cellavista microscope system (Hoffman-La Roche, Basel, Switzerland).

NPC differentiation

Murine NPCs were differentiated for 8 days [85]. Briefly, cells were plated at 200,000 cells/well in a poly-D-lysine/laminin-coated plate in either full growth factor media (20 ng/ml of EGF and FGF2; proliferative conditions) or in media with only 5 ng/ml FGF2. After 2 days, the proliferative wells and the 2d differentiation wells were harvested while the 4d and 8d wells received a complete media change to media with no growth factors added. At day 4, the 4d wells were harvested and the 8d wells received a ½ media change with no growth factors added. A ½ media change was repeated on day 6 and the remaining wells were harvested on day 8.

RNA harvesting and conversion to cDNA

Cells were removed from the plate using Accutase Cell Dissociation Reagent (Invitrogen) then centrifuged at 400 g for 5 min. The cell pellet was stored at −80 °C until later RNA extraction. RNA extraction was performed using the RNeasy Mini Kit (Qiagen, Venlo, Netherlands) as per manufacturer instructions. The resulting RNA was quantified using a nanodrop spectrophotometer and RNA purity was confirmed using A260/A280 ratios. 500 ng of RNA was treated with DNase I as per manufacturer instructions (Invitrogen) to eliminate any genomic DNA contamination and then converted to cDNA using SuperScript III first-strand synthesis system (Invitrogen) as per manufacturer instructions. cDNA was diluted 1:5 in water.

Real-time quantitative PCR

2 μl of cDNA was quantified in duplicate for each sample using LightCycler 480 SYBR Green I (Roche) on a LightCycler 480 II as per manufacturer instructions. Cycling conditions were: 15 min at 95 °C, 45 cycles of [15 s at 94 °C, 25 s at 58 °C, 20 s at 72 °C]. Melt curve cycles immediately followed and were: 5 s at 95 °C, 1 min at 65 °C and then gradual temperature rise to 97 °C at a rate of 0.11 °C/s followed by 30s at 40 °C. GDF3 levels were normalized to MAPK3 [86] as a reference gene because MAPK3 has been shown not to change with differentiation in contrast to many other standard housekeeping genes such as actin, which change dramatically during the differentiation process [87]. Melt curve analysis was performed to verify primer specificity and all primers were tested in a dilution series before use. Data is displayed as fold change above proliferative condition mRNA levels using 2^(ΔΔCt) values.

Primer sequences were obtained from the MIT/Harvard PrimerBank.

GDF3 fwd: 5' ATGCAGCCTTATCAACGGCTT
GDF3 rev: 5' AGGCGCTTTCTCTAATCCCAG
GDF3 PrimerBankID: 6679979a1

MAPK3 fwd: 5' TCCGCCATGAGAATGTTATAGGC
MAPK3 rev: 5' GGTGGTGTTGATAAGCAGATTGG
MAPK3 PrimerBankID: 21489933a1

Abbreviations

AD: Alzheimer's disease; BMP: bone morphogenetic protein; BrdU: bromodeoxyuridine; Dcx: doublecortin; FTLD: frontotemporal lobar degeneration; GDF: growth-differentiation factor; GO: gene ontology; MMSE: mini-mental state examination; NPC: neural progenitor cells; SNP: single nucleotide polymorphism; svPPA: semantic-variant primary progressive aphasia.

Competing interest

R-PH and RH work for RayBiotech and provided custom slides at a discounted rate. No other competing interests exist.

Authors' contributions

PAJ extracted the array images, wrote the code to analyze the array data, and made all figures. KML, EDK, and RA, performed the *in vivo* GDF3 confirmation experiments. MB, HJ, RN, SP, and C-HS performed the plasma preparation, the array development, the array incubation and scanning. BV and LAF performed the GWAS analysis. R-PH and RH made substantial contributions to conception and design, and provided reagents for the array development. BFB, ALB, NF, NRG-R, AK, DSK, RCP, RR, SGY, EH, and BLM collected plasma samples for this study and provided pathological and neurological diagnostic expertise. EH and EM provided fresh brain tissue for GDF WB experiments and diagnosed the samples pathology. MH performed the semantic similarity analysis. AL and AP performed the mRNA expression analysis. PAJ, MB, and TWC conceived the experiments. PAJ, TI, and TWC wrote the manuscript. All authors read, revised critically for important intellectual content and approved the final version of the manuscript.

Acknowledgments

This work was supported by National Institutes of Health (NIH) grants R01AG045034 (TW-C), R01GM084279 (TI), P01HG005062 (TI), P30MH062261 (TI), P41GM103504 (TI), P50AG016574 (Mayo Clinic ADRC), U01AG006786 (BFB, DSK, RCP), R01AG038791 (ALB), P50AG023501 (BLM), P01AG019724 (BLM), P01AG16573 (EH), AG5131/AG/NIA (EM), AG18440/AG/NIA (EM) The Consortium for Frontotemporal Dementia (TW-C), Anonymous (TW-C), The Veterans Administration (TW-C), Tau Research Consortium (ALB), Alzheimer's Drug Discovery Foundation (ALB), Bluefield Project (ALB). This research was conducted partially, while PAJ was an Ellison Medical Foundation/AFAR Postdoctoral Fellow. The funders had no role in study design, data collection and analysis, decision to publish, or preparation of the manuscript. This study's contents are solely the responsibility of the authors and do not necessarily represent the official views of the National Institute on Aging or NIH. Guangdong Innovative Research Team Program (201001s0104659419) (RPH).

Author details

[1]Department of Neurology and Neurological Sciences, Stanford University School of Medicine, Stanford, CA, USA. [2]Institute of Chemistry and Biochemistry, Free University Berlin, Berlin, Germany. [3]Departments of Bioengineering and Medicine, University of California San Diego, La Jolla, CA, USA. [4]Department of Medicine (Biomedical Genetics), Boston University Schools of Medicine, Boston, MA, USA. [5]RayBiotech, Guangzhou, China. [6]RayBiotech, Norcrosse, GA, USA. [7]Department of Neurology, Mayo Clinic, Rochester, MN, USA. [8]Department of Neurology, University of California San Francisco, San Francisco, CA, USA. [9]Departments of Neurology, Ophthalmology, Genetics and Genomics, Epidemiology, and Biostatistics, Boston University Schools of Medicine and Public Health, Boston, MA, USA. [10]Department of Neuroscience, Mayo Clinic, Jacksonville, FL, USA. [11]Department of Neurology, Mayo Clinic, Jacksonville, FL, USA. [12]Departments of Pharmacology and Nutritional Sciences and Sanders-Brown Center on Aging, University of Kentucky, Lexington, KY, USA. [13]Department of Computer Science and Engineering, University of California San Diego, La Jolla, CA, USA. [14]Genetics and Pharmacogenomics, Merck Research Laboratories, West Point, PA, USA. [15]Department of Pathology, University of California San Diego, La Jolla, CA, USA. [16]Center for Tissue Regeneration, Repair and Restoration, VA Palo Alto Health Care System, Palo Alto, CA, USA. [17]Present address: Biology Department, Eastern Connecticut State University, Willimantic, CT, USA. [18]Present address: Roche Pharma Research and Early Development, NORD DTA, Roche Innovation, Center Basel, Basel, Switzerland.

References

1. Rifai N, Gillette MA, Carr SA. Protein biomarker discovery and validation: the long and uncertain path to clinical utility. Nat Biotechnol. 2006;24:971–83.
2. Mallick P, Kuster B. Proteomics: a pragmatic perspective. Nat Biotechnol. 2010;28:695–709.
3. Kiddle SJ, Sattlecker M, Proitsi P, Simmons A, Westman E, Bazenet C, Nelson SK, Williams S, Hodges A, Johnston C, Soininen H, Kłoszewska I, Mecocci P, Tsolaki M, Vellas B, Newhouse S, Lovestone S, Dobson RJB. Candidate blood proteome markers of Alzheimer's disease onset and progression: a systematic review and replication study. J Alzheimers Dis. 2014;38:515–31.
4. Jaeger PA, Villeda SA, Berdnik D, Britschgi M, Wyss-Coray T. Focused plasma proteomics for the study of brain aging and neurodegeneration. In: Coppola G, editor. The OMICS: Applications in Neuroscience. New York: Oxford Univ. Press; 2014. p. 183–91.
5. Snowden J, Neary D, Mann D. Frontotemporal lobar degeneration: clinical and pathological relationships. Acta Neuropathol. 2007;114:31–8.
6. Hodges JR, Mitchell J, Dawson K, Spillantini MG, Xuereb JH, McMonagle P, Nestor PJ, Patterson K. Semantic dementia: demography, familial factors and survival in a consecutive series of 100 cases. Brain. 2010;133:300–6.
7. Miller ZA, Rankin KP, Graff-Radford NR, Takada LT, Sturm VE, Cleveland CM, Criswell LA, Jaeger PA, Stan T, Heggeli KA, Hsu SC, Karydas A, Khan BK, Grinberg LT, Gorno-Tempini M-L, Boxer AL, Rosen HJ, Kramer JH, Coppola G, Geschwind DH, Rademakers R, Seeley WW, Wyss-Coray T, Miller BL. TDP-43 frontotemporal lobar degeneration and autoimmune disease. J Neurol Neurosurg Psychiatr. 2013;84:956–62.
8. La Joie R, Landeau B, Perrotin A, Bejanin A, Egret S, Pélerin A, Mézenge F, Belliard S, de La Sayette V, Eustache F, Desgranges B, Chételat G. Intrinsic connectivity identifies the hippocampus as a main crossroad between Alzheimer'sand semantic dementia-targeted networks. Neuron. 2014;81:1417–28.
9. Jaeger PA. Cytokine and Leukocyte Profiling Reveal Pro-Inflammatory and Autoimmune Features in Frontotemporal Dementia Patients. http://dx.doi.org/10.1101/049791.
10. Folstein MF, Folstein SE, McHugh PR. "Mini-mental state." A practical method for grading the cognitive state of patients for the clinician. J Psychiatr Res. 1975;12:189–98.
11. de La Fuente A. From 'differential expression' to 'differential networking' – identification of dysfunctional regulatory networks in diseases. Trends Genet. 2010;26:326–33.
12. Eisen MB, Spellman PT, Brown PO, Botstein D. Cluster analysis and display of genome-wide expression patterns. Proc Natl Acad Sci U S A. 1998;95:14863–8.
13. Huang DW, Sherman BT, Lempicki RA. Systematic and integrative analysis of large gene lists using DAVID bioinformatics resources. Nat Protoc. 2009;4:44–57.
14. Huang DW, Sherman BT, Lempicki RA. Bioinformatics enrichment tools: paths toward the comprehensive functional analysis of large gene lists. Nucleic Acids Res. 2009;37:1–13.
15. Lewis RD, Perry MJ, Guschina IA, Jackson CL, Morgan BP, Hughes TR. CD55 deficiency protects against atherosclerosis in ApoE-deficient mice via C3a modulation of lipid metabolism. Am J Pathol. 2011;179:1601–7.
16. Wada H, Ura S, Kitaoka S, Satoh-Asahara N, Horie T, Ono K, Takaya T, Takanabe-Mori R, Akao M, Abe M, Morimoto T, Murayama T, Yokode M, Fujita M, Shimatsu A, Hasegawa K. Distinct characteristics of circulating vascular endothelial growth factor-a and C levels in human subjects. PLoS ONE. 2011;6, e29351.
17. Eickelberg O, Pansky A, Koehler E, Bihl M, Tamm M, Hildebrand P, Perruchoud AP, Kashgarian M, Roth M. Molecular mechanisms of TGF-(beta) antagonism by interferon (gamma) and cyclosporine A in lung fibroblasts. FASEB J. 2001;15:797–806.

18. Strickertsson JAB, Døssing KBV, Aabakke AJM, Nilsson H-O, Hansen TVO, Knigge U, Kjær A, Wadström T, Friis-Hansen L. Interferon-γ inhibits ghrelin expression and secretion via a somatostatin-mediated mechanism. World J Gastroenterol. 2011;17:3117–25.
19. Shibanuma M, Mashimo J, Mita A, Kuroki T, Nose K. Cloning from a mouse osteoblastic cell line of a set of transforming-growth-factor-beta 1-regulated genes, one of which seems to encode a follistatin-related polypeptide. Eur J Biochem. 1993;217:13–9.
20. Britschgi M, Rufibach K, Huang SLB, Clark CM, Kaye JA, Li G, Peskind ER, Quinn JF, Galasko DR, Wyss-Coray T. Modeling of pathological traits in Alzheimer's disease based on systemic extracellular signaling proteome. Mol Cell Proteomics. 2011;10:M111. 008862.
21. Ray S, Britschgi M, Herbert C, Takeda-Uchimura Y, Boxer A, Blennow K, Friedman LF, Galasko DR, Jutel M, Karydas A, Kaye JA, Leszek J, Miller BL, Minthon L, Quinn JF, Rabinovici GD, Robinson WH, Sabbagh MN, So YT, Sparks DL, Tabaton M, Tinklenberg J, Yesavage JA, Tibshirani R, Wyss-Coray T. Classification and prediction of clinical Alzheimer's diagnosis based on plasma signaling proteins. Nat Med. 2007;13:1359–62.
22. Zhang B, Gaiteri C, Bodea L-G, Wang Z, McElwee J, Podtelezhnikov AA, Zhang C, Xie T, Tran L, Dobrin R, Fluder E, Clurman B, Melquist S, Narayanan M, Suver C, Shah H, Mahajan M, Gillis T, Mysore J, MacDonald ME, Lamb JR, Bennett DA, Molony C, Stone DJ, Gudnason V, Myers AJ, Schadt EE, Neumann H, Zhu J, Emilsson V. Integrated systems approach identifies genetic nodes and networks in late-onset Alzheimer's disease. Cell. 2013; 153:707–20.
23. Naj AC, Jun G, Beecham GW, Wang L-S, Vardarajan BN, Buros J, Gallins PJ, Buxbaum JD, Jarvik GP, Crane PK, Larson EB, Bird TD, Boeve BF, Graff-Radford NR, De Jager PL, Evans D, Schneider JA, Carrasquillo MM, Ertekin-Taner N, Younkin SG, Cruchaga C, Kauwe JSK, Nowotny P, Kramer P, Hardy J, Huentelman MJ, Myers AJ, Barmada MM, Demirci FY, Baldwin CT, et al. Common variants at MS4A4/MS4A6E, CD2AP, CD33 and EPHA1 are associated with late-onset Alzheimer's disease. Nat Genet. 2011.
24. Podtelezhnikov AA, Tanis KQ, Nebozhyn M, Ray WJ, Stone DJ, Loboda AP. Molecular insights into the pathogenesis of Alzheimer's disease and its relationship to normal aging. PLoS ONE. 2011;6, e29610.
25. Wyss-Coray T, Lin C, Yan F, Yu GQ, Rohde M, McConlogue L, Masliah E, Mucke L. TGF-beta1 promotes microglial amyloid-beta clearance and reduces plaque burden in transgenic mice. Nat Med. 2001;7:612–8.
26. Town T, Laouar Y, Pittenger C, Mori T, Szekely CA, Tan J, Duman RS, Flavell RA. Blocking TGF-β–Smad2/3 innate immune signaling mitigates Alzheimer-like pathology. Nat Med. 2008.
27. Burke RM, Norman TA, Haydar TF, Slack BE, Leeman SE, Blusztajn JK, Mellott TJ. BMP9 ameliorates amyloidosis and the cholinergic defect in a mouse model of Alzheimer's disease. Proc Natl Acad Sci U S A. 2013;110:19567–72.
28. Hexige S, Guo J, Ma L, Sun Y, Liu X, Ma L, Yan X, Li Z, Yu L. Expression pattern of growth/differentiation factor 3 in human and murine cerebral cortex, hippocampus as well as cerebellum. Neurosci Lett. 2005;389:83–7.
29. Levine AJ, Brivanlou AH. GDF3, a BMP inhibitor, regulates cell fate in stem cells and early embryos. Development. 2006;133:209–16.
30. Levine AJ, Brivanlou AH. GDF3 at the crossroads of TGF-beta signaling. Cell Cycle. 2006;5:1069–73.
31. Tykwinska K, Lauster R, Knaus P, Rosowski M. Growth and differentiation factor 3 induces expression of genes related to differentiation in a model of cancer stem cells and protects them from retinoic acid-induced apoptosis. PLoS ONE. 2013;8, e70612.
32. Calloni R, Cordero EAA, Henriques JAP, Bonatto D. Reviewing and updating the major molecular markers for stem cells. Stem Cells Dev. 2013;22:1455–76.
33. Li Q, Liu X, Wu Y, An J, Hexige S, Ling Y, Zhang M, Yang X, Yu L. The conditioned medium from a stable human GDF3-expressing CHO cell line, induces the differentiation of PC12 cells. Mol Cell Biochem. 2011;359:115–23.
34. Villeda SA, Luo J, Mosher KI, Zou B, Britschgi M, Bieri G, Stan TM, Fainberg N, Ding Z, Eggel A, Lucin KM, Czirr E, Park J-S, Couillard-Després S, Aigner L, Li G, Peskind ER, Kaye JA, Quinn JF, Galasko DR, Xie XS, Rando TA, Wyss-Coray T. The ageing systemic milieu negatively regulates neurogenesis and cognitive function. Nature. 2011;477:90–4.
35. Lu T, Aron L, Zullo J, Pan Y, Kim H, Chen Y, Yang T-H, Kim H-M, Drake D, Liu XS, Bennett DA, Colaiácovo MP, Yankner BA. REST and stress resistance in ageing and Alzheimer's disease. Nature. 2014;507:448–54.
36. Kidder BL, Yang J, Palmer S. Stat3 and c-Myc genome-wide promoter occupancy in embryonic stem cells. PLoS ONE. 2008;3, e3932.
37. Spalding KL, Bergmann O, Alkass K, Bernard S, Salehpour M, Huttner HB, Boström E, Westerlund I, Vial C, Buchholz BA, Possnert G, Mash DC, Druid H, Frisén J. Dynamics of hippocampal neurogenesis in adult humans. Cell. 2013;153:1219–27.
38. Tsai K-J, Tsai Y-C, Shen C-KJ. G-CSF rescues the memory impairment of animal models of Alzheimer's disease. J Exp Med. 2007;204:1273–80.
39. Ma Q-H, Futagawa T, Yang W-L, Jiang X-D, Zeng L, Takeda Y, Xu R-X, Bagnard D, Schachner M, Furley AJ, Karagogeos D, Watanabe K, Dawe GS, Xiao Z-C. A TAG1-APP signalling pathway through Fe65 negatively modulates neurogenesis. Nat Cell Biol. 2008;10:283–94.
40. Sattlecker M, Kiddle SJ, Newhouse S, Proitsi P, Nelson S, Williams S, Johnston C, Killick R, Simmons A, Westman E, Hodges A, Soininen H, Kłoszewska I, Mecocci P, Tsolaki M, Vellas B, Lovestone S, Dobson RJB, Consortium TA. Alzheimer's disease biomarker discovery using SOMAscan multiplexed protein technology. Alzheimers Dement. 2014;10:724–34.
41. Zhao X, Lejnine S, Spond J, Zhang C, Ramaraj TC, Holder DJ, Dai H, Weiner R, Laterza OF. A candidate plasma protein classifier to identify Alzheimer's disease. J Alzheimers Dis. 2015;43:549–63.
42. Wang J, Li M, Deng Y, Pan Y. Recent advances in clustering methods for protein interaction networks. BMC Genomics. 2010;11:S10.
43. Dalton L, Ballarin V, Brun M. Clustering algorithms: on learning, validation, performance, and applications to genomics. Curr Genomics. 2009;10:430–45.
44. Schnoes AM, Ream DC, Thorman AW, Babbitt PC, Friedberg I. Biases in the experimental annotations of protein function and their effect on Our understanding of protein function space. PLoS Comput Biol. 2013;9, e1003063.
45. Dutkowski J, Ono K, Kramer M, Yu M, Pratt D, Demchak B, Ideker T. NeXO Web: the NeXO ontology database and visualization platform. Nucleic Acids Res. 2013;42:D1269–74.
46. Kramer M, Dutkowski J, Yu M, Bafna V, Ideker T. Inferring gene ontologies from pairwise similarity data. Bioinformatics. 2014;30:i34–42.
47. O'Bryant SE, Xiao G, Barber R, Reisch J, Doody R, Fairchild T, Adams P, Waring S, Diaz-Arrastia R, for the Texas Alzheimer's Research Consortium. A serum protein-based algorithm for the detection of Alzheimer disease. Arch Neurol. 2010;67:1077–81.
48. Hu WT, Chen-Plotkin A, Arnold SE, Grossman M, Clark CM, Shaw LM, Mccluskey L, Elman L, Karlawish J, Hurtig HI, Siderowf A, Lee VM-Y, Soares H, Trojanowski JQ. Biomarker discovery for Alzheimer"s disease, frontotemporal lobar degeneration, and Parkinson"s disease. Acta Neuropathol. 2010;120:385–99.
49. Craig-Schapiro R, Kuhn M, Xiong C, Pickering EH, Liu J, Misko TP, Perrin RJ, Bales KR, Soares H, Fagan AM. Multiplexed immunoassay panel identifies novel CSF biomarkers for Alzheimer's disease diagnosis and prognosis. PLoS ONE. 2011;6, e18850.
50. Soares HD, Potter WZ, Pickering E, Kuhn M, Immermann FW, Shera DM, Ferm M, Dean RA, Simon AJ, Swenson F, Siuciak JA, Kaplow J, Thambisetty M, Zagouras P, Koroshetz WJ, Wan HI, Trojanowski JQ, Shaw LM, Biomarkers Consortium Alzheimer's Disease Plasma Proteomics Project. Plasma biomarkers associated with the apolipoprotein E genotype and Alzheimer disease. Arch Neurol. 2012;69:1310–7.
51. Ringman JM, Elashoff D, Geschwind DH, Welsh BT, Gylys KH, Lee C, Cummings JL, Cole GM. Plasma signaling proteins in persons at genetic risk for Alzheimer disease: influence of APOE genotype. Arch Neurol. 2012;69:757–64.
52. Doecke JD, Laws SM, Faux NG, Wilson W, Burnham SC, Lam C-P, Mondal A, Bedo J, Bush AI, Brown B, De Ruyck K, Ellis KA, Fowler C, Gupta VB, Head R, Macaulay SL, Pertile K, Rowe CC, Rembach A, Rodrigues M, Rumble R, Szoeke C, Taddei K, Taddei T, Trounson B, Ames D, Masters CL, Martins RN, Alzheimer's Disease Neuroimaging Initiative, Australian Imaging Biomarker and Lifestyle Research Group. Blood-based protein biomarkers for diagnosis of Alzheimer disease. Arch Neurol. 2012;69:1318–25.
53. Hu WT, Holtzman DM, Fagan AM, Shaw LM, Perrin R, Arnold SE, Grossman M, Xiong C, Craig-Schapiro R, Clark CM, Pickering E, Kuhn M, Chen Y, Van Deerlin VM, Mccluskey L, Elman L, Karlawish J, Chen-Plotkin A, Hurtig HI, Siderowf A, Swenson F, Lee VM-Y, Morris JC, Trojanowski JQ, Soares H, Initi ADN. Plasma multianalyte profiling in mild cognitive impairment and Alzheimer disease. Neurology. 2012;79:897–905.
54. Leung V, Gillis J, Raboud J, Cooper C, Hogg RS, Loutfy MR, Machouf N, Montaner JSG, Rourke SB, Tsoukas C, Klein MB, CANOC Collaboration. Predictors of CD4:CD8 ratio normalization and its effect on health outcomes in the era of combination antiretroviral therapy. PLoS ONE. 2013;8:e77665.
55. Llano DA, Devanarayan V, Simon AJ, ADNI. Evaluation of plasma proteomic data for Alzheimer disease state classification and for the prediction of progression from mild cognitive impairment to Alzheimer disease. Alzheimer Dis Assoc Disord. 2013;27:233–43.

56. Guo L-H, Alexopoulos P, Wagenpfeil S, Kurz A, Perneczky R, Neuroimaging AD. Plasma proteomics for the identification of Alzheimer disease. Alzheimer Dis Assoc Disord. 2013;27:337–42.
57. Burnham SC, Faux NG, Wilson W, Laws SM, Ames D, Bedo J, Bush AI, Doecke JD, Ellis KA, Head R, Jones G, Kiiveri H, Martins RN, Rembach A, Rowe CC, Salvado O, Macaulay SL, Masters CL, Villemagne VL, Initiative ARSDN, Australian Imaging BALSRG. A blood-based predictor for neocortical Ab burden in Alzheimer's disease: results from the AIBL study. Mol Psychiatry. 2013;19:519–26.
58. Delaby C, Gabelle A, Blum D, Schraen-Maschke S, Moulinier A, Boulanghien J, Séverac D, Buée L, Rème T, Lehmann S. Central nervous system and peripheral inflammatory processes in Alzheimer's disease: biomarker profiling approach. Front Neurol. 2015;6:103.
59. Lehallier B, Essioux L, Gayan J, Alexandridis R, Nikolcheva T, Wyss-Coray T, Britschgi M, for the Alzheimer's Disease Neuroimaging Initiative. Combined plasma and cerebrospinal fluid signature for the prediction of midterm progression from mild cognitive impairment to Alzheimer disease. JAMA Neurol. 2015;1.
60. Chiam JTW, Dobson RJB, Kiddle SJ, Sattlecker M. Are blood-based protein biomarkers for Alzheimer's disease also involved in other brain disorders? A systematic review. J Alzheimers Dis. 2015;43:303–14.
61. McKhann GM, Knopman DS, Chertkow H, Hyman BT, Jack Jr CR, Kawas CH, Klunk WE, Koroshetz WJ, Manly JJ, Mayeux R, Mohs RC, Morris JC, Rossor MN, Scheltens P, Carillo MC, Thies B, Weintraub S, Phelps CH. The diagnosis of dementia due to Alzheimer's disease: recommendations from the national institute on aging and the Alzheimer's association workgroup. Alzheimers Dement. 2011;1–7.
62. Gorno-Tempini ML, Hillis AE, Weintraub S, Kertesz A, Mendez M, Cappa SF, Ogar JM, Rohrer JD, Black S, Boeve BF, Manes F, Dronkers NF, Vandenberghe R, Rascovsky K, Patterson K, Miller BL, Knopman DS, Hodges JR, Mesulam MM, Grossman M. Classification of primary progressive aphasia and its variants. Neurology. 2011;76:1006–14.
63. Eisen M, de Hoon M. Cluster 3.0 Manual. 2002. p. 1–34.
64. Storey JD. A direct approach to false discovery rates - Storey - 2002 - Journal of the Royal Statistical Society: Series B. J R Stat Soc Ser B. 2002;64:479–98.
65. Montojo J, Zuberi K, Rodriguez H, Kazi F, Wright G, Donaldson SL, Morris Q, Bader GD. GeneMANIA Cytoscape plugin: fast gene function predictions on the desktop. Bioinformatics. 2010;26:2927–8.
66. Shannon P, Markiel A, Ozier O, Baliga NS, Wang JT, Ramage D, Amin N, Schwikowski B, Ideker T. Cytoscape: a software environment for integrated models of biomolecular interaction networks. Genome Res. 2003;13:2498–504.
67. Schaefer CF, Anthony K, Krupa S, Buchoff J, Day M, Hannay T, Buetow KH. PID: the Pathway Interaction Database. Nucleic Acids Res. 2009;37(Database):D674–9.
68. Croft D, O'Kelly G, Wu G, Haw R, Gillespie M, Matthews L, Caudy M, Garapati P, Gopinath G, Jassal B, Jupe S, Kalatskaya I, Mahajan S, May B, Ndegwa N, Schmidt E, Shamovsky V, Yung C, Birney E, Hermjakob H, D'Eustachio P, Stein L. Reactome: a database of reactions, pathways and biological processes. Nucleic Acids Res. 2010;39(Database):D691–7.
69. Joshi-Tope G. Reactome: a knowledgebase of biological pathways. Nucleic Acids Res. 2004;33(Database issue):D428–32.
70. Croft D, Mundo AF, Haw R, Milacic M, Weiser J, Wu G, Caudy M, Garapati P, Gillespie M, Kamdar MR, Jassal B, Jupe S, Matthews L, May B, Palatnik S, Rothfels K, Shamovsky V, Song H, Williams M, Birney E, Hermjakob H, Stein L, D'Eustachio P. The reactome pathway knowledgebase. Nucleic Acids Res. 2013;42:D472–7.
71. Wu G, Feng X, Stein L. A human functional protein interaction network and its application to cancer data analysis. Genome Biol. 2010;11:R53.
72. Chatr-aryamontri A, Breitkreutz BJ, Oughtred R, Boucher L, Heinicke S, Chen D, Stark C, Breitkreutz A, Kolas N, O'Donnell L, Reguly T, Nixon J, Ramage L, Winter A, Sellam A, Chang C, Hirschman J, Theesfeld C, Rust J, Livstone MS, Dolinski K, Tyers M. The BioGRID interaction database: 2015 update. Nucleic Acids Res. 2015;43:D470–8.
73. Turner B, Razick S, Turinsky AL, Vlasblom J, Crowdy EK, Cho E, Morrison K, Donaldson IM, Wodak SJ. iRefWeb: interactive analysis of consolidated protein interaction data and their supporting evidence. Database. 2010; 2010:baq023–3.
74. Ashburner M, Ball CA, Blake JA, Botstein D, Butler H, Cherry JM, Davis AP, Dolinski K, Dwight SS, Eppig JT, Harris MA, Hill DP, Issel-Tarver L, Kasarskis A, Lewis S, Matese JC, Richardson JE, Ringwald M, Rubin GM, Sherlock G, Consortium GO. Gene ontology: tool for the unification of biology. Nat Genet. 2000;25:25–9.
75. The Gene Ontology Consortium. Gene ontology consortium: going forward. Nucleic Acids Res. 2015;43:D1049–56.
76. Kanehisa M, Goto S. KEGG: Kyoto encyclopedia of genes and genomes. Nucleic Acids Res. 2000;28:27–30.
77. Mi H, Muruganujan A, Casagrande JT, Thomas PD. Large-scale gene function analysis with the PANTHER classification system. Nat Protoc. 2013;8:1551–66.
78. Ideker T, Krogan NJ. Differential network biology. Mol Syst Biol. 2012;8:565.
79. Yu G, Li F, Qin Y, Bo X, Wu Y, Wang S. GOSemSim: an R package for measuring semantic similarity among GO terms and gene products. Bioinformatics. 2010;26:976–8.
80. Halekoh U, Højsgaard S. The R package geepack for generalized estimating equations. J Stat Softw. 2006.
81. Chen M-H, Yang Q. GWAF: an R package for genome-wide association analyses with family data. Bioinformatics. 2010;26:580–1.
82. Willer CJ, Li Y, Abecasis GR. METAL: fast and efficient meta-analysis of genomewide association scans. Bioinformatics. 2010;26:2190–1.
83. Li J, Ji L. Adjusting multiple testing in multilocus analyses using the eigenvalues of a correlation matrix. Heredity (Edinb). 2005;95:221–7.
84. Liu JZ, McRae AF, Nyholt DR, Medland SE, Wray NR, Brown KM, AMFS Investigators, Hayward NK, Montgomery GW, Visscher PM, Martin NG, Macgregor S. A versatile gene-based test for genome-wide association studies. Am J Hum Genet. 2010;87:139–45.
85. Babu H, Claasen J-H, Kannan S, Rünker AE, Palmer T, Kempermann G. A protocol for isolation and enriched monolayer cultivation of neural precursor cells from mouse dentate gyrus. Front Neurosci. 2011;5.
86. Gurok U, Steinhoff C, Lipkowitz B, Ropers H-H, Scharff C, Nuber UA. Gene expression changes in the course of neural progenitor cell differentiation. J Neurosci. 2004;24:5982–6002.
87. Castaño Z, Kypta RM. Housekeeping proteins: limitations as references during neuronal differentiation. Open Neurosci J. 2008;2.

Alzheimer's disease-like APP processing in wild-type mice identifies synaptic defects as initial steps of disease progression

Mickael Audrain[1,2,3], Romain Fol[1,2,3], Patrick Dutar[4†], Brigitte Potier[4†], Jean-Marie Billard[4†], Julien Flament[3,5], Sandro Alves[1,3], Marie-Anne Burlot[1,2,3], Gaelle Dufayet-Chaffaud[1,3], Alexis-Pierre Bemelmans[3,6], Julien Valette[3,6], Philippe Hantraye[3,5,6], Nicole Déglon[7,8], Nathalie Cartier[1,3*] and Jérome Braudeau[1,3]

Abstract

Background: Alzheimer's disease (AD) is the most frequent form of dementia in the elderly and no effective treatment is currently available. The mechanisms triggering AD onset and progression are still imperfectly dissected. We aimed at deciphering the modifications occurring *in vivo* during the very early stages of AD, before the development of amyloid deposits, neurofibrillary tangles, neuronal death and inflammation. Most current AD models based on Amyloid Precursor Protein (APP) overproduction beginning from *in utero*, to rapidly reproduce the histological and behavioral features of the disease within a few months, are not appropriate to study the early steps of AD development. As a means to mimic *in vivo* amyloid APP processing closer to the human situation in AD, we used an adeno-associated virus (AAV)-based transfer of human mutant APP and Presenilin 1 (PS1) genes to the hippocampi of two-month-old C57Bl/6 J mice to express human APP, without significant overexpression and to specifically induce its amyloid processing.

Results: The human APP, βCTF and Aβ42/40 ratio were similar to those in hippocampal tissues from AD patients. Three months after injection the murine Tau protein was hyperphosphorylated and rapid synaptic failure occurred characterized by decreased levels of both PSD-95 and metabolites related to neuromodulation, on proton magnetic resonance spectroscopy (^{1}H-MRS). Astrocytic GLT-1 transporter levels were lower and the tonic glutamatergic current was stronger on electrophysiological recordings of CA1 hippocampal region, revealing the overstimulation of extrasynaptic N-methyl D-aspartate receptor (NMDAR) which precedes the loss of long-term potentiation (LTP). These modifications were associated with early behavioral impairments in the Open-field, Y-maze and Morris Mater Maze tasks.

Conclusions: Altogether, this demonstrates that an AD-like APP processing, yielding to levels of APP, βCTF and Aβ42/Aβ40 ratio similar to those observed in AD patients, are sufficient to rapidly trigger early steps of the amyloidogenic and Tau pathways *in vivo*. With this strategy, we identified a sequence of early events likely to account for disease onset and described a model that may facilitate efforts to decipher the factors triggering AD and to evaluate early neuroprotective strategies.

Keywords: Alzheimer's disease early stages, Aβ ratio, Human samples, Animal model, Extrasynaptic NMDAR, Synaptic failure

* Correspondence: nathalie.cartier@inserm.fr
Nathalie Cartier and Jérome Braudeau indicates joint last authors.
[†]Equal contributors
[1]INSERM UMR1169, Université Paris-Sud, Université Paris-Saclay, Orsay 94100, France
[3]CEA, DSV, I2BM, MIRCen, Fontenay-aux-Roses 92265, France
Full list of author information is available at the end of the article

Background

Alzheimer's disease (AD) is characterized by amyloid deposits, intracellular neurofibrillary tangles, neuronal loss and a progressive decline in cognitive function [1, 2]. Much progress has been made towards understanding the physiopathology of the disease, mostly through studies of transgenic mice designed to reproduce, as closely as possible, the histological and behavioral features of AD [3, 4].

AD is multifactorial, but the abnormal processing of Amyloid Precursor Protein (APP) is a key element in its development [5]. The physiological functions of APP are unclear, but it has been shown to play crucial roles in spine density, morphology and plasticity [6]. The injection of anti-APP antibodies into the rat brain is known to induce behavioral impairments [7, 8]. Furthermore, APP knockout mice have very low levels of dendritic complexity [9]. Altogether, this suggests that APP has an important physiological role associated with synaptic plasticity as well as trophic properties. Overexpression of wild-type (WT) APP and various mutant forms has been used as a means to model AD in many transgenic mouse lines [10, 11]. In most of these transgenic strains, the significant increase in APP production beginning *in utero* may trigger consequences that are not likely mimicking the biochemical deficit observed in AD. Interestingly, Saito and coworkers recently described a new APP knock-in model without APP overproduction [12]. This model reproduces the cognitive deficits and amyloid plaques of AD, but unfortunately does not provide information about changes occurring early in the development of the pathology.

If the role of amyloid component is crucial, the role of amyloid plaque deposition in disease development is currently a matter of debate [13]. The presence of plaques is a diagnostic criterion for AD, but several studies have suggested that the accumulation of amyloid deposits may have a protective function [14]. Moreover, an absence of plaque has been reported in patients with familial AD and mutant forms of APP [15], whereas abundant Aβ plaques have been found in brain samples from elderly patients without clinical dementia [16–19]. Plaques appear many years after disease onset and they cannot, therefore, be responsible for the early events in AD development [20]. By contrast, soluble Aβ may play an important role in the synaptic and cognitive impairments observed in the early stages of AD [21]. The use of transgenic models displaying higher levels of APP and cleavage products compared to the human situation and inducing artificial phenotypes in few months is therefore likely to be inappropriate for studies of the initial phases of AD. The levels of Aβ produced in these models are much higher than those observed in patients and may have toxic effects unrelated to the early phases of AD. In addition, the negative outcomes of recent clinical trials have fueled debate about the validity of overexpression models. Indeed, most of the therapeutic strategies previously tried and largely unsuccessful, have been tested in such transgenic models. There is a growing body of evidence suggesting that amyloid plaques and tangles occur late in disease progression. Therefore, the development of pertinent protective or disease-modifying therapeutic strategies based on the decrease of these markers does not seem to fit well [22, 23]. These compelling observations demonstrate the need to develop new alternative models of AD more closely mimicking the human disease and in particular the early events in its development.

The present study is an attempt at developing such an alternative model involving the production, *in vivo,* in the mouse hippocampus, of moderate levels of amyloid derivatives, resembling as closely as possible the pattern of expression observed in the hippocampus of human AD patients to study the consequences of initial amyloid pathway engagement. We used this modelling strategy to analyze the events potentially contributing to AD development before the appearance of late hallmarks of the disease, such as amyloid deposits, neurofibrillary tangles and neuronal death. The injection of AAV vectors carrying mutated forms of human APP and PS1 into the mouse hippocampus led to the stable production [24, 25] of APP, βCTF and Aβ peptides, at levels similar to those observed in the hippocampus from AD patients and significantly lower than those present in the hippocampus of APP/PS1ΔE9 transgenic mice. The data generated demonstrate the importance of the Aβ42/Aβ40 ratio, which has already been identified as a relevant biomarker in AD patients [26], together with early changes in synaptic functions, Tau phosphorylation and cognitive deficits. These modifications were observed in the absence of plaque formation, or any sign of inflammation, atrophy and/or neuronal death. They were nevertheless capable of inducing cellular changes, such as the abnormal activation of extrasynaptic NMDARs and a decrease in the levels of neuromodulation-associated metabolites, causing memory impairment. These results suggest that APP processing in a limited number of neurons, as recently observed in sporadic forms of AD [27], may be sufficient to trigger an impairment of hippocampal-dependent behavior.

Results

Injections of the AAV-APP and AAV-PS1 vectors lead to APP and PS1 transgenes expression in the hippocampus of wild-type mice, from one month after injection

We generated AAV vectors encoding human mutant full-length PS1M146L and human mutant APPSL. These vectors were injected bilaterally into the stratum lacunosum of the hippocampus of eight-week-old C57BL/6 J mice. We used the AAVrh.10 capsid, which is known to transduce the central nervous system and the hippocampus efficiently [28]. We studied four groups of animals: non-injected wild-type mice (non-injected WT mice), mice receiving the AAV-CAG-PS1M146L vector (AAV-PS1 mice), mice receiving the AAV-CAG-APPSL vector (AAV-APP mice) and mice receiving a co-injection of both vectors (AAV-APP/PS1 mice, Fig. 1a). To monitor vector-mediated APP and PS1 expression, mice were killed one month after injection. Western blot analysis of whole hippocampus revealed comparable full-length PS1 (PS1 FL) expression in the four groups, despite a trend to increase in AAV-PS1 and AVV-APP/PS1 mice (Fig. 1b and c). Interestingly, 30 kDa PS1 N-terminal fragment (PS1 NTF) was mainly detectable in AAV-PS1 and AAV-APP/PS1 hippocampi (Fig. 1b and d). This PS1 NTF production confirms the endoproteolysis of exogenous PS1 FL which is essential for the formation of the PS1 active site responsible for the formation the Aβ species [29]. AAV-APP and AAV-APP/PS1 mice showed exogenous human APP expression with higher amount in the AAV-APP mice hippocampi (6E10 antibody, Fig. 1b and e). By contrast, the total amount of APP (exogenous human + endogenous murine forms, APP C-ter antibody) did not differ significantly between non-injected WT, AAV-PS1 and AAV-APP/PS1 mice (Fig. 1b and f). Immunohistochemical analyses of hippocampal sections using an APP C-ter antibody revealed a noticeable overexpression of APP only in the AAV-APP mice and observed in the CA2 layer and in the subiculum subfield of the hippocampus (Fig. 1g). Consistent with the result on total APP expression (see Fig. 1f), the human APP expression in the AAV-APP/PS1 group (see Fig. 1e) was not sufficient to be detected by immunohistochemistry. Double-immunostaining with the NeuN antibody confirmed that essentially neurons were transduced by the vectors. No transduction of astrocytes or microglia was observed (data not shown). Analysis of serial anteroposterior coronal sections demonstrated widespread APP C-ter immunoreactivity in the hippocampus from -0.94 mm to -2.46 mm from the Bregma (Fig. 1h-l). Subcellular clustering of human APP was observed in transduced neurons (Fig. 1m). By contrast, staining with the 4G8 antibody, which detects both APP full length and Aβ, yielded a diffuse signal from the intracellular compartment and extracellular medium, suggesting that APP or its cleavage products like Aβ species, may diffuse out of the transduced cells into the adjacent parenchymal space (Fig. 1m).

Amyloidogenic processing of human APP in AAV-APP/PS1 mice promotes Tau phosphorylation, 3 months after injection

To confirm the production of human Aβ, we evaluated the processing of human APP in non-injected WT, AAV-PS1, AAV-APP and AAV-APP/PS1 mice three months after vector injection. βCTF, the first cleavage product of the amyloidogenic pathway [30] was quantified by ELISA (Fig. 2a). AAV-APP mice produced larger amounts of human βCTF than non-injected WT, AAV-PS1 and also AAV-APP/PS1 mice (p = 0.045). We then quantified the production of the sAPPβ fragment, which is also produced by Bace1 activity, and found a linear relationship between the levels of this fragment and βCTF production (Fig. 2b; Spearman correlation test, r^2 = 0.85, p = 0.0034). Next, we evaluated Bace1 levels and activity. We did not observe any modification between the four groups (data not shown). As observed for the human βCTF, no human Aβ42 was detected in non-injected WT and AAV-PS1 mice. Interestingly, larger amounts of Aβ42 were detected in AAV-APP/PS1 mice than in AAV-APP mice (Fig. 2c), and there was an inverse correlation between βCTF and Aβ42 levels between AAV-APP and AAV-APP/PS1 mice (Fig. 2d; Spearman correlation test, r^2 = 0.65, p = 0.03). These results suggest that, in AAV-APP/PS1 mice, human βCTF is cleaved by the exogenous PS1 to produce larger amounts of Aβ42 peptide. This production/diffusion was restricted to the hippocampus and was not observe in cortical areas (data not shown). We then investigated the ratios of the amounts of the various Aβ species. Aβ42/Aβ40 and Aβ42/Aβ38 ratios were significantly higher in AAV-APP/PS1 compared to AAV-APP mice (Fig. 2e and f; $p <$ 0.001). Despite production of both Aβ42 and Aβ40, no amyloid deposit was detected in the cortex and hippocampus of AAV-PS1, AAV-APP or AAV-APP/PS1 mice by staining with either Thioflavin S, Congo red or other amyloid antibodies (data not shown). We also carried out immunostaining for GFAP and Iba1 to analyze the potential astrocytic (GFAP) and microglial (Iba1) responses induced by amyloid APP processing. No recruitment of astrocytes or microglia, or change in cellular morphology suggestive of activation process was observed three months after injection (data not shown). We then investigated the potential impact of the amyloidogenic pathway on phosphorylation of the endogenous Tau protein. ELISA (AT270, Thr181) demonstrated significant increase in Tau phosphorylation in AAV-APP/PS1 mice three months after injection compared to non-injected WT, AAV-PS1 and AAV-APP mice (Fig. 2g; p = 0.04). By contrast, no modification of total Tau amount was observed in these four groups suggesting a modification of Tau kinase/phosphatase balance in AAV-APP/PS1 mice (Fig. 2h).

Similar levels of human APP and amyloid derivatives are observed in the hippocampus of AAV-APP/PS1 mice and AD patients

We compared the levels of APP and amyloid derivatives in non-injected WT, AAV-PS1, AAV-APP and AAV-APP/PS1 mice (3 months after injection i.e. in five-

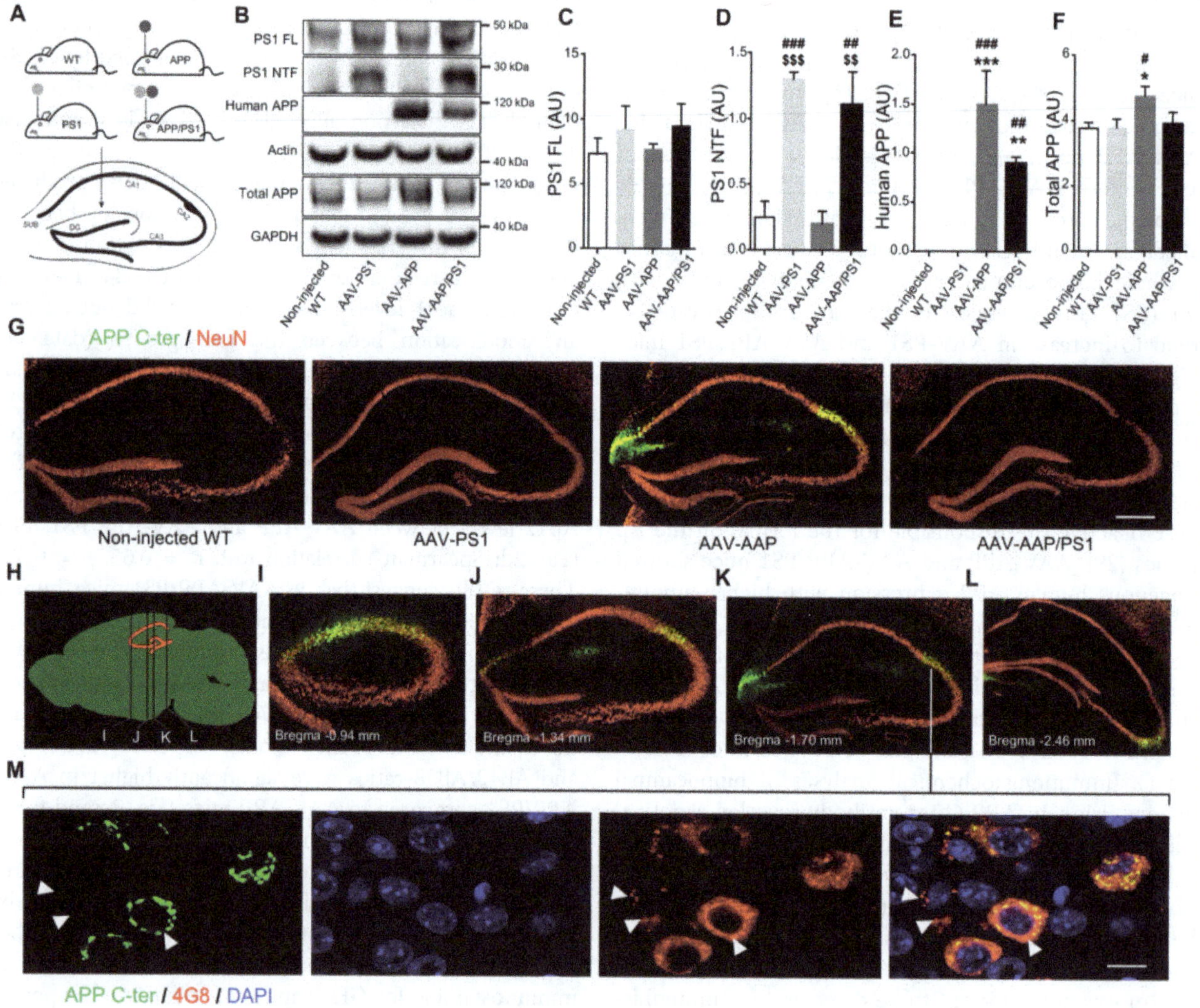

Fig. 1 Stereotactic injection of AAV vectors induces the neuronal expression of human APP and PS1 in the hippocampus of C57BL/6 J mice, 1 month after injection. C57Bl/6 J mice (all males) were injected at 8 weeks of age either with AAV-CAG-PS1M146L (AAV-PS1 mice, $n = 4$), AAV-CAG-APPSL (AAV-APP mice, $n = 4$) or both vectors at the same doses as for the other two groups (AAV-APP/PS1 mice, $n = 4$). Non-injected WT mice ($n = 4$) were also analyzed. Mice were killed one month later for analyses. **a** Upper panel: schematic representation of the four groups used. Bottom panel: coronal diagram showing the injection site and the architecture of the mouse hippocampus. **b** Representative western blots showing the expression of PS1 (full length: PS1 FL and N-terminal fragment: PS1 NTF), human APP (6E10 antibody) and total APP (murine + human forms; APP C-ter antibody) confirming transgene expression 1 month after injection. All western blots were performed on the whole hippocampus (TBS-Tx soluble fraction). **c-f** Densitometric analyses of western blots showing the expression of PS1 FL (**c**), PS1 NTF (**d**), human APP (**e**) and total APP (**f**) in the four groups hippocampi 1 month after injection. Note that despite the expression of human APP in the AAV-APP/PS1 group, no significant difference in total APP levels was found between non-injected, AAV-PS1 and AAV-APP/PS1 groups. Bars represent means ± SEM and data were normalized with respect to GAPDH. Statistical analysis was performed by one-way ANOVA followed by Tukey's post-hoc test where ###, *** and $$$ denote $p < 0.001$ versus non-injected WT mice, AAV-PS1 mice and AAV-APP mice respectively. ##, ** and $$ denote $p < 0.01$; # and * denote $p < 0.05$. **g** High magnification of a hippocampal coronal section of each group showing neuronal layers (NeuN antibody, red) and the APP expression (APP C-ter antibody, green). Note that the human APP expression in the AAV-APP/PS1 group (see Fig. 1e) is not sufficient to exceed a threshold detectable by immunohistochemistry. The exogenous APP is essentially detected into two areas: the CA2 and subiculum. Scale bar represents 500 μm. **h** Scheme representing antero-posterior coordinates of coronal sections depicted in (**i-l**). **i-l** Immunostaining of APP (APP C-ter antibody, green) and NeuN (*red*) at different antero-posterior coordinates in AAV-APP mice coronal sections. **m** Magnified confocal images of an AAV-APP mouse section with double immunofluorescence staining showing the location of APP (APP C-ter antibody, *green*) and the diffusion of Aβ indicated by arrow heads (4G8 antibody, red) in the CA2 layer. *Blue*: DAPI. Scale bar represents 10 μm

month-old mice) with those present in the hippocampus of human controls and AD patients (five age-matched controls + five AD Braak 6/Thal 5 patients) and in APP/PS1ΔE9 transgenic mice [31]. Human APP content was found to be lower in AD cases than in age-matched controls, even after normalization for neuronal NeuN

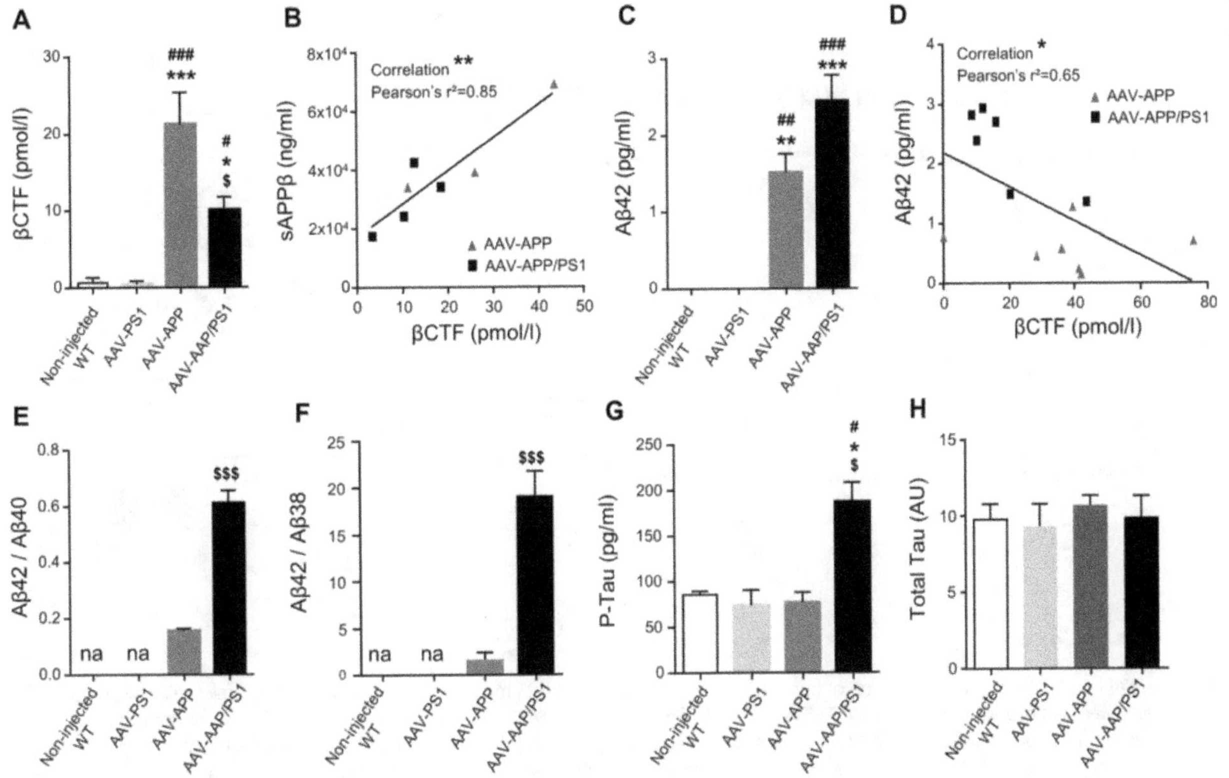

Fig. 2 Exogenous human APP is processed following the amyloidogenic pathway, 3 months after injection. C57Bl/6 J mice (all males) were injected at 8 weeks of age either with AAV-CAG-PS1M146L (AAV-PS1 mice), AAV-CAG-APPSL (AAV-APP mice) or both vectors at the same doses as for the other two groups (AAV-APP/PS1 mice, n = 7-8 mice per group). Non-injected WT mice (n = 4) were also analyzed. Mice were killed three months later for analyses of whole hippocampi. **a** Comparative analysis of TBS-Tx soluble human βCTF levels by ELISA. Note that βCTF levels follow the same pattern of expression than for the human APP in the four different groups (see Fig. 1e). Bars represent means ± SEM. Statistical analysis was performed by one-way ANOVA with Tukey's post-hoc test where ###, *** denote $p < 0.001$ versus non-injected WT and AAV-PS1 mice. #, * and $ denote $p < 0.05$. **b** Correlation between TBS-Tx soluble human βCTF and sAPPβ levels between AAV-APP and AAV-APP/PS1 mice (n = 7). Linear regression analysis confirms the engagement in the amyloidogenic pathway. Correlation analysis was performed with Pearson's parametric correlation test: **$p < 0.01$. **c** Comparative analysis of TBS-Tx soluble human Aβ42 levels by MSD immunoassay showing higher levels in AAV-APP/PS1 mice (n = 6-8 mice per group). Bars indicate means ± SEM. Statistical analysis was performed by one-way ANOVA followed by Tukey's post-hoc test where ###, *** denote $p < 0.001$ versus non-injected WT mice and AAV-PS1 mice. ## and ** denote $p < 0.01$. **d** Correlation between TBS-Tx soluble human Aβ42 and βCTF levels between AAV-APP and AAV-APP/PS1 (n = 13). Correlation analysis was performed with Pearson's parametric correlation test: *$p < 0.05$. **e-f** Representation of Aβ42/40 (**e**) and Aβ42/38 (**f**) ratios determined by multiplex MSD immunoassay (n = 4 mice per group). Bars indicate means ± SEM. Statistical analysis was performed by one-way ANOVA followed by Tukey's post-hoc test where $$$ denotes $p < 0.001$ versus AAV-APP mice. na = not applicable. **g** Comparative analysis of TBS-Tx soluble murine phosphorylated Tau protein (AT270, Thr181) by ELISA. Bars indicate means ± SEM. Statistical analysis was performed by one-way ANOVA followed by Tukey's post-hoc test where #, * and $ denote $p < 0.05$ versus non-injected WT mice, AAV-PS1 mice and AAV-APP mice respectively. **h** Densitometric analyses of western blots showing the expression of the total Tau protein in each group (n = 4 mice per group). Bars represent means ± SEM and data were normalized with respect to GAPDH

marker expression (p = 0.03), suggesting a higher rate of APP processing in sporadic forms of AD (Fig. 3a and b; Additional file 1: Figure S1). The amount of human APP present in the hippocampus of AAV-APP/PS1 mice was similar to that observed in the hippocampus of AD patients. By contrast, much larger amounts of human APP were found in five-month-old APP/PS1ΔE9 mice (Fig. 3a and b, $p < 0.0001$). Interestingly, total amount of APP was not significantly modified by virus injection compared to non-injected WT mice and in contrast to 5 months old APP/PS1ΔE9 who displayed a two-fold accumulation (p = 0.0011, Fig. 3c and d). We then evaluated metabolites released by the amyloidogenic pathway into the hippocampus of mice receiving AAV injections and compared it to those found in APP/PS1ΔE9 transgenic mice at different ages and human AD patients. We used 14 and 16-month-old APP/PS1ΔE9 mice because we detected behavioral deficits in these mice from 14-month-old of age (internal data). βCTF levels which tend to increase in AD patients compared to human controls, were similar in AAV-APP/PS1 mice and in AD patients. Interestingly, these levels were significantly lower

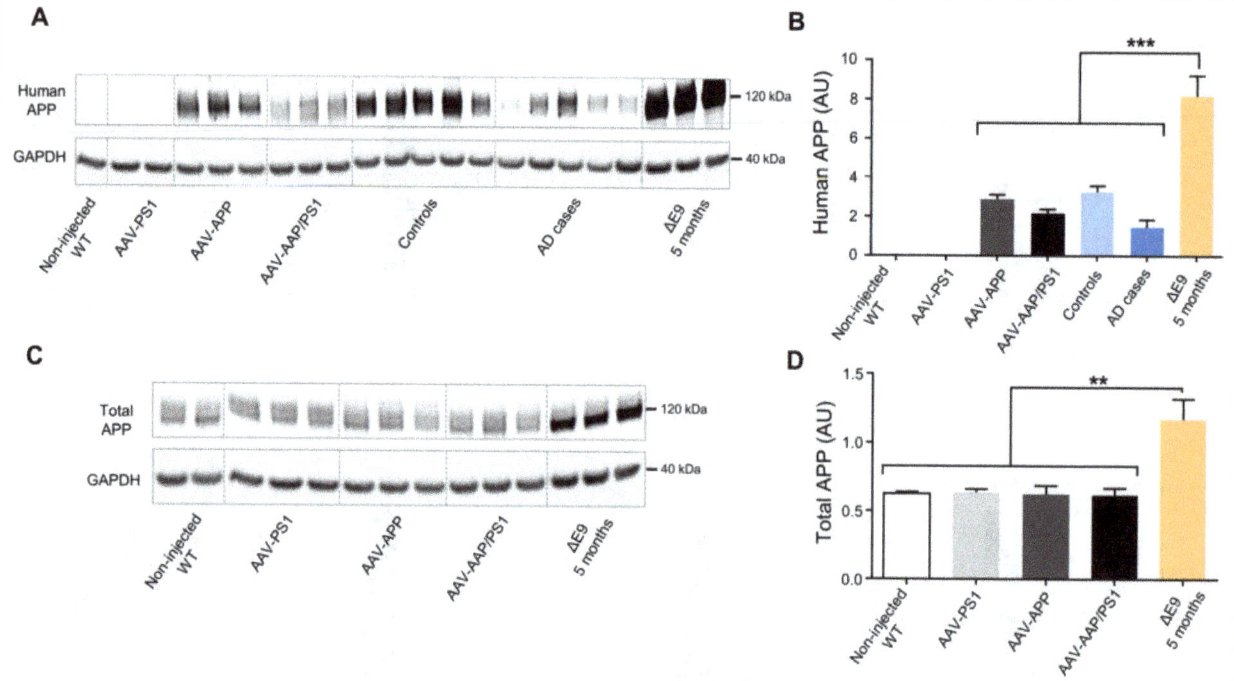

Fig. 3 AAV-APP/PS1 mice show a production of human APP similar to AD patients, 3 months after injection. C57Bl/6 J mice (all males) were injected at 8 weeks of age either with AAV-CAG-PS1M146L (AAV-PS1 mice, $n = 4$), AAV-CAG-APPSL (AAV-APP mice, $n = 4$) or both vectors at the same doses as for the other two groups (AAV-APP/PS1 mice, $n = 4$). Non-injected WT mice ($n = 4$) and transgenic APP/PS1ΔE9 mice were also used and all animals were killed at 5 months of age. Human samples were obtained from late-onset AD cases (Braak 6, Thal 5) and age-matched controls. The hippocampus was the structure analyzed for all samples. **a** Representative western blot of human APP (6E10 antibody) between AAV injected mice ($n = 3$ per group), human samples ($n = 5$ per group) and transgenic APP/PS1ΔE9 mice ($n = 3$). **b** Densitometric analyses of the antibody immunoreactivity shown in panel (**a**). Bars represent means ± SEM and data were normalized with respect to GAPDH. Statistical analysis was performed by one-way ANOVA with Tukey's post-hoc test: $***p < 0.001$. Note that AAV-APP/PS1 mice and human AD cases have similar levels. **c** Representative western blot of total APP (APP C-ter antibody) between non-injected WT, AAV injected and APP/PS1ΔE9 mice. **d** Densitometric analyses of the antibody immunoreactivity shown in panel **c**. Bars represent means ± SEM and data were normalized with respect to GAPDH. Statistical analysis was performed by one-way ANOVA with Tukey's post-hoc test: $**p < 0.01$

compared to both 14 and 16-month-old APP/PS1ΔE9 mice (Fig. 4a; $p < 0.0001$). In AAV-APP/PS1 injected mice, a tendency towards larger amounts of Aβ42 than in human controls was observed, but Aβ42 levels were lower than those in patients with advanced AD and APP/PS1ΔE9 mice at 5 months of age (Fig. 4b). Furthermore, Aβ40 levels were significantly higher in APP/PS1ΔE9 mice compared to other groups and increased with aging in these animals (Fig. 4c). Numerous studies have established the ratio of Aß42 to Aß40 as an important factor in determining the toxicity of Aβ in vivo [32]. We confirmed that Aβ42/Aβ40 ratios were significantly different between human controls and AD patients (Fig. 4d). Interestingly, these ratios were similar between AD patients and AAV-APP/PS1 mice, but significantly different in APP/PS1ΔE9 mice, which had a particularly low Aβ42/Aβ40 ratio. Together, these results indicate that co- injection of the AAV-APP and AAV-PS1 vectors into the hippocampus of normal mice leads to an overall pattern of amyloid processing close to that observed in the hippocampus of AD patients and contrasts to that of APP/PS1ΔE9 mice. Based on results obtained during analysis of APP processing and because AAV-PS1 mice and non-injected WT mice appeared similar in all analyses (see Figs. 1, 2, 3 and 4), we decided to use AAV-PS1 mice as an injected control group for further characterizations.

NMR spectroscopy shows changes to the neurochemical profile of the hippocampus in AAV-APP/PS1 mice

Proton magnetic resonance spectroscopy (^{1}H-MRS) has been shown to detect modifications in AD patients [33]. Using a 11.7 T scanner, we acquired ^{1}H-MRS spectra *in vivo* from the right and left hippocampi of AAV-PS1 and AAV-APP/PS1 mice, three months after injection, to evaluate the early consequences of APP processing on hippocampal metabolites. We determined the concentrations of seven metabolites from spectra: GABA, glutamine (Gln), glutamate (Glu), taurine (T), N-acetyl-aspartate + N-acetyl-aspartyl-glutamate (tNAA), myo-inositol (Ins) and glycerophosphocholine + phosphocholine + choline (tCho). Macromolecules and lipids were not included in

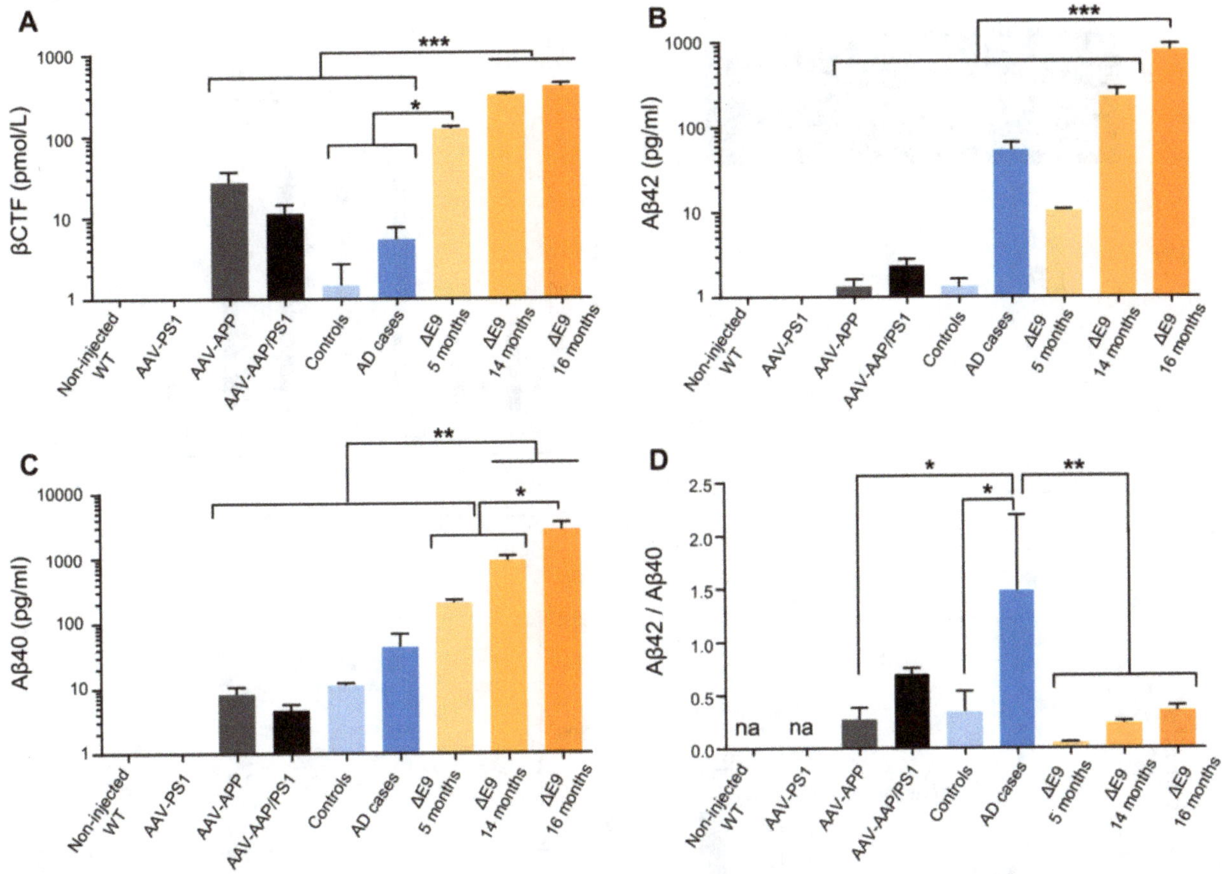

Fig. 4 AAV-APP/PS1 mice show a production of amyloid derivatives similar to AD patients, 3 months after injection. C57Bl/6 J mice (all males) were injected at 8 weeks of age either with AAV-CAG-PS1M146L (AAV-PS1 mice, *n* = 4), AAV-CAG-APPSL (AAV-APP mice, *n* = 4) or both vectors at the same doses as for the other two groups (AAV-APP/PS1 mice, *n* = 4). Non-injected WT mice (*n* = 4) and transgenic APP/PS1ΔE9 mice at 5 (*n* = 3), 14 (*n* = 8) and 16 (*n* = 8) months of age were also used. Human samples were obtained from late-onset AD cases (Braak 6, Thal 5) and age-matched controls. The hippocampus was the structure analyzed for all samples. **a** Comparative analysis of TBS-Tx soluble human βCTF levels by ELISA. Statistical analysis was performed by one-way ANOVA with Tukey's post-hoc test: $^{***}p < 0.001$. A logarithmic scale was used. Note that AAV-APP/PS1 mice and human AD cases have similar levels. **b-c** Quantification (6E10 based MSD immunoassay detecting human Aβ species) of TBS-Tx soluble human Aβ42 (**b**) and Aβ40 (**c**). Statistical analysis was performed by one-way ANOVA with Tukey's post-hoc test: $^{***}p < 0.001$, $^{**}p < 0.01$. Note that AAV-APP/PS1 injected mice show higher levels of Aβ42 compared to human controls and reduced levels compared to late stage human cases. **d** Representation of the Aβ42/40 ratio. Note that no significant difference was detectable between AAV-APP/PS1 mice and human AD cases

the study and the values obtained were expressed as ratios relative to creatine + phosphocreatine (tCr) (Fig. 5a). A two-way Anova with repeated measure revealed a group effect ($p = 0.04$). The concentration values obtained were generally lower in AAV-APP/PS1 than in AAV-PS1 mice, in absence of significant individual difference for each metabolite (Group x Metabolite interaction effect ($p = 0.13$)). Among studied metabolites, levels of metabolites related to neuromodulation (GABA, Gln, Glu, T and tNAA) were globally lower in AAV-APP-PS1 mice (Fig. 5b, group effect: $p = 0.002$). By contrast, metabolites not associated with neuromodulation (Ins, tCho) were not affected by co-injection of the AAV-APP and AAV-PS1 vectors. These results suggest that there is a decrease in the global pool of metabolites involved in neurotransmission processes in AAV-APP-PS1 mice. They also rule out the possibility of a single metabolite being entirely responsible for changes, at this stage and in this model. In this way, the absence of increased concentration of glutamate excluded glutamate induced excitotoxicity.

AAV-APP/PS1 mice present early extrasynaptic deficits

A loss of synaptic contacts in the hippocampus is one of the major early neuropathological findings in AD patients [34]. Moreover, deficiencies in glutamate transport have been shown to be associated with AD [35]. We assessed the functionality of glutamatergic synapses by electrophysiological analyses on hippocampal slices. The long-term potentiation (LTP) of glutamate synaptic transmission was first evaluated in mice three months

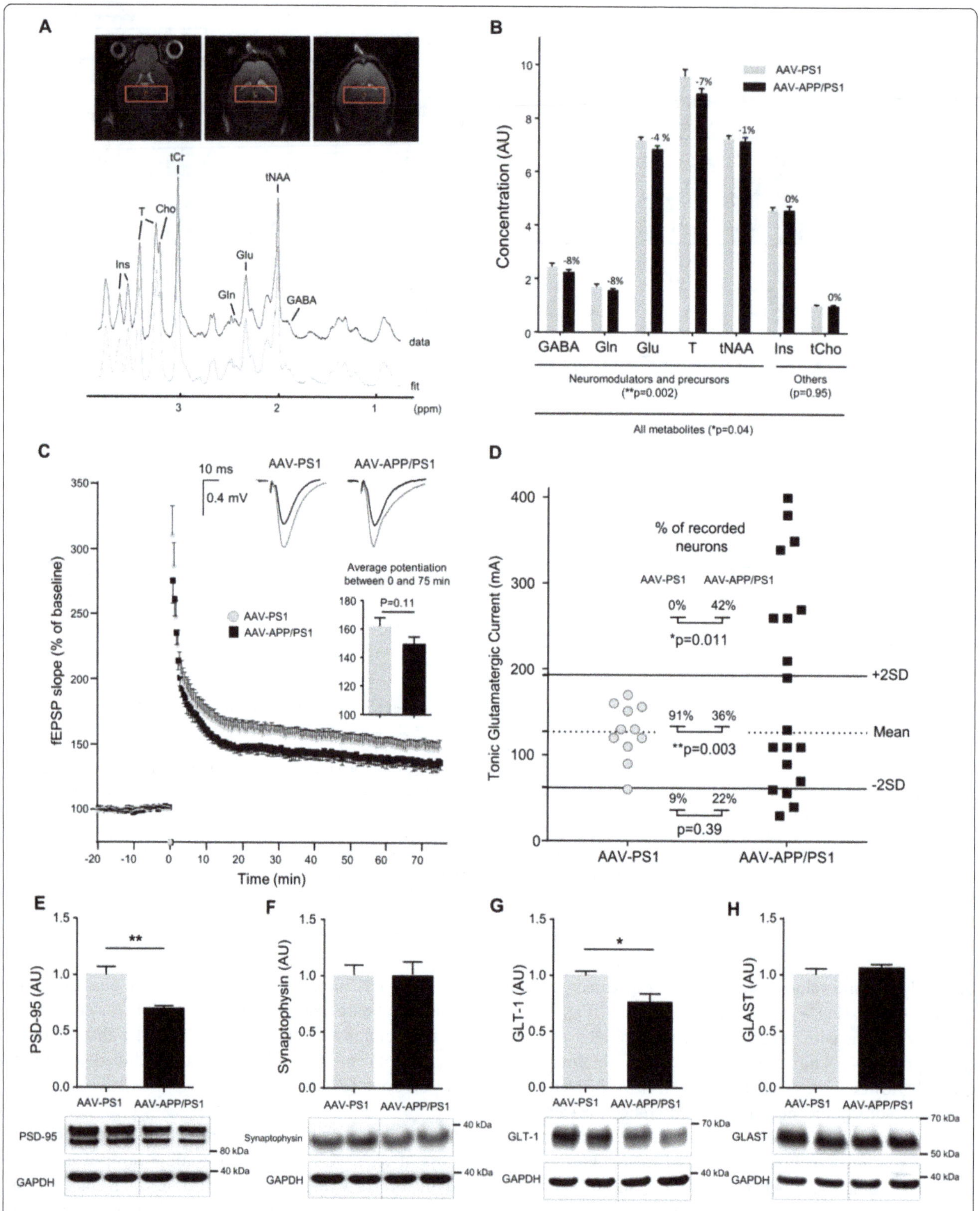

Fig. 5 (See legend on next page.)

(See figure on previous page.)

Fig. 5 AAV-APP/PS1 mice present synaptic defects, 3 months after injection. C57Bl/6 J mice (all males) were injected at 8 weeks of age either with AAV-CAG-PS1M146L (AAV-PS1 mice used as an injected control group, *n* = 10) or AAV-CAG-APPSL + AAV-CAG-PS1M146L (AAV-APP/PS1 mice, *n* = 10). Mice were used for *in-vivo* (**a**-**b**) and *ex-vivo* (**c**-**d**) recording three months later. **a** *Top* panel: localization of the spectroscopic volume of 7.2 mm x 2 mm x 2.6 mm encompassing both. Hippocampi of each mouse. Bottom panel: representative ^{1}H-MR spectrum acquired from the hippocampus of a mouse 3 months after injection. **b** Concentrations of seven metabolites were determined from spectra: GABA, Gln, Glu, T, tNAA, Ins and tCho. Macromolecules and lipids were not included in the study and the values obtained were expressed as ratios relative to tCr (*n* = 10-11 per group). Bars represent means ± SEM. Statistical analysis was performed by two-way ANOVA with experimental group and metabolites as effects. Note that metabolite levels were significantly lower in AAV-APP/PS1 mice (experimental group effect: $p = 0.04$). A selective analysis of metabolites linked to neuromodulation and precursors (GABA, Gln, Glu, T, tNAA) increased the significance of the difference between both groups (experimental group effect: $p = 0.002$). **c** Long-term potentiation (LTP) over 75 min induced by high-frequency stimulation. The inset graphs represent for each group an example of unit field excitatory postsynaptic potentials (fEPSP) before (black line) and after (gray line) LTP induction. The inset histogram shows average potentiation. Bars represent means ± SEM (*n* = 15-16 slices from *n* = 10 mice per group). Statistical analysis was performed with Student's t-test. **d** Scatter diagram showing the tonic glutamatergic current recorded at a holding potential of +40 mV (whole cell patch-clamp of CA1 pyramidal cells, *n* = 11-19/group from *n* = 10 mice per group). Normal response was characterized in a range comprised between AAV-PS1 mean +/- 2SD. Analysis of AAV-APP/PS1 profile revealed a decrease of number of neurons with normal response (Chi^2 test: $p = 0.003$) in association with an increase of neurons with an high level of Tonic glutamatergic current (Chi^2 test: $p = 0.011$) suggesting this current was stronger in the AAV-APP/PS1 group. **e**-**h** Western blot analysis of PSD-95, Synaptophysin, GLT-1 and GLAST. Bars represent means ± SEM and data were normalized with respect to GAPDH. Student's t-test was used for statistical analysis: *$p < 0.05$

after injection. A trend towards a decrease in LTP expression following high-frequency stimulation but not theta burst stimulation was found to be linked to the co-expression of APP_{SL} and $PS1_{M146L}$ (Fig. 5c; $p = 0.11$). Beside, we recorded the tonic current generated in CA1 pyramidal cells by the ambient levels of glutamate acting on extrasynaptic NMDA receptors (NMDAR). The amplitude of the tonic current was significantly greater in the AAV-APP/PS1 mice and characterized by a significant dispersion of current amplitude suggesting greater disorganization of the synapse in this population than in the more homogeneous AAV-PS1 or AAV-APP mouse groups (Fig. 5d). Indeed, no difference was observed between the AAV-PS1 and AAV-APP groups (Additional file 2: Figure S2). Synaptic dysfunction occurs early in AD [34] and brains of AD patients have been shown to contain abnormally low levels of synaptic proteins [36]. We compared the levels of the PSD-95 and synaptophysin synaptic markers in the hippocampus of AAV-PS1 and AAV-APP/PS1 mice. PSD-95 levels were significantly lower in AAV-APP/PS1 than AAV-PS1 mice ($p = 0.007$), while synaptophysin was not modified (Fig. 5e and f). Next we investigated the contribution of extrasynaptic glutamate receptor uptake further, by assessing the expression of two astrocytic glutamate transporters, GLT-1 and GLAST. AAV-APP/PS1 mice were found to have significantly lower levels of GLT-1 ($p = 0.003$), with no difference in GLAST levels (Fig. 5g and h).

AAV-APP/PS1 mice develop early cognitive deficits

Most transgenic mouse models of AD reproduce cognitive impairments relevant to the human disease. In most of these models, progressive deficits are associated with excessive Aβ production at an advanced age [3]. We evaluated weather moderate amyloid production in AAV-APP-PS1 mice could be associated with early cognitive dysfunctions. We used AAV-PS1 as control group since previous studies demonstrated that mutant PS1 overexpression in mouse hippocampus did not induce cognitive abnormalities in Morris Water Maze [37] nor in Y-Maze tasks [38], and APP processing profile was similar in WT animals and AAV-PS1 animals (see Figs. 1, 2, 3 and 4). In the Open-field task a decreased distance travelled across time suggests habituation to the novel environment as classically described [39]. Distance travelled during task was similar between AAV-PS1 and AAV-APP/PS1 mice confirming no motor abnormality in our experimental AD mouse model (Fig. 6a). Interestingly, AAV-APP/PS1 mice displayed a much higher periphery/center ratio than AAV-PS1 mice. This difference in behavior may either reflect changes in emotional behavior when faced to a new environment or an increase in anxiety (Fig. 6b; $p = 0.02$). Similarly to Open-field, both groups showed habituation during the Ymaze task, confirmed by a decrease of distance travelled across time (Fig. 6c). No motor impairment was observed in AAV-PS1 and AAV-APP/PS1 mice. Furthermore, a trend towards short term memory impairment was observed in AAV-APP/PS1 mice that spent less time than AAV-PS1 mice exploring the new arm of the maze (Fig. 6d; $p = 0.08$). Finally, we assessed spatial learning and memory, using the Morris Water Maze task. The travelled distance to find the hidden platform was not different between both groups over time (Fig. 6e) with no difference during this learning phase (data not shown). Interestingly, AAV-PS1 mice spent longer in the target quadrant than AAV-APP/PS1 mice (Fig. 5f and g) in both the four-hour ($p = 0.054$) and the 72-h ($p = 0.0085$) probe tests indicating an alteration in memory retention in AAV-APP/PS1 mice. Thus, AAV-PS1 mice displayed a spatial bias in the target quadrant during both the 4-h (target

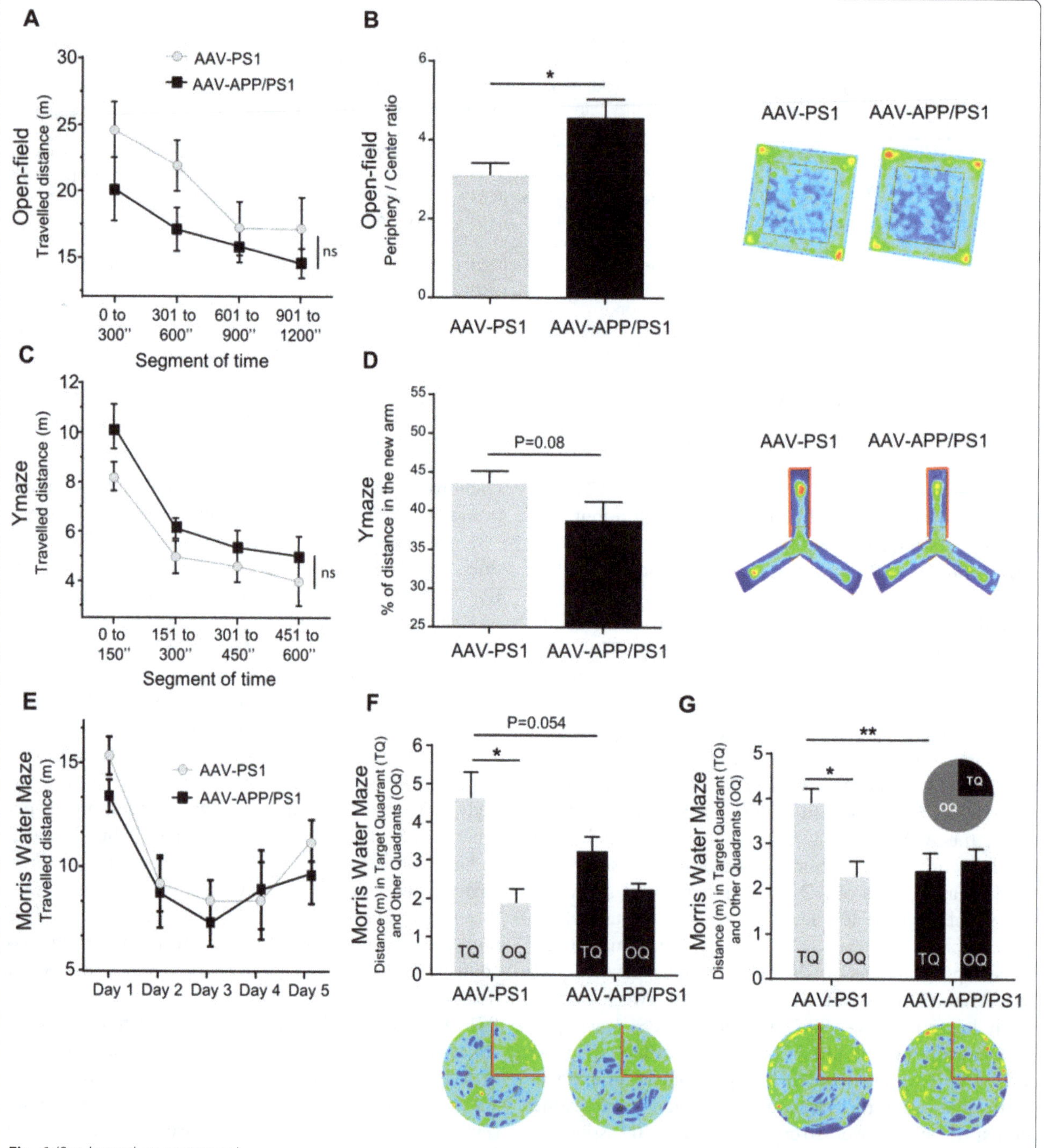

Fig. 6 (See legend on next page.)

(See figure on previous page.)

Fig. 6 AAV-APP/PS1 mice present memory impairments, 3 months after injection. C57Bl/6 J mice (all males) were injected at 8 weeks of age either with AAV-CAG-PS1M146L (AAV-PS1 mice used as an injected control group, $n = 8$) or AAV-CAG-APPSL + AAV-CAG-PS1M146L (AAV-APP/PS1 mice, $n = 8$) and behavioral analyses were performed three months later. **a** Open-field assay. Travelled distance during the Open-field task showing no significant difference between both groups. **b** *Left* panel: time in periphery/time in center ratio showing a change in emotional behavior when faced to a new environment in the AAV-APP/PS1 group (n = 7-8 mice per group). Bars represent means ± SEM. Statistical analysis was performed with Student's t-test: $*p < 0.05$. Right panel: group occupancy plots for visualizing the areas in which the animals spent the most time during the test. **c** Y-maze assay. Travelled distance during the Y-Maze task showing no significant difference between both groups during the test session. **d** Left panel: percentage of distance in the new arm showing that AAV-APP/PS1 mice spent less time in the new arm than the other groups ($p = 0.08$; n = 7-8 mice per groups). Bars represent means ± SEM. Statistical analysis was performed with Student's t-test. *Right* panel: group occupancy plots for visualizing the areas in which the animals spent the most time during the test. The arm circled in red is the new arm. **e** Morris Water Maze assay. Travelled distance during the Morris Water Maze task showing no significant difference between both groups during the five training days. **f-g** Probe trial performance at 4 h (**f**) and 72 h (**g**) after the last training session. TQ = target quadrant that housed the platform during the training sessions. OQ = mean of distance covered in the other three quadrants. Note that AAV-APP/PS1 mice were impaired in comparison to AAV-PS1 mice confirmed by no preference for the trained target quadrant. Bars represent means ± SEM. A two way ANOVA was used with experimental group and quadrant as main effects: $*p < 0.05$, $**p < 0.01$

quadrant TQ vs. mean of other quadrants OQ; $p = 0.031$) and 72-h (TQ vs. OQ; $p = 0.023$) probe tests, confirming their preserved spatial memory. By contrast, AAV-APP/PS1 mice did not spend more time in the target quadrant in either the four-hour (TQ vs. OQ; $p = 0.06$) or the 72-h (TQ vs. OQ; $p = 0.69$) probe trial, confirming an absence of efficient memorization of platform position. These data suggest that co-injection of both vectors triggers detectable memory impairment as soon as three months after injection.

Discussion

Alzheimer's disease (AD) is a complex condition. To improve our understanding of the physiopathology of the disease and design new therapeutic strategies, it is crucial to get access to the initial phases of its development. We aimed at recapitulating *in vivo* key features that are suspected to account for triggering AD, more specifically an increased Aβ42/Aβ40 ratio, while avoiding major APP overexpression. The importance of the Aβ ratio in the disease onset above their absolute levels has been already proposed [40] and the absence of APP overproduction is increasingly being recognized as an important factor to take into account when modeling AD [12]. Towards this goal, we developed an alternative approach to existing models, involving a single co-administration of two AAV vectors encoding human mutated APP (APP_{sl}) and PS1 ($PS1_{M146L}$) in adult wild-type mice hippocampi.

Transgenic mice expressing WT form of the 695-amino acid isoform of APP do not develop AD-like phenotype nor behavioral impairment [41, 42] in contrast to APP751 transgenic mice which have strong learning deficits at 12 months of age [11]. Therefore, the APP751 isoform seems more interesting to trigger an AD-like phenotype. In order to specifically enhance amyloidogenic APP processing, we decided to express the APP751 isoform including the Swedish and London mutations [43]. We simultaneously expressed PS1 with the M146L mutation to increase the specificity of the 42-specific γ-secretase cleavage [44]. Thus, the co-expression of PS1 (PS1M146L) with APP751SL resulted in an increased production of Aβ with an Aβ42/Aβ40 ratio similar to the one observed in AD patients. Interestingly, increase of APP cleavage products was not associated with amyloid deposition, neurofibrillary tangles and neuronal loss.

AAV-APP/PS1 mice display cognitive impairment as early as three months post-injection. These memory deficiencies reflect a global impairment of neuronal activity, as suggested by ^{1}H-MRS, showing the levels of metabolites related to neurotransmission expressed in the hippocampus globally reduced. These result highlights that there is an early response of neurons to the APP processing affecting their functionality.

To get further insight in the understanding of this neuronal dysfunction, we used electrophysiological recordings on the CA1 layer to characterize synaptic consequences of moderate soluble Aβ42 production. We observed an enhancement of the tonic glutamatergic current generated in CA1 pyramidal cells of AAV-APP/PS1 mice. Two types of N-methyl D-aspartate receptors (NMDARs) have been described (synaptic and extrasynaptic), the tonic current resulting mostly from the activation of the extrasynaptic subgroup, stimulated by ambient glutamate present outside the synaptic cleft [45, 46]. As we did not observe an increase of glutamate synthesis by ^{1}H-MRS, the higher tonic current observed in AAV-APP/PS1 mice may reflect the accumulation of glutamate in the extrasynaptic space. There are two possible explanations for this possible accumulation. First, lower levels of glutamate transporters, such as GLT-1, may result in weaker levels of glutamate uptake by astrocytes [35]. Second, lower levels of scaffolding proteins, such as PSD-95, may lead to the internalization of synaptic NMDARs, resulting in the preferential activation of extrasynaptic ones [47]. AAV-APP/PS1 mice display these features since they express significantly lower levels of GLT-1 and PSD-95. No decrease of GLAST, the second most important glutamate transporter, was observed which might suggest that GLAST expression could be decreased later in the course of the disease [48]. This hypothesis is not surprising, in light of published data about GLT-1 and PSD-95 dysfunctions, which may play an important role in synaptic dysfunction and, thus, in the pathogenesis of AD [49, 50]. To our knowledge, we show for the first time that an impairment of the extrasynaptic compartment could precede sustained alterations of the synaptic compartment associated with LTP deficits, during the early stage of AD progression. We also showed that a subtle loss of neuronal integrity in the hippocampus is sufficient to trigger deleterious effects before actual neuronal death occurs. Despite diffusion properties of Aβ42 [51], no amyloid peptide have been detected outside the hippocampus excluding an Aβ42 direct effect far from its hippocampal production area. By contrast, Aβ altered hippocampus functions could lead to a less efficient communication between hippocampal neurons and connected structures especially cortex and amygdala. This network dysfunction could be responsible of cognitive modifications especially during memory formation [52, 53] or emotional behaviors [54].

In addition to these consequences, AAV-APP/PS1 mice displayed higher levels of Tau phosphorylation (thr181, AT270 antibody) compared to the other groups. It has been reported that soluble Aβ and extrasynaptic NMDAR activation contribute to Tau protein phosphorylation [55, 56]. Our results are consistent with these previous reports. The pattern of Tau phosphorylation was shown to be correlated with the multiple steps of neurofibrillary tangle development [57]. Thr181 immunoreactivity is detected earlier than thr212/Ser214 (AT100 antibody) or ser199/ser202/thr205 (AT8 antibody) immunoreactivity. We could not detect some AT8 or AT100 positive cells (data not shown), suggesting that the modifications observed in AAV-APP/PS1 mice might be compared to early phases of AD in humans. These data suggest that the moderate AD-like APP processing engagement observed in AAV-APP/PS1 mice is sufficient to trigger the Tau pathway engagement.

A particular feature in our experimental strategy is the localized production of human APP and its cleavage products. Contrasting with the ubiquitous overproduction of human APP in mouse transgenic lines, injection of AAV-APP and AAV-PS1 vectors in the stratum lacunosum moleculare region, leads to the transduction of neurons in restricted regions of the hippocampus (CA2 and the subiculum). Interestingly, this pattern of expression may mimic the genomic mosaicism recently described in AD, in which an increase in copy number was observed for the APP gene in a limited number of neurons, in sporadic forms of AD [27]. The presence of rare neurons with APP amplification may be sufficient to trigger a dysregulation of APP processing with aging. Our findings also point to this direction. The second particular feature in our experimental design is the co-injection of the PS1 vector. Indeed, we demonstrated that AAV-APP injection alone was not sufficient to induce hippocampal alteration. Thus, despite the production of βCTF, Aβ40 and Aβ42 in AAV-APP mouse hippocampus, no change in the levels of phosphorylated Tau, PSD-95, GLT-1 or tonic current were observed, compared to the AAV-APP/PS1 group. There are two possible reasons for this difference between the AAV-APP and AAV-APP/PS1 groups. First, APP acts as a trophic factor [58] and an increase in the levels of this molecule may increase neuron viability [59], countering Aβ toxicity. Second, the Aβ42/Aβ40 ratios in the AAV-APP/PS1 group were highly similar to those found in AD patients and different from those of the AAV-APP group or human controls.

Our data raise several questions. This configuration, with no plaque nor tangle and with levels of APP cleavage products close to the human hippocampal condition, is sufficient to induce cognitive impairment three months after injection. It takes about 13 months to obtain an equivalent defect in APP/PS1ΔE9 mice [60]. This delayed cognitive impairment may result from the trophic roles of APP and the low Aβ42/Aβ40 ratio observed in 5- to 16-month-old APP/PS1ΔE9 mice. These findings confirm the greater importance of the Aβ ratio rather than the absolute amounts of Aβ42 and Aβ40 [40] to induce synaptic and extrasynaptic impairments. Finally, neurons may become brittle, leading to cognitive impairments, with defects in emotional behavior and long-term memory.

Conclusions

This study reports the development of a novel mouse model focusing on the early consequences of the amyloid processing of APP with similarities to human AD cases. Our results support the importance of the Aβ42/Aβ40 ratio to trigger initial neuronal dysfunctions *in vivo*. All mechanisms described here are consistent with memory impairments in the earliest stages of the clinical disease beginning with subtle changes in the efficacy of hippocampal synapses, before amyloid deposition and neuronal loss. It appears that minimal dysregulation of amyloidogenic pathway is sufficient to set up synaptic, and notably extrasynaptic dysfunctions, potential first step towards the full AD phenotype. Using animal models closely mimicking the human disease in terms of APP and APP cleavage products and focusing on early stages of AD development may increase our understanding of disease onset. This model may ultimately make it possible to identify early biomarkers of AD while evaluating relevant neuroprotective therapeutic strategies.

Methods

Plasmid design and vector production

We used a double-mutant human APP751 cDNA containing the Swedish and London mutations (codon optimized and containing a Kozak sequence; GeneArt, Life Technologies, Saint Aubin, France), and a human PS1 cDNA containing the M146L mutation (pENTR4-PS1-S182M146L). The APP_{SL} and PS1M146L sequences were cloned in an AAV2 plasmid with CAG promoter to generate the AAV2-CAG-APPSL or -CAG-PS1M146L. AAV vectors were produced as previously described [61], except that the AAV packaging plasmid was replaced with a plasmid construct containing the *rep* gene of AAV2 and the *cap* gene of AAVrh10.

Human brain samples

Postmortem samples were obtained from brains collected as part of the Brain Donation Program of the GIE-Neuro-CEB Brain Bank. Autopsies were carried out by accredited pathologists, after informed consent had been obtained from the relatives, in accordance with French Bioethics laws. Five hippocampal samples from five patients with sporadic forms of AD (male and female; Braak 6 Thal 5; aged between 69 and 89 years, with a postmortem interval (PMI) of 30 to 59 h) and five hippocampus samples from five age-matched control subjects (male and female, aged between 69 and 92 years, PMI of 6 to 63 h) were used in this study.

Animals

We used 90 male C57Bl/6 J mice (eight-week-old; SARL JanvierLabs, Le Genest Saint Isle, France) and 19 male APP/PS1ΔE9 mice [31]. All experiments were conducted in accordance with ethical standards and French and European regulations (Directive 2010/63/EU).

Stereotactic injections of AAVs

Mice were anesthetized by an intraperitoneal injection of ketamine/xylazine (0.1/0.05 g/kg body weight) and placed in a stereotactic frame (Stoelting, Wood Dale, IL, USA). Stereotactic intracerebral injections of AAVs into the hippocampi of both hemispheres were performed, using the following coordinates: antero-posterior: -2 mm, lateral: ± 1 mm, ventral: -2 mm relative to bregma. We injected 2 μl of viral preparation into each site (5 x 10^8 vg/site and 10^9 vg/site for AAV-PS1 and AAV-APP vectors, respectively) at a rate of 0.2 μl/min. Four groups were designed, a non-injected wild-type (non-injected WT mice) and three injected groups: AAV-CAG-PS1M146L (AAV-PS1 mice), AAV-CAG-APPSL (AAV-APP mice), AVV-CAG-APPSL + AAV10-CAG-$PS1_{M146L}$ (AAV-APP/PS1 mice).

Tissue collection and sample preparation

Mice were anesthetized with ketamine/xylazine and transcardially perfused with 20 ml ice-cold phosphate-buffered saline (PBS). One hemisphere was post-fixed by incubation for 48 h in 4 % PFA, cryoprotected in 30 % sucrose in PBS and cut into 40 μm sections with a freezing microtome (Leica) for histological analyses. The contralateral hemisphere was dissected for isolation of the hippocampus and cortex. Samples were homogenized in a lysis buffer (150 mM NaCl and 1 % Triton in Tris-buffered saline, referenced as TBS-Tx) containing phosphatase (Pierce) and protease (Roche) inhibitors and centrifuged for 20 min at 15000 g. The same procedure was applied to human samples (GIE NeuroCEB Brain Bank).

ELISA

The Aβ extracted was quantified with the MSD Human Aβ42 V-PLEX Kit and the triplex Aβ Peptide Panel 1 (6E10) V-PLEX Kit (Meso Scale Diagnostics, Rockville, USA). βCTF was determined with the IBL Human APP βCTF Assay Kit (IBL International GmbH, Hamburg, Germany). Hyperphosphorylated Tau was determined with the Innogenetics Phospho-Tau 181P kit (Fujirebio Europe, Ghent, Belgium). sAPPβ was determined with the MSD sAPPalpha/sAPPbeta Kit. ELISA was performed according to the kit manufacturer's instructions in each case.

Western blotting

Equal amounts of protein (30 μg) were separated by electrophoresis in NuPAGE Bis-Tris Gels (Life Technologies) and transferred to nitrocellulose membranes. The membranes were hybridized with various primary antibodies (APP 6E10, 1/500, Covance; PS1, 1/1000, Millipore; APP C-ter, 1/500, Millipore; Actin, 1/2000, Abcam; GAPDH, 1/1000 Abcam; Total Tau, 1/1000, Santa Cruz; PSD-95, Invitrogen, 1/2000; Synaptophysin, Santa Cruz, 1/200; GAD65, Abcam, 1/2000; GLT-1, 1/1000, Frontier Science; GLAST, 1/1000, Frontier Science; NeuN, Millipore, 1/1000). Various secondary antibodies was also used (ECL Anti-rabbit Horseradish Peroxidase linked, 1/2000, GE Healthcare; ECL Anti-mouse Horseradish Peroxidase linked, 1/2000, GE Healthcare; ECL Anti-rat Horseradish Peroxidase linked, 1/2000, GE Healthcare).

Immunohistochemistry and image acquisition

Cryosections were washed with 0.25 % Triton in PBS and saturated by incubation (0.25 % Triton in PBS/5 % goat serum). They were then incubated with primary antibodies (APP C-ter, 1/500, Millipore; NeuN-Biotin, 1/1000, Millipore; 4G8-Biotin, 1/1000, Covance). Images were taken with a Nikon Eclipse Ti Microscope or a

Leica TCS SP8 confocal microscope and analyzed with ImageJ software (NIH).

Behavioral assessment

Open-field

The apparatus consisted of an open-topped, clear Plexiglas box measuring 50 x 50 x 38 cm placed in a room with controlled dim lighting (25 lux) and constant white noise at 60 dB. The mice were placed in the center of the arena and a video recording was made over a period of five minutes. The behavior of the animals was analyzed from this video. The arena was divided into a central region (20 x 20 cm) and a peripheral region, and the time spent in the center and periphery of the open field was measured. The ratio of time spent in the periphery to that spent in the center was calculated as an index of emotional behavior.

Ymaze

The apparatus consisted of three identical arms separated by 120°. Each arm of the Y maze was 37 cm long, and 8 cm wide, with 12.5 cm-high opaque walls. Various extra maze cues were placed on the surrounding walls. One arm of the Y-maze was blocked and the subject was allowed to explore the other two arms for 10 min. The starting position was varied pseudorandomly, between the three arms. The animal was then returned to its home cage. Fifteen minutes later, the mouse was placed in the maze again, this time with all three arms open, and allowed to explore for an additional five minutes. The distance traveled and the number of times the mouse entered each arm were measured both during initial exposure to the maze and during testing.

Morris water maze

Experiments were performed in a tank 120 cm in diameter and 50 cm deep, filled with opacified water kept at 21 °C and equipped with a platform 10 cm in diameter, kept submerged 1 cm below the surface of the water. Visual clues were positioned around the pool, to provide the mouse with spatial landmarks, and luminosity was maintained at 350 lux. The mice were initially exposed to a learning phase, which consisted of daily sessions (three trials per session) on five consecutive days. The starting position was varied pseudorandomly, between the four cardinal points. A mean interval of 15 min was left between trials. The trial was considered to have ended when the animal reached the platform. A 60-s cutoff was used, after which the mice were gently guided to the platform. Once on the platform, the animals were allowed to rest for 30 s before being returned to their cage. Long-term spatial memory was assessed 72 h after the last training trial (fifth day), in a probe trial in which the platform was no longer available. Animals were monitored with ANY-maze video tracking software (Stoelting Co, Wood Dale, USA).

***Ex vivo* electrophysiology**

Mice were anesthetized with halothane and decapitated. The brain was rapidly removed from the skull and placed in chilled (0–3 °C) artificial cerebrospinal fluid (ACSF) containing 124 mM NaCl, 3.5 mM KCl, 1.5 mM $MgSO_4$, 2.5 mM $CaCl_2$, 26.2 mM $NaHCO_3$, 1.2 mM NaH_2PO_4, 11 mM glucose. Transverse slices (300–400 µm thick) were cut with a vibratome and placed in ACSF in a holding chamber, at 27 °C, for at least one hour before recording. Each slice was individually transferred to a submersion-type recording chamber and submerged in ACSF continuously superfused and equilibrated with 95 % O_2, 5 % CO_2.

The biophysical properties of the tonic current generated by the activation of extrasynaptic NMDA receptors with ambient glutamate were evaluated. Whole-cell patch-clamp recordings of CA1 pyramidal cells were performed at room temperature, with borosilicate patch pipettes (5 MΩ) filled with 140 mM $CsCH_4O_3S$, 6 mM CsCl, 2 mM $MgCl_2$, 10 mM HEPES, 1.1 mM EGTA, 5 mM QX-314 5, 4 mM ATP, (pH 7.3; 290 mosm). Transmembrane currents were acquired and filtered through an amplifier (AxoPatch 1-D, Axon Instruments), stored on a computer and digitized with WinLTP software for analysis [62]. The tonic current was recorded at a holding potential of +40 mV, in the presence of TTX (1 µM), NBQX (10 µM), and bicuculline (10 µM), to isolate the NMDA component of the holding current (hc). After the recording of a stable control hc for three to five minutes, APV (50 µM) was added to the superfusion medium. The hc fell to a new stable value under the effect of APV, and the difference between the control hc and that recorded in the presence of APV determined the amplitude of the tonic current.

Two kinds of electrically induced long-term potentiation (LTP) were studied: a strong, saturating LTP consisting of 3x100 Hz (3x 100 pulses, 1 s, with 20 s between pulses), and a weaker stimulation, theta-burst stimulation (TBS), mimicking the natural stimulation at the theta frequency from the medial septum to the hippocampus, consisting of five trains of four 100 Hz pulses each, separated by 200 ms and delivered at the test intensity. The sequence was repeated three times, with an interburst interval of 10s. Testing with a single pulse was resumed for 60 min (TBS) or 75 min (3x100 Hz), to determine the level of LTP.

Proton magnetic resonance spectroscopy (^{1}H-MRS)

Magnetic Resonance Imaging and Magnetic Resonance Spectroscopy were performed with a horizontal 11.7 T scanner (Bruker, Ettlingen, Germany) and a quadrature cryoprobe was used for radiofrequency transmission and reception. A 37.4 μl voxel (7.2 × 2 × 2.6 mm^3) was placed over both hemispheres, such that it contained essentially hippocampal tissue (Fig. 5), and the signal of this voxel was then averaged over 10 min. T_2-weighted images were acquired with a 2D TurboRARE sequence (80 × 80 $μm^2$ in-plane resolution, and 300 μm slice thickness) and manually segmented to measure hippocampal volume. ^{1}H-MRS acquisitions were performed with a LASER sequence, with echo time (TE)/repetition time (TR) = 20/5000 ms and a 10 kHz bandwidth for the hyperbolic secant pulses. LCModel was used to determine metabolite concentrations. The macromolecule (MM) spectrum of a control mouse was determined by metabolite nulling and included in the base set for LCModel. The following metabolites were systematically quantified (Cramér-Rao lower limits <5 % in all experiments): total choline (glycerophosphocholine + phosphocholine + choline, tCho), total creatine (creatine + phosphocreatine, tCr), glutamate (Glu), glutamine (Gln), myo-inositol (Ins), N-acetyl-aspartate + N-acetyl-aspartyl-glutamate (NAA + NAAG, tNAA), taurine (T) and γ-aminobutyric acid (GABA). Metabolite concentrations were normalized with respect to 8 mM tCr.

Statistical analysis

Data are expressed as mean ± SEM. Statistical analyses were performed with GraphPad Prism (GraphPad Software, La Jolla, CA, USA) or Statistica (StatSoft, Inc., Tulsa, OK, USA) software. One-way ANOVA and Tukey's *post-hoc* test were used to determine the significance of differences between groups. Student's *t* test was used when only two groups were analyzed (AAV-PS1 vs AAV-APP/PS1), except for tonic glutamatergic current recording, for which Chi^2 tests were used. Two-way ANOVA with repeated measure using Group and Metabolite as effect factors, was used for NMR spectroscopy analysis.

Additional files

Additional file 1: Figure S1. APP is processed in sporadic AD cases. Human samples were obtained from late-onset AD cases (Braak 6, Thal 5) and age-matched controls (n = 5 per group). The hippocampus was the studied structure. (**A**) Western blot analysis of NeuN. (**B**) Densitometric analyses of western blots showing the expression of human APP in the hippocampus of human controls and AD cases (n = 5 per group). Bars represent means ± SEM, and data were normalized with respect to GAPDH. Statistical analyses were performed with Student's t-test: $**p <$ 0.01. (**C**) Densitometric analyses of **A**, showing the expression of NeuN in the hippocampus of human controls and AD cases (n = 5 per group). Bars represent means ± SEM, and data were normalized with respect to GAPDH. Statistical analyses were performed with Student's t-test: $*p <$ 0.05. (**D**) Representation of the APP/NeuN ratio following densitometric analyses of the corresponding western blots (n = 5 per group). Note that APP seems to be processed in sporadic AD cases. Bars represent means ± SEM and data were normalized with respect to GAPDH. Statistical analyses were performed with Student's t-test: $*p < 0.05$.

Additional file 2: Figure S2. AAV-PS1 and AAV-APP mice do not exhibit neuronal defects in terms of PSD-95, GLT-1 and tonic glutamatergic current. C57Bl/6 J mice (all males) were injected at 8 weeks of age either with AAV-CAG-PS1M146L (AAV-PS1 mice) or AAV-CAG-APPSL (AAV-APP mice). Mice were killed three months later for analyses. (**A**) Western blot of PSD-95 and GLT-1 (n = 3-4 per group). (**B**) Densitometric analyses of the antibody immunoreactivities shown in panel **A**. (**C**) Tonic glutamatergic current recorded at a holding potential of +40 mV by the whole-cell patch-clamping of CA1 pyramidal cells. No significant difference in tonic glutamatergic current intensity was observed between the AAV-PS1 and AAV-APP groups (whole cell patch-clamp of CA1 pyramidal cells, n = 11/group from n = 10 mice per group).

Abbreviations

AAV: Adeno-associated virus; Aβ: β-amyloid peptide; AD: Alzheimer's disease; APP: Amyloid precursor protein; βCTF: β-carboxy-terminal fragment; ELISA: Enzyme-linked immunosorbent assay; NMDAR: N-methyl-D-aspartate receptor; PS1: Presenilin 1.

Competing interest

The authors have no competing financial interests to declare.

Authors' contributions

MA, NC and JB carried out the design of the study and wrote the manuscript. MA and JB performed biochemical, behavioral, histological and statistical analyses. RF, SA, MAB and GDC participated in the biochemical analyses and helped to draft the manuscript. PD, BP and JMB performed the electrophysiological recording and helped to design the study and draft the manuscript. JF and JV performed the MRI analyses. APB helped with the viral production. PH and ND helped to draft the manuscript. All authors read and approved the final manuscript.

Acknowledgments & funding

We thank Charlène Joséphine, Noëlle Dufour and Gwenaëlle Auregan for viral vector production, Françoise Fouquet for ThioS staining and Karine Cambon for advice concerning animal behavior. This work was supported by DIM Biotherapies, *région Ile-de-France*, IDEX Paris Saclay, INSERM Transfert and by a grant from "Investissement d'Avenir - ANR-11-INBS-0011" - NeurATRIS: A Translational Research Infrastructure for Biotherapies in Neurosciences. Human postmortem samples were obtained from the GIE-Neuro-CEB brain bank, which is run by a consortium of patients' associations.

Author details

[1]INSERM UMR1169, Université Paris-Sud, Université Paris-Saclay, Orsay 94100, France. [2]Université Paris Descartes, Paris, France. [3]CEA, DSV, I2BM, MIRCen, Fontenay-aux-Roses 92265, France. [4]INSERM UMR894, Centre de Psychiatrie et Neurosciences, Université Paris Descartes, Sorbonne Paris Cité, Paris, France. [5]INSERM UMS27, Fontenay-aux-Roses 92265, Université Paris-Sud, Université Paris-Saclay, Orsay 94100, France. [6]CNRS UMR9199, Fontenay-aux-Roses 92265, Université Paris-Sud, Université Paris-Saclay, Orsay 94100, France. [7]Department of Clinical Neurosciences, Laboratory of Cellular and Molecular Neurotherapies, Lausanne University Hospital, Lausanne, Switzerland. [8]Neuroscience Research Center, Laboratory of Cellular and Molecular Neurotherapies, Lausanne University Hospital, Lausanne, Switzerland.

References

1. Selkoe DJ. Alzheimer's disease: genes, proteins, and therapy. Physiol Rev. 2001;81(2):741–66.
2. Hardy J, Allsop D. Amyloid deposition as the central event in the aetiology of Alzheimer's disease. Trends Pharmacol Sci. 1991;12(10):383–8.

3. Lee JE, Han PL. An update of animal models of Alzheimer disease with a reevaluation of plaque depositions. Exp Neurobiol. 2013;22(2):84–95. doi:10.5607/en.2013.22.2.84.
4. Oddo S, Caccamo A, Shepherd JD, Murphy MP, Golde TE, Kayed R, et al. Triple-transgenic model of Alzheimer's disease with plaques and tangles. Neuron. 2003;39(3):409–21. doi:10.1016/s0896-6273(03)00434-3.
5. Jonsson T, Atwal JK, Steinberg S, Snaedal J, Jonsson PV, Bjornsson S, et al. A mutation in APP protects against Alzheimer's disease and age-related cognitive decline. Nature. 2012;488(7409):96–9. doi:10.1038/nature11283.
6. Hick M, Herrmann U, Weyer SW, Mallm JP, Tschape JA, Borgers M, et al. Acute function of secreted amyloid precursor protein fragment APPsalpha in synaptic plasticity. Acta Neuropathol. 2015;129(1):21–37. doi:10.1007/s00401-014-1368-x.
7. Doyle E, Bruce MT, Breen KC, Smith DC, Anderton B, Regan CM. Intraventricular infusions of antibodies to amyloid-beta-protein precursor impair the acquisition of a passive avoidance response in the rat. Neurosci Lett. 1990;115(1):97–102.
8. Huber G, Martin JR, Loffler J, Moreau JL. Involvement of amyloid precursor protein in memory formation in the rat: an indirect antibody approach. Brain Res. 1993;603(2):348–52.
9. Weyer SW, Zagrebelsky M, Herrmann U, Hick M, Ganss L, Gobbert J, et al. Comparative analysis of single and combined APP/APLP knockouts reveals reduced spine density in APP-KO mice that is prevented by APPsalpha expression. Acta Neuropathol Commun. 2014;2:36. doi:10.1186/2051-5960-2-36.
10. Hsiao K, Chapman P, Nilsen S, Eckman C, Harigaya Y, Younkin S, et al. Correlative memory deficits, abeta elevation, and amyloid plaques in transgenic mice. Science. 1996;274(5284):99–102.
11. Moran PM, Higgins LS, Cordell B, Moser PC. Age-related learning deficits in transgenic mice expressing the 751-amino acid isoform of human beta-amyloid precursor protein. Proc Natl Acad Sci U S A. 1995;92(12):5341–5.
12. Saito T, Matsuba Y, Mihira N, Takano J, Nilsson P, Itohara S, et al. Single App knock-in mouse models of Alzheimer's disease. Nat Neurosci. 2014;17(5):661–3. doi:10.1038/nn.3697.
13. DaRocha-Souto B, Scotton TC, Coma M, Serrano-Pozo A, Hashimoto T, Sereno L, et al. Brain oligomeric beta-amyloid but not total amyloid plaque burden correlates with neuronal loss and astrocyte inflammatory response in amyloid precursor protein/tau transgenic mice. J Neuropathol Exp Neurol. 2011;70(5):360–76. doi:10.1097/NEN.0b013e318217a118.
14. Cheng IH, Scearce-Levie K, Legleiter J, Palop JJ, Gerstein H, Bien-Ly N, et al. Accelerating amyloid-beta fibrillization reduces oligomer levels and functional deficits in Alzheimer disease mouse models. J Biol Chem. 2007;282(33):23818–28. doi:10.1074/jbc.M701078200.
15. Tomiyama T, Nagata T, Shimada H, Teraoka R, Fukushima A, Kanemitsu H, et al. A new amyloid beta variant favoring oligomerization in Alzheimer's-type dementia. Ann Neurol. 2008;63(3):377–87. doi:10.1002/ana.21321.
16. Storandt M, Mintun MA, Head D, Morris JC. Cognitive decline and brain volume loss as signatures of cerebral amyloid-beta peptide deposition identified with Pittsburgh compound B: cognitive decline associated with Abeta deposition. Arch Neurol. 2009;66(12):1476–81. doi:10.1001/archneurol.2009.272.
17. Morris JC, Roe CM, Grant EA, Head D, Storandt M, Goate AM, et al. Pittsburgh compound B imaging and prediction of progression from cognitive normality to symptomatic Alzheimer disease. Arch Neurol. 2009;66(12):1469–75. doi:10.1001/archneurol.2009.269.
18. Gibson PH. Form and distribution of senile plaques seen in silver impregnated sections in the brains of intellectually normal elderly people and people with Alzheimer-type dementia. Neuropathol Appl Neurobiol. 1983;9(5):379–89.
19. Mackenzie IR, McLachlan RS, Kubu CS, Miller LA. Prospective neuropsychological assessment of nondemented patients with biopsy proven senile plaques. Neurology. 1996;46(2):425–9.
20. Selkoe DJ. Alzheimer's disease is a synaptic failure. Science. 2002;298(5594):789–91. doi:10.1126/science.1074069.
21. Klein WL, Krafft GA, Finch CE. Targeting small abeta oligomers: the solution to an Alzheimer's disease conundrum? Trends Neurosci. 2001;24(4):219–24.
22. Salloway S, Sperling R, Fox NC, Blennow K, Klunk W, Raskind M, et al. Two phase 3 trials of bapineuzumab in mild-to-moderate Alzheimer's disease. N Engl J Med. 2014;370(4):322–33. doi:10.1056/NEJMoa1304839.
23. Cummings JL, Morstorf T, Zhong K. Alzheimer's disease drug-development pipeline: few candidates, frequent failures. Alzheimers Res Ther. 2014;6(4):37. doi:10.1186/alzrt269.
24. During MJ, Young D, Baer K, Lawlor P, Klugmann M. Development and optimization of adeno-associated virus vector transfer into the central nervous system. Methods Mol Med. 2003;76:221–36.
25. Tenenbaum L, Chtarto A, Lehtonen E, Velu T, Brotchi J, Levivier M. Recombinant AAV-mediated gene delivery to the central nervous system. J Gene Med. 2004;6 Suppl 1:S212–22. doi:10.1002/jgm.506.
26. Sauvee M, DidierLaurent G, Latarche C, Escanye MC, Olivier JL, Malaplate-Armand C. Additional use of abeta(4)(2)/abeta(4)(0) ratio with cerebrospinal fluid biomarkers P-tau and abeta(4)(2) increases the level of evidence of Alzheimer's disease pathophysiological process in routine practice. JAD. 2014;41(2):377–86. doi:10.3233/JAD-131838.
27. Bushman DM, Kaeser GE, Siddoway B, Westra JW, Rivera RR, Rehen SK et al. Genomic mosaicism with increased amyloid precursor protein (APP) gene copy number in single neurons from sporadic Alzheimer's disease brains. eLife. 2015;4. doi:10.7554/eLife.05116
28. Zerah M, Piguet F, Colle MA, Raoul S, Deschamps JY, Deniaud J et al. Intracerebral gene therapy using AAVrh.10-hARSA recombinant vector to treat patients with early-onset forms of metachromatic leukodystrophy: preclinical feasibility and safety assessments in non-human primates. Hum Gene Ther Clin Dev. 2015. doi:10.1089/humc.2014.139
29. Wanngren J, Franberg J, Svensson AI, Laudon H, Olsson F, Winblad B, et al. The large hydrophilic loop of presenilin 1 is important for regulating gamma-secretase complex assembly and dictating the amyloid beta peptide (Abeta) Profile without affecting Notch processing. J Biol Chem. 2010;285(12):8527–36. doi:10.1074/jbc.M109.055590.
30. Hardy JA, Higgins GA. Alzheimer's disease: the amyloid cascade hypothesis. Science. 1992;256(5054):184–5.
31. Jankowsky JL, Fadale DJ, Anderson J, Xu GM, Gonzales V, Jenkins NA, et al. Mutant presenilins specifically elevate the levels of the 42 residue beta-amyloid peptide in vivo: evidence for augmentation of a 42-specific gamma secretase. Hum Mol Genet. 2004;13(2):159–70. doi:10.1093/hmg/ddh019.
32. Sweeney MD, Sagare AP, Zlokovic BV. Cerebrospinal fluid biomarkers of neurovascular dysfunction in mild dementia and Alzheimer's disease. J Cereb Blood Flow Metab. 2015;35(7):1055–68. doi:10.1038/jcbfm.2015.76.
33. Murray ME, Przybelski SA, Lesnick TG, Liesinger AM, Spychalla A, Zhang B, et al. Early Alzheimer's disease neuropathology detected by proton MR spectroscopy. J Neurosci. 2014;34(49):16247–55. doi:10.1523/JNEUROSCI.2027-14.2014.
34. Scheff SW, Price DA, Schmitt FA, DeKosky ST, Mufson EJ. Synaptic alterations in CA1 in mild Alzheimer disease and mild cognitive impairment. Neurology. 2007;68(18):1501–8. doi:10.1212/01.wnl.0000260698.46517.8f.
35. Masliah E, Alford M, DeTeresa R, Mallory M, Hansen L. Deficient glutamate transport is associated with neurodegeneration in Alzheimer's disease. Ann Neurol. 1996;40(5):759–66. doi:10.1002/ana.410400512.
36. Proctor DT, Coulson EJ, Dodd PR. Reduction in post-synaptic scaffolding PSD-95 and SAP-102 protein levels in the Alzheimer inferior temporal cortex is correlated with disease pathology. JAD. 2010;21(3):795–811. doi:10.3233/JAD-2010-100090.
37. Schneider I, Reverse D, Dewachter I, Ris L, Caluwaerts N, Kuiperi C, et al. Mutant presenilins disturb neuronal calcium homeostasis in the brain of transgenic mice, decreasing the threshold for excitotoxicity and facilitating long-term potentiation. J Biol Chem. 2001;276(15):11539–44. doi:10.1074/jbc.M010977200.
38. Duff K, Eckman C, Zehr C, Yu X, Prada CM, Perez-tur J, et al. Increased amyloid-beta42(43) in brains of mice expressing mutant presenilin 1. Nature. 1996;383(6602):710–3. doi:10.1038/383710a0.
39. Walker JM, Fowler SW, Miller DK, Sun AY, Weisman GA, Wood WG, et al. Spatial learning and memory impairment and increased locomotion in a transgenic amyloid precursor protein mouse model of Alzheimer's disease. Behav Brain Res. 2011;222(1):169–75. doi:10.1016/j.bbr.2011.03.049.
40. Karran E, Mercken M, De Strooper B. The amyloid cascade hypothesis for Alzheimer's disease: an appraisal for the development of therapeutics. Nat Rev Drug Discov. 2011;10(9):698–712. doi:10.1038/nrd3505.
41. Quon D, Wang Y, Catalano R, Scardina JM, Murakami K, Cordell B. Formation of beta-amyloid protein deposits in brains of transgenic mice. Nature. 1991;352(6332):239–41. doi:10.1038/352239a0.
42. Higgins LS, Catalano R, Quon D, Cordell B. Transgenic mice expressing human beta-APP751, but not mice expressing beta-APP695, display early Alzheimer's disease-like histopathology. Ann N Y Acad Sci. 1993;695:224–7.
43. Sinha S, Lieberburg I. Cellular mechanisms of beta-amyloid production and secretion. Proc Natl Acad Sci U S A. 1999;96(20):11049–53.

44. Sudoh S, Kawamura Y, Sato S, Wang R, Saido TC, Oyama F, et al. Presenilin 1 mutations linked to familial Alzheimer's disease increase the intracellular levels of amyloid beta-protein 1-42 and its N-terminally truncated variant(s) which are generated at distinct sites. J Neurochem. 1998;71(4):1535–43.
45. Jabaudon D, Shimamoto K, Yasuda-Kamatani Y, Scanziani M, Gahwiler BH, Gerber U. Inhibition of uptake unmasks rapid extracellular turnover of glutamate of nonvesicular origin. Proc Natl Acad Sci U S A. 1999;96(15):8733–8.
46. Le Meur K, Galante M, Angulo MC, Audinat E. Tonic activation of NMDA receptors by ambient glutamate of non-synaptic origin in the rat hippocampus. J Physiol. 2007;580(Pt. 2):373–83. doi:10.1113/jphysiol.2006.123570.
47. Li S, Jin M, Koeglsperger T, Shepardson NE, Shankar GM, Selkoe DJ. Soluble Abeta oligomers inhibit long-term potentiation through a mechanism involving excessive activation of extrasynaptic NR2B-containing NMDA receptors. J Neurosci. 2011;31(18):6627–38. doi:10.1523/JNEUROSCI.0203-11.2011.
48. Schallier A, Smolders I, Van Dam D, Loyens E, De Deyn PP, Michotte A, et al. Region- and age-specific changes in glutamate transport in the AbetaPP23 mouse model for Alzheimer's disease. JAD. 2011;24(2):287–300. doi:10.3233/JAD-2011-101005.
49. Scimemi A, Meabon JS, Woltjer RL, Sullivan JM, Diamond JS, Cook DG. Amyloid-beta1-42 slows clearance of synaptically released glutamate by mislocalizing astrocytic GLT-1. J Neurosci. 2013;33(12):5312–8. doi:10.1523/JNEUROSCI.5274-12.2013.
50. Talantova M, Sanz-Blasco S, Zhang X, Xia P, Akhtar MW, Okamoto S, et al. Abeta induces astrocytic glutamate release, extrasynaptic NMDA receptor activation, and synaptic loss. Proc Natl Acad Sci U S A. 2013;110(27):E2518–27. doi:10.1073/pnas.1306832110.
51. Epelbaum S, Youssef I, Lacor PN, Chaurand P, Duplus E, Brugg B, et al. Acute amnestic encephalopathy in amyloid-beta oligomer-injected mice is due to their widespread diffusion in vivo. Neurobiol Aging. 2015;36(6):2043–52. doi:10.1016/j.neurobiolaging.2015.03.005.
52. Czajkowski R, Jayaprakash B, Wiltgen B, Rogerson T, Guzman-Karlsson MC, Barth AL, et al. Encoding and storage of spatial information in the retrosplenial cortex. Proc Natl Acad Sci U S A. 2014;111(23):8661–6. doi:10.1073/pnas.1313222111.
53. Radwanska K, Schenatto-Pereira G, Ziolkowska M, Lukasiewicz K, Giese KP. Mapping fear memory consolidation and extinction-specific expression of JunB. Neurobiol Learn Mem. 2015;125:106–12. doi:10.1016/j.nlm.2015.08.007.
54. Dejean C, Courtin J, Rozeske RR, Bonnet MC, Dousset V, Michelet T, et al. Neuronal circuits for fear expression and recovery: recent advances and potential therapeutic strategies. Biol Psychiatry. 2015;78(5):298–306. doi:10.1016/j.biopsych.2015.03.017.
55. Tackenberg C, Grinschgl S, Trutzel A, Santuccione AC, Frey MC, Konietzko U, et al. NMDA receptor subunit composition determines beta-amyloid-induced neurodegeneration and synaptic loss. Cell Death Dis. 2013;4, e608. doi:10.1038/cddis.2013.129.
56. Tokutake T, Kasuga K, Yajima R, Sekine Y, Tezuka T, Nishizawa M, et al. Hyperphosphorylation of Tau induced by naturally secreted amyloid-beta at nanomolar concentrations is modulated by insulin-dependent Akt-GSK3beta signaling pathway. J Biol Chem. 2012;287(42):35222–33. doi:10.1074/jbc.M112.348300.
57. Augustinack JC, Schneider A, Mandelkow E-M, Hyman BT. Specific tau phosphorylation sites correlate with severity of neuronal cytopathology in Alzheimer's disease. Acta Neuropathol. 2001;103(1):26–35. doi:10.1007/s004010100423.
58. Caldwell JH, Klevanski M, Saar M, Muller UC. Roles of the amyloid precursor protein family in the peripheral nervous system. Mech Dev. 2013;130(6-8):433–46. doi:10.1016/j.mod.2012.11.001.
59. Kogel D, Deller T, Behl C. Roles of amyloid precursor protein family members in neuroprotection, stress signaling and aging. Exp Brain Res. 2012;217(3-4):471–9. doi:10.1007/s00221-011-2932-4.
60. Volianskis A, Kostner R, Molgaard M, Hass S, Jensen MS. Episodic memory deficits are not related to altered glutamatergic synaptic transmission and plasticity in the CA1 hippocampus of the APPswe/PS1deltaE9-deleted transgenic mice model of ss-amyloidosis. Neurobiol Aging. 2010;31(7):1173–87. doi:10.1016/j.neurobiolaging.2008.08.005.
61. Berger A, Lorain S, Josephine C, Desrosiers M, Peccate C, Voit T, et al. Repair of Rhodopsin mRNA by spliceosome-mediated RNA trans-splicing: a new approach for autosomal dominant retinitis pigmentosa. Mol Ther. 2015. doi:10.1038/mt.2015.11.
62. Anderson WW, Collingridge GL. The LTP Program: a data acquisition program for on-line analysis of long-term potentiation and other synaptic events. J Neurosci Methods. 2001;108(1):71–83.

12

Dynamic presenilin 1 and synaptotagmin 1 interaction modulates exocytosis and amyloid β production

Katarzyna Marta Zoltowska[1], Masato Maesako[1], Iryna Lushnikova[2], Shuko Takeda[1], Laura J. Keller[1], Galina Skibo[2], Bradley T. Hyman[1] and Oksana Berezovska[1*]

Abstract

Background: Alzheimer's disease (AD)-linked protein, presenilin 1 (PS1), is present at the synapse, and the knock-out of presenilin in mice leads to synaptic dysfunction. On the other hand, synaptic activity was shown to influence PS1-dependent generation of distinct amyloid β (Aβ) species. However, the precise nature of these regulations remains unclear. The current study reveals novel role of PS1 at the synapse, and deciphers how PS1 and synaptic vesicle-associated protein, synaptotagmin 1 (Syt1) modulate each other functions in neurons via direct activity-triggered interaction. Additionally, the therapeutic potential of fostering PS1-Syt1 binding is investigated as a synapse-specific strategy for AD prevention.

Methods: PS1-based cell-permeable peptide targeting PS1-Syt1 binding site was designed to inhibit PS1-Syt1 interaction in neurons. PS1 conformation, synaptic vesicle exocytosis and trafficking were assayed by fluorescence lifetime imaging microscopy (FLIM), glutamate release/synaptopHluorin assay, and fluorescence recovery after photobleaching, respectively. Syt1 level and interaction with PS1 in control and sporadic AD brains were determined by immunohistochemistry and FLIM. AAV-mediated delivery of Syt1 into mouse hippocampi was used to investigate the therapeutic potential of strengthening PS1-Syt1 binding in vivo. Statistical significance was determined using two-tailed unpaired Student's t-test, Mann-Whitney's *U*-test or two-way ANOVA followed by a Bonferroni's post-test.

Results: We demonstrate that targeted inhibition of the PS1-Syt1 binding in neurons, without changing the proteins' expression level, triggers "pathogenic" conformational shift of PS1, and consequent increase in the Aβ42/40 ratio. Moreover, our data indicate that PS1, by binding directly to Syt1, regulates synaptic vesicle trafficking and facilitates exocytosis and neurotransmitter release. Analysis of human brain tissue revealed that not only Syt1 levels but also interactions between remaining Syt1 and PS1 are diminished in sporadic AD. On the other hand, overexpression of Syt1 in mouse hippocampi was found to potentiate PS1-Syt1 binding and promote "protective" PS1 conformation.

Conclusions: The study reports novel functions of PS1 and Syt1 at the synapse, and demonstrates the importance of PS1-Syt1 binding for exocytosis and safeguarding PS1 conformation. It suggests that reduction in the Syt1 level and PS1-Syt1 interactions in AD brain may present molecular underpinning of the pathogenic PS1 conformation, increased Aβ42/40 ratio, and impaired exocytosis.

Keywords: Presenilin 1, Synaptotagmin 1, Synapse, Exocytosis, Amyloid β, Alzheimer's disease

* Correspondence: oberezovska@mgh.harvard.edu
[1]Department of Neurology, MassGeneral Institute for Neurodegenerative Disease, Massachusetts General Hospital, Harvard Medical School, 114 16th Street, Rm. 2006, 02129 Charlestown, MA, USA
Full list of author information is available at the end of the article

Background

Aberrant amyloid β (Aβ) generation resulting in increased Aβ42/total ratio, and loss of cortical and hippocampal synapses have been established as important contributors to Alzheimer's disease (AD) pathophysiology [1–8]. However, amyloid deposition and reduced levels of synaptic proteins found in postmortem human brain tissue do not reveal the early stage molecular events preceding the observed pathology, and do not allow to determine dynamic functional relationship between the synaptic impairments and Aβ generating machinery.

The amyloid precursor protein (APP) and its processing enzymes, β-secretase 1 (BACE1) and presenilin 1 (PS1)/γ-secretase, are abundantly present at the synaptic terminals [9–12], enabling local production of Aβ. The generation of the longer Aβ42/43 species readily forming toxic oligomers is influenced by the PS1/γ-secretase conformational state [13–20]. Fluorescence lifetime imaging microscopy (FLIM) and real-time Förster resonance energy transfer (FRET) assays of the PS1 domain arrangement demonstrated that PS1 exists in a dynamic equilibrium of conformational states. Although the assays do not address the detailed structural rearrangements within the PS1 molecule, they can reliably distinguish between the normal, so-called "open" and pathogenic, named "closed" PS1 conformations. These are characterized by greater and smaller distance, respectively, between the fluorophores labeling different PS1 domains. "Open" and "closed" PS1 conformations correspond to lower and higher ratio of the Aβ42 to Aβ40 peptides, respectively [12, 15, 21, 22]. However, the precise molecular mechanisms altering the arrangement of the PS1 domains in neurons remain unknown.

Although the role of PS1 in Aβ generation has received the greatest attention, presenilin knockout studies have suggested that PS1 may also be involved in neurotransmission [23, 24]. However, the exact role of the "undisturbed" PS1, expressed at the physiological level, and the specific molecular mechanism of its involvement in synaptic vesicle release remain unexplored.

It has recently been reported that both APP [25, 26] and PS1 interact with the pre-synaptic protein synaptotagmin 1 (Syt1) [12], a calcium sensor in synaptic vesicle exocytosis and neurotransmitter release [27–29]. Moreover, knock-down of Syt1 in PC12 cell line was found to alter APP processing and reduce Aβ generation [12, 25]. However, Syt1 knock-down also impaired subcellular compartmentalization of PS1 and BACE1, resulting in decreased maturation and stability of BACE1, and diminished γ-secretase activity [12, 25]. Therefore, the significance of the direct PS1-Syt1 binding per se, as well as functional outcomes of the disrupted PS1-Syt1 interaction for synaptic physiology and/or their relevance to AD pathology remain unknown.

In the current study we investigate in detail the functional interplay between PS1 and Syt1 by selectively targeting the PS1-Syt1 binding using PS1-based cell-permeable peptide corresponding to the PS1-Syt1 interaction site, without altering the proteins' expression level. Using complementary cell/molecular biology approaches and functional assays, we present evidence that calcium influx-induced binding between PS1 and Syt1 is essential for regulation of the synaptic vesicle trafficking along neuronal processes, promotion of exocytosis and neurotransmitter release. Moreover, we provide direct evidence that Syt1 binding to PS1 is important for maintenance of the protective PS1 conformation in neurons, and for determination of the local, synaptic pool of Aβ species. Finally, we demonstrate that not only Syt1 levels but also proximity between the remaining Syt1 and PS1 is decreased in sporadic AD brain, and that overexpression of Syt1 in vivo has potential to promote PS1-Syt1 interaction, and to stabilize the protective, "open" PS1 conformation.

Methods

Human brain tissue

The medial temporal cortex of the sporadic Alzheimer's disease (sAD) patients (92.25 ± 4.52 years old) with neuropathologically confirmed Braak V-VI stage, and age- (90.75 ± 1.60 years old) and post mortem interval-matched control tissue was obtained from the Massachusetts Alzheimer's Disease Research Center Brain Bank. For the immunohistochemical analysis, medial temporal lobe specimens were fixed for 48 h with 4% paraformaldehyde (PFA) and cut into 50 μm coronal sections using a sliding freezing microtome (Leica SM 2000R, Bannockburn, IL).

Animal research

Syt1-V5 expression in vivo in hippocampi of wild type male C57BL/6 mice was achieved using stereotaxic injection (stereotaxic coordinates from bregma: 3.1 mm posterior; 2.8 mm lateral and 2.5 mm depth from brain surface) of adeno-associated viruses serotype 2/8 (AAV2/8) carrying hSyn. Syt1-V5 or control, empty, expression plasmids. One month after the AAV2/8 injection, the mice were sacrificed.

The mice were euthanized using CO_2 asphyxiation and perfused intracardially with phosphate-buffered saline (PBS). The brains were dissected, fixed by immersion in 4% PFA, 15% glycerol (Sigma-Aldrich, Saint Louis, MO) in PBS and cryoprotected using 30% glycerol in PBS. Prior to immunostaining, the brains were cut on freezing sliding microtome (Leica SM 2000R, Bannockburn, IL) into 35 μm-thick coronal sections.

Cell culture

Rat pheochromacytoma cell line (PC12) was a kind gift from Dr. Amy B. Harkins (St. Louis University School of

Medicine, St. Louis, MO) [30]. The PC12 cells were cultured in RPMI Medium 1640 supplemented with 10% heat-inactivated horse serum, 5% fetal bovine serum (FBS) (ThermoScientific, Waltham, MA) in a 37 °C, 5% CO_2 incubator. Transfections were performed using lipofectamine 3000 (ThermoScientific, Waltham, MA) according manufacturer's protocol.

Mouse embryonic fibroblasts (MEF) with *PSEN1* and *PSEN2* knock-out (PS DKO) and MEF PS DKO stably expressing PS1 wt or PS1 Δe9 were kind gifts from Dr. Bart De Strooper [31]. The cells were maintained in OptiMEM supplemented with 5% fetal bovine serum (FBS) (ThermoScientific, Waltham, MA) in a 37 °C, 5% CO_2 incubator. Transfections were performed using lipofectamine LTX with Plus reagent (ThermoScientific, Waltham, MA) according manufacturer's protocol.

Mixed cortical primary neurons from 16 to 18 embryonic-day-old embryos were enzymatically dissociated using papain dissociation system (Worthington Biochemical Corporation, Lakewood, NJ). The neuronal cultures were maintained in Neurobasal medium supplemented with 2% B27 supplement, 1% GlutaMax, and 1% penicilin/streptomycin mix (ThermoScientific, Waltham, MA) in a 37 °C, 5% CO_2 incubator. The neurons were transfected using lipofectamine 2000 (ThermoScientific, Waltham, MA) following the supplier's protocol.

Chemicals and treatments

Calcium influx was induced by 15-min application of 50 mM KCl (Sigma-Aldrich, Saint Louis, MO) for neurons and PC12 cell line, or of 5 μM A23187 calcium ionophore (Sigma-Aldrich, Saint Louis, MO) for MEFs.

PS1-Syt1 interactions were blocked by incubating primary neurons for 2 h at 37 °C with 5 μM of cell-permeable peptide (CPP), we named PS1-LNT. The PS1-LNT was obtained by fusing 47–57 amino acids (aa) from HIV1 TAT protein (YGRKKRRQRRR) with the N-terminal portion of the cytosolic PS1 loop domain through a GGG linker. A peptide comprising 47–57 aa from HIV1 TAT fused to a scramble sequence ENSFRFLADIFPAKAFPV RFE through a GGG linker was used as a negative control. The peptides were synthesized at the MGH peptide/protein core facility https://researchcores.partners.org/pepcor/about.

Expression plasmids

Human wild type (wt) presenilin 1 (PS1) was cloned into pcDNA™3.1. (+) (ThermoScientific, Waltham, MA). The PS1 sequence was tagged with an N-terminal FLAG and His tags to facilitate detection of exogenous versus endogenous PS1.

The His-FLAG-huPS1 construct (PS1 del265-279) was created by introducing 15 aa deletion within the huPS1 sequence using a QuickChange site-directed mutagenesis kit (Stratagene, La Jolla, CA) according to the manufacturer's recommendation.

Human wt synaptotagmin 1 (Syt1) was cloned into pcDNA™ 6 V5 Myc expression vector (ThermoScientific, Waltham, MA).

Plasmids encoding vesicular glutamate transporter 1 (vGlut1) fused with pH-sensitive GFP (synaptophluorin (SypHy)), eGFP-tagged synaptophysin (eGFP-Syp) and eGFP-tagged tubulin (eGFP-Tub) were kind gifts from Dr Pamela McLean (Mayo Clinic, Jacksonville, FL).

Cytotoxicity assay

Cytotoxicity was analyzed using lactate dehydrogenase (LDH) cytotoxicity assay (Roche, Indianapolis, IN). Briefly, conditioned medium was collected from the respective wells, mixed with the assay solution, incubated for 20 min in the dark, and the absorbance at 490 nm was measured using a spectrophotometer. For a positive control, cells were incubated for 45 min at 37 °C with 1% Triton X (TX)-100.

ELISA for Aβ40 and Aβ42

Intracellular or secreted level of Aβ was quantified using human/rat Aβ40 and Aβ42 (high-sensitive) enzyme-linked immunosorbent assay (ELISA) kits (Wako, Japan) according to the manufacturer's protocol. The Aβ levels detected in the conditioned medium or cell lysates (determined in [pmol]), were normalized to the total amount of protein extracted from the respective cells (quantified in [g]) using BCA protein assay (Pierce, Rockford, IL).

Glutamate release assay

Glutamate release was stimulated by application of 50 mM KCl in Hank's balanced salt solution after 2-h pre-treatment with scramble or PS1-LNT peptides. The glutamate uptake was inhibited by the addition of *DL*-threo-β-benzyloxyaspartate (DL-TBOA), an excitatory amino acid transporters 1 and 2 (EAAT1, EAAT2) inhibitor [32]. The level of glutamate in the conditioned medium was determined using Amplex Glutamate assay (ThermoScientific, Waltham, MA) according to the manufacturer's protocol. Overnight pre-treatment with 37 nM tetanus toxin (TeTx) was used as a control.

NanoOrange protein quantitation

The total amount of protein in the conditioned medium collected from neurons pre-treated for 2 h with scramble or PS1-LNT peptides, and stimulated for 15 min with 50 mM KCl was determined using NanoOrange protein quantitation assay (ThermoScientific, Waltham, MA), according the manufacturer's protocol. Briefly, the serum-free conditioned medium was diluted 100 times in NanoOrange reagent, and the mixtures were heated at

95 °C for 10 min protected from light. The samples were cooled down to room temperature, and the fluorescence, corresponding to the total amount of protein in the samples, was measured using Wallac Victor 2 plate reader (PerkinElmer, Waltham, MA) with filters and settings allowing excitation at 485 nm and capturing the emission at 590 nm. Standard curve was generated by serial dilution of the bovine serum albumin (BSA) in the NanoOrange reagent.

Exocytosis assay

The exocytosis was monitored using a previously established protocol [33, 34]. Briefly, the primary neurons were transfected with a construct encoding a pH-sensitive reporter of synaptic vesicle exocytosis, synaptophluorin (SypHy). The acidic pH of the synaptic vesicles results in quenching of the SypHy fluorescence. During the exocytosis event the pH-sensor is exposed to the extracellular neutral pH, which results in the dequenching of the SypHy signal. The SypHy was excited using 488 nm Argon laser at low power, 4–6% to reduce photobleaching and phototoxicity, and the fluorescence was monitored at 63x magnification using time-lapse recording with 3 s interval on Zeiss 510 Meta laser scanning confocal microscope equipped with ZEN 2009 software. First, five frames were collected before the stimulus to determine the baseline SypHy fluorescence in cells pre-treated for 2 h with the scramble or PS1-LNT peptides at 5 μM concentration. Then exocytosis was triggered by 50 mM KCl stimulation, and the subsequent frames were acquired immediately following the KCl application. The laser intensity and photomultiplier parameters (PMTs) were adjusted to avoid saturation of the signal on both pre- and post-stimulus images. The fluorescence intensity of the SypHy pre- and post-stimulus was analyzed using ImageJ 1.46c software. The region of interests (ROIs) were selected around the spatially resolved SypHy-positive puncta corresponding to synaptic terminals.

Fluorescence recovery after photobleaching (FRAP)

The 12-14 DIV neurons were transfected with plasmids encoding eGFP-synaptophysin (eGFP-Syp) as a fluorescent reporter of synaptic vesicles or eGFP-tubulin (eGFP-Tub) as a control. For the imaging the culture medium was substituted with Hank's balanced salt solution (HBSS) (ThermoScientific, Waltham, MA), and the cell culture dishes were placed on an imaging stage in the microscope environmental chamber (37 °C, 5% CO_2). The eGFP was excited using 488 nm Argon laser at low power (2–4%) to avoid photobleaching during the time-lapse imaging; the emitted light was passed through a band pass emission filter. Five pre-bleach images at 63x magnification with 2x zoom were recorded to determine the baseline fluorescence intensity of the target protein. Then, the eGFP-Syp or eGFP-Tub fluorescence was photobleached within the selected ROIs using 75 iterations with 100% 488 nm Argon laser, and the imaging was continued for 90 s using time-lapse recording with 1-s intervals. Three ROIs were recorded and analyzed: bleached, control (not bleached), and background. The fluorescence intensities of the selected ROIs were measured using ImageJ 1.46c software.

The recorded data were analyzed with Microsoft Excel 2007 and GraphPad Prism 5 software. Following the background subtraction, the intensity of the bleached ROI was normalized to its initial pre-bleach intensity (calculated as an average of the 5 pre-bleach frames) and to the intensity of the control, not bleached region. Then the data were further normalized in respect to the intensities immediately after bleaching (value = 0, full scale normalization). In order to determine the statistical difference between the conditions, the mean fluorescence recovery 10 s post-bleach was compared using unpaired Student's t-test.

Analysis of the spine density and spine morphology

Mouse primary neurons at 12–14 DIV were transfected with pcDNA-eGFP. Two days post-transfection the neurons were pre-treated for 2 h with scramble or PS1-LNT peptides and depolarized for 15 min with 50 mM KCl. The spine density and morphology were examined using the LSM 510 Zeiss confocal microscope equipped with the 488 nm excitation laser. The images were captured at 63x magnification, and consisted of a *z*-stack of pictures taken at 0.5 μm intervals, and then projected into one image. The images were analyzed using NeuronStudio software [35]. The spine density was calculated by dividing the number of spines by the length of the corresponding neurite. In addition, the spines were categorized into three morphological classes: mushroom, stubby and thin using an algorithm implemented in the NeuronStudio application. 30 neurites per condition from eight independent experiments were analyzed.

Immunoprecipitation (IP)

Cells were lysed in 1% 3-[(3-cholamidopropyl) dimethylammonio]-2-hydroxy-1-propanesulfonate (CHAPS) buffer (50 mM HEPES, 100 mM NaCl, pH 7.4 and 1% CHAPS) supplemented with HALT protease and phosphatase inhibitor cocktails (ThermoScientific, Waltham, MA) by pipetting up-and-down, passing through a 37-gauge needle and rotating for 1 h at 4 °C. The lysates were centrifuged at 14,000xg for 15 min and the supernatants were collected for the IP. Total protein in the samples was measured using ThermoScientific Pierce BCA Protein Assay (ThermoScientific, Waltham, MA). The aliquots of the supernatant containing equal protein amount were incubated with 3 μg of the respective antibody or normal IgG, as a negative control, with end-over-end rotation over night at 4 °C. Subsequently, 30 μl of Protein G Dynabeads (ThermoScientific, Waltham, MA) were added to the samples and incubated with end-over-end rotation for 10 min at room temperature. The beads were collected using a magnetic tube rack, washed twice with the 1% CHAPS buffer and once with the wash buffer containing 50 mM HEPES, 100 mM NaCl, pH7.4. The protein was eluted by 5-min boiling in 25 μl 2x LDS, 1x reducing agent buffer (ThermoScientific, Waltham, MA).

Immobilized metal affinity chromatography (IMAC)

IMAC technique was used to pull down His-PS1 and endogenous Syt1 complexes from PC12 cells transfected with His-tagged PS1 wt or PS1 del265-279. Briefly, 24 h following the transfection the cells were stimulated for 15 min with 50 mM KCl, harvested and lysed in a buffer containing 50 mM HEPES, 100 mM NaCl, protease inhibitors (Roche, Indianapolis, Indiana) and 1% CHAPS. The lysates were incubated for 1 h at 4 °C and centrifuged at 14,000xg for 15 min to collect the soluble fractions. Protein concentration in each sample was determined using a BCA assay (ThermoScientific, Waltham, MA) according the manufacturer's recommendations. The samples with equal amount of protein were supplemented with 20 mM imidazole to reduce non-specific binding, and were incubated for 2 min with 30 μl MagneHis Ni-Particles (Promega, Madison, WI). Following the incubation, the beads were washed 3 times with the lysis buffer, and the protein was eluted with the elution buffer provided with the MagneHis Ni-Particles, containing 500 mM imidazole.

In vitro PS1-Syt1 binding assay

Syt1 tagged with V5 and His was overexpressed in PS DKO MEF cells. The protein was extracted from the cells using a lysis buffer containing 50 mM HEPES, 100 mM NaCl, protease inhibitors (Roche, Indianapolis, Indiana) and 1% TX-100, and was immobilized on the MagneHis Ni-Particles (Promega, Madison, WI) by 2-min incubation in the presence of 20 mM imidazole to reduce non-specific binding. Subsequently, 30 μl of the Syt1-V5-His bound beads were added to the mouse brain lysates containing 2 mg of total protein and prepared in a buffer containing 50 mM HEPES, 100 mM NaCl, protease inhibitors (Roche, Indianapolis, Indiana), 1% CHAPS, 20 mM imidazole, 2 mM $CaCl_2$. 100 μg of PS1-LNT or scramble, as a negative control, peptides were added to the samples. Additional negative controls included Syt1-V5-His bound beads incubated with the lysis buffer only, or empty beads incubated with the mouse brain lysates. The mixtures were incubated overnight at 4 °C with end-over-end rotation. Then, the beads were washed 3 times with the 1% CHAPS-based lysis buffer, and the attached protein was eluted with the elution buffer provided with the MagneHis Ni-Particles, containing 500 mM imidazole.

Western blotting

The proteins were resolved by electrophoresis on 4–12% Bis-Tris NuPage polyacrylamide gels (ThermoScientific, Waltham, MA) and transferred to nitrocellulose membranes (GE Healthcare Lifesciences, Pittsburgh, PA) using the BioRad system. Proteins were detected by immunoblotting with specific primary and corresponding IRdye680/800- or HRP-conjugated secondary antibodies. The membranes were developed using Odyssey Infrared Imaging System (Li-COR, Lincoln, NE) or ECL Western Blotting Substrate (Pierce, Rockford, IL), respectively. The exposure times were adjusted to avoid signal saturation. The relative amounts of the proteins were measured by densitometry using ImageStudio Lite Ver 5.2 or ImageJ 1.46c software, respectively.

Immunocytochemistry (ICC) and immunohistochemistry (IHC)

Cultured cells or brain tissue slices were fixed with 4% PFA, permeabilized using 0.1% TX-100 or 0.4% TX-100, respectively, and non-specific binding of the antibodies was blocked by incubation with 1.5% normal donkey serum (Jackson ImmunoResearch Labs, West Grove, PA). The permeabilized and blocked samples were incubated with primary antibodies overnight at 4 °C. Excess antibodies were washed off and the samples were incubated with corresponding Alexa Fluor 488- or Cy3-conjugated secondary antibodies for 1 h at room temperature. To visualize actin cytoskeleton, the cells were incubated with fluorophore-conjugated phalloidin (ThermoScientific, Waltham, MA) according to the manufacturer's protocol. The medium was supplemented with 4′, 6-diamidino-2-phenylindole dihydrochloride (DAPI) when visualization of nuclei was required. The slides were mounted with VectaShield mounting medium (Vector Laboratories, Inc., Burlingame, CA).

Antibodies

The following primary antibodies were used: anti-APP CT (A8717, Sigma-Aldrich, St. Louis, MO); anti-β-amyloid, 17–24 (clone 4G8) (800701, BioLegend, San Diego, CA); anti-PS1 NT raised against the N terminus of PS1 (APS11) (ab15456, Abcam, Cambridge, MA); anti-PS1 CT raised against the C-terminus of PS1 (mAb5643, Cell Signaling Technology, Danvers, MA); anti-PS1 loop raised against the loop domain between transmembrane domains 6 and 7 of PS1 (E2000Y) (ab76083, Abcam, Cambridge, MA); anti-Syt1 (AB5600, Millipore, Temecula, CA); anti-Gapdh (mAb2118, Cell Signaling Technology, Danvers, MA); anti-MAP2 (ab5392, Abcam, Cambridge, MA); anti-His (ab18184,

Abcam, Cambridge, MA); anti-V5 (ab9116, Abcam, Cambridge) and anti-FLAG M2 (F1804, Sigma-Aldrich, St. Louis, MO). Alexa Fluor 488 (ThermoScientific, Waltham, MA) and Cy3-labeled corresponding secondary antibodies (Jackson ImmunoResearch, West Grove, PA) were used for confocal microscopy imaging, and IRDye680/800- (Li-COR, Lincoln, NE) or HRP- (Jackson ImmunoResearch, West Grove, PA) conjugated ones were used for western blotting.

Fluorescent lifetime imaging microscopy (FLIM)

The proximity between PS1 and Syt1 or PS1 NT and PS1 loop domain was evaluated by a previously validated Förster Resonance Energy Transfer (FRET)-based fluorescence lifetime imaging microscopy (FLIM) assay [22, 36, 37]. The samples were immunostained with the following pairs of primary antibodies: a) anti-PS1 NT (APS11) (ab15456, Abcam, Cambridge, MA) and anti-Syt1 (AB5600, Millipore, Temecula, CA) or anti-FLAG M2 (F1804, Sigma-Aldrich, St. Louis, MO) and anti-Syt1 for analysis of PS1-Syt1 interaction; b) anti-PS1 NT (APS11) and anti-PS1 loop (EP2000Y) (ab76083, Abcam, Cambridge, MA) for the analysis of PS1 conformation. Alexa Fluor 488 (AF488) and Cy3-labeled corresponding secondary antibodies were used as the donor and acceptor fluorophores, respectively. AF488 donor fluorophore was excited using pulsing Chameleon Ti:Sapphire laser (Coherent Inc., Santa Clara, CA) (two-photon excitation at 780 nm or 800 nm wavelength, respectively). The baseline lifetime ($t1$) of the AF488 donor fluorophore in the absence of the Cy3 acceptor was used as a negative control. The donor lifetimes were determined using a high-speed photomultiplier tube (MCP R3809; Hamamatsu, Bridgewater, NJ) and a fast time-correlated single-photon counting acquisition board (SPC-830; Becker & Hickl, Berlin, Germany). Bright fluorophores were chosen, and prolonged image acquisition at low laser power was applied in order to acquire sufficient number of photons for accurate curve fitting, without photobleaching of the samples. The lack of photobleaching was established by the lack of noticeable decrease in the count rate during acquisition time, and was confirmed by analysis of the fluorescence intensity in pre- and post-acquisition confocal images. Typically, 1,000–5,000 photons per analyzed pixel (within the selected intensity-thresholded region of interest (ROI)) were acquired. If necessary, binning was applied to increase the signal to noise ratio. The data were analyzed using SPCImage software (Becker & Hickl, Berlin, Germany). The analysis was performed on a cell-by-cell basis, and the threshold was adjusted in order to exclude the low intensity background fluorescence. The ROIs were selected by outlining the neurons, and the average fluorescence lifetimes per neuron were determined. Two analysis modes were applied: two component analysis for cells in vitro and mouse tissue and three component analysis for human brain tissue to account for the presence of autofluorescence, as described previously [38]. The lifetimes of the "non-FRET" donor (t_1), and if applicable of the autofluorescence (t_3), were "fixed" and the remaining lifetime reflecting the presence of FRET was calculated by the system as the t_2 value. This approach allows the exclusion of the "non-FRETing" components, and thus reliable quantification of the relative distances between the fluorophores, irrespectively of their absolute amounts. Moreover, it significantly improves the accuracy of the multicomponent analysis [39]. The fluorescence lifetime of the "non-FRETing" donor, determined independently in every single experiment was ~2.5 ns. Of note, the 4.1 ns has been reported for the unconjugated Alexa Fluor 488 dye. However, conjugation of the dye to the antibody results in the reduction in its fluorescence lifetime [40]. To calculate $\%E_{FRET}$ the following equation was used: $\%E_{FRET} = 100^*(t_1\text{-}t_2)/t_1$.

The calculated lifetimes t_2 were displayed on a 128×128 pixel matrix to create the pseudocoloured images where green-to-red pixels represent shorter lifetimes, indicative of short distance between the fluorophores, whereas blue pixels correspond to longer lifetimes, indicative of a greater distance between the donor and the acceptor. In the images, the lifetimes were weighted by intensity, and a threshold was adjusted to exclude dim pixels. Importantly, all the analyses and the display parameters were kept constant in each experiment, providing the most accurate quantification of the acquired data.

Electron microscopy

Electron microscopy was applied to analyze the size and distribution of the synaptic vesicles in mouse primary neurons in vitro. The 12-14 DIV neuronal cultures were fixed with ice-cold 2% PFA and 0.2% glutaraldehyde (Sigma-Aldrich, St. Louis, MO) for 1 h at 4 °C. Then the cells were washed three times with 0.1M phosphate buffer pH 7.4 (PB), stained with 1% OsO_4 in 0.1 M PB for 1 h, dehydrated in graded ethanol series and flat-embedded in EPON (Fluka). Ultrathin (50–60 nm thick) sections were cut with an ultratome (LKB 8800, Sweden), stained for 20 min with 5% uranyl acetate and 30 s in lead citrate, and examined using a JEM100-CX transmission electron microscope (Japan). The images, taken at magnifications of x19,000, were scanned with a flatbed scanner at 600 dpi and 256 gray levels. Quantitative image analysis was carried out using the ImageJ 1.46c software.

Statistics

Statistics were calculated with Microsoft Office Excel 2007. The graphs were prepared with GraphPad® Prism 5 (GraphPad Prism Software inc., La Jolla, CA). Gaussian distribution of the data was determined using D'Agostino & Pearson omnibus normality test. The F statistics were calculated to determine the variance equality. Subsequently, a standard two-tailed unpaired Student's t-test or Welch t-test was calculated for the normally distributed data and Mann-Whitney's *U*-test for the data, which did not meet the latter criterion. Glutamate release, cytotoxicity and frequency distribution of synaptic vesicles data were analyzed using two-way ANOVA followed by a Bonferroni's post-test. A *p*-value of <0.05 was considered a predetermined threshold for statistical significance.

Results

Peptide corresponding to the N-terminal fragment of the L6-7 domain of PS1 inhibits PS1-Syt1 interaction

Our previous data suggest that the interaction site between presenilin 1 (PS1) and synaptotagmin 1 (Syt1) is potentially located within the N-terminal part of the PS1 cytosolic loop domain between 6th and 7th transmembrane helices (L6-7) [12]. First, to confirm that this region is indeed critical for the PS1-Syt1 binding, fifteen amino acid deletion (del265-279) was introduced within the PS1 sequence (Fig. 1a). The construct was expressed in PC12 cells, and the proximity between PS1 and Syt1 was analyzed using antibody-based fluorescence lifetime imaging microscopy (FLIM) assay in 15-min 50 mM KCl stimulated cells. N-terminal PS1 FLAG-tag was used for PS1 detection to selectively visualize exogenous mutant PS1. Reduced Förster resonance energy transfer (FRET) efficiency indicates that the PS1 deletion mutant shows reduced binding to Syt1, as compared to the wild type (wt) PS1 (Fig. 1b and Additional file 1), supporting the importance of the PS1 aa 265-279 for PS1-Syt1 interaction.

These findings were further validated by a complementary approach: immobilized metal affinity chromatography (IMAC), designed for selective isolation of the His-tagged proteins. PC12 cells were transiently transfected with His-tagged wt or del265-279 mutant PS1, stimulated for 15 min with 50 mM KCl, and His-PS1 and endogenous Syt1 complexes were analyzed. We found that deletion of the amino acids 265–279 within the PS1 sequence significantly inhibits the PS1-Syt1 binding (Fig. 1c).

Of note, the PS1-Syt1 interaction is not dependent on the PS1 endoproteolysis, as demonstrated by successful pull-down of His-V5-tagged Syt1-PS1 wt as well as His-V5-Syt1-PS1Δe9, lacking the endoproteolysis site, complexes from PS double knock-out mouse embryonic fibroblasts (PS DKO MEF) stably expressing respective PS1 variants and transiently transfected with His-V5-Syt1 (Fig. 1d).

Based on these data, we designed a peptide corresponding to the N-terminus of the PS1 loop domain (PS1-LNT) to inhibit the PS1-Syt1 binding. The fragment was fused with positively charged TAT HIV1 epitope to enable cell permeability. In addition, for the initial experiments aiming to monitor the peptide intracellular delivery, PS1-LNT was conjugated with the fluorescein isothiocyanate (FITC) (Fig. 2a).

As shown in Fig. 2, PS1-LNT-FITC at 5 μM can efficiently permeate the cells within 2-h incubation (Fig. 2b) without causing any toxicity (Fig. 2c). We also determined that PS1-LNT does not alter PS1 endoproteolysis, as demonstrated by the lack of significant changes in PS1 NTF and PS1 CTF generation (Fig. 2d).

Next, to assess if the PS1-LNT can inhibit the target interaction, we monitored proximity between endogenous PS1 and Syt1 in intact primary neurons. For this, the cells were pre-treated for 2 h with PS1-LNT or scramble peptide as a control, stimulated for 15 min with 50 mM KCl or H_2O vehicle, immunostained with anti-PS1 NT and anti-Syt1 antibodies, and relative proximity between the fluorescently labeled proteins was determined by FLIM. PS1-LNT did not have any noticeable effect on the PS1-Syt1 interaction in the absence of KCl stimulation, due to relatively low intracellular calcium concentration and minimal spontaneous activity of the in vitro cultured primary neurons [41]. Thus, observed calcium-dependent PS1-Syt1 binding is relatively scarce at the basal condition, as visualized by the occasional red pixels on the pseudo-colored FLIM images (Fig. 3a). As expected, KCl-mediated synchronous calcium influx increased the relative FRET efficiency (PS1-Syt1 proximity) by $29.53 \pm 5.15\%$, $p < 0.0001$ in scramble peptide pre-treated cells, similarly to that in non-pre-treated neurons [12] (Fig. 3a and Additional file 1). However, KCl failed to increase the E_{FRET} in the PS1-LNT pre-treated neurons (Fig. 3a and Additional file 1). These data demonstrate that the effect of the PS1-LNT peptide is the most pronounced in the KCl(+) condition, when it reduces the efficiency of the PS1-Syt1 binding.

The ability of the PS1-LNT peptide to impede calcium-dependent PS1-Syt1 interaction was further confirmed using a complementary approach: IMAC in vitro PS1-Syt1 binding assay. His-V5-Syt1, extracted from the PS DKO MEF cells transiently transfected with His-V5-Syt1, was immobilized on the beads, and the beads were incubated with mouse brain lysates, supplemented with 2 mM Ca^{2+}, in the presence of scramble or PS1-LNT peptide. Binding of the endogenous PS1 to the immobilized His-V5-Syt1 was observed only in the presence of scramble peptide, and was blocked by the presence of PS1-LNT (Fig. 3b).

Together, these data confirm the ability of PS1-LNT peptide to inhibit calcium-triggered PS1-Syt1 interaction in primary neurons.

PS1-Syt1 interaction modulates PS1 conformation and Aβ secretion

We have previously demonstrated that PS1/γ-secretase exists in a dynamic equilibrium of the distinct conformational states, so called "closed" and "open", as determined

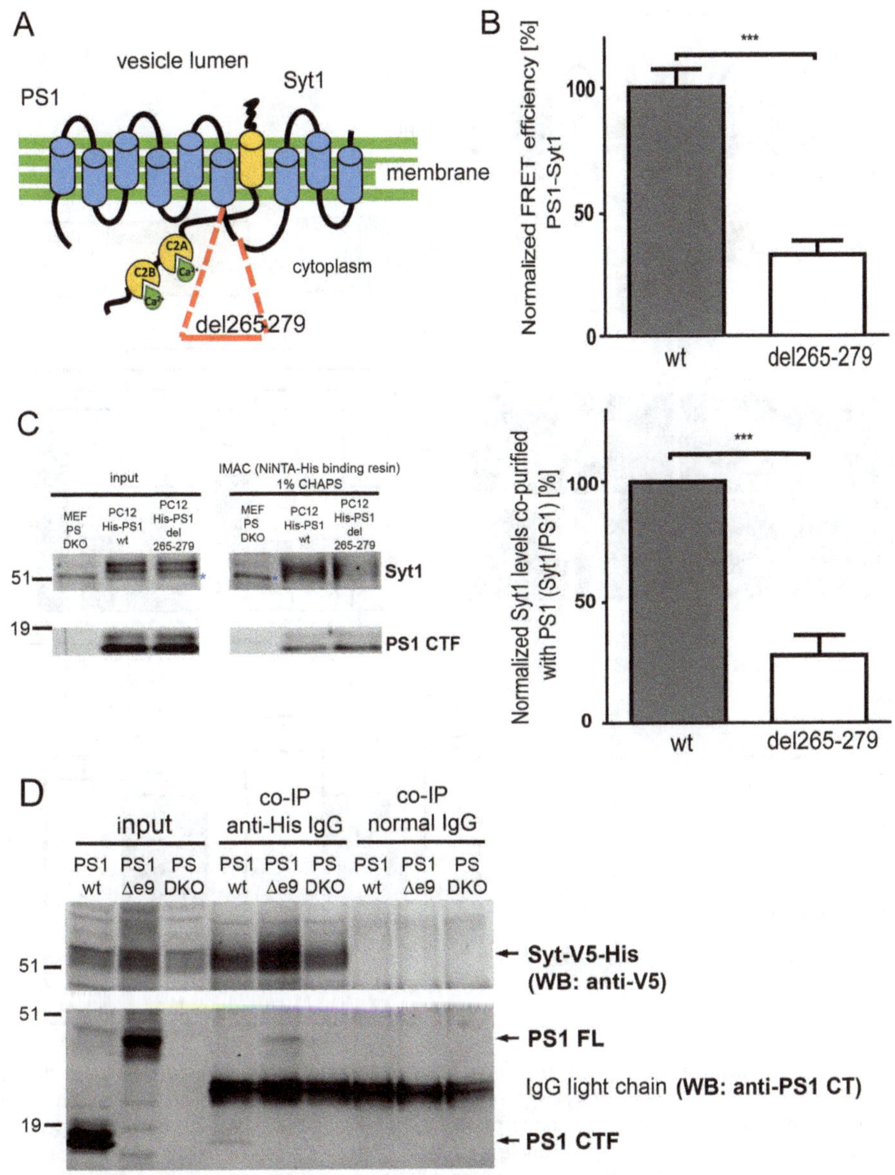

Fig. 1 Determination of Syt1-interacting region within PS1 sequence. **a** Schematic presents the PS1-Syt1 complex and the 15-amino acid deletion within the PS1 L6-7 sequence (del265-279). **b** Deletion within the L6-7 domain of PS1 inhibits PS1-Syt1 interaction. PC12 cells transfected with FLAG-tagged wild type (wt) or del265-279 PS1 were immunostained with anti-FLAG and anti-Syt1 antibodies, followed by fluorescently conjugated secondary antibodies, and analyzed by FLIM. The graph shows normalized FRET efficiency between fluorescently labeled endogenous Syt1 and overexpressed PS1 in PC12 cells stimulated for 15 min with 50 mM KCl. The data are presented as mean ± SEM, $n = 38$ for PS1 wt, and $n = 33$ for PS1 del265-279, n = total number of cells analyzed in 3 independent experiments. Statistical significance was determined using two-tailed unpaired Student's t-test, ***$p < 0.001$. The fluorescence lifetimes and corresponding FRET efficiency values are specified in the Additional file 1. **c** Syt1 co-purifies more efficiently with His-PS1 wt than with His-PS1 del265-279. Overexpressed His-tagged PS1 and endogenous Syt1 complexes extracted from PC12 cells following 15-min 50 mM KCl application were purified using immobilized metal affinity chromatography (IMAC) and analyzed by western blotting; unspecific bands are marked with blue asterisks. PS double knock-out (PS DKO) mouse embryonic fibroblasts (MEF) cells were used as a negative control. The adjacent graph presents quantification of the Syt1 levels co-purified with PS1. The data are presented as mean ± SEM, $n = 3$; two-tailed unpaired Student's t-test, ***$p < 0.001$. **d** PS1 with the deleted exon 9 (PS1Δe9) interacts with Syt1. PS DKO and PS DKO cells stably expressing PS1 wt or PS1Δe9 were transiently transfected with His-V5-Syt1 and incubated for 15 min with 5 μM A23187 calcium ionophore. Anti-His antibody or normal mouse IgG as a control were used for the immunoprecipitation, and anti-V5 and anti-PS1 CT antibodies were applied for the immunodetection. The experiment was performed three times

by varied distances between the fluorescently labeled PS1 N-terminus and PS1-C-terminus/loop domains. The conformation of PS1 affects the position of the γ-secretase cleavage site on amyloid precursor protein (APP), and hence impacts generation of the different amyloid β (Aβ) species. Close PS1 domain arrangement, "closed"

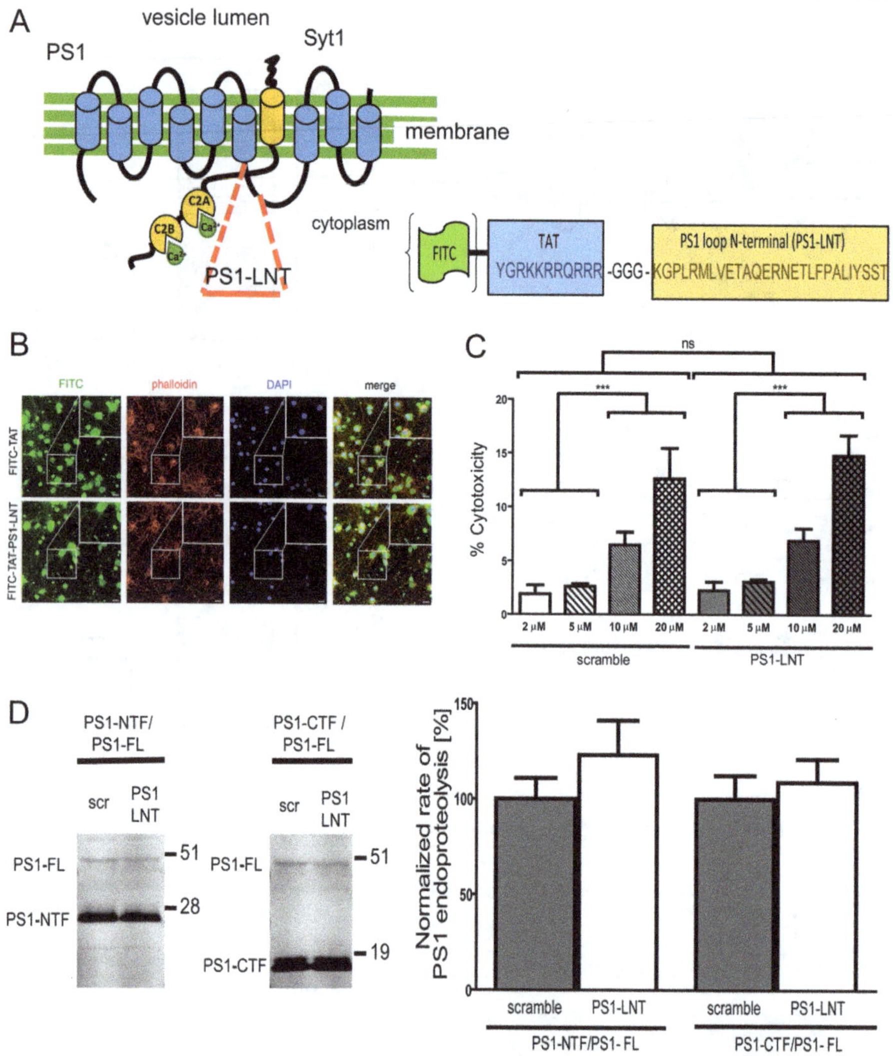

Fig. 2 Design of the cell-permeable peptide and its application in primary neurons. **a** Schematic representation of the PS1-Syt1 complex. The PS1 fragment used for the design of the cell-permeable peptide to inhibit the PS1-Syt1 interaction is indicated in red. The adjacent image presents the fusion of the HIV1 TAT domain with the respective PS1 fragment. For initial experiments the peptide was conjugated with fluorescein (FITC) to visualize intracellular delivery. Scramble peptide was used as a control. **b** Representative images demonstrate successful delivery of 5 μM TAT-FITC and TAT-PS1-LNT-FITC (green) peptides to the primary neurons after two-hour incubation. The cells were counterstained with phalloidin (red) and DAPI (blue) to visualize the actin cytoskeleton and the nuclei, respectively; scale bar 10 μm; the magnified inserts demonstrate efficient entry of the FITC-labeled peptides into neuronal cell bodies and processes. **c** Analysis of the cytotoxicity of the scramble and PS1-LNT peptides in neurons after two-hour incubation at the respective concentrations. The % cytotoxicity was determined using lactase dehydrogenase (LDH) activity assay. The data are normalized to the 1% TX-100 condition, considered to cause 100% toxicity. There is negligible toxicity of scramble and PS1-LNT peptides used at 2 μM and 5 μM final concentrations. The data are presented as mean ± SEM, $n = 37$ for 5 μM, $n = 13$ for 10 μM and $n = 7$ for the remaining conditions. Statistical significance was determined using two-tailed unpaired Student's t-test, ***$p < 0.001$. **d** Representative western blot shows efficient endoproteolysis of the full length PS1 (PS1-FL) to yield PS1-NTF and PS1-CTF in control and PS1-LNT pre-treated neurons. The graph presents quantification of the optical density of the respective bands. The ratio between PS1-CTF or PS1-NTF and PS1-FL was used to estimate endoproteolysis efficiency. The data are presented as mean ± SEM, $n = 7$. Statistical significance was determined using two-tailed unpaired Student's t-test, ns $p > 0.05$

conformation, correlates with the increased Aβ42/40 ratio [12, 15, 21, 22].

To determine the role of the PS1-Syt1 interaction in the modulation of PS1 conformation and Aβ production, PS1 conformation was assayed in non-stimulated and KCl-stimulated neurons, pre-treated with PS1-LNT or scramble peptide, using antibody based FLIM. The 15-min KCl application triggered an increase in the FRET efficiency, indicative of the shorter distance between the fluorophores labeling PS1 NT and loop domains, in both scramble and PS1-LNT pre-treated neurons, consistent with the previous data for non-pre-treated cells [12].

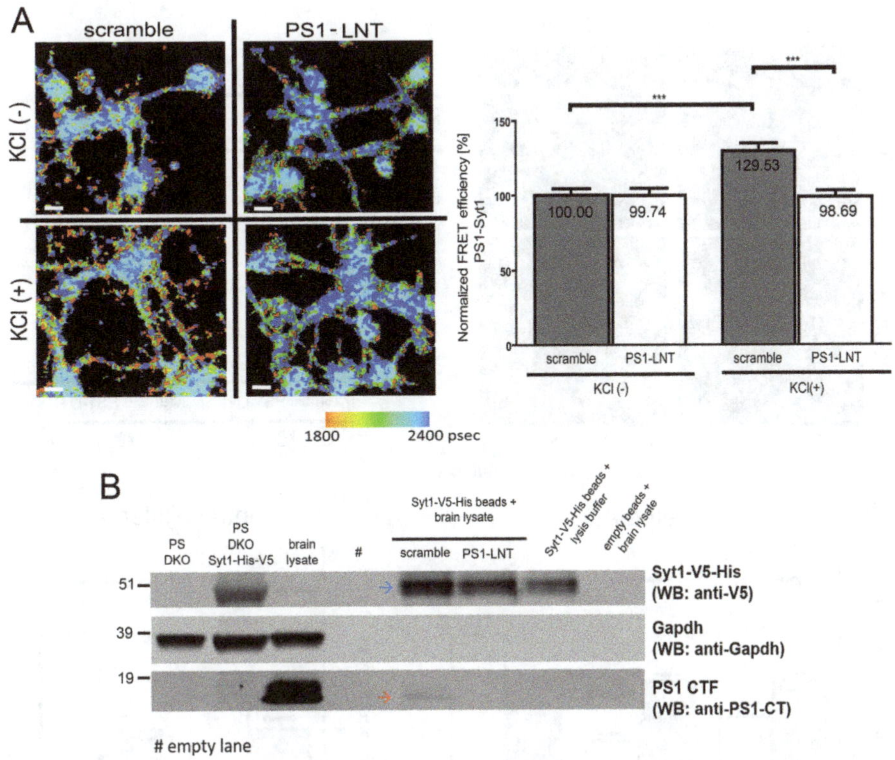

Fig. 3 Inhibition of calcium-induced PS1-Syt1 interactions in primary neurons using PS1-LNT peptide. **a** The PS1-Syt1 proximity in neurons pre-treated with PS1-LNT or scramble peptide at the basal (KCl(-)) conditions or after 15-min depolarization with 50 mM KCl was determined by FLIM. The neurons were immunostained with anti-PS1 N-terminus (NT) and anti-Syt1 antibodies, followed by fluorescently conjugated secondary antibodies. The change in FRET efficiency was used to estimate relative change in the proximity between PS1 and Syt1. The pseudo-colored image presents the lifetime of the donor fluorophore in picoseconds. The orange-red pixels indicate shorter lifetimes reflecting closer proximity between the fluorescently labeled PS1 and Syt1; scale bar 10 μm. The graph shows normalized FRET efficiency between PS1 and Syt1. Note, PS1-LNT-mediated inhibition of the calcium-induced PS1-Syt1 interaction in neurons. The data are presented as mean ± SEM, $n = 64$ for scramble KCl (-), $n = 70$ for PS1-LNT KCl (-), $n = 68$ for scramble KCl (+) and $n = 70$ for PS1-LNT KCl (+), n = total number of neurons analyzed in 3 independent experiments. Statistical significance was determined using two-tailed unpaired Student's t-test, ***$p < 0.001$. The fluorescence lifetimes and corresponding FRET efficiency values are shown in the Additional file 1. **b** In vitro IMAC analysis demonstrates successful inhibition of the PS1 binding to Syt1 by the PS1-LNT peptide. His-V5-Syt1 expressed in PS DKO cells was purified and immobilized on the beads using immobilized metal affinity chromatography, IMAC. The beads were incubated with mouse brain lysate in the presence of scramble or PS1-LNT peptide. The blue arrow indicates bands corresponding to the Syt1 immobilized on the beads. The red arrow shows the band corresponding to PS1 CTF bound to the immobilized Syt1 in the presence of scramble peptide only. Gapdh immunobloting was used as control. $n = 3$ independent experiments

Interestingly, this increase was significantly higher in the PS1-LNT pre-treated neurons, where binding to the Syt1 was blocked, compared to the scramble/control cells (Fig. 4a and Additional file 1). This suggests that Syt1 via binding to PS1 lessens the strong, "pathogenic" closure of the PS1 conformation caused by high calcium.

To test whether inhibition of the PS1-Syt1 interaction would affect Aβ production/secretion, the Aβ42 and Aβ40 levels in the conditioned medium of the PS1-LNT and control pre-treated neurons were measured. We found that inhibition of the interaction between PS1 and Syt1 results in a significant increase in the Aβ42/40 ratio, although individual levels of the Aβ40 and Aβ42 were reduced (Fig. 4b).

The reduced Aβ levels in the conditioned medium could be a consequence of the changed APP expression and/or processing, or impaired Aβ secretion. To distinguish between these possibilities, we evaluated the levels of APP full length (APP-FL) and APP C-terminal fragments (APP-CTFs) in KCl-stimulated scramble and PS1-LNT pre-treated neurons. No accumulation of the APP-CTFs was observed upon the inhibition of the PS1-Syt1 binding, suggestive of the lack of alterations in the overall PS1/γ-secretase activity (Additional file 2).

To explore if the observed decrease in the Aβ amount in the conditioned medium is indeed a consequence of the impaired Aβ secretion, we measured intracellular Aβ42 and Aβ40 levels in the control or PS1-LNT pre-treated, KCl-stimulated neurons (Fig. 4c). An increased amount of the intracellular Aβ42 and Aβ40 was detected in the cells pre-treated with PS1-LNT compared to the control, suggesting that inhibition of the PS1-Syt1

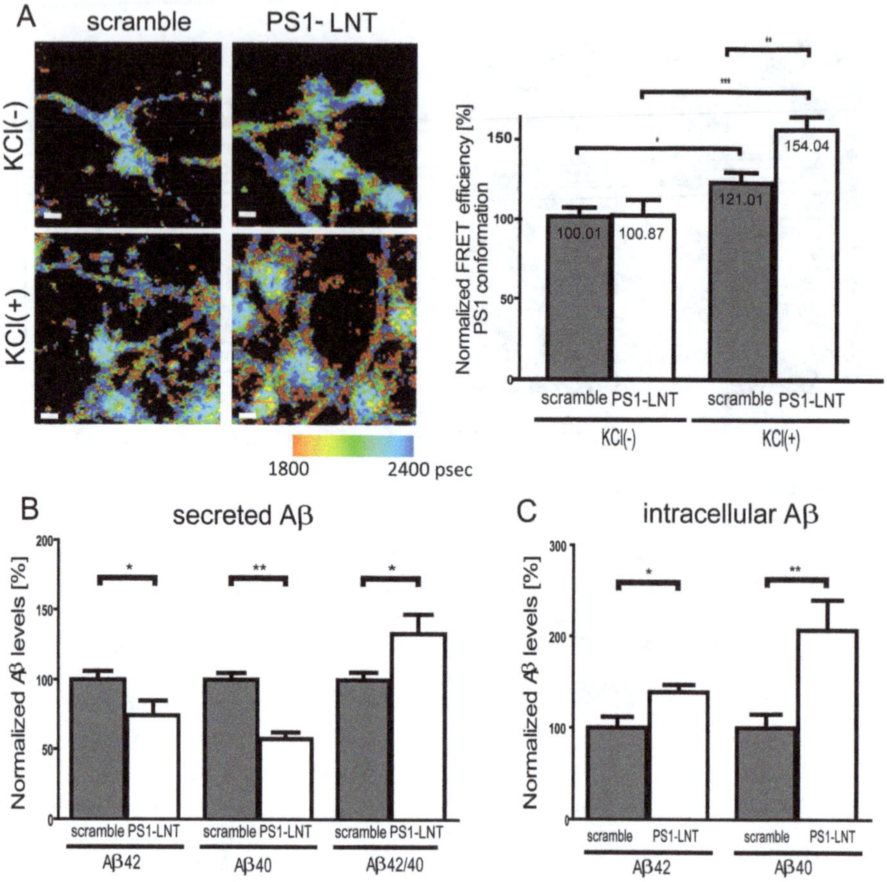

Fig. 4 Activity-driven PS1-Syt1 interaction stabilizes open PS1 conformation and modulates Aβ production/secretion. **a** The conformation of endogenous PS1 in primary neurons pre-treated with PS1-LNT or scramble peptide at basal (KCl(-)) and high calcium (upon 15-min 50 mM KCl stimulation) conditions was determined by FLIM assay, monitoring proximity between PS1 N-terminus and PS1 loop domain. Cells were immunostained with anti-PS1 NT and anti-PS1 loop antibodies, followed by fluorescently conjugated secondary antibodies. The pseudo-colored images present the donor fluorophore lifetime in picoseconds. The orange-red pixels indicate PS1 in "closed" conformation; scale bar 10 μm. The adjacent graph presents normalized FRET efficiency between PS1-NT and PS1 cytosolic loop. The KCl stimulation shifts PS1 to "closed" conformation in both scramble and PS1-LNT pre-treated neurons but the shift is greater in the PS1-LNT conditions. The data are presented as mean ± SEM, $n = 64$ for scramble (KCl(-)), $n = 57$ for PS1-LNT (KCl(-)), $n = 59$ for scramble (KCl(+)) and $n = 65$ for PS1-LNT (KCl(+)), n = number of neurons analyzed in 3 independent experiments. Statistical significance was determined using two-tailed unpaired Student's t-test, $^{**}p < 0.01$. The fluorescence lifetimes and corresponding FRET efficiency values are shown in the Additional file 1. **b** The graph presents relative Aβ40, Aβ42 levels and Aβ42/40 ratio in conditioned medium collected from the neurons pre-treated with PS1-LNT and depolarized with KCl to induce calcium influx. The values, determined by ELISA, were normalized to the scramble treated cells. The data are presented as mean ± SEM, n = 19-26. Statistical significance was determined using two-tailed unpaired Student's t-test, $^{*}p < 0.05$, $^{**}p < 0.01$. **c** The graph presents relative Aβ40 and Aβ42 levels in cell lysates prepared from the neurons used in (**b**). The values were normalized to the scramble treated cells. The data are presented as mean ± SEM, n = 7-12. Statistical significance was determined using two-tailed unpaired Student's t-test, $^{*}p < 0.05$, $^{**}p < 0.01$

binding may result in aberrant exocytosis. These results were further supported by double-immunostaining of neurons with the anti-β-amyloid antibody 4G8, recognizing both Aβ and APP, and anti-microtubule associated protein 2 (MAP2) antibody as an internal control. Since we did not see difference in the APP-FL and APP-CTFs between the scramble and PS1-LNT pre-treated cells, increased 4G8 fluorescence intensity in PS1-LNT pre-treated cells (Additional file 3) suggests accumulation of the intracellular Aβ.

Next, we determined whether PS1-LNT impaired exocytosis is specific for Aβ or represents more general phenomena. Multiple proteins are released from neurons in an activity-dependent exocytosis controlled by synaptic proteins [42–44]. Thus, we used an accurate and ultrasensitive NanoOrange assay to monitor changes in the total protein concentration in the conditioned medium of neurons pre-treated for 2 h with PS1-LNT or scramble peptide, and stimulated with 50 mM KCl for 15 min. Indeed, the amount of total protein detected in the conditioned medium of PS1-LNT pre-treated neurons was significantly reduced, compared to that of scramble pre-treated cells (Fig. 5a). This further supports overall impairment of exocytosis/secretion after the inhibition of the Syt1-PS1 binding.

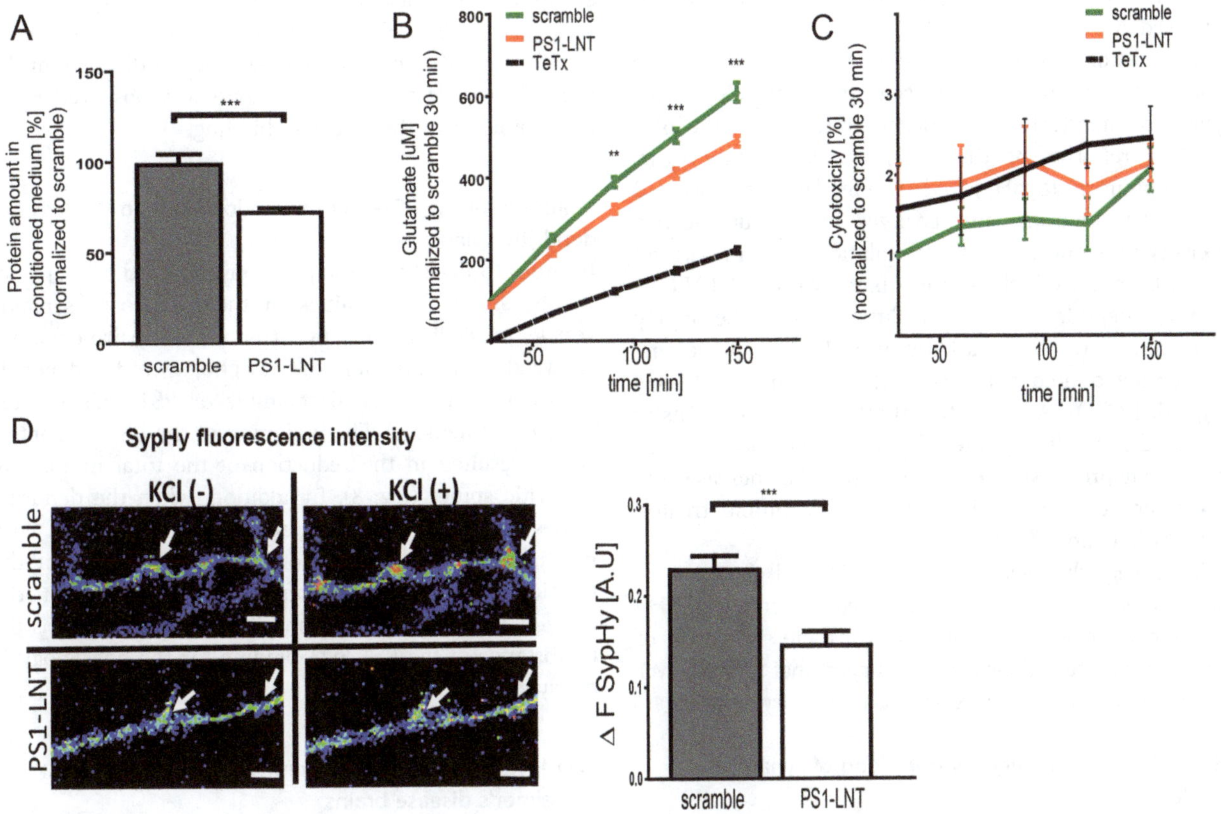

Fig. 5 PS1-Syt1 interaction modulates exocytosis/neurotransmitter release. **a** The graph presents the quantification of the total protein amount in the conditioned medium collected from neurons plated at 1.5×10^6 cells/well, pre-treated for 2 h with scramble and PS1-LNT peptides, and stimulated for 15 min with 50 mM KCl. The protein secreted by the PS1-LNT pre-treated neurons is shown as a percent of the protein secreted by the scramble peptide pre-treated cells; mean ± SEM, $n = 12$. Statistical significance was determined using two-tailed unpaired Student's t-test, $***p < 0.001$. **b** The graph presents relative amounts of glutamate in the conditioned medium collected from neurons pre-treated for 2 h with PS1-LNT, scramble peptide or exocytosis inhibitor, tetanus toxin (TeTx), and depolarized using 50 mM KCl in the presence of the DL-TBOA, an inhibitor of the glutamate transporters EAAT1 and EAAT2. The data are presented as mean ± SEM, $n = 31$ for scramble and PS1-LNT, $n = 6$ for TeTx. Statistical significance was determined using two-way ANOVA followed by Bonferroni's post-test, $**p < 0.01$, $*** < 0.001$. **c** The graph presents relative level of lactate dehydrogenase activity, indicative of the potential cytotoxicity of the applied treatment, in primary neurons pre-treated with PS1-LNT or scramble peptide for 2 h and depolarized using 50 mM KCl in the presence of the DL-TBOA for the duration of the assay. The data are presented as mean ± SEM, $n = 7$. Statistical significance was determined using two-way ANOVA followed by Bonferroni's post-test. No significant toxicity of the applied treatments was observed. **d**, The pseudocolor-coded images present synaptophluorin (SypHy) fluorescence at the synaptic puncta in neurons pre-treated for 2 h with PS1-LNT or scramble peptide. The red spots indicate high fluorescence intensity corresponding to the high level of exocytosis observed immediately after the 50 mM KCl stimulation; scale bar 5 μm. The adjacent bar graph demonstrates the quantification of the increase in SypHy fluorescence at the synaptic ROIs in response to the depolarizing stimulus in the scramble and PS1-LNT pre-treated neurons. The data are presented as mean ± SEM, $n = 263$ for scramble and $n = 255$ for PS1-LNT, n = number of synaptic puncta analyzed in 4 independent experiments. Statistical significance was determined using Mann-Whitney's *U*-test, $***p < 0.01$

PS1-Syt1 interaction stimulates exocytosis and neurotransmitter release in primary neurons

Syt1 is primarily expressed at the synapse and calcium influx has been shown to predominantly trigger PS1-Syt1 interaction at the synaptic loci [12]. This rises a possibility that PS1-Syt1 binding may modulate synaptic vesicle exocytosis and neurotransmitter release. Therefore, to examine whether the PS1-Syt1 interaction indeed modulates synaptic exocytosis we monitored the level of secreted glutamate over the 150-min time course in the conditioned medium of KCl-stimulated neurons pre-treated for 2 h with 5 μM of either PS1-LNT or scramble peptides. A blocker of the excitatory amino acid transporters 1 and 2 (EAAT1, EAAT2), DL-threo-beta-benzyloxyaspartate (DL-TBOA), was used to inhibit glutamate re-uptake. The inhibition of the PS1-Syt1 binding by PS1-LNT resulted in a significant reduction of the glutamate level in the conditioned medium (Fig. 5b), suggesting importance of the PS1-Syt1 interaction for glutamate secretion/exocytosis. Overnight pre-treatment of the neurons with tetanus toxin (TeTx), a commonly used potent inhibitor of the exocytosis [45], markedly diminished glutamate release, and served as an assay control. Importantly, the described reductions in glutamate release in the

PS1-LNT and TeTx pre-treated neurons were not due to increased cytotoxicity (Fig. 5c).

The role of PS1-Syt1 interactions in synaptic vesicle exocytosis was further assessed using an alternative approach, monitoring fluorescence intensity of the pH-sensitive reporter of the synaptic vesicle exocytosis, synaptophluorin (SypHy) [33]. The SypHy was expressed in 13 DIV neurons, and changes in its fluorescence intensity pre- and post-KCl stimulation were monitored in real time in live cells pre-incubated with PS1-LNT or scramble peptide. No marked differences in the SypHy expression were observed between PS1-LNT and scramble peptide treated neurons at the baseline conditions (Fig. 5d, KCl(-)). As expected, the fluorescence intensity increased immediately after the KCl application, indicative of synaptic vesicle exocytosis, but the increase was less prominent in PS1-LNT than in scramble treated neurons (Fig. 5d, KCl(+)).

Collectively, the decreased level of Aβ and glutamate in the conditioned medium, and reduced rise in the SypHy fluorescence in KCl-stimulated neurons after inhibition of the PS1-Syt1 interactions strongly suggest that the PS1-Syt1 binding may help upkeep exocytosis in primary neurons.

PS1-Syt1 binding influences trafficking of synaptic vesicles

To further address the role of PS1-Syt1 interaction in synaptic physiology, the mobility of synaptic vesicles along the processes was investigated using fluorescence recovery after photobleaching (FRAP) of the eGFP-synaptophysin (eGFP-Syp). eGFP-Syp has been previously reported to be predominantly expressed in axons and to co-localize with the other synaptic vesicle markers [46, 47]. The neurons expressing eGFP-Syp were pre-treated with 5 μM scramble or PS1-LNT peptides for 2 h and stimulated for 15 min with 50 mM KCl to promote PS1-Syt1 interaction. The inhibition of the PS1-Syt1 binding by PS1-LNT led to decreased recovery rate of the eGFP-Syp fluorescence (Fig. 6a,b), suggestive of compromised synaptic vesicle movement in PS1-LNT vs. scramble peptide pre-treated cells. Of note, FRAP of the eGFP-tubulin, which served as a negative control, was not altered by the PS1-LNT pre-treatment (Fig. 6c,d).

Inhibition of PS1-Syt1 interaction leads to alterations in the synaptic vesicle morphology and distribution

To determine if PS1-LNT interference with the PS1-Syt1 binding may lead to ultrastructural alterations at the synapse, we performed electron microscopy (EM) analysis of the synaptic vesicle size, density and distance from the active zone in primary neurons pre-treated for 2 h with scramble or PS1-LNT peptide, and stimulated for 15 min with 50 mM KCl (Fig. 7). A population of significantly larger synaptic vesicles and reduced overall synaptic vesicle density were detected in synaptic terminals of the PS1-LNT pre-treated neurons compared to the control. Moreover, an increase in the distance of the synaptic vesicle to the active zone was observed upon the inhibition of the PS1-Syt1 binding.

Inhibition of the PS1-Syt1 interaction leads to the loss of dendritic spines

In order to investigate the pathophysiological relevance of the observed abnormalities in the exocytosis, synaptic vesicle trafficking and ultrastructural impairments, we analyzed the number and the morphology of the dendritic spines in KCl-stimulated scramble or PS1-LNT peptide pre-treated neurons. The inhibition of the PS1-Syt1 interaction resulted in the reduction of the total number of dendritic spines (Fig. 8). In addition, when the dendritic spines were classified according to their shape into mushroom-shaped, stubby or thin, the decrease in the fraction of mushroom spines was apparent in the PS1-LNT pre-treated neurons. This further reaffirms the importance of the PS1-Syt1 binding for the physiology of the synapse.

Syt1 level and PS1-Syt1 proximity are decreased in Alzheimer's disease brains

Synaptic defects, impaired exocytosis, and pathogenic change in the PS1 conformation were reported to occur in AD [38, 48–51]. Since our data show that these were affected by the inhibition of the PS1-Syt1 interaction, we analyzed Syt1 protein expression and the relative proximity between PS1 and Syt1 in medial temporal cortex from sporadic AD (sAD) cases with neuropathologically confirmed Braak stage V-VI, and in age- and post mortem interval (PMI)-matched control subjects. The number and fluorescence intensity of the Syt1-positive puncta were significantly decreased in sAD brains (Fig. 9a).

To determine if the proximity between the remaining Syt1 and PS1 is also altered in sAD, we employed an antibody-based FLIM assay. FLIM approach determines the fluorophore lifetime, which is an intrinsic biophysical property of a fluorophore, and hence does not depend on the absolute amounts of the donor and the acceptor in the sample [36, 52, 53]. Therefore, despite significant reduction in the absolute levels of synaptic proteins in AD brain, FLIM is uniquely suited to report the relative distance between the remaining Syt1 and PS1. Longer lifetimes of the donor fluorophore, indicative of the lower FRET efficiency, stemming from reduced proximity between the fluorescently labeled PS1 and Syt1, were recorded in sAD compared to control cases (Fig. 9b and Additional file 1). This indicates that in addition to decreased Syt1 level, the interaction between Syt1 and PS1/γ-secretase in sAD brains is also significantly reduced.

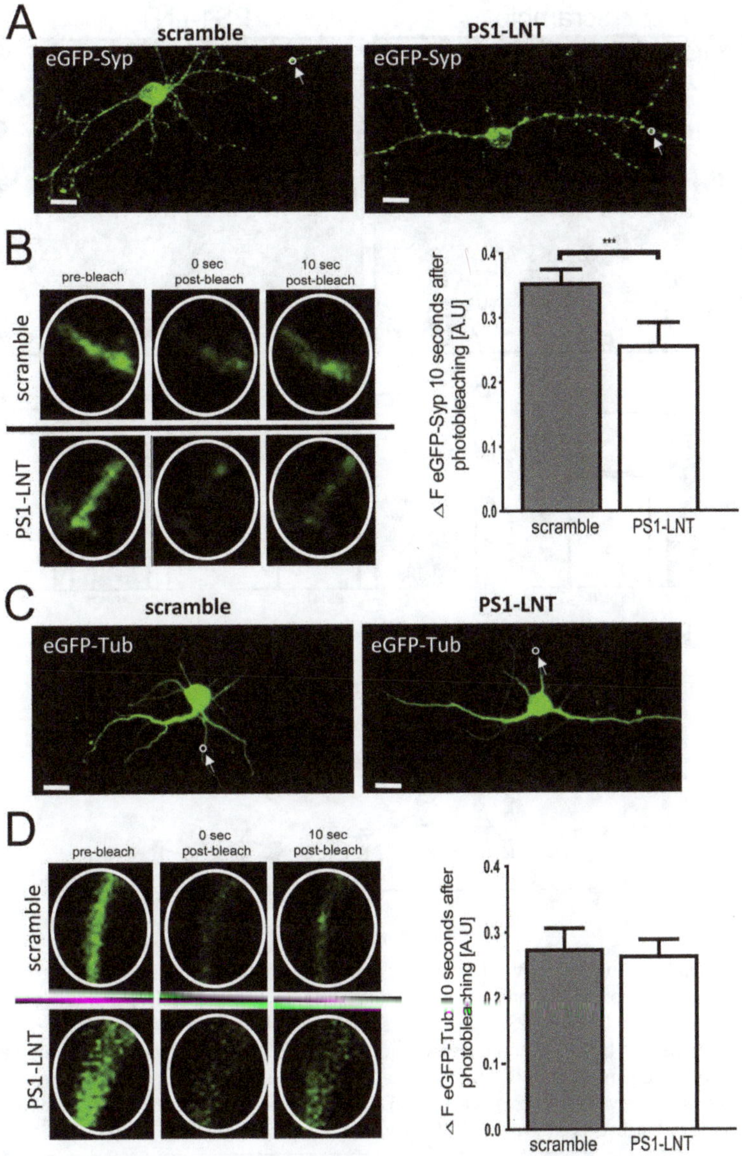

Fig. 6 PS1-Syt1 interaction modulates synaptic vesicle trafficking. **a** Fluorescent images show distribution of the eGFP-synaptophysin (eGFP-Syp) in primary neurons pre-treated for 2 h with scramble and PS1-LNT peptides. Note increased fluorescence intensity in synaptic puncta along the processes. The arrows point to the example region of interests (ROIs) used for the photobleaching experiments; scale bar 15 μm. **b** Fluorescence recovery after photobleaching (FRAP) experiments demonstrate impaired motion of synaptic vesicle proteins in the PS1-LNT pre-treated neurons. The fluorescent images present 5 μm-diameter ROIs recorded in eGFP-Syp expressing neurons pre-treated for 2 h with scramble or PS1-LNT peptides, and stimulated for with 50 mM KCl. Three ROIs are analyzed for each condition: pre-bleach, immediately after bleach and 10 s after bleach. The adjacent bar graph demonstrates the quantification of the eGFP-Syp fluorescence recovered within 10 s post-bleach. The data are presented as mean + SEM, $n = 36$. Statistical significance was determined using unpaired Student's t-test, $^{***}p < 0.001$. **c** Fluorescent images present distribution of the eGFP-tubulin (eGFP-Tub) in primary neurons pre-treated with scramble and PS1-LNT peptides. The arrows point to the ROIs used for the photobleaching experiments; scale bar 15 μm. **d** Control FRAP experiments demonstrate no alterations in eGFP-tubulin fluorescence recovery after photobleaching in neurons pre-treated for 2 h with PS1-LNT or scramble peptides, and stimulated with 50 mM KCl for 15 min. The fluorescent images present 5 μm-diameter ROIs recorded in eGFP-Tub expressing neurons pre-treated with scramble or PS1-LNT peptides. The data are presented as mean + SEM, $n = 19$. Statistical significance was determined using unpaired Student's t-test

Syt1 overexpression in vivo in mouse brain promotes protective "open" PS1 conformation

To investigate whether overexpression of Syt1 in vivo in mouse hippocampi would promote the PS1-Syt1 interaction, and thus support the protective "open" PS1 conformation, we employed adeno-associated virus (AAV2/8)-mediated delivery of the Syt1-V5 or empty vector control plasmids into the hippocampi of wild type C57BL/6 mice. To minimize variability between the animals Syt1-V5 was expressed in one hemisphere and an

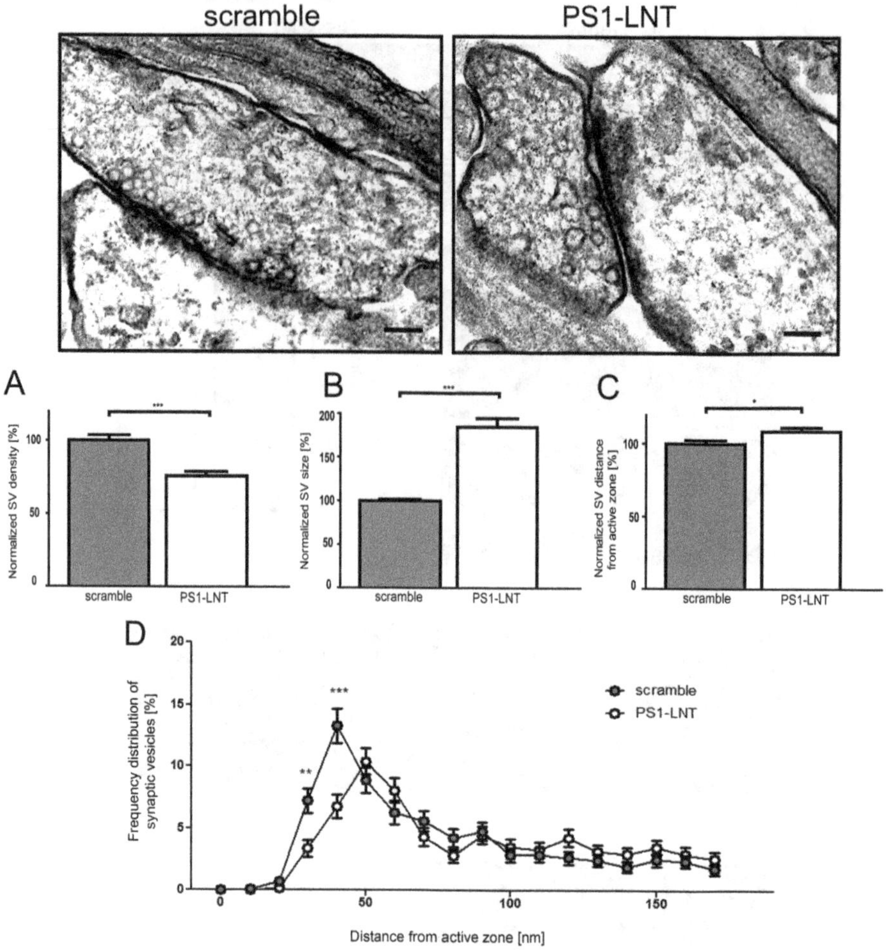

Fig. 7 Inhibition of PS1-Syt1 binding leads to the alterations in synaptic vesicle morphology and distribution. Representative electron micrographs show synaptic vesicles within the synapses of the primary neurons pre-treated for 2 h with scramble or PS1-LNT peptides, and stimulated for 15 min with 50 mM KCl. Enlarged synaptic vesicles in the PS1-LNT treated synapses are shown by red asterisks. Scale bar 100 nm. The graphs show the quantification of: **a** synaptic vesicle size; **b** density; and **c** distance from the active zone. The data are normalized to scramble-treated cells and presented as mean ± SEM, $n = 100$, n = total number of synapses analyzed in three independent experiments. Graph (**d**) presents the frequency distribution of the synaptic vesicles within individual synapses as a function of the distance from the active zone. Statistical significance was determined using two-tailed unpaired Student's t-test (**a**, **b**, **c**) or two-way ANOVA followed by Bonferroni's post-test (**d**), $^{*}p < 0.05$, $^{**}p < 0.01$, $^{***}p < 0.001$

empty vector was delivered to the contralateral side (Fig. 10a). One month post-injection the brains were dissected and the Syt1-V5 expression in the targeted hemisphere was confirmed by immunostaining with anti-V5 antibody (Fig. 10b). We found that increased Syt1 expression promoted the interaction between PS1 and Syt1, as determined by antibody-based FLIM assay (Fig. 10c and Additional file 1).

Next, we analyzed if increased Syt1 expression and its interaction with PS1 would promote "open" PS1 conformation in vivo. Significantly decreased FRET efficiency, indicative of a longer distance between fluorescently labeled PS1 N-terminus and large cytosolic loop domain, was observed in the hemisphere injected with the AAV2/8-Syt1-V5 compared to the contralateral control hemisphere (Fig. 10d and Additional file 1). This reaffirms that Syt1 expression in vivo helps sustain protective "open" PS1 conformation and might be worth exploring therapeutically.

Discussion

By using targeted inhibition of the presenilin 1 (PS1) and synaptotagmin 1 (Syt1) binding, without affecting the proteins' expression levels, we provide evidence of the reciprocal relationship between PS1 and synaptic vesicle protein Syt1, by showing that PS1 and Syt1 modulate each other's functions. Furthermore, we found that proximity between the Syt1 and PS1 is significantly reduced in sporadic Alzheimer's disease (sAD) brain, indicating physiological relevance of the PS1-Syt1 interaction, and suggesting that disrupted interaction may contribute to the synaptic pathology that starts early in the disease.

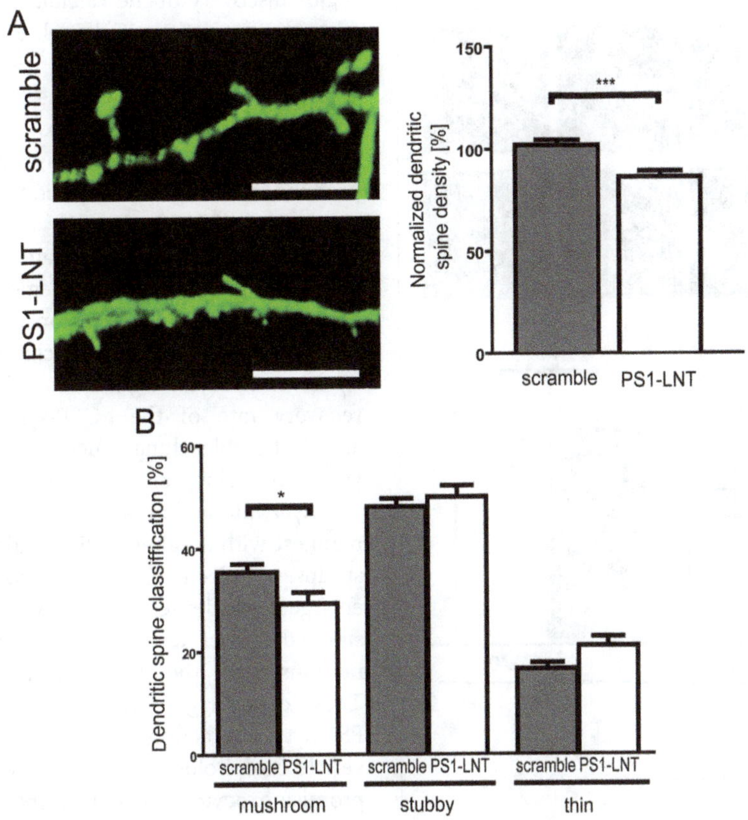

Fig. 8 Inhibition of PS1-Syt1 interaction alters the number and the morphology of dendritic spines. **a** Representative images of the dendritic spines in GFP overexpressing neurons, pre-treated for 2 h with scramble or PS1-LNT peptides, and stimulated for 15 min with 50 mM KCl. Scale bar 5 μm. The adjacent bar graph shows the quantification of the dendritic spine density. The values are normalized to the scramble treated cells. The data are presented as mean ± SEM, $n = 30$, n = number of neurites analyzed per condition in 8 independent experiments. Statistical significance was determined using two-tailed unpaired Student's t-test, $^{***}p < 0.01$. **b** The bar graph presents quantitative analysis of the relative contribution of the mushroom, stubby and thin dendritic spines to the total spine number in neurons shown in (**a**). The data are presented as mean ± SEM, $n = 50$ for scramble and $n = 43$ for PS1-LNT, n = number of images acquired per condition in 8 independent experiments. Statistical significance was determined using two-way ANOVA followed by a Bonferroni's post-test, $^{*}p < 0.05$

A link between abnormal neuronal/synaptic activity and Aβ accumulation has been reported [54–56] although the precise molecular mechanisms regulating synaptic Aβ generation and release remain elusive. We found that blocking KCl-triggered PS1-Syt1 interaction affected both the type of Aβ species generated and their release, without affecting overall γ-secretase activity or APP processing. First, targeted, peptide-based inhibition of the PS1-Syt1 binding exacerbated KCl-induced shift of PS1 towards the pathogenic "closed" state, and caused concurrent increase in the Aβ42/40 ratio. This suggests that Syt1 may serve as a protective factor stabilizing "open" PS1/γ-secretase conformation at the synapse at high calcium conditions. Second, we found that inhibition of the interaction between PS1 and Syt1 resulted in the reduced overall protein secretion and neurotransmitter release, and increased accumulation of the intracellular Aβ, indicating that PS1 may be involved in Syt1-mediated vesicle trafficking and exocytosis in primary neurons.

The potential role of PS1 at the synapse beyond γ-secretase activity remains poorly understood. The compromised neurotransmission has been observed in conditional pre- but not post-synaptic PS double knock-out neurons (PS cDKO), proposing a role of PS1 in the modulation of neurotransmitter release [23]. Since PS1 interacts with the ryanodine receptor (RyR) [57], and PS cDKO mice present reduced RyR level [58], the impaired neurotransmission in PS cDKO neurons has been attributed to the aberrant calcium release through RyR [23]. On the other hand, γ-secrease activity-dependent PS1 involvement in regulation of the spontaneous neurotransmitter release was also shown in PS1 knock-out neurons [24]. However, given the pleiotropic effect of protein knock-out and considering multiple functions of presenilins, as shown by the global PS1-dependent transcriptome changes [59], PS1 knock-out approach does not provide evidence of the direct involvement of PS1 in synaptic vesicle exocytosis/neurotransmission.

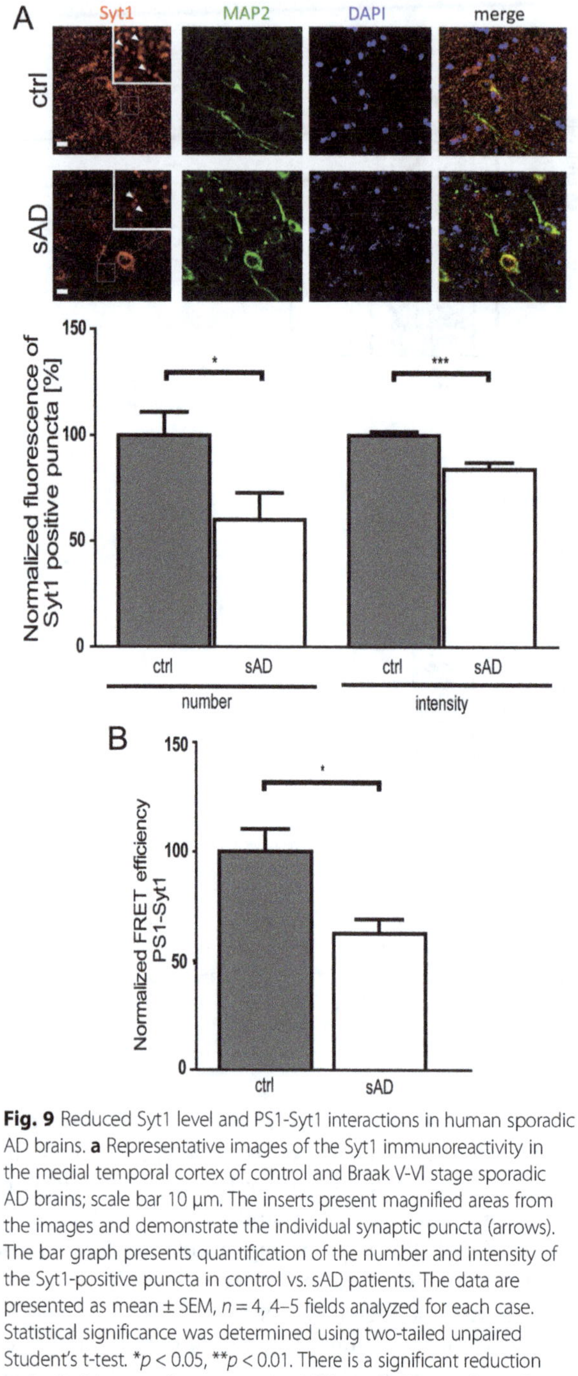

Fig. 9 Reduced Syt1 level and PS1-Syt1 interactions in human sporadic AD brains. **a** Representative images of the Syt1 immunoreactivity in the medial temporal cortex of control and Braak V-VI stage sporadic AD brains; scale bar 10 μm. The inserts present magnified areas from the images and demonstrate the individual synaptic puncta (arrows). The bar graph presents quantification of the number and intensity of the Syt1-positive puncta in control vs. sAD patients. The data are presented as mean ± SEM, $n = 4$, 4–5 fields analyzed for each case. Statistical significance was determined using two-tailed unpaired Student's t-test. $*p < 0.05$, $**p < 0.01$. There is a significant reduction in the Syt1 immunofluorescence in sAD brains. **b** FLIM analysis of PS1-Syt1 interactions in medial temporal cortex of control vs. sAD presents reduced PS1-Syt1 binding in sAD. The tissue was immunostained with anti-PS1 NT (APS11) and anti-Syt1 antibodies, and relative proximity between the fluorescently labeled proteins was determined by FLIM. There is significant reduction in the FRET efficiency between PS1 and Syt1, indicative of a greater distance between the molecules, in sAD brains. The data are presented as mean ± SEM, $n = 4$; 20–25 neurons analyzed for each case. Statistical significance was determined using Mann-Whitney's *U*-test. $*p < 0.05$. The fluorescence lifetimes and corresponding FRET efficiency values are shown in the Additional file 1

Our discovery of the calcium-regulated PS1 interaction with the synaptic vesicle release protein, Syt1, further alluded to the possibility that PS1 may play an important regulatory role at the synapse. Since Syt1 is directly involved in calcium-triggered exocytosis that depends on its precise, sequential interactions with the SNARE complex proteins, allowing vesicle fusion to occur and exocytosis to proceed [27–29, 60, 61], we hypothesized that PS1 binding to Syt1 may modulate this process. Consistent with this idea, our findings demonstrate that targeted inhibition of the PS1 interaction with one of the members of synaptic vesicle release machinery diminishes the activity driven exocytosis/glutamate release. Moreover, reduced recovery rate of the eGFP-synaptophysin fluorescence after photobleaching suggests compromised synaptic vesicle trafficking along the neuronal processes when the PS1-Syt1 interaction is impeded. These impairments may manifest with an altered distribution of the vesicles at the synapses. Indeed, electron microscopy analysis revealed enlarged, less densely packed synaptic vesicles that are positioned farther from the active zone in KCl-stimulated neurons after the inhibition of the PS1-Syt1 binding. These data suggest that PS1-LNT interference with the PS1-Syt1 interaction may lead to alterations in synaptic vesicle morphology/distribution at the synapse and compromise exocytosis. It is plausible that PS1 via the direct interaction with Syt1 regulates its structural flexibility and/or presentation of specific motifs on Syt1 necessary for the interaction with other synaptic partners crucial for synaptic vesicle exocytosis [62–65]. On the other hand, accumulation of the enlarged vesicles might indicate that the PS1-Syt1 binding regulates the Syt1-dependent mechanisms controlling synaptic vesicle size [66]. Of note, analogous structural abnormalities in the synaptic vesicles have been observed in Syt1 knock-out synapses [67, 68], but not in the Syt1 calcium-binding motif mutants [67], indicating that this is not a Syt1 calcium-binding defect.

The impairments in the exocytosis and neurotransmitter release at the pre-synapse due to the inhibition of the PS1-Syt1 interaction lead to the concomitant reduction in the number of dendritic spines, and mushroom spines in particular. This finding is consistent with the previous observations of decreased spine density in vivo following the expression of potent exocytosis inhibitors [69] and in AD models, as reviewed in [70, 71]. Together, with our findings of the detrimental effect of PS1-LNT blocking peptide treatment on PS1 conformation, Aβ42/40 ratio and intracellular Aβ accumulation, this further supports the beneficial role of the PS1-Syt1 interaction for synaptic wellbeing.

The described pathophysiological changes were detected in vitro upon profound but relatively short-lasting inhibition of the PS1-Syt1 binding. It is plausible that chronic, lasting over decades inhibition of the PS1-Syt1 interaction, even if

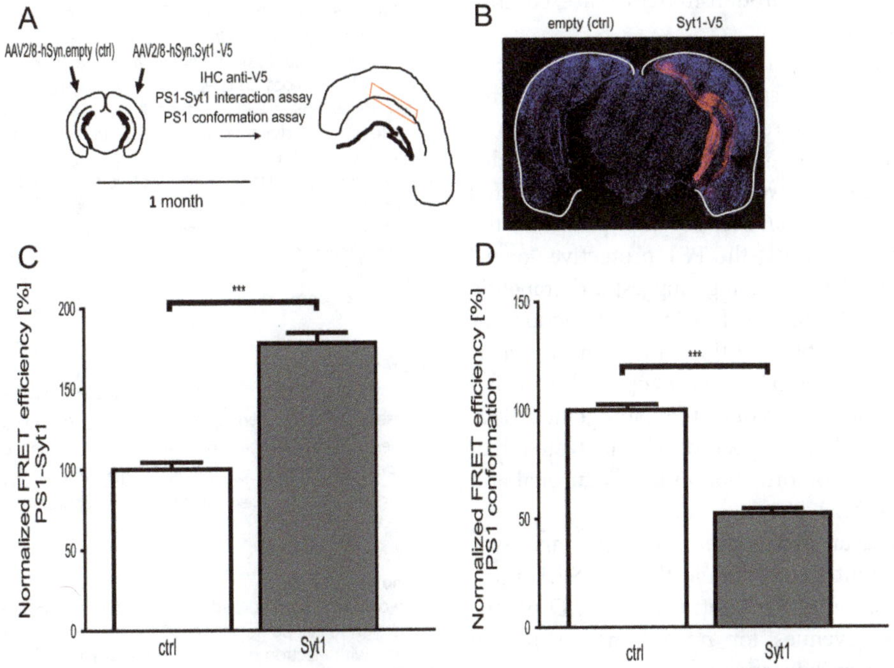

Fig. 10 Syt1 overexpression in vivo increases PS1-Syt1 interactions and promotes open PS1 conformation in mouse brain. **a** Schematic representation of the experimental design. Bilateral injection of AAV2/8-hSyn1. Syt1-V5 or empty plasmid to the contralateral hemisphere was performed. One month after the injections the brains were dissected and subjected to immunofluorescence analysis. **b** The fluorescent images demonstrate successful expression of Syt1-V5 in mouse brain one month after the AAV2/8-hSyn1. Syt1-V5 injection. The tissue was immunostained with anti-V5 antibody and corresponding Cy3-conjugated secondary antibody. **c, d** The bar graphs present FLIM assays of the PS1-Syt1 interactions and PS1 conformation in mouse hippocampi injected with AAV2/8-hSyn1. Syt1-V5 or empty vector as a control. The tissue was immunostained with anti-PS1 NT and anti-Syt1 for the PS1-Syt1 interaction assay, or anti-PS1 NT and anti-PS1 loop antibodies for the PS1 conformation assay, followed by respective fluorescently labeled secondary antibodies. There is a significant increase in the PS1-Syt1 binding and a shift towards protective "open" conformation of PS1 in the hemispheres transduced with AAV2/8-hSyn1. Syt1-V5. The data are presented as mean ± SEM, $n = 721$-723 neurons for PS1-Syt1 interaction and $n = 573$-586 for PS1 conformation were analyzed in 5 mice. Statistical significance was determined using Mann-Whitney's *U*-test, $^{***}p < 0.001$. The fluorescence lifetimes and corresponding FRET efficiency values are shown in the Additional file 1

more subtle, would lead to the neuronal circuitry dysfunction, and ultimately to AD. In accordance, several studies have reported changes in the synaptic physiology and exocytosis, such as alterations in RCAN1-mediated modulation of exocytosis in AD [49, 51] or exocytosis impairments in the cells from APP/PS1 mouse model of AD [50].

Synaptic dysfunction/loss is one of the major neuropathological feature of the disease, and the strongest correlate of the disease progression [1–3, 7, 48, 72]. The described protective Syt1 function might be compromised in AD brains, since, in agreement with other reports, we found reduced levels of Syt1 in sAD brains (this study and [7, 73]). Intriguingly, reduced Syt1 level in the brain is followed by its concomitant decrease in the cerebrospinal fluid and plasma neuronal-derived exosomes, raising the prospect for Syt1 being used as a potential biomarker for synaptic AD pathology [74, 75].

Furthermore, by applying fluorescence lifetime imaging microscopy, we found that the proximity between the remaining Syt1 and PS1 is also reduced in the disease. Of note, we have observed that the PS1-Syt1 interaction in mouse brain increases during normal aging (unpublished data). Therefore, it is possible that the PS1-Syt1 proximity is also higher in normal aged human brain (perhaps as a compensatory mechanism) but not in the sporadic AD brain. There is an array of factors that could potentially affect the baseline PS1-Syt1 interaction in aged brain. Despite the lack of PS1 mutations, the wild type PS1 in sAD brain presents structural alteration, i.e. pathogenic "close" conformation that is linked to elevated Aβ42/40 ratio [38, 76, 77]. Therefore, it is possible that conformational changes in PS1 might result in reduced binding to Syt1. It is also possible that reduction in the PS1-Syt1 binding can occur early, before the onset of symptoms, since ~30% decrease in the PS1-Syt1 interaction is observed in 9 month old Tg2576 AD mice without synaptic loss and before the appearance of amyloid plaque pathology (unpublished data). Together with other factors, the impaired PS1-Syt1 binding may weaken the synapse via local increase in the Aβ42/40 ratio and deficits in the overall protein exocytosis/neurotransmitter release, contributing to the synaptic loss.

Finally, since reduced Syt1 level and diminished PS1-Syt1 binding have a detrimental effect on PS1 conformation, we reasoned that overexpression of Syt1 in vivo in the brain might induce the protective "open" PS1 subdomain architecture. Indeed, we found that AAV-mediated delivery of the Syt1 into mouse hippocampi promotes the PS1-Syt1 binding, and impels the PS1 protective "open" conformational state. These findings suggest a therapeutic potential through fostering the PS1-Syt1 interaction for AD treatment. It is possible that this strategy may constitute a synapse-specific complementary approach to using GSMs. GSMs are known to reduce the pathogenic Aβ42/40 ratio [78–80], and a number of GSMs tested had promoted "open" PS1 conformation in both neuronal and non-neuronal cells [21, 22, 81].

Collectively, the data reveal novel role of PS1 and Syt1 at the synapse; present a reduction in the PS1-Syt1 interactions as potential molecular contributor to AD pathogenesis; and open avenues for novel synapse-specific AD-targeting therapeutic interventions.

Conclusions

The study reveals novel role of presenilin 1 (PS1) and synaptotagmin 1 (Syt1) at the synapse. It demonstrates that PS1 and Syt1 can influence each other function via direct interaction. Furthermore, it reports that the PS1-Syt1 binding is reduced in sporadic Alzheimer's disease (sAD) brains, which may contribute to the abnormal PS1/γ-secretase conformation, increased amyloid β (Aβ) 42/40 ratio, and impaired neurotransmitter release. The findings in this study indicate that fostering PS1-Syt1 interaction might serve as a novel synapse-specific therapeutic approach for AD. In summary, the reported data point towards novel mechanism regulating synaptic physiology and relative generation of the longer to shorter Aβ species, describe new pathogenic mechanisms of AD, and propose novel therapeutic target for the disease.

Additional files

Additional file 1: Fluorescence lifetime and corresponding FRET efficiency values recorded in the FLIM assays. The table summarizes the mean ± SEM fluorescence lifetimes and corresponding, calculated FRET efficiencies for the all presented FLIM analyses. (XLSX 14 kb)

Additional file 2: Inhibition of PS1-Syt1 interaction does not affect APP expression and APP-CTF levels. The representative western blot demonstrates levels of APP-FL, APP-CTFs and Gapdh, as a loading control, in the protein lysates extracted from primary neurons pre-treated with scramble or PS1-LNT peptides for 2 h and stimulated for 15 min with 50 mM KCl. The adjacent graph shows the quantification of the APP-FL levels relative to Gapdh, and APP processing rate as an APP-CTFs/APP-FL ratio. The values were normalized to the scramble pre-treated cells. The data are presented as mean ± SEM, $n = 10$-11. Statistical significance was determined using two-tailed unpaired Student's t-test, ns $p > 0.05$. (TIF 3734 kb)

Additional file 3: Inhibition of the PS1-Syt1 interaction leads to intraneuronal Aβ accumulation. The representative images demonstrate immunofluorescent staining of primary neurons pre-treated with scramble or PS1-LNT peptides, and depolarized for 15 min with 50 mM KCl. Anti-MAP2 (red) and anti-β-amyloid 17–24, clone 4G8 (green) antibodies were used; scale bar 10 μm. The adjacent graph presents the quantification of the fluorescent intensity of Aβ/APP normalized to the MAP2 fluorescence. The values were normalized to the scramble treated cells. The data are presented as mean ± SEM, $n = 105$ for scramble and $n = 96$ for PS1-LNT, n = number of neurons analyzed in 4 independent experiments. Statistical significance was determined using two-tailed unpaired Student's t-test, ***$p < 0.001$. (TIF 5598 kb)

Abbreviations

Aβ: Amyloid β; APP: Amyloid precursor protein; fAD: Familial Alzheimer's disease; FLIM: Fluorescence lifetime imaging microscopy; FRAP: Fluorescence recovery after photobleaching; FRET: Förster resonance energy transfer; PS1: Presenilin 1; sAD: Sporadic Alzheimer's disease; SypHy: Synaptophluorin; fluorescent reporter of exocytosis; Syt1: Synaptotagmin 1; wt: Wild type

Acknowledgements

We would like to acknowledge Ashok Khatri (MGH, Boston) for the advice on the design of cell permeable peptides; Ms. Kateryna Smozhanyk for technical support with electron microscopy experiments; and MGH ADRC (Dr. Hyman, Director) for providing human brain tissue.

Funding

This work was supported by the National Institutes of Health (AG15379 and AG044486 to OB).

Authors' contributions

KMZ designed, performed and analyzed the experiments; MM performed the APP processing analysis and discussed the data; IL and GS performed and analyzed the electron microscopy experiments, and discussed the data; ST participated in the design and carrying out of the in vivo studies; LJK provided assistance with co-IP experiments; BTH discussed the data; OB conceived the study, participated in its design and coordination; KMZ and OB wrote the manuscript. All authors read and approved the final manuscript.

Authors' information

Not applicable.

Competing interests

The authors declare that they have no competing interests.

Author details

Department of Neurology, MassGeneral Institute for Neurodegenerative Disease, Massachusetts General Hospital, Harvard Medical School, 114 16th Street, Rm. 2006, 02129 Charlestown, MA, USA. [2]Department of Cytology, Bogomoletz Institute of Physiology, National Academy of Sciences of Ukraine, 4 Bogomoletz Street, 01024 Kyiv, Ukraine.

References

1. DeKosky ST, Scheff SW. Synapse loss in frontal cortex biopsies in Alzheimer's disease: correlation with cognitive severity. Ann Neurol. 1990;27:457–64.
2. DeKosky ST, Scheff SW, Styren SD. Structural correlates of cognition in dementia: quantification and assessment of synapse change. Neurodegeneration. 1996;5:417–21.

3. Masliah E, Mallory M, Hansen L, DeTeresa R, Alford M, Terry R. Synaptic and neuritic alterations during the progression of Alzheimer's disease. Neurosci Lett. 1994;174:67–72.
4. Selkoe DJ. Alzheimer's disease is a synaptic failure. Science. 2002;298:789–91.
5. Hardy J, Allsop D. Amyloid deposition as the central event in the aetiology of Alzheimer's disease. Trends Pharmacol Sci. 1991;12:383–8.
6. Selkoe DJ, Hardy J. The amyloid hypothesis of Alzheimer's disease at 25 years. EMBO Mol Med. 2016;8:595–608.
7. Lassmann H, Weiler R, Fischer P, Bancher C, Jellinger K, Floor E, Danielczyk W, Seitelberger F, Winkler H. Synaptic pathology in Alzheimer's disease: immunological data for markers of synaptic and large dense-core vesicles. Neuroscience. 1992;46:1–8.
8. Tan MG, Lee C, Lee JH, Francis PT, Williams RJ, Ramirez MJ, Chen CP, Wong PT, Lai MK. Decreased rabphilin 3A immunoreactivity in Alzheimer's disease is associated with Abeta burden. Neurochem Int. 2014;64:29–36.
9. Kandalepas PC, Sadleir KR, Eimer WA, Zhao J, Nicholson DA, Vassar R. The Alzheimer's beta-secretase BACE1 localizes to normal presynaptic terminals and to dystrophic presynaptic terminals surrounding amyloid plaques. Acta Neuropathol. 2013;126:329–52.
10. Del Prete D, Lombino F, Liu X, D'Adamio L. APP is cleaved by Bace1 in pre-synaptic vesicles and establishes a pre-synaptic interactome, via its intracellular domain, with molecular complexes that regulate pre-synaptic vesicles functions. PLoS One. 2014;9, e108576.
11. Schedin-Weiss S, Caesar I, Winblad B, Blom H, Tjernberg LO. Super-resolution microscopy reveals gamma-secretase at both sides of the neuronal synapse. Acta Neuropathol Commun. 2016;4:29.
12. Kuzuya A, Zoltowska KM, Post KL, Arimon M, Li X, Svirsky S, Maesako M, Muzikansky A, Gautam V, Kovacs D, et al. Identification of the novel activity-driven interaction between synaptotagmin 1 and presenilin 1 links calcium, synapse, and amyloid beta. BMC Biol. 2016;14:25.
13. Somavarapu AK, Kepp KP. The dynamic mechanism of presenilin-1 function: Sensitive gate dynamics and loop unplugging control protein access. Neurobiol Dis. 2016;89:147–56.
14. Uemura K, Farner KC, Nasser-Ghodsi N, Jones P, Berezovska O. Reciprocal relationship between APP positioning relative to the membrane and PS1 conformation. Mol Neurodegener. 2011;6:15.
15. Berezovska O, Lleo A, Herl LD, Frosch MP, Stern EA, Bacskai BJ, Hyman BT. Familial Alzheimer's disease presenilin 1 mutations cause alterations in the conformation of presenilin and interactions with amyloid precursor protein. J Neurosci. 2005;25:3009–17.
16. Fernandez MA, Klutkowski JA, Freret T, Wolfe MS. Alzheimer presenilin-1 mutations dramatically reduce trimming of long amyloid beta-peptides (Abeta) by gamma-secretase to increase 42-to-40-residue Abeta. J Biol Chem. 2014;289:31043–52.
17. Fukumori A, Steiner H. Substrate recruitment of gamma-secretase and mechanism of clinical presenilin mutations revealed by photoaffinity mapping. EMBO J. 2016.
18. Li N, Liu K, Qiu Y, Ren Z, Dai R, Deng Y, Qing H. Effect of Presenilin Mutations on APP Cleavage; Insights into the Pathogenesis of FAD. Front Aging Neurosci. 2016;8:51.
19. Chavez-Gutierrez L, Bammens L, Benilova I, Vandersteen A, Benurwar M, Borgers M, Lismont S, Zhou L, Van Cleynenbreugel S, Esselmann H, et al. The mechanism of gamma-Secretase dysfunction in familial Alzheimer disease. EMBO J. 2012;31:2261–74.
20. Okochi M, Tagami S, Yanagida K, Takami M, Kodama TS, Mori K, Nakayama T, Ihara Y, Takeda M. gamma-secretase modulators and presenilin 1 mutants act differently on presenilin/gamma-secretase function to cleave Abeta42 and Abeta43. Cell Rep. 2013;3:42–51.
21. Lleo A, Berezovska O, Herl L, Raju S, Deng A, Bacskai BJ, Frosch MP, Irizarry M, Hyman BT. Nonsteroidal anti-inflammatory drugs lower Abeta42 and change presenilin 1 conformation. Nat Med. 2004;10:1065–6.
22. Uemura K, Lill CM, Li X, Peters JA, Ivanov A, Fan Z, DeStrooper B, Bacskai BJ, Hyman BT, Berezovska O. Allosteric modulation of PS1/gamma-secretase conformation correlates with amyloid beta(42/40) ratio. PLoS One. 2009;4:e7893.
23. Zhang C, Wu B, Beglopoulos V, Wines-Samuelson M, Zhang D, Dragatsis I, Sudhof TC, Shen J. Presenilins are essential for regulating neurotransmitter release. Nature. 2009;460:632–6.
24. Pratt KG, Zhu P, Watari H, Cook DG, Sullivan JM. A novel role for {gamma}-secretase: selective regulation of spontaneous neurotransmitter release from hippocampal neurons. J Neurosci. 2011;31:899–906.
25. Gautam V, D'Avanzo C, Berezovska O, Tanzi RE, Kovacs DM. Synaptotagmins interact with APP and promote Abeta generation. Mol Neurodegener. 2015;10:31.
26. Fanutza T, Del Prete D, Ford MJ, Castillo PE, D'Adamio L. APP and APLP2 interact with the synaptic release machinery and facilitate transmitter release at hippocampal synapses. elife. 2015;4, e09743.
27. Sudhof TC. The synaptic vesicle cycle. Annu Rev Neurosci. 2004;27:509–47.
28. Chapman ER. How does synaptotagmin trigger neurotransmitter release? Annu Rev Biochem. 2008;77:615–41.
29. Tucker WC, Chapman ER. Role of synaptotagmin in Ca2 + -triggered exocytosis. Biochem J. 2002;366:1–13.
30. Roden WH, Papke JB, Moore JM, Cahill AL, Macarthur H, Harkins AB. Stable RNA interference of synaptotagmin I in PC12 cells results in differential regulation of transmitter release. Am J Physiol Cell Physiol. 2007;293:C1742–52.
31. Herreman A, Hartmann D, Annaert W, Saftig P, Craessaerts K, Serneels L, Umans L, Schrijvers V, Checler F, Vanderstichele H, et al. Presenilin 2 deficiency causes a mild pulmonary phenotype and no changes in amyloid precursor protein processing but enhances the embryonic lethal phenotype of presenilin 1 deficiency. Proc Natl Acad Sci U S A. 1999;96:11872–7.
32. Shimamoto K, Lebrun B, Yasuda-Kamatani Y, Sakaitani M, Shigeri Y, Yumoto N, Nakajima T. DL-threo-beta-benzyloxyaspartate, a potent blocker of excitatory amino acid transporters. Mol Pharmacol. 1998;53:195–201.
33. Royle SJ, Granseth B, Odermatt B, Derevier A, Lagnado L. Imaging phluorin-based probes at hippocampal synapses. Methods Mol Biol. 2008;457:293–303.
34. Dreosti E, Lagnado L. Optical reporters of synaptic activity in neural circuits. Exp Physiol. 2011;96:4–12.
35. Rodriguez A, Ehlenberger DB, Dickstein DL, Hof PR, Wearne SL. Automated three-dimensional detection and shape classification of dendritic spines from fluorescence microscopy images. PLoS One. 2008;3:e1997.
36. Yasuda R. Imaging spatiotemporal dynamics of neuronal signaling using fluorescence resonance energy transfer and fluorescence lifetime imaging microscopy. Curr Opin Neurobiol. 2006;16:551–61.
37. Zoltowska KM, Maesako M, Berezovska O. Interrelationship between changes in the amyloid beta 42/40 ratio and presenilin 1 conformation. Mol Med. 2016;22.
38. Wahlster L, Arimon M, Nasser-Ghodsi N, Post KL, Serrano-Pozo A, Uemura K, Berezovska O. Presenilin-1 adopts pathogenic conformation in normal aging and in sporadic Alzheimer's disease. Acta Neuropathol. 2013;125:187–99.
39. Walsh AJ, Sharick JT, Skala MC, Beier HT. Temporal binning of time-correlated single photon counting data improves exponential decay fits and imaging speed. Biomed Optics Express. 2016;7:1385–99.
40. Bacskai BJ, Skoch J, Hickey GA, Allen R, Hyman BT. Fluorescence resonance energy transfer determinations using multiphoton fluorescence lifetime imaging microscopy to characterize amyloid-beta plaques. J Biomed Opt. 2003;8:368–75.
41. Penn Y, Segal M, Moses E. Network synchronization in hippocampal neurons. Proc Natl Acad Sci U S A. 2016;113:3341–6.
42. Shimojo M, Courchet J, Pieraut S, Torabi-Rander N, Sando 3rd R, Polleux F, Maximov A. SNAREs Controlling Vesicular Release of BDNF and Development of Callosal Axons. Cell Rep. 2015;11:1054–66.
43. Petoukhov E, Fernando S, Mills F, Shivji F, Hunter D, Krieger C, Silverman MA, Bamji SX. Activity-dependent secretion of progranulin from synapses. J Cell Sci. 2013;126:5412–21.
44. Poo MM. Neurotrophins as synaptic modulators. Nat Rev Neurosci. 2001;2:24–32.
45. Van Vliet BJ, Sebben M, Dumuis A, Gabrion J, Bockaert J, Pin JP. Endogenous amino acid release from cultured cerebellar neuronal cells: effect of tetanus toxin on glutamate release. J Neurochem. 1989;52:1229–39.
46. Nakata T, Terada S, Hirokawa N. Visualization of the dynamics of synaptic vesicle and plasma membrane proteins in living axons. J Cell Biol. 1998;140:659–74.
47. Stagi M, Dittrich PS, Frank N, Iliev AI, Schwille P, Neumann H. Breakdown of axonal synaptic vesicle precursor transport by microglial nitric oxide. J Neurosci. 2005;25:352–62.
48. Ferrer I, Marti E, Tortosa A, Blasi J. Dystrophic neurites of senile plaques are defective in proteins involved in exocytosis and neurotransmission. J Neuropathol Exp Neurol. 1998;57:218–25.
49. Keating DJ, Dubach D, Zanin MP, Yu Y, Martin K, Zhao YF, Chen C, Porta S, Arbones ML, Mittaz L, Pritchard MA. DSCR1/RCAN1 regulates vesicle

exocytosis and fusion pore kinetics: implications for Down syndrome and Alzheimer's disease. Hum Mol Genet. 2008;17:1020–30.
50. de Diego AM, Lorrio S, Calvo-Gallardo E, Garcia AG. Smaller quantal size and faster kinetics of single exocytotic events in chromaffin cells from the APP/PS1 mouse model of Alzheimer's disease. Biochem Biophys Res Commun. 2012;428:482–6.
51. Ermak G, Morgan TE, Davies KJ. Chronic overexpression of the calcineurin inhibitory gene DSCR1 (Adapt78) is associated with Alzheimer's disease. J Biol Chem. 2001;276:38787–94.
52. Berezin MY, Achilefu S. Fluorescence lifetime measurements and biological imaging. Chem Rev. 2010;110:2641–84.
53. Berezovska O, Bacskai BJ, Hyman BT. Monitoring proteins in intact cells. Sci Aging Knowledge Environ. 2003;2003:PE14.
54. Cirrito JR, Yamada KA, Finn MB, Sloviter RS, Bales KR, May PC, Schoepp DD, Paul SM, Mennerick S, Holtzman DM. Synaptic activity regulates interstitial fluid amyloid-beta levels in vivo. Neuron. 2005;48:913–22.
55. Kamenetz F, Tomita T, Hsieh H, Seabrook G, Borchelt D, Iwatsubo T, Sisodia S, Malinow R. APP processing and synaptic function. Neuron. 2003;37:925–37.
56. Li X, Uemura K, Hashimoto T, Nasser-Ghodsi N, Arimon M, Lill CM, Palazzolo I, Krainc D, Hyman BT, Berezovska O. Neuronal activity and secreted amyloid beta lead to altered amyloid beta precursor protein and presenilin 1 interactions. Neurobiol Dis. 2013;50:127–34.
57. Rybalchenko V, Hwang SY, Rybalchenko N, Koulen P. The cytosolic N-terminus of presenilin-1 potentiates mouse ryanodine receptor single channel activity. Int J Biochem Cell Biol. 2008;40:84–97.
58. Wu B, Yamaguchi H, Lai FA, Shen J. Presenilins regulate calcium homeostasis and presynaptic function via ryanodine receptors in hippocampal neurons. Proc Natl Acad Sci U S A. 2013;110:15091–6.
59. Mirnics K, Korade Z, Arion D, Lazarov O, Unger T, Macioce M, Sabatini M, Terrano D, Douglass KC, Schor NF, Sisodia SS. Presenilin-1-dependent transcriptome changes. J Neurosci. 2005;25:1571–8.
60. Maximov A, Tang J, Yang X, Pang ZP, Sudhof TC. Complexin controls the force transfer from SNARE complexes to membranes in fusion. Science. 2009;323:516–21.
61. Stevens CF, Sullivan JM. The synaptotagmin C2A domain is part of the calcium sensor controlling fast synaptic transmission. Neuron. 2003;39:299–308.
62. Brewer KD, Bacaj T, Cavalli A, Camilloni C, Swarbrick JD, Liu J, Zhou A, Zhou P, Barlow N, Xu J, et al. Dynamic binding mode of a Synaptotagmin-1-SNARE complex in solution. Nat Struct Mol Biol. 2015;22:555–64.
63. Wang S, Li Y, Ma C. Synaptotagmin-1 C2B domain interacts simultaneously with SNAREs and membranes to promote membrane fusion. elife. 2016;5.
64. Evans CS, He Z, Bai H, Lou X, Jeggle P, Sutton RB, Edwardson JM, Chapman ER. Functional analysis of the interface between the tandem C2 domains of synaptotagmin-1. Mol Biol Cell. 2016;27:979–89.
65. de Wit H, Walter AM, Milosevic I, Gulyas-Kovacs A, Riedel D, Sorensen JB, Verhage M. Synaptotagmin-1 docks secretory vesicles to syntaxin-1/SNAP-25 acceptor complexes. Cell. 2009;138:935–46.
66. Poskanzer KE, Fetter RD, Davis GW. Discrete residues in the c(2)b domain of synaptotagmin I independently specify endocytic rate and synaptic vesicle size. Neuron. 2006;50:49–62.
67. Loewen CA, Royer SM, Reist NE. Drosophila synaptotagmin I null mutants show severe alterations in vesicle populations but calcium-binding motif mutants do not. J Comp Neurol. 2006;496:1–12.
68. Reist NE, Buchanan J, Li J, DiAntonio A, Buxton EM, Schwarz TL. Morphologically docked synaptic vesicles are reduced in synaptotagmin mutants of Drosophila. J Neurosci. 1998;18:7662–73.
69. Heimer-McGinn V, Murphy AC, Kim JC, Dymecki SM, Young PW. Decreased dendritic spine density as a consequence of tetanus toxin light chain expression in single neurons in vivo. Neurosci Lett. 2013;555:36–41.
70. Dorostkar MM, Zou C, Blazquez-Llorca L, Herms J. Analyzing dendritic spine pathology in Alzheimer's disease: problems and opportunities. Acta Neuropathol. 2015;130:1–19.
71. Tackenberg C, Ghori A, Brandt R. Thin, stubby or mushroom: spine pathology in Alzheimer's disease. Curr Alzheimer Res. 2009;6:261–8.
72. Terry RD. Cell death or synaptic loss in Alzheimer disease. J Neuropathol Exp Neurol. 2000;59:1118–9.
73. Sze CI, Bi H, Kleinschmidt-DeMasters BK, Filley CM, Martin LJ. Selective regional loss of exocytotic presynaptic vesicle proteins in Alzheimer's disease brains. J Neurol Sci. 2000;175:81–90.
74. Davidsson P, Jahn R, Bergquist J, Ekman R, Blennow K. Synaptotagmin, a synaptic vesicle protein, is present in human cerebrospinal fluid: a new biochemical marker for synaptic pathology in Alzheimer disease? Mol Chem Neuropathol. 1996;27:195–210.
75. Goetzl EJ, Kapogiannis D, Schwartz JB, Lobach IV, Goetzl L, Abner EL, Jicha GA, Karydas AM, Boxer A, Miller BL. Decreased synaptic proteins in neuronal exosomes of frontotemporal dementia and Alzheimer's disease. FASEB J. 2016.
76. Ingelsson M, Fukumoto H, Newell KL, Growdon JH, Hedley-Whyte ET, Frosch MP, Albert MS, Hyman BT, Irizarry MC. Early Abeta accumulation and progressive synaptic loss, gliosis, and tangle formation in AD brain. Neurology. 2004;62:925–31.
77. Szaruga M, Veugelen S, Benurwar M, Lismont S, Sepulveda-Falla D, Lleo A, Ryan NS, Lashley T, Fox NC, Murayama S, et al. Qualitative changes in human gamma-secretase underlie familial Alzheimer's disease. J Exp Med. 2015;212:2003–13.
78. Golde TE, Koo EH, Felsenstein KM, Osborne BA, Miele L. gamma-Secretase inhibitors and modulators. Biochim Biophys Acta. 1828;2013:2898–907.
79. Bursavich MG, Harrison BA, Blain JF. Gamma Secretase Modulators: New Alzheimer's Drugs on the Horizon? J Med Chem. 2016;59:7389–409.
80. Kounnas MZ, Danks AM, Cheng S, Tyree C, Ackerman E, Zhang X, Ahn K, Nguyen P, Comer D, Mao L, et al. Modulation of gamma-secretase reduces beta-amyloid deposition in a transgenic mouse model of Alzheimer's disease. Neuron. 2010;67:769–80.
81. Ohki Y, Higo T, Uemura K, Shimada N, Osawa S, Berezovska O, Yokoshima S, Fukuyama T, Tomita T, Iwatsubo T. Phenylpiperidine-type gamma-secretase modulators target the transmembrane domain 1 of presenilin 1. EMBO J. 2011;30:4815–24.

Downregulating ANP32A rescues synapse and memory loss via chromatin remodeling in Alzheimer model

Gao-Shang Chai[1,2†], Qiong Feng[1,2†], Zhi-Hao Wang[1,2], Yu Hu[1,2], Dong-Sheng Sun[1,2], Xiao-Guang Li[1,2], Dan Ke[1,2], Hong-Lian Li[1,2*], Gong-Ping Liu[1,2,3*] and Jian-Zhi Wang[1,2,3*]

Abstract

Background: The impairment of histone acetylation is causally linked to the cognitive decline in Alzheimer's disease (AD). In addition to histone acetyltransferases (HATs) and histone deacetylases (HDACs), inhibitor of acetyltransferases (INHAT) can also regulate histone acetylation. As a key component of INHAT, level of ANP32A is selectively upregulated in the brain of AD patients. Here we investigated whether downregulating ANP32A can rescue AD-like synapse and memory deficits.

Methods: RFP-labeled lentiviral ANP32A-shRNA was infused stereotaxically into the hippocampal CA3 region of the human tau transgenic mice (termed htau). The spatial learning and memory were assessed by Morris water maze (MWM). The synaptic function was measured by electrophysiological recording and the spine density was detected by Golgi staining. RT-PCR and Western blotting were used to detect the mRNA and protein levels.

Results: Elevation of ANP32 in htau transgenic mice was correlated with learning deficits, while the hippocampal infusion of lenti-siANP32A to downregulate ANP32A in 12 m-old htau mice could rescue memory loss. Further studies demonstrated that downregulating ANP32A restored synapse morphology and the function. In the brain of htau mice, the acetylated histone decreased while knockdown ANP32A unmasked histone for a robust acetylation with reduced INHAT complex formation. Downregulating of ANP32A also attenuated AD-like tau hyperphosphorylation. Finally, several AD-associated risk factors, including tau accumulation, β-amyloid and H_2O_2 exposure, increased ANP32A by activating CCAAT/enhancer binding protein β (C/EBPβ).

Conclusion: We conclude that downregulating ANP32A rescues synaptic plasticity and memory ability by reducing INHAT formation and unmasking histone for hyperacetylation. Our findings reveal novel mechanisms for AD memory loss and potential molecular markers for protection.

Keywords: Alzheimer's disease, ANP32A, Histone acetylation, Synapse, Memory

Background

Synapse impairment and memory deficit are hallmark pathology and symptom of Alzheimer's disease (AD), while the underlying mechanisms are currently unclear. Recent studies suggest that epigenetic modifications, particularly histone acetylation in the nervous system, play a critical role in regulating gene expression for long-term memory [1]. The chromatin remodeling *via* histone acetylation is a key mechanism to control gene expression [2]. Histone acetylation diminishes the electrostatic affinity between neighboring histones and the DNA, and consequently promotes a more open chromatin structure that allows for transcription of the memory-related genes [3].

Acetylation and deacetylation of histone is catalyzed by histone acetyltransferases (HATs) and histone deacetylases (HDACs), respectively. Reduced histone acetylation has been observed in animal models of neurodegenerative

* Correspondence: lihonglian@hust.edu.cn; liugp111@mail.hust.edu.cn; wangjz@mails.tjmu.edu.cn
†Equal contributors
[1]Department of Pathophysiology, School of Basic Medicine, Tongji Medical College, Huazhong University of Science and Technology, Wuhan 430030, China
Full list of author information is available at the end of the article

diseases including AD, which are characterized by cognitive decline [4]. So far, most studies aimed at pharmacologically increasing histone acetylation for therapeutic purpose mainly focused on approaches manipulating activity of HATs or HDACs. However, histone acetylation is also suppressed by a cellular complex termed inhibitor of acetyltransferases (INHAT) through histone-masking, in which INHAT binds to histones and masks their access to HAT [5, 6].

As key components of INHAT, the levels of ANP32A (also termed as I_1^{PP2A}) and SET (also termed as I_2^{PP2A}) are selectively upregulated in the brain regions affected with neurofibrillary pathology in AD [7–10]. Both ANP32A and SET are endogenous PP2A inhibitors, so that a causal association of ANP32A or SET with tau hyperphosphorylation has been reported [7, 8, 11]. However, whether and how ANP32A plays a role in the memory impairment of AD has not been reported.

In the present study, we found that downregulating C/EBPβ-associated elevation of ANP32A rescues synaptic plasticity and cognitive functions by unmasking histone for a robust acetylation in a well-recognized mouse model of AD.

Methods

Materials, cell culture and PP2A activity assay

All the antibodies used in this study are listed in Additional file 1: Table S1. Aβ peptide preparation, cell culture and PP2A activity assay, and the plasmids used in the present study please see Additional file 2.

Animals

Human tau transgenic mice (STOCK Mapttml (EGFP) Klt Tg (MAPT)8cPdav/J) were purchased from Jackson lab. All animal experiments were performed according to the 'Policies on the Use of Animals and Humans in Neuroscience Research' revised and approved by the Society for Neuroscience in 1995, and the animal study was approved by the Academic Review Board of Tongji Medical College, Huazhong University of Science and Technology.

Production and brain infusion of lentiviral constructs

The ANP32A-shRNA sequence is CGGATTTATTTA GAGCTGC, and it was cloned into LentiLox 3.7. The RFP sequence was driven by a cytomegalovirus (CMV) promoter and terminated using polyadenylation signal in the 3' long terminal repeat (LTR). The 3rd generation packaging systems was used for lentiviral production. These vectors include: pMDLg/pRRE (gag/pol elements), pRSV-REV, and pMD.G (env elements). The RFP-labeled lentiviral ANP32A-shRNA (LV-siANP) and the scrambled control (LV-siC) were constructed according to the standard procedure. The recombinant lentivirus was produced by transient transfection of HEK293T cells using the calcium phosphate method; the virus was harvested at 48 h and 72 h posttransfection and purified by centrifugation at 4 °C. The titer of the virus was 2×10^9 TU/ml. The in vivo knockdown efficiency was measured by Western blotting and RT-PCR after injection of the virus into the hippocampal CA3 of mice brains.

For brain injections, male 11 m-old htau mice, or 11 m-old wild-type littermates, were positioned respectively in a stereotaxic instrument, then 2 μl LV-siANP32A (htau-siANP), LV-siC (htau-siC) were bilaterally injected into the hippocampal CA3 region (AP ±2.0, ML -1.5, DV -2.0) at a rate of 0.50 μl/min. The needle was left in place for ~3 min before being withdrawn. All mice were kept at 24 ± 2 °C on daily 12 h light-dark cycles with ad libitum access to food and water. The injection did not significantly increase the death rate or change the normal activity of the mice compared with the non-injected controls. The hippocampal CA3 region was used for the biochemical measurements.

Behavioral tests

Four weeks after brain infusion of the viral vectors, the spatial learning and memory were assessed by Morris water maze (MWM) test [12, 13]. For spatial learning, mice were trained in water maze to find a hidden platform for 6 consecutive days, 4 trials per day with a 30 s interval from 14:00 to 20:00 pm. On each trial, the mice started from one of the four quadrants facing the wall of the pool and ended when the animal climbed on the platform. If the mice did not locate the platform within 60 s, they were guided to the platform. The swimming path and the time used to find the platform (latency) or pass through the previous platform quadrant were recorded each day by a video camera fixed to the ceiling, 1.5 m from the water surface. The camera was connected to a digital-tracking device attached to an IBM computer. The spatial memory was tested 1 day after the last training. The longer a mouse stayed in the previous platform-located quadrant, the better it scored the spatial memory.

Real time PCR

Total RNA (3 μg in 25 μl), isolated using TrizolTM (Invitrogen, CA), was reversely transcribed and the produced cDNA (1 μl) was used for real time PCR with primer sets: 5'-CAAACAATACCGAAGGGCACAG-3' and 5'-AAGAGGGCTAGATAATCAGAAGACAGA-3' for synaptophysin, 5'- CTTTGCTTGTTTATTTTGCTTC-3' and 5'-CCAATGTGTTTATCTGTGACTG-3' for synapsin I, 5'-TATGCTCTTTGGGTCAGTCTCGTT-3' and 5'- GTC CCTTTATCCTCCGTCTTTCTT-3' for NR2B, 5'- TCAA GGAAAGCAGAAGGGGAAA-3' and 5'-TGTGGAATG GAATGATAGGCGA-3' for NR2A, 5'-CACATGTAGCC

GGAGTGATG-3' and, 5'-CACTCAAGAGGATGGGG AAA-3' for GluR1, 5'-ATTTCGGGTAGGGATGGTTC-3' and 5'-ACCATCCTTCACTGGCATTC-3' for GluR2, 5'-CACGTTTTCTCGGTAGGCATT-3' and 5'- AGGG GACCTGGAAGTATTGGC-3' for ANP32A, and 5'-AG CCTTCCTTCTTGGGTAT-3' and 5'-GCTCAGTAACA GTCCGCCTA-3' for β-actin.

Golgi impregnation and dendritic morphology analysis

For Golgi stain, the mice were anesthetized and then perfused transcardially with 4% paraformaldehyde, and brain tissue was processed as described [14]. Individual sections were incubated overnight at room temperature in water solution of 3.5% $K_2Cr_2O_7$ and 0.4% OsO_4. The sections were then sandwiched in two glass slides and incubated in 1% $AgNO_{3(aq)}$ for 5 h at room temperature in dark. Then the slide assemblies were dismantled in water and the sections were mounted on gel-coated slides (0.5% porcine gelatin), dehydrated in a series of graded ethanol rinses, cleared with Histoclear, and cover slipped with cytoseal. The images were taken using Olympus BX60 (Tokyo).

The spine density was determined in the segments of dendrites at a distance of 190-210 μm (distal) from the soma. To acquire images for spine analysis, the dendritic segments were imaged under bright-field illumination on a Zeiss Axioimager microscope with a 63× oil immersion objective, and spine morphology was analyzed according to a previously reported method [15], which does not assess spine density in a 3 dimensional manner but focuses on spines paralleled to the plane of section. Although the method may underestimate the total number of spines, it facilitates a direct comparison of treatment groups when they are analyzed in an identical manner. Image J software was used to calculate linear spine density [16], which was presented as the number of spines per 10 μm of dendrite length. On the basis of morphology, spines were classified into thin (spines with a long neck and a visible small head) and mushroom (big spines with a well-defined neck and a very voluminous head) spines. Data from 5-7 neurons were averaged per animal and used in further statistical analysis.

Electrophysiological analysis

Mice brains were cut into horizontal sections of 400 μm thickness by a vibration microtome in cold artificial cerebrospinal fluid (aCSF) containing (in mM) NaCl 126, KCl 2.5, $NaHCO_3$ 26, NaH_2PO_4 1.25, $CaCl_2$ 2, $MgCl_2$ 2, glucose 10, equilibrated with 95% O_2 and 5% CO_2. Then the hippocampal slices were transferred into oxygen-enriched artificial cerebrospinal fluid (aCSF) to recover for 30 min. Individual slices were laid down over an 8×8 array of planar microelectrodes, each 50×50 mm in size, with an interpolar distance of 450 mm (MED-P5455; Alpha MED Sciences, Kadoma, Japan) and kept submerged in aCSF (4 ml/min; 30 °C) with a nylon mesh glued to a platinum ring. Voltage signals were acquired using the MED64 System (Alpha MED Sciences). Field excitatory postsynaptic potentials (fEPSPs) were recorded from CA3 in hippocampus by stimulating mossy fibers. Stimulation intensity was adjusted to evoke fEPSP amplitudes that were 30 % of maximal size. Long-term potentiation was induced by applying 1 train of high-frequency stimulation (100 Hz, 1 second duration at test strength). Paired-pulse facilitation (PPF) was examined by applying pairs of pulses, which were separated by 50–300 ms intervals.

Western blotting

Western blotting was performed as described previously [17]. Mice were decapitated after the spatial memory retention test. The hippocampal CA3 region (where virus infected), cortex and cerebellum were rapidly removed and homogenized at 4 °C using a Teflon glass homogenizer with 50 mM Tris-HCl (pH 7.4), 150 mM NaCl, 10 mM NaF, 1 mM Na_3VO_4, 5 mM EDTA, 2 mM benzamidine, and 1 mM phenylmethylsulfonyl fluoride. The extract was mixed with sample buffer (3:1, v/v) containing 200 mM Tris-HCl (pH 7.6), 8% SDS, 40% glycerol, 40 mM dithiothreitol, then boiled for 10 min. The proteins were separated by 10% SDS-polyacrylamide gel electrophoresis and transferred to nitrocellulose membranes. The membranes were blocked with 5% non-fat milk dissolved in TBSTween-20 (50 mM Tris-HCl (pH 7.6), 150 mM NaCl, 0.2% Tween-20) for 1 h and probed with primary antibody at 4 °C overnight. Finally, the blots were incubated with anti rabbit or anti-mouse IgG conjugated to IRDyeTM (800CW) for 1 h at 15-25 °C and visualized using the Odyssey Infrared Imaging System (Licor biosciences, Lincoln, NE, USA).

Immunohistochemistry

In brief, mice were sacrificed and perfused through aorta with 100 ml 0.9 % NaCl followed by 400 ml phosphate buffer containing 4 % paraformaldehyde. Brains were removed and postfixed in perfusate overnight and then cut into sections (20 μm) with a vibratome (Leica, Nussloch, Germany; S100, TPI). Free floating sections were blocked with 3% H_2O_2 in anhydrous methanol for 30 min and nonspecific sites were blocked with bovine serum albumin (BSA) for 30 min at room temperature. Sections were then incubated overnight at 4 °C with primary antibodies. Immunoreaction was developed using HistostainTM-SP kits and visualized with diaminobenzidine (brown color). For each primary antibody, 3-5 consecutive sections from each brain were used. The images were observed using a microscope (Olympus BX60, Tokyo, Japan).

Immunoprecipitation

The protein extracts from mouse hippocampal CA3 region injected with virus were subsequently incubated for overnight at 4 °C with the precipitating antibodies. Twenty microliters of a 1:1 suspension of protein G-Sepharose beads was added to the mixture and incubated for 2 h at 4 °C with gentle rotation. The beads were collected by centrifugation and washed extensively with cell lysis buffer. The bound proteins were dissociated by boiling the beads in 2×Laemmli sample buffer and separated by SDS-polyacrylamide gel electrophoresis (SDS-PAGE).

Statistical analysis

The data was expressed as mean±SD or mean±SEM (for animal behavior measurement) and statistical comparisons were performed using SPSS 12.0 statistical software (SPSS Inc., Chicago, Illinois). Student's unpaired t-test, and one-way analysis of variance procedure followed by Bonferroni' s post hoc test, or two-way repeated measures ANOVA and Bonferroni' s post hoc test were used to determine the statistical significance of means.

Results

ANP32A elevation is correlated with learning deficit in htau mice

ANP32A is significantly increased in the AD brains [7, 8], but the role of ANP32A in learning and memory is not known. We observed by Morris water maze (MWM) test that the human tau transgenic mice (htau) show learning deficits at 12 m but not at 4 m and 8 m-old compared with the age-matched wild-type littermates (Fig. 1a–c). Interestingly, the htau mice show significant elevation of ANP32A only at 12 m but not at 4 m and 8 m-old, and the increase was only detected in the hippocampus and cortex but not in cerebellum (Fig. 1d–i), the latter is not directly involved in learning and memory. A remarkable increase of ANP32A protein level was also detected by immunohistochemical staining in hippocampal CA3 of 12 m-old htau mice (Fig. 1j). These data indicate that ANP32A may play a role in learning performance.

Downregulating ANP32A rescues memory in htau mice

To test whether knockdown ANP32A could rescue memory deficits, we constructed lentivirus co-expressing ANP32A shRNA (LV-siANP) or the scrambled control shRNA (LV-siC), and injected the virus into the hippocampal CA3 of 11 m-old htau transgenic mice (Fig. 2a). Four weeks after the injection, a robust virus transfection was seen by direct fluorescent imaging (Fig. 2b), and the knockdown efficiency was confirmed by the significantly reduced protein and mRNA levels of ANP32A in hippocampal CA3 of htau mice measured by Western blotting (Fig. 2c and d), RT-PCR (Fig. 2e) and immunohistochemical staining (Fig. 2f). With ANP32A knockdown, the improved learning ability was shown by the reduced escape latency during 6 days training trials (Fig. 2g); and a remarkably improved memory was also detected at day 7 by removed the platform, demonstrated by the decreased latency to reach the target quadrant, the increased time crossings and time spent in the target quadrant (Fig. 2h–k). Swimming behavior was similar among the groups (Fig. 2l and m). These data together demonstrate that arresting ANP32A elevation in hippocampal CA3 can rescue learning and memory decline in htau transgenic mice.

Downregulating ANP32A preserves synaptic morphology and the functions

To explore the underlying mechanisms of knockdown ANP32A improving cognitive functions, we first measured the synaptic transmission by electrophysiological recording in the acute brain slices. We observed that the slope of fEPSP in 12 m-old htau mice was decreased compared with the age-matched littermates, while downregulation of ANP32A by LV-siANP32A significantly increased fEPSP slope when compared with the LV-C control mice (Fig. 3a and b). Using a paired-pulse protocol to determine the paired-pulse facilitation (PPF) of the fEPSP at mossy fiber-CA3 circuit, we did not find significant difference among three groups (Fig. 3c), indicating knockdown ANP32 did not significantly affect the presynaptic functions.

The spine generation and mushroom spine formation play a crucial role in learning and memory. Significant reduction of mushroom and thin-shaped spines was also detected in hippocampus of 12 m-old htau transgenic mice, while knockdown of ANP32A restored the spine density (Fig. 3d–f).

To verify the molecular mechanisms underlying the altered synapse morphology, we measured the levels of synapse-associated proteins. We observed that the protein (Fig. 4a and b) and mRNA (Fig. 4c) levels of presynaptic proteins including synaptophysin (Syp) and synapsin I (Syn1) and postsynaptic proteins including N-methyl-D-aspartate receptor type 2A (NR2A) and N-methyl-D-aspartate receptor type 2B (NR2B), AMPA receptor subunits GluR1 and GluR2 were decreased in 12 m-old htau mice compared with the age-matched control mice, while knockdown ANP32A with LV-siANP32A restored the protein and mRNA levels of these synaptic proteins in htau mice to the control levels. These data together

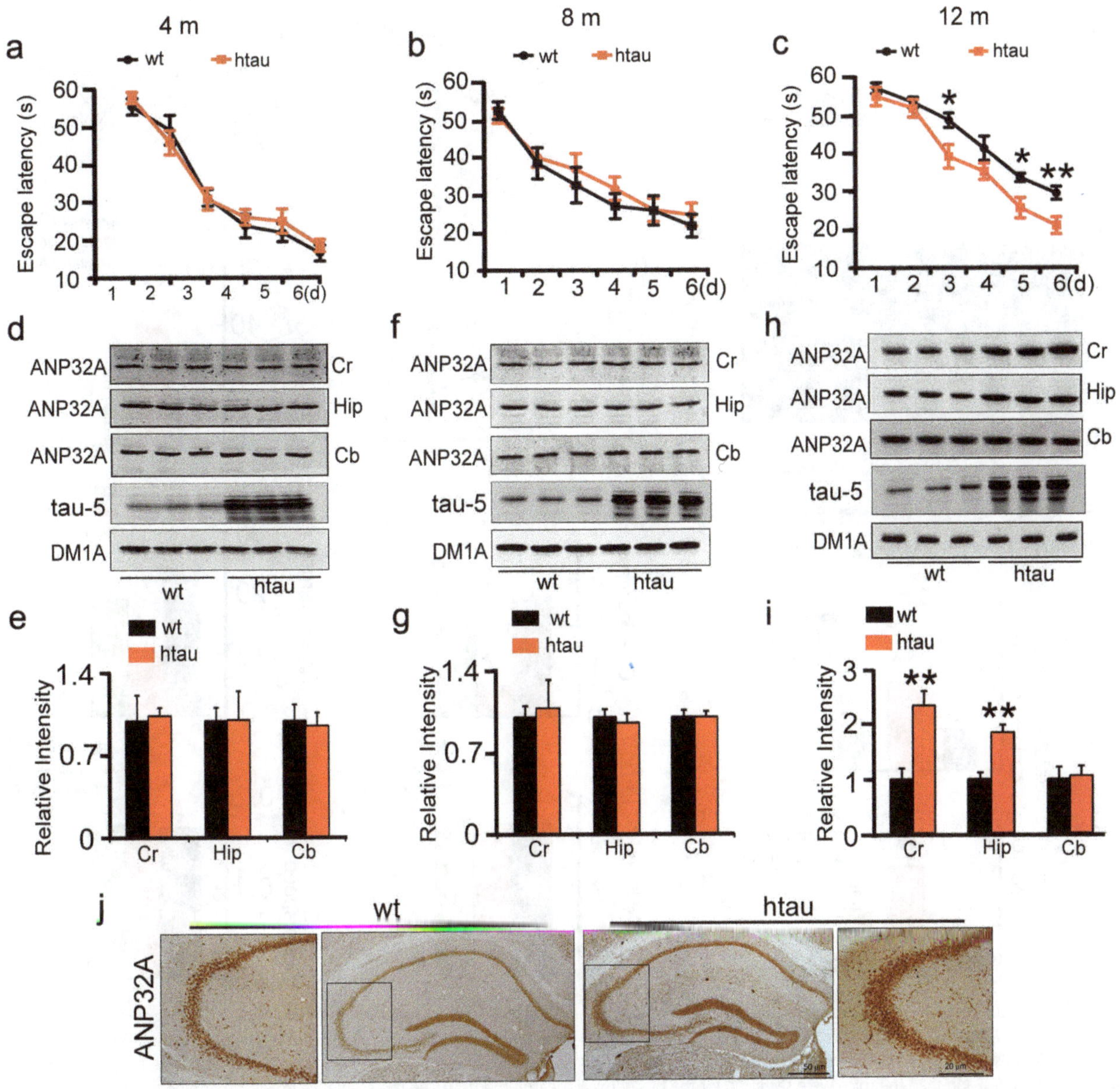

Fig. 1 ANP32A elevation is correlated with learning deficit in htau mice. **a–c** Only the 12 m- but not 4 m- and 8 m-old htau transgenic mice show increased latency during 6 days learning trials in MWM test when compared with the age-matched wild-type (wt) littermates (a: wt, n=10, htau, n=9; b: wt, n=15, htau, n=12; c: n=9 each group). Data were presented as mean ± s.e.m. *, p<0.05, **, p<0.01 *vs* wt (one-way repeated measures ANOVA and Bonferroni' s post hoc test). **d–i** Only the 12 m- but not 4 m- and 8 m-old htau mice show increased ANP32A level in cortex (Cr) and hippocampus (Hip) compared with the wt littermates, and no difference of ANP32A was detected in cerebellum (Cb) measured by Western blotting. Tubulin probed by DM1A was used as a loading control. Data were presented as mean ± SD. **, p<0.01 *vs* wt (Unpaired Student's t-test (two-tailed)). **j** The representative images of ANP32A in hippocampus measured by immunohistochemical staining (n=3-6 slices from 3 mice for each group)

suggest that downregulating ANP32A efficiently rescues the synapse impairments in htau transgenic mice.

Knockdown ANP32A restores histone acetylation by blocking INHAT formation

Histone acetylation regulates expression of synaptic proteins [18]. The acetylation of H3 at K9 and K14 (H3K9, H3K14) and H4 at K5 and K12 (H4K5, H4K12) were significantly decreased in 12 m-old htau mice compared with the age-matched littermates, while knockdown ANP32A restored the acetylated levels of H3 and H4 without changing the total level of H3 and H4 subunits (Fig. 5).

ANP32A and SET can bind histone to form an inhibitory complex (i.e., INHAT) that masks the histone acetylation

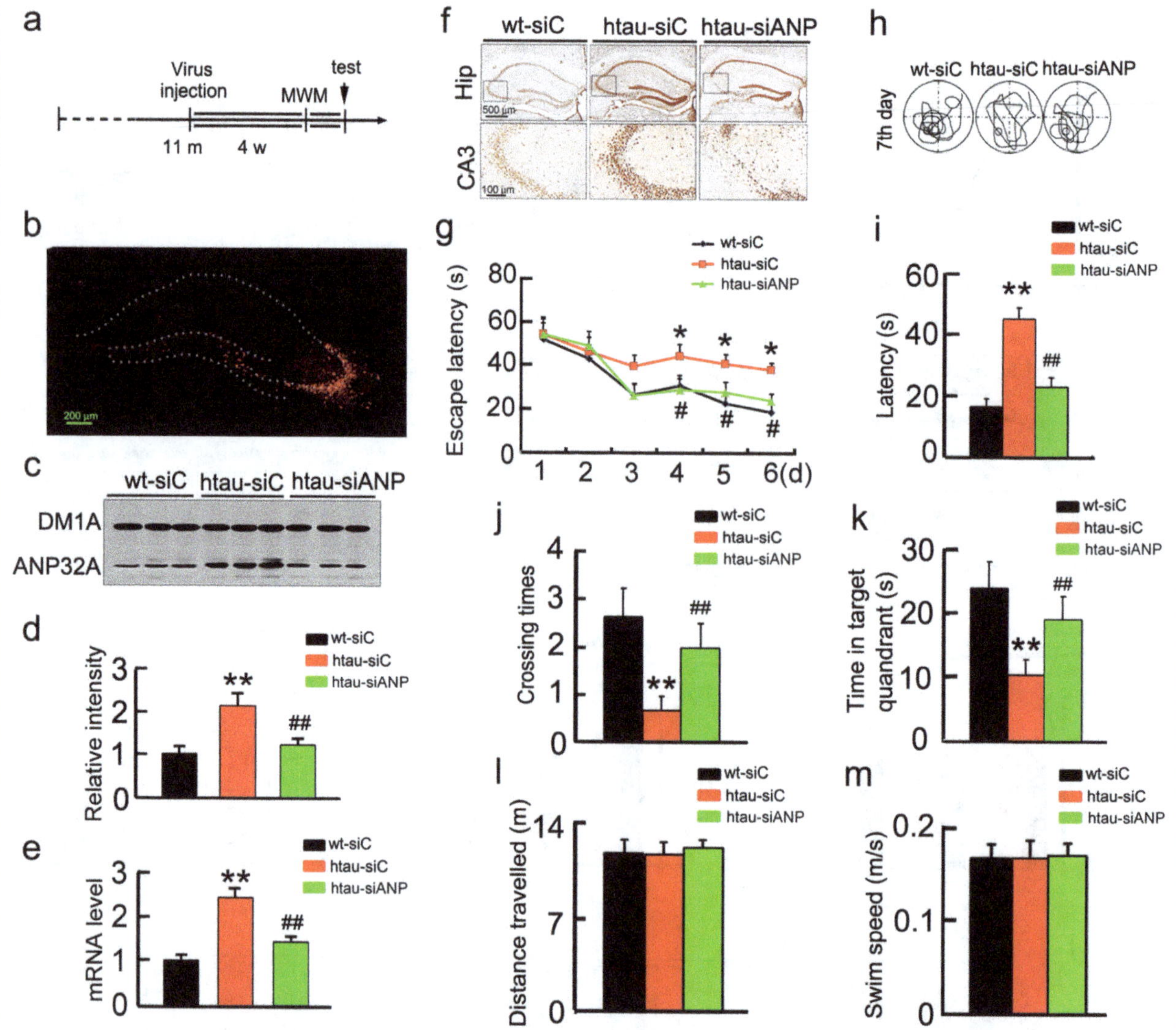

Fig. 2 Downregulating ANP32A improves spatial learning and memory in htau mice. **a** Schematics of the procedure. Lentivirus co-expressing RFP and ANP32A shRNA (siANP) or the scrambled control shRNA (siC) (2×10^9 TU/ml) were stereotaxically injected into the hippocampal CA3 of 11 m-old htau mice (htau-siC and htau-siANP) or the age-matched wild-type littermates (wt-siC). One month later, learning and memory were detected in Morris water maze (MWM) and then the mice were sacrificed for the biochemical measurements. **b** The representative image confirming expression of the injected lentivirus in hippocampal CA3. **c, d** The knockdown efficiency of ANP32A protein in hippocampal CA3 measured by Western blotting and quantitative analysis. Data were presented as mean ± SD (two-way ANOVA followed by Bonferroni' s post hoc test). **e** The knockdown efficiency of ANP32 mRNA in the hippocampal CA3 detected by RT-PCR. Data were presented as mean ± SD (two-way ANOVA followed by Bonferroni' s post hoc test). **f** The knockdown efficiency of ANP32A protein in hippocampal CA3 measured by immunohistochemistry. **g** Arresting ANP32A overexpression improves spatial learning shown by the reduced escape latency in htau mice measured in MWM. Data were presented as mean ± s.e.m (two-way repeated measures ANOVA followed by Bonferroni' s post hoc test). **h** The representative swimming traces of the mice recorded in the maze after removed the platform in 7th day. **i–k** Arresting ANP32A overexpression improves spatial memory shown by the reduced latency to reach the platform quadrant (i), the increased crossing times in the platform site (j) and time spent in the target quadrant (k) measured at day 7 by removed the platform ($n = 11$ each group). Data were presented as mean ± SD (two-way ANOVA followed by Bonferroni' s post hoc test). **l, m** Arresting ANP32A overexpression did not change the distance travelled (l) and swimming speed (m) of the mice in water maze task (two-way ANOVA followed by Bonferroni' s post hoc test). *, $p<0.05$; **, $p<0.01$ *vs* wt-siC; #, $p<0.05$; ##, $p<0.01$ *vs* htau-siC

by HAT [5]. To verify the mechanisms underlying the inhibited histone acetylation by ANP32A, we first examined the interaction of ANP32A with histone by immunoprecipitation assay. An increased association of H3 or H4 with ANP32A was observed in htau mice compared with the control mice, while siANP32A reduced the interaction of ANP32A with H3 or H4 (Fig. 6a and b). Knockdown ANP32A also decreased interaction of ANP32A, H3 and

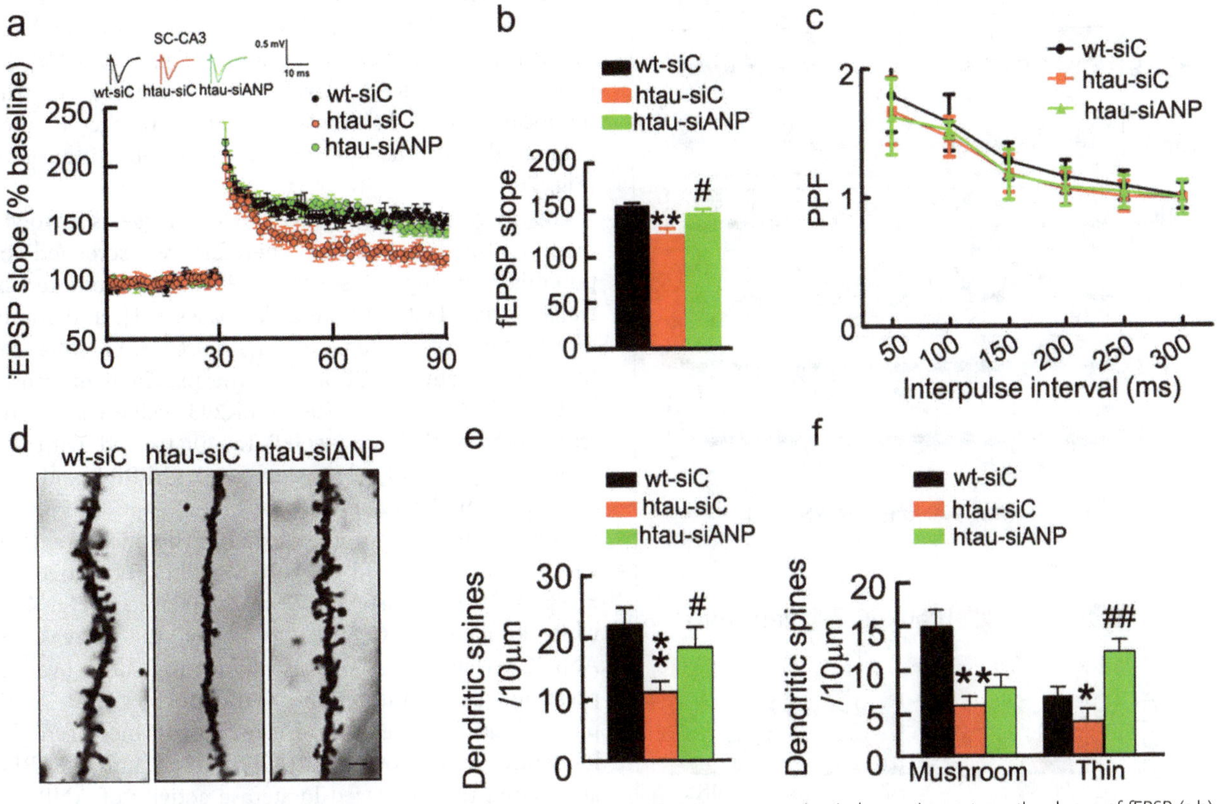

Fig. 3 Downregulating ANP32A improves synaptic plasticity. **a–c** Arresting ANP32A overexpression in htau mice restores the slopes of fEPSP (a,b) with no influence on paired-pulse ratio (c) in hippocampal CA3 by stimulating mossy fibers. (*n*=7-8 slices from 4 mice for each group). **d–f** Arresting ANP32A overexpression in htau mice restores total, thin- and mushroom-shaped spines in the hippocampal CA3 neurons (at least 20 neurons from six to seven mice per group were analyzed by the Sholl). Bar=5 μm. Data were presented as mean ± SD. *, $p<0.05$, **, $p<0.01$ *vs* wt-siC; #, $p<0.05$; ##, $p<0.01$ *vs* htau-siC (two-way ANOVA followed by Bonferroni' s post hoc test)

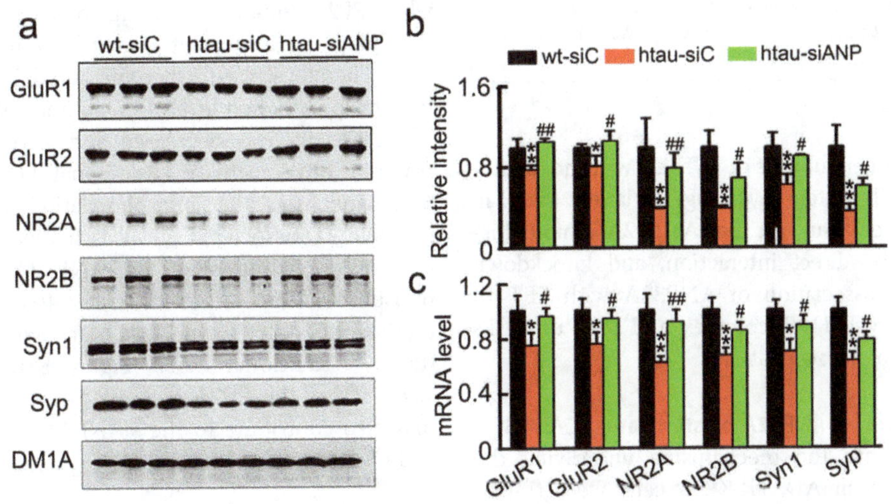

Fig. 4 Downregulating ANP32A increases expression of synapse-related proteins. **a**, **b** Arresting ANP32A overexpression in htau mice increases the level of several synaptic proteins in hippocampal CA3, detected by Western blotting. **c** Arresting ANP32A overexpression in htau mice increases mRNA level of several synaptic proteins in the hippocampal CA3, detected by RT-PCR. Data were presented as mean ± SD. *, $p<0.05$, **, $p<0.01$ *vs* wt-siC; #, $p<0.05$; ##, $p<0.01$ *vs* htau-siC (two-way ANOVA followed by Bonferroni' s post hoc test)

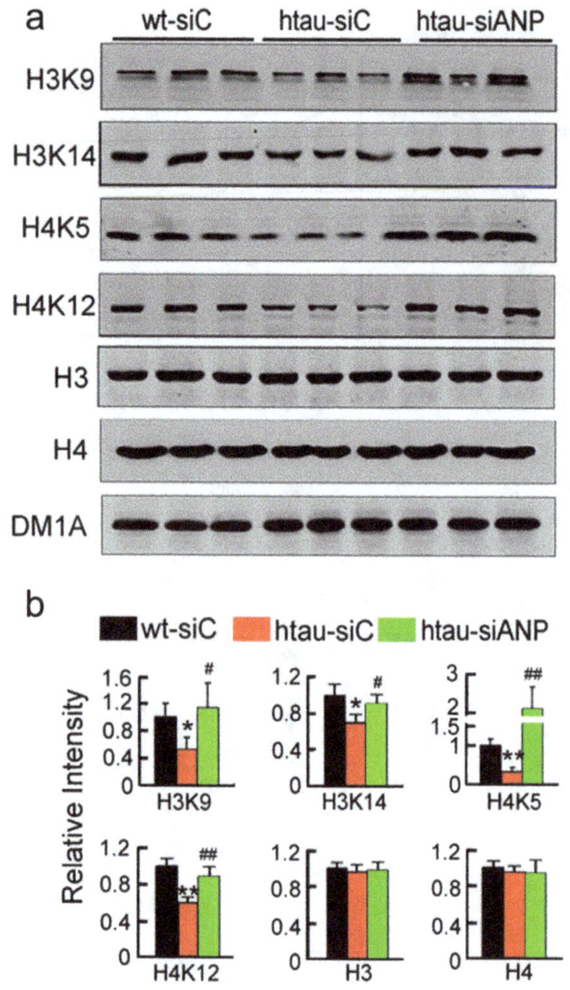

Fig. 5 Downregulating ANP32A increases histone acetylation. **a**, **b** Arresting ANP32A overexpression in htau mice increases levels of the acetylated histone in the hippocampal CA3 subset, measured by Western blotting. Data were presented as mean ± SD. *, $p<0.05$, **, $p<0.01$ *vs* wt-siC; #, $p<0.05$; ##, $p<0.01$ *vs* htau-siC (two-way ANOVA followed by Bonferroni' s post hoc test)

H4 with SET, another subunit of INHAT with no significant change of SET protein level (Fig. 6c, lane 2 and 3 in the Input). These data suggest that ANP32A inhibits histone acetylation by direct interaction, and knockdown ANP32A reduces association of ANP32A with SET to form the inhibitory INHAT complex and thus unmasks the histone for a robust acetylation.

AD-risk factors increase ANP32A by stimulating C/EBPβ

To gain insight into the mechanisms underlying the increased ANP32A in AD, HEK293 cells were transiently transfected with pIRES-eGFP-Tau40 or its vector pIRES-eGFP plasmid (Fig. 7a), treated with Aβ oligomers (Fig. 7b) or hydrogen peroxide (H_2O_2) (Fig. 7c), the recognized precipitating factors of AD [19, 20]. We observed that htau accumulation, $A\beta_{1-42}$ or H_2O_2 treatments induced significant increases of ANP32A protein (Fig. 7a–c,e) and mRNA (Fig. 7f). ANP32A protein and mRNA levels also increased in the hippocampus of 12-month old htau transgenic mice compared with the age-matched wild-type littermates (Fig. 7d–f).

The increase of ANP32A mRNA suggests involvement of the transcription, therefore, we screened for potential binding sites of the ANP32A promoter in transcription factor binding databases [21], and found a well-conserved element for the CCAAT/enhancer binding protein-β (C/EBPβ) in the proximal promoter region of ANP32A. After HEK293 cells transiently transfected with pIRES-eGFP-Tau40, treated with Aβ oligomers or H_2O_2, levels of total C/EBPβ and the phosphorylated C/EBPβ at Thr238/188 (pC/EBPβ, the activated site) were found significantly increase (Fig. 7a–c), and total C/EBPβ and the phosphorylated C/EBPβ also increased in 12-m htau mice (Fig. 7d), while knockdown C/EBPβ attenuated the increase of ANP32A (Fig. 7g–j). We also found that htau overexpression by transfection with pIRES-eGFP-Tau40 plasmid or H_2O_2 exposure significantly increased the luciferase activity of ANP32A promoter, and siC/EBPβ attenuated the increased luciferase activity of ANP32A induced by htau overexpression (Fig. 7k). These data indicate that AD-related toxic stimuli can increase ANP32A gene transcription with the mechanisms involving C/EBPβ activation.

Knockdown ANP32A reverses tau phosphorylation by activating PP2A

ANP32A is an endogenous inhibitor of PP2A [22], while PP2A inhibition leading to tau hyperphosphorylation plays an important role in AD neurodegeneration [23]. Therefore, we further measured PP2A activity and tau phosphorylation levels in htau mice. We observed that PP2A activity was decreased and ANP32A knockdown restored PP2A activity (Additional file 3: Figure S1a). Simultaneously, the phosphorylation level of tau at multiple AD-associated sites was significantly increased in htau mice, while silencing ANP32A attenuated tau phosphorylation at Ser231/262/404 and increased unphosphorylated tau level at Ser195/198/199/202 (tau-1) (Additional file 3: Figure S1b, c). These data suggest that the PP2A-assocaited tau dephosphorylation may also contribute to the siANP32A-improved learning and memory in htau mice.

Discussion

ANP32A is significantly increased in the AD brains [8]. Here we found that protein level of ANP32A was inversely correlated with spatial learning ability in AD

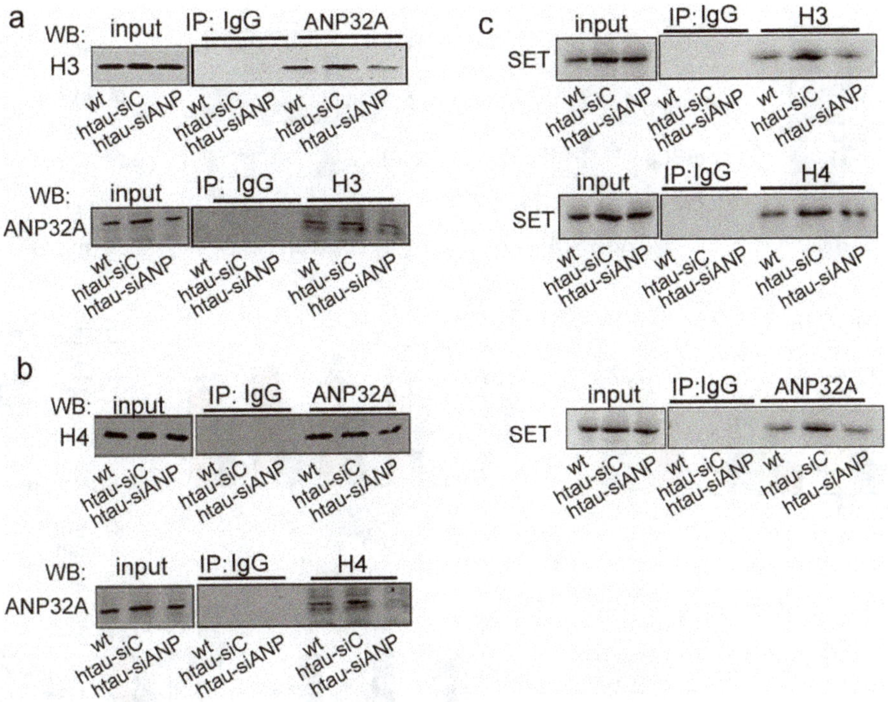

Fig. 6 Downregulating ANP32A decreases formation of INHAT complex. **a** The association level between ANP32A and histone 3 (H3) increased in hippocampal CA3 of htau mice, while siANP32A reduced the interaction detected by co-immunoprecipitation using antibodies as indicated on the blots. **b** The association level between ANP32A and histone 4 (H4) increased in hippocampal CA3 of htau mice, while siANP32A reduced the interaction detected by co-immunoprecipitation. **c** The association levels between SET and H3 or H4 or ANP32A increased in hippocampal CA3 of htau mice, while siANP32A reduced the interaction detected by co-immunoprecipitation

mice, knockdown ANP32A rescues learning and memory with preservation of synaptic plasticity. As a subunit of INHAT, ANP32A knockdown can decrease formation of INHAT and thus unmask histone for acetylation that lead to an increased expression of synaptic proteins. The increased synaptic proteins can remodel the synaptic plasticity and ameliorate cognitive deficits (Fig. 8). These findings reveal that ANP32A plays a critical role in learning and memory, and arresting ANP32A elevation in hippocampus may represent a promising therapeutic approach for preserving the cognitive capacity in AD.

The impairment of histone acetylation is causally linked to the cognitive decline in AD [4, 24]. In addition to HATs and HDACs that respectively regulate histone acetylation and deacetylation, INHAT, a complex composed of three essential subunits, TAF-Iα, SET/TAF-Iβ and ANP32A, also affects the acetylation level of histone [5]. INHAT regulates histone acetylation by binding to histones thereby preventing their access to HATs [5]. ANP32A, a key subunit of INHAT, can regulate histone acetylation [6] or the expression of neurofilament light chain by modulating histone acetylation [25], and histone 3 (H3) and H4 acetylation regulates expression of synaptic protein [18]. Here, we show for the first time that ANP32A negatively regulates the expression of a set of synaptic proteins including glutamate receptor subunits GluR1, GluR2, NR2A and NR2B, and as well as Syp and Syn1 *via* suppressing histone acetylation and ANP32A elevation is associated with cognitive impairment in an AD model. Several studies have demonstrated that, genes related to synaptic plasticity such as GluR1, GluR2, NR2A and NR2B, and Syp and Syn1 are downregulated in human AD brains [26–30]. Our results indicate that suppression of histone acetylation induced by the upregulated ANP32A at least contributes to the cognitive decline in AD.

Histone binding is a prerequisite for ANP32A to inhibit HAT activity. Recent study found that ANP32A INHAT domains, a major HAT inhibitory domain of ANP32A residing between amino acids 151 and 180, are responsible for histone binding, HAT inhibitory activity, and repression of transcription. The relative IC_{50} values of the synthesized ANP32A peptide representing ANP32A INHAT domain toward the individual histones H2B, H2A, H3, and H4 ranged between 0.6 and 1.5 μM. Although isolated ANP32A

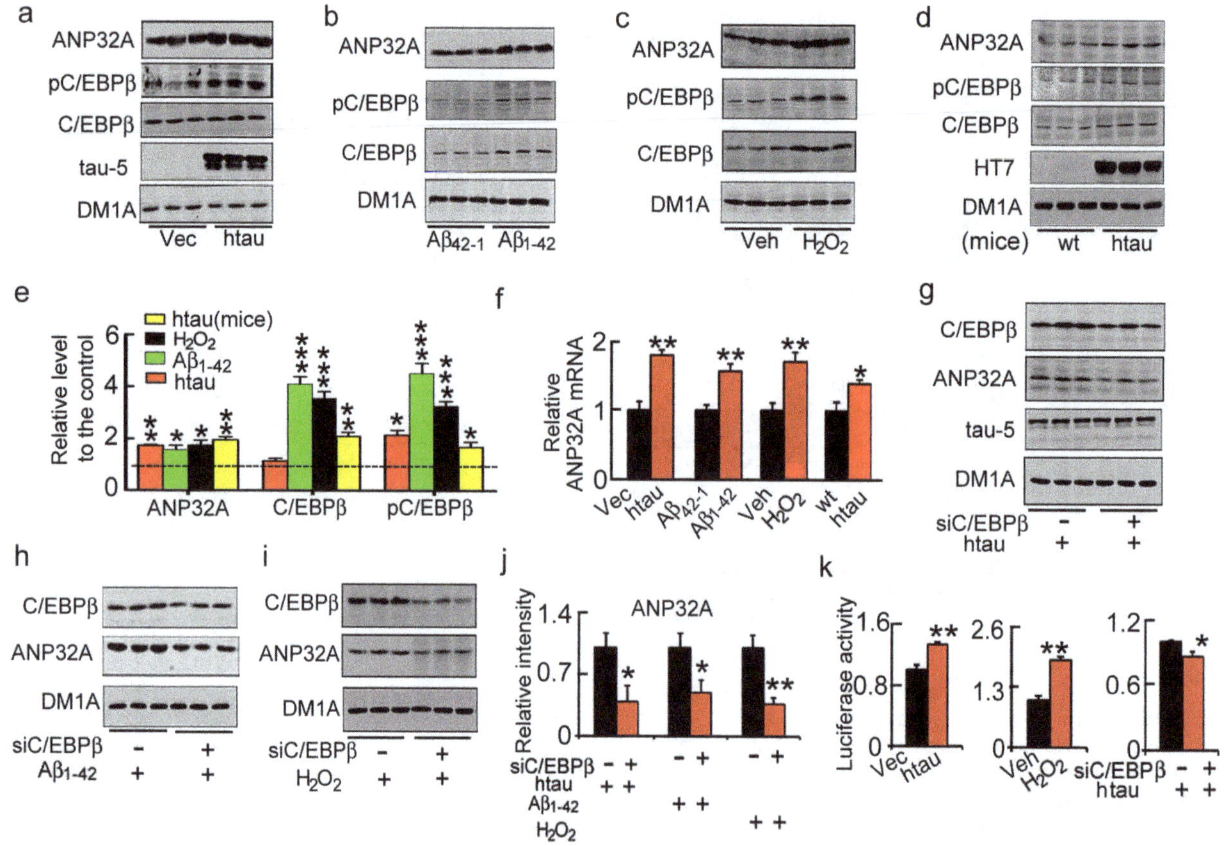

Fig. 7 AD-risk factors increase ANP32A *via* activating C/EBPβ. **a** Overexpressing htau in HEK293 cells increased protein level of ANP32A with elevation of total and the phosphorylated transcription factor C/EBPβ (pC/EBPβ) measured by Western blotting, the empty vector (Vec) was transfected as control. **b**, **c** Treatment of HEK293 cells with $A\beta_{1-42}$ (5 μM, 24 h) or H_2O_2 (50 μM, 40 min) increased protein level of ANP32A with elevation of total and the pC/EBPβ, and the scrambled $A\beta_{42-1}$ (b) or sterile water (veh, vehicle) (c) was used as control. **d** ANP32A with C/EBPβ and pC/EBPβ levels increased in the hippocampus of 12-month old htau mice compared with the age-matched wild-type (wt) littermates. **e** The quantitative analysis of ANP32A, C/EBPβ and pC/EBPβ level in a-d. The broken line indicates the control level received by the empty vector, $A\beta_{42-1}$, wt or the vehicle. '—' presents the relative level of control (Vec, $A\beta_{42-1}$, wt or the vehicle). **f** Overexpression of htau and treatment with $A\beta_{1-42}$ (5 μM, 24 h) or H_2O_2 (50 μM, 40 min) increased mRNA level of ANP32A in HEK293 cells, and ANP32A mRNA level also increased in the hippocampus of 12-m old htau mice, detected by RT-PCR. **g**–**j** Simultaneous downregulation of C/EBPβ by expressing siC/EBPβ for 48 h attenuated the htau–, $A\beta_{1-42}$–and H_2O_2–induced elevation of ANP32A protein in HEK293 cells, detected by Western blotting and quantitative analysis. **k** Overexpression of htau or H_2O_2 treatment increased luciferase activity of ANP32A in HEK293 cells, while simultaneous knockdown of C/EBPβ reduced the luciferase activity. Data were presented as mean ± SD. *, $p<0.05$, **, $p<0.01$ *vs* Vec, $A\beta_{42-1}$, wt or the vehicle (Unpaired Student's *t*-test (two-tailed))

has a high affinity to bind to and inhibit acetylation of histone H2B and H3, this H2B preference is lost when ANP32A is incorporated into the INHAT complex, which predominantly binds to and inhibits acetylation of histones H3 and H4 [5, 6]. Based on the above reasons, we measured the interaction between ANP32A and H3 or H4. We found that knockdown ANP32A decreased the binding protein level with H3 or H4, and increased the acetylated levels of H3K9, H3K14, H4K5 and H4K12. We also found that knockdown ANP32A decreased the interaction of ANP32A with SET and reduced the binding levels of SET with H3 and H4. These findings suggest that knockdown ANP32A not only inhibits INHAT complex formation, but also decreases the interaction of INHAT with histone.

We also identified in the present study that the expression of ANP32A is regulated by C/EBPβ *via* binding to a well-conserved recognition element in the proximal promoter region of ANP32A. C/EBPβ is a transcription factor that belongs to the C/EBP family, which plays a central role in cell differentiation and cell lineage definition, as well as in inflammation control [31]. Of note, C/EBPβ is increased in the brains of AD patients and the AD transgenic animal models [32, 33]. It is conceivable that the upregulation of ANP32A in AD may be a result of the increased C/EBPβ. Interestingly, we find that different type of AD-associated stressors (e.g. tau overexpression,

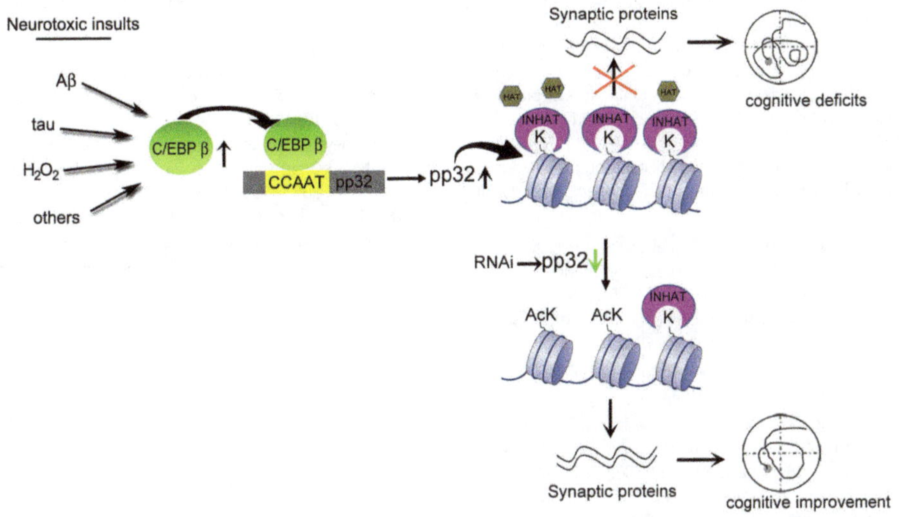

Fig. 8 The proposed working model by which ANP32A regulates synaptic plasticity and cognitive function. The neurotoxic insults, such as htau accumulation, or Aβ-fibrils or H_2O_2 overproduction, activate C/EBPβ by increasing its protein level and promoting its phosphorylation at Thr238/188. The activated C/EBPβ binds to its responsive element (CCAAT box) in the proximal ANP32A promoter region, and thus stimulates the expression of ANP32A. Then ANP32A interacts with SET to form INHAT, which masks histones for acetylation by HAT. Hypo-acetylation of histone inhibits transcription of synapse-associated proteins, leading to cognitive deficits. Arresting ANP32A overproduction unmasks histone for a robust acetylation, and thus increases the transcription of synaptic plasticity-related proteins to preserve learning and memory capacities

Aβ exposure, and oxidative stress) can increase the levels of total and the phosphorylated C/EBPβ. This result indicates that upregulation of C/EBPβ may represent a common pathway leading to overexpression of ANP32A, followed by impairment of histone acetylation and cognitive deficits.

Conclusion

Taken together, our study establishes that arresting ANP32A elevation in AD mice rescues the cognitive functions by unmasking histone for a robust acetylation and thus increasing expression of synapse-associated proteins with reconstruction of synapse morphology and the functions.

Abbreviations

AD: Alzheimer's disease; C/EBPβ: CCAAT/enhancer binding protein-β; HATs: Histone acetyltransferases; HDACs: Histone deacetylases; htau mice: Human tau transgenic mice; INHAT: Inhibitor of acetyltransferases; MWM: Morris water maze; NR2A: N-methyl-D-aspartate receptor type 2A; NR2B: N-methyl-D-aspartate receptor type 2B; Syp: Synaptophysin; Syn1: Synapsin I

Acknowledgements

Not applicable.

Funding

This work was supported by grants from the Natural Science Foundation of China (81471303, 81528007, 81601121 and 91132305), and from the Ministry of Science and Technology of China (2016YFC1305801).

Authors' contribution

This study was initiated and designed by JZW, GPL and GSC; JZW and GPL directed and coordinated the study; GSC and QF performed major animal behavior studies, virus injections, Western blotting and immunohistochemistry; ZHW and DSS performed brain slice electrophysiology recordings, and collected and analyzed the data; YH and XGL performed part of the animal behavior studies, immunohistochemistry and Western blotting; QF and GSC analyzed the data; DK helped to collect and analyze the data; HLL performed immunohistochemistry and helped to interpret the results and commented on the manuscript. GPL and JZW wrote the manuscript. All authors read and approved the final manuscript.

Competing interests

The authors declare that they have no competing interests.

Author details

[1]Department of Pathophysiology, School of Basic Medicine, Tongji Medical College, Huazhong University of Science and Technology, Wuhan 430030, China. [2]the Collaborative Innovation Center for Brain Science, Key Laboratory of Ministry of Education of China for Neurological Disorders, Tongji Medical College, Huazhong University of Science and Technology, Wuhan 430030, China. [3]Co-innovation Center of Neuroregeneration, Nantong University, Nantong, JS 226001, China.

References

1. Kosik KS, Rapp PR, Raz N, Small SA, Sweatt JD, Tsai LH. Mechanisms of age-related cognitive change and targets for intervention: epigenetics. J Gerontol A Biol Sci Med Sci. 2012;67:741–6.
2. Jenuwein T, Allis CD. Translating the histone code. Science. 2001;293:1074–80.
3. Brownell JE, Allis CD. Special HATs for special occasions: linking histone acetylation to chromatin assembly and gene activation. Curr Opin Genet Dev. 1996;6:176–84.
4. Gräff J, Kim D, Dobbin MM, Tsai LH. Epigenetic regulation of gene expression in physiological and pathological brain processes. Physiol Rev. 2011;91:603–49.
5. Seo SB, McNamara P, Heo S, Turner A, Lane WS, Chakravarti D. Regulation of histone acetylation and transcription by INHAT, a human cellular complex containing the set oncoprotein. Cell. 2001;104:119–30.
6. Seo SB, Macfarlan T, McNamara P, Hong R, Mukai Y, Heo S, et al. Regulation of histone acetylation and transcription by nuclear protein pp32, a subunit of the INHAT complex. J Biol Chem. 2002;277:14005-14010.

7. Tsujio I, Zaidi T, Xu J, Kotula L, Grundke-Iqbal I, Iqbal K. Inhibitors of protein phosphatase-2A from human brain structures, immunocytological localization and activities towards dephosphorylation of the Alzheimer type hyperphosphorylated tau. FEBS Lett. 2005;579:363–72.
8. Tanimukai H, Grundke-Iqbal I, Iqbal K. Upregulation of inhibitors of protein phosphatase-2A in Alzheimer's disease. Am J Pathol. 2005;166:1761–71.
9. Zhang Y, Ma RH, Li XC, Zhang JY, Shi HR, Wei W, et al. Silencing [Formula: see text] Rescues Tau Pathologies and Memory Deficits through Rescuing PP2A and Inhibiting GSK-3β Signaling in Human Tau Transgenic Mice. Front Aging Neurosci. 2014;6:123.
10. Liu GP, Wei W, Zhou X, Shi HR, Liu XH, Chai GS, et al. Silencing PP2A inhibitor by lenti-shRNA interference ameliorates neuropathologies and memory deficits in tg2576 mice. Mol Ther. 2013;21:2247–57.
11. Li M, Damuni Z. I_1^{PP2A} and I_2^{PP2A}. Two potent protein phosphatase 2A-specific inhibitor proteins. Methods Mol Biol. 1998;93:59–66.
12. Morris RG, Garrud P, Rawlins JN, O'Keefe J. Place navigation impaired in rats with hippocampal lesions. Nature. 1982;297:681–3.
13. Nagahara AH, Merrill DA, Coppola G, Tsukada S, Schroeder BE, Shaked GM, et al. Neuroprotective effects of brain-derived neurotrophic factor in rodent and primate models of Alzheimer's disease. Nat Med. 2009;15:331–7.
14. Woolley CS, McEwen BS. Estradiol mediates fluctuation in hippocampal synapse density during the estrous cycle in the adult rat. J Neurosci. 1992;12(7):2549–54.
15. Magariños AM, Li CJ, Gal Toth J, Bath KG, Jing D, Lee FS, et al. Effect of brain-derived neurotrophic factor haploinsufficiency on stress-induced remodeling of hippocampal neurons. Hippocampus. 2011;21:253–64.
16. Spires-Jones TL, Kay K, Matsouka R, Rozkalne A, Betensky RA, Hyman BT. Calcineurin inhibition with systemic FK506 treatment increases dendritic branching and dendritic spine density in healthy adult mouse brain. Neurosci Lett. 2011;487:260–3.
17. Zhang CE, Wei W, Liu YH, Peng JH, Tian Q, Liu GP, et al. Hyperhomocysteinemia increases beta-amyloid by enhancing expression of gamma-secretase and phosphorylation of amyloid precursor protein in rat brain. Am J Pathol. 2009;174:1481–91.
18. Gräff J, Rei D, Guan JS, Wang WY, Seo J, Hennig KM, et al. An epigenetic blockade of cognitive functions in the neurodegenerating brain. Nature. 2012;483:222–6.
19. Markesbery WR, Carney JM. Oxidative alterations in Alzheimer's disease. Brain Pathol. 1999;9:133–46.
20. Yankner BA. Mechanisms of neuronal degeneration in Alzheimer's disease. Neuron. 1996;16:921–32.
21. Sandelin A, Alkema W, Engstrom P, Wasserman WW, Lenhard B. JASPAR: an open-access database for eukaryotic transcription factor binding profiles. Nucleic Acids Res. 2004;32:D91–4.
22. Li M, Makkinje A, Damuni Z. Molecular identification of I1PP2A, a novel potent heat-stable inhibitor protein of protein phosphatase 2A. Biochemistry. 1996;35:6998–7002.
23. Tanimukai H, Kudo T, Tanaka T, Grundke-Iqbal I, Iqbal K, Takeda M. Novel therapeutic strategies for neurodegenerative disease. Psychogeriatrics. 2009;9:103–9.
24. Peleg S, Sananbenesi F, Zovoilis A, Burkhardt S, Bahari-Javan S, Agis-Balboa RC, et al. Altered histone acetylation is associated with age-dependent memory impairment in mice. Science. 2010;328:753–6.
25. Kular RK, Cvetanovic M, Siferd S, Kini AR, Opal P. Neuronal differentiation is regulated by leucine-rich acidic nuclear protein (LANP), a member of the inhibitor of histone acetyltransferase complex. J Biol Chem. 2009;284:7783–92.
26. Wakabayashi K, Narisawa-Saito M, Iwakura Y, Arai T, Ikeda K, Takahashi H, et al. Phenotypic down-regulation of glutamate receptor subunit GluR1 in Alzheimer's disease. Neurobiol Aging. 1999;20:287–95.
27. Counts SE, He B, Che S, Ginsberg SD, Mufson EJ. Galanin fiber hyperinnervation preserves neuroprotective gene expression in cholinergic basal forebrain neurons in Alzheimer's disease. J Alzheimers Dis. 2009;18(4):885–96.
28. Bi H, Sze CI. N-methyl-D-aspartate receptor subunit NR2A and NR2B messenger RNA levels are altered in the hippocampus and entorhinal cortex in Alzheimer's disease. J Neurol Sci. 2002;200:11–8.
29. Callahan LM, Vaules WA, Coleman PD. Quantitative decrease in synaptophysin message expression and increase in cathepsin D message expression in Alzheimer disease neurons containing neurofibrillary tangles. J Neuropathol Exp Neurol. 1999;58:275–87.
30. Mufson EJ, Counts SE, Ginsberg SD. Gene expression profiles of cholinergic nucleus basalis neurons in Alzheimer's disease. Neurochem Res. 2002;27:1035–48.
31. Nerlov C. The C/EBP family of transcription factors: a paradigm for interaction between gene expression and proliferation control. Trends Cell Biol. 2007;17:318–24.
32. Strohmeyer R, Shelton J, Lougheed C, Breitkopf T. CCAAT-enhancer binding protein-β expression and elevation in Alzheimer's disease and microglial cell cultures. PLoS One. 2014;9:e86617.
33. Ramberg V, Tracy LM, Samuelsson M, Nilsson LN, Iverfeldt K. The CCAAT/enhancer binding protein (C/EBP) δ is differently regulated by fibrillar and oligomeric forms of the Alzheimer amyloid-β peptide. J Neuroinflammation. 2011;8:34.

14

Late onset Alzheimer's disease genetics implicates microglial pathways in disease risk

Anastasia G. Efthymiou and Alison M. Goate*

Abstract

Alzheimer's disease (AD) is a highly heritable complex disease with no current effective prevention or treatment. The majority of drugs developed for AD focus on the amyloid cascade hypothesis, which implicates Aß plaques as a causal factor in the disease. However, it is possible that other underexplored disease-associated pathways may be more fruitful targets for drug development. Findings from gene network analyses implicate immune networks as being enriched in AD; many of the genes in these networks fall within genomic regions that contain common and rare variants that are associated with increased risk of developing AD. Of these genes, several (including *CR1, SPI1, the MS4As, TREM2, ABCA7, CD33,* and *INPP5D*) are expressed by microglia, the resident immune cells of the brain. We summarize the gene network and genetics findings that implicate that these microglial genes are involved in AD, as well as several studies that have looked at the expression and function of these genes in microglia and in the context of AD. We propose that these genes are contributing to AD in a non-Aß-dependent fashion.

Keywords: Alzheimer's disease, Genetics, Microglia, Myeloid

Background

AD is a chronic, incurable, neurodegenerative disease that affects an estimated 5.4 million people in the United States [1]. It is a complex disease that is highly heritable, and several genes have been found to be associated with risk for developing AD. Early onset AD (EOAD), diagnosed in individuals who are under the age of 65 years, accounts for a small percentage of all AD cases (5–10%). Mutations in three genes, *APP* [2], *PSEN1* [3, 4], and *PSEN2* [5, 6], are associated with autosomal dominant AD (ADAD), a subset of EOAD [7]. This has led to the prevailing mechanistic theory for AD: the amyloid cascade hypothesis [8]. However, no therapies that target this pathway have yet been successful in preventing the development of or ameliorating the effects of this disease in humans. Late onset AD (LOAD) shares the same clinical and pathological features of early onset AD, but is diagnosed in individuals who are over the age of 65 years. The most important genetic risk factor for the development of LOAD and sporadic EOAD is presence of the E4 variant of the *APOE* gene (*APOE4*) [9, 10].

Clinically, AD manifests as a gradual and unrelenting decline of memory [11]. Patients are diagnosed based on a variety of cognitive factors, but confirmation of an AD diagnosis can only be made by observing the underlying neuropathology. As such, people who are suffering from AD may be misdiagnosed with other forms of dementia, and vice versa, thereby reducing the power of clinical trials and the effectiveness of treatment.

Memory loss in AD is accompanied by neuronal loss and the accumulation of extracellular Aß plaques and intracellular neurofibrillary tangles of hyperphosphorylated Tau. In ADAD, the accumulation of Aß plaques results from improper processing of APP, which may be a consequence of mutations within the *APP* gene itself, or in associated factors such as *PSEN1* and *PSEN2*. In LOAD and sporadic AD, there is no evidence of improper APP processing that leads to amyloid accumulation. However, there is evidence that the clearance of Aß is disrupted [12].

Research on LOAD has shown that there is a slow accumulation of Aß in the brain for up to twenty years before the manifestation of any cognitive symptoms. It is

* Correspondence: alison.goate@mssm.edu
Department of Neuroscience, Ronald M. Loeb Center for Alzheimer's disease, Icahn School of Medicine at Mount Sinai, 1425 Madison Ave, New York, NY 10029, USA

possible that this prodromal state of AD may be an effective therapeutic target, and limiting the accumulation of Aß may halt the development of further symptoms. Biomarkers for AD, including amyloid imaging and monitoring cerebrospinal fluid levels for Aß and Tau, are currently used to inform diagnosis. However, in a clinical setting, they can only be utilized after cognitive symptoms have already become apparent. Understanding how these biomarkers exist in non-demented individuals will be important to inform our future diagnosis and treatment of disease (e.g. Do all non-demented individuals with amyloid accumulation develop clinical AD and if so over what time period?). Similarly, accumulation of Tau is characteristic of other neurodegenerative diseases and is also observed in elderly non-demented individuals. Understanding the natural course of this accumulation will be important to advise therapy.

Current knowledge about the neuropathologic and genetic information informs current theories about the development and progression of AD. However, there are still no good therapies for its prevention or treatment. A possible explanation is that there may be other pathways that are also disrupted in AD, which are not accounted for in the current version of the amyloid cascade hypothesis, and which could serve as more efficient therapeutic targets and/or should be part of combination therapies.

Early descriptions of AD include additional neuropathological features, including gliosis and neuroinflammation, the contributions of which are under investigation. The presence of these features implicates microglia, the resident immune cell type in the brain, in AD pathology. However, these observations do not indicate, for example, whether microglia accumulation around plaques is a consequence or cause of disease [13, 14]. Recently, genetic studies have implicated microglial function as a causal factor in LOAD, as opposed to merely a biological response [15].

In recent years, genome-wide association studies (GWAS), whole genome sequencing (WGS), and gene-expression network analysis have uncovered gene networks and common and rare genetic variants that are associated with LOAD. These genes are involved in previously understudied pathways, including cholesterol metabolism, endocytosis, and innate immunity [16]. The GWAS findings and gene expression network analysis both implicate immune and microglial networks as important players in the development and progression of AD (Fig. 1). However, the exact contribution of microglia is not well understood. Genetic and early functional studies suggest that microglia may directly contribute to AD pathology [13]. This review highlights several genes identified in these studies that confer risk for AD and are involved in innate immunity. By looking at the role of microglia in AD, we may uncover novel therapeutic targets to help treat this disease.

AD GWAS studies

AD genetics implicate microglial and immune genes as being important players in the development and progression

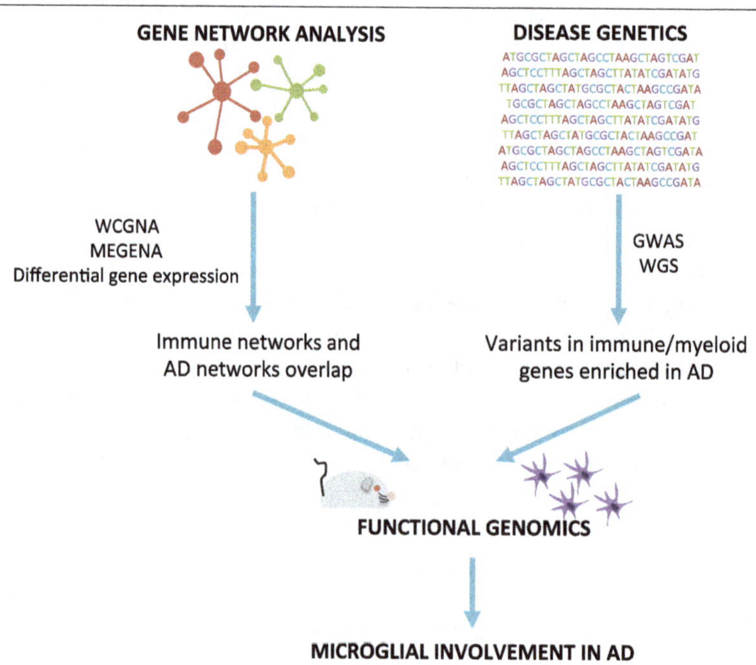

Fig. 1 Framework of support for microglia involvement in LOAD. Findings from gene network analysis and disease genetics converge to show enriched immune and myeloid contributions in AD. These findings are verified through functional genomics using cell and animal models to determine the contribution of these genes to LOAD pathology

of disease. These investigations include genome-wide association studies (GWAS), which must then be validated through functional genomics approaches and large-scale sequencing projects. In this section we will discuss the genes identified in AD GWAS studies and how these genes support the involvement of microglia.

Choose wisely: population sample and size in GWAS studies

GWAS are used to simultaneously examine millions of genetic variants in tens or hundreds of thousands of individuals to identify variants that are associated with a particular trait or disease state. The most common study design for AD GWAS is a comparison of unrelated disease cases with unrelated elderly non-demented controls from the same population. Importantly, GWAS identify regions of the genome (loci) that exhibit association with a trait rather than specific genes. Indeed, some loci may contain a single gene while others can contain many genes (Table 1). The challenge is to then fine-map these loci to identify specific genes that contain causal functional variants and to understand the mechanisms of pathogenesis leading to increased or decreased risk for disease.

GWAS are most frequently performed in populations of European origin, but can be very informative if conducted in multiple populations due to the differences in linkage-disequilibrium (LD) structure across different groups. Some loci may show stronger effects in specific populations (e.g. *ABCA7* in African Americans [17]), which can aid in identification of functional variants, but generally LD differences help to narrow the region of association, particularly in African ancestry populations [18].

The importance of sample size cannot be overestimated in GWAS. Meta-analysis of multiple GWAS is commonly used to increase sample size and greatly increase the number of loci discovered and validated as associated with disease [19]. In AD, GWAS with samples of 5000 cases or less could only identify the *APOE* locus as a region associated with disease [20]. Studies with sample sizes of 6000 identified three loci, which were then replicated in larger cohorts [21–23]. Once sample size increased to near 10,000 cases, several loci could be identified and replicated. In 2013 a meta-analyses of >70,000 samples conducted by the International Genomics of Alzheimer's Project (IGAP) in Caucasian populations has identified more than 20 genetic loci that are associated with AD [24]. In contrast, a GWAS conducted in an African American population with less than 2000 cases identified only one locus outside of the APOE region (*ABCA7*) to be associated with AD [17].

Sample size can also compensate for restricted phenotype data, as shown in a recent study using family history of AD as a proxy in the UK Biobank dataset, which identified several novel loci associated with AD [25]. This study, which included over 100,000 individuals, was described as a genome-wide association study by proxy (GWAX) and replaced disease cases with their first-degree relatives. Despite the absence of a disease phenotype, this study was still able to replicate the main

Table 1 AD-risk loci identified through genome-wide analyses (GWAS and GWAX) [24, 25]

SNP	Chr	Reported gene	Additional genes in locus
rs6656401	1	*CR1*	
rs6733839	2	*BIN1*	
rs35349669	2	*INPP5D*	*NGEF, NEU2*
rs190982	5	*MEF2C*	*LOC645323, MIR9-2*
rs2074612[a]	5	*SCIMP*	*ZNF594, RABEP1, USP6*
rs9271192	6	*HLA-DRB5–HLA-DRB1*	*C6orf10, HLA-DRB5, HLA-DRB6, HLA-DRB1, HLA-DQA1, HCG23, BTNL2, HLA-DRA, HLA-DQB1, HLA-DQA2, HLA-DQB2, HLA-DOB, TAP1, TAP2, PSMB8, PSMB9*
rs10948363	6	*CD2AP*	*GPR111, GPR115*
rs2718058	7	*NME8*	*GPR141*
rs1476679	7	*ZCWPW1*	*TRIM4, GJC3, AZGP1, AZGP1P1, ZKSCAN1, ZSCAN21, ZNF3, COPS6, MCM7, C7orf59, GPC2, STAG3, GATS, PVRIG, SPDYE3, PMS2P1, PILRA, PILRB, PPP1R35, MEPCE, NYAP1, SAP25, AGFG2, LRCH4, ZASP, LRCH4, FBXO24, PCOLCE-AS1*
rs11771145	7	*EPHA1*	*CLCN1, FAM131B, ZYX, TAS2R60, LOC285965, TAS2R41*
rs28834970	8	*PTK2B*	*STMN4, TRIM35, CHRNA2, EPHX2*
rs9331896	8	*CLU*	*PTK2B, CHRNA2, EPHX2, SCARA3, CCDC25, ESCO2, PBK*
rs7920721[a]	10	*ECHDC3*	
rs10838725	11	*CELF1*	*ARFGAP2, PACSIN3, DDB2, ACP2, MADD, MYBPC3, SPI1, SLC39A13, PSMC3, RAPSN, PTPMT1, KBTBD4, NDUFS3, C1QTNF4, MTCH2, AGBL2, FNBP4, NUP160*
rs983392	11	*MS4A6A*	*PLAC1L, MS4A3, MS4A2, MS4A4A, MS4A6E*
rs10792832	11	*PICALM*	*CCDC83*
rs11218343	11	*SORL1*	
rs17125944	14	*FERMT2*	*ERO1L, PSMC6, STYX, GNPNAT1*
rs10498633	14	*SLC24A4*	*RIN3*
rs59685680[a]	15	*SPPL2A*	*TRPM7, USP50*
rs77493189[a]	17	*HBEGF*	*HBEGF*
rs4147929	19	*ABCA7*	*CFD, MED16, PRTN3, R3HDM4, KISS1R, ELANE, ARID3A, TMEM259, GRIN3B, WDR18, HMHA1, CNN2, POLR2E, SBNO2, GPX4, ATP5D, MIDN, CIRBP, EFNA2*
rs7274581	20	*CASS4*	*CSTF1, RTFDC1, GCNT7, FAM209A, FAM209B*

Disease-associated SNPs that have reached genome-wide significance for each locus are labeled, along with their chromosome, the closest gene (that which is reported) and additional genes within the locus
[a]identified in GWAX

findings from earlier smaller studies and identify four novel loci due to the number of samples involved. This removes an important barrier for identifying disease-associated loci through genetic screens by increasing the population from which "cases" can be obtained.

Know what you're getting: GWAS results and limitations

It is common practice to display GWAS data in Manhattan plots, with chromosome location on the x-axis and degree of association (as $-\log_{10}(p\text{-value})$) on the y-axis, with each data-point representing one single nucleotide polymorphism (SNP). SNPs whose *p*-values are lower than the genome-wide significance cutoff of 10^{-8} are considered significant, and often labeled with the gene that is closest to that locus. However, it is important to note that this labeling based on *proximity* of the most significant SNP to a gene in that locus does not necessarily mean that the disease-associated SNP has any functional interaction or influence on that gene. In fact, it is possible that the genes affected by these variants are many kilobases away. Additionally, it is hard to distinguish SNPs with high LD, indicating the possibility that the actual SNP that confers risk for developing the disease is not the one determined to be most significant by GWAS. Table 1 displays 25 AD-risk loci that have been detected through GWAS meta-analyses, along with all genes within the nearest recombination hotspots of the most significant SNP in that locus. Additional studies will have to be conducted to conclude which gene is affected by that variant.

Validating GWAS results with functional genomics

The limitations presented by GWAS necessitate functional validation of all target loci in order to determine which gene is affected by these variants or other variants in LD, the effect of the variant on gene expression and function, and subsequently, the effect of the variant on the disease state. This can be done by first fine-mapping the region using computational approaches, which integrate information including transcription factor binding sites, chromatin state, DNA methylation, splicing, and gene expression, to prioritize SNPs and determine which is most likely to have a functional effect and on what gene. Fine-mapping should be followed by in vitro and in vivo studies that seek to validate the SNP-gene pair and to determine their effects in appropriate models. Several examples of functional genomics have been conducted for putative AD-risk genes, including *SPI1* [26] and *CD33* [27], discussed below.

Many of the loci identified through GWAS do not contain genes that are highly expressed in whole brain tissues, impeding our ability to fine-map these loci and assess their contribution to disease. It is possible that this is a result of the heterogeneity of cell types in these samples. Microglia share a similar developmental lineage, gene expression pattern, and function with other peripheral immune cells of the myeloid lineage. Because these gene expression signatures are conserved, there are two ways of interpreting these data. First; microglia contribute to the etiology of AD, and second; peripheral myeloid cells, such as monocytes and macrophages, could be contributing alone, or in combination with microglia, to the observed immune effect. The connection of these cells to other peripheral myeloid cells can be exploited to learn more about the underlying neuropathology of LOAD. Previous work by Raj et al. profiled purified monocytes from a young and healthy population and looked at their gene expression patterns for enrichment across multiple diseases [28]. They found that AD susceptibility alleles are enriched among expression quantitative trait loci (eQTLs) in monocytes but not in T cells. This suggests that monocytes could be used as a proxy to examine the effects of microglia in AD.

AD-risk genes in microglia

The importance of validating GWAS hits with functional genomics cannot be understated. However, despite the absence of thorough and complete functional studies, integrating information from multiple sources can provide evidence in support of specific genes and pathways. Below, we describe several genes that are present within AD-risk loci, are expressed in microglia, associate with other microglial or immune genes through co-expression analysis, and have previously been shown to be associated with AD in human or animal studies. We also discuss several other genes that have been detected in GWAS and may be involved in these same pathways, which still need to be supported with additional evidence.

Genes identified through common variants in GWAS

CR1

Complement receptor 1 (CR1) is a glycoprotein expressed on immune-related cells, including microglia. Its encoding gene, *CR1*, is located on chromosome 1q32 and is represented by four different alleles that vary in size, transcript, and frequency among populations [29]. The *CR1* locus has been identified through GWAS as a risk factor for AD [21], and complement factors are highly expressed in AD brain [30, 31]. The AD-risk SNP identified in IGAP, rs6656401, falls within an intronic region of *CR1*, with SNPs in high LD spanning the entire length of *CR1* [32]. Another LOAD-associated SNP, rs3818361 (($r^2 > 0.8$ with rs6656401), was reported to be strongly associated with disease in *APOE4* carriers [21]. Both SNPs are associated with low *CR1* expression in brain tissue and neurons, and higher expression in monocytes [33].

CR1 plays a major role in regulating immune activation through the complement cascade and acts as the main receptor for the complement protein C3b [34]. The complement cascade is known to mediate microglial activity, including pruning of synapses [35]. Aβ has been shown to activate the complement system through an association with C1q, which binds to CR1 [36–39]. Increased CR1 is associated with more active microglia, and blocking CR1 impedes microglial ability to phagocytose Aβ [40]. However, given that CR1 is expressed in several cell types in the brain and in peripheral immune cells it is unclear whether the genetic effects of CR1 on AD are mediated through functional effects in a specific cell type or through all cells in which it is expressed [29].

CELF1/SPI1

The IGAP meta-analysis identified the SNP rs10838725 to be a risk factor for AD, and this variant is present within an intronic region of the gene *CELF1* [24]. However, LD in this region is extensive, and there are multiple genes that could be affected by the identified AD risk SNP (Table 1). One of these genes, *SPI1*, has been implicated in LOAD through network analysis [41]. Additional studies suggest that PU.1, a transcription factor encoded by the gene *SPI1*, is a central hub in an AD gene network and is associated with AD pathology [41, 42].

SPI1 is highly expressed in immune cells, macrophages, and microglia, which share a developmental lineage [43, 44]. Further analyses of GWAS data and fine mapping of this locus by Huang et al., indicate that *SPI1* is the gene affected in this locus [26]. Fine-mapping identified 5 variants associated with AD and *SPI1* expression in myeloid cells, including macrophages and monocytes. These variants are located within PU.1 binding sites or a miR-569 binding site within the 3′ UTR of *SPI1*, consistent with potential effects on gene expression. Colocalization analyses of this GWAS locus with variants that influence gene expression suggest that *SPI1*, rather than other nearby genes including *CELF1* and *MYBPC3*, is most likely the gene in this locus contributing to LOAD [26].

The PU.1 cistrome, which includes transcription factor binding sites throughout the entire genome, is also enriched in AD [26]. Chromatin immunoprecipitation (ChIP)-Seq data from myeloid cells shows that PU.1 binds *TYROBP, MS4As, INPP5D, TREM2*, and *CD33*, suggesting that it regulates their gene expression. These recent findings regarding *SPI1* emphasize the importance of verifying genetic targets through a variety of functional genomics approaches.

MS4A family

The membrane-spanning 4-domain subfamily A (*MS4A*) gene cluster is present on chromosome 11q12 and includes eighteen genes spanning approximately 600kb [45–47]. Multiple GWAS in European and Asian populations have implicated several genes within the MS4A cluster in AD, including *MS4A4A*, *MS4A4E, MS4A6A*, and *MS4A6E* [23, 48–51]. The IGAP meta-analysis identified rs983392, upstream of *MS4A6A* and downstream of *MS4A2,* as an AD-risk SNP that is associated with reduced LOAD risk. This SNP is associated with chromatin marks that confer low transcription in brain tissues and neuronal cells, and is associated with enhancers and active transcription sites in peripheral primary human monocytes [33]. Another SNP, rs670139, lies between *MS4A4A* and *MS4A6A* and is associated with increased LOAD risk. The LD between these two SNPs is between $0.4 < r^2 < 0.6$, suggesting they may be having independent effects.

The exact function of these transmembrane proteins is unknown, although they have been implicated in mediating calcium influx, regulating endocytosis, trafficking, and signaling [52], and may act as chemoreceptors [53]. However, their ligand binding partners and downstream signaling cascades have not yet been fully described. High levels of expression of *MS4A6A* in AD brains is associated with increased Braak tangle and plaque scores, indicating advanced disease pathology [30]. While most loci appear to have similar effects in *APOE4*$^+$ and *APOE4*$^-$ AD patients, the *MS4A* signal is stronger in *APOE4*$^-$ subjects [54].

MS4As are expressed in microglia and macrophages within the brain, and are also highly expressed in peripheral immune cells. Several of the *MS4A*s, including *MS4A4A* and *MS4A6A*, contain binding regions for the transcription factor PU.1, which is also selectively expressed in myeloid cells and has been implicated in AD. Work by Huang, et al., has shown that changes in expression level of *Spi1*, the gene encoding PU.1 in mouse, correlate with similar expression changes in *Ms4a4a and Ms4a6d* (mouse ortholog to *MS4A6A*) in BV2 microglial cell lines [26]. Further experiments will have to be done to determine the exact function of the *MS4As* and which genes within this family are involved in AD.

Genes identified through sequencing strategies and rare variants

Sequencing strategies generate high-coverage data of different genetic loci to identify rare variants that are not seen through standard GWAS. Rare variants in two genes, *ABCA7* and *TREM2*, have a strong and replicated association with AD, and are described below.

ABCA7

ATP-binding cassette transporter A7 (ABCA7) is a membrane transporter. *ABCA7* is located on chromosome 19p13.3, and common SNPs in this locus have been implicated in LOAD through GWAS. Additionally, this locus contains several rare variants that have been identified by sequencing studies. GWAS in European and African Americans have implicated the chromosomal region including *ABCA7* [17, 24]. Indeed this locus contains the only SNPs to reach genome-wide significance in a GWAS of African Americans apart from those in the APOE locus [17]. One of these SNPs identified in Europeans, rs3764650, is located within an intronic region of *ABCA7*. It is associated with T-box transcription factor binding sites and myeloid-related transcription factors such as CEBPD [33]. The AD-risk SNP identified in African Americans, rs115550680, is also found in an intronic region of *ABCA7* and is in high LD ($r^2 > 0.8$) with variants identified in European populations. Both SNPs are associated with weak transcription in the brain and strong transcription in myeloid cells [33].

ABCA7 is expressed in microglia, and is associated with increased risk of LOAD. ABCA7 is known to transfer phospholipids to apolipoproteins [55], including APOE and APOJ/CLU, and it is possible that mutations in this protein may be affecting AD though this pathway [56–58]. However, *ABCA7* has also been implicated as a modulator of microglial function by its association with microglial phagocytosis and clearance [16]. Multiple rare coding variants in *ABCA7* confer loss of function, resulting in increased risk of AD [59–62]. Indeed, targeted resequencing of *ABCA7* in African Americans with low or high risk alleles at this locus led to the identification of a 44 bp deletion, which results in a frameshift mutation and increased AD risk. However, a recent follow-up study of *ABCA7* mutations challenges the assertion that all of these variants are loss of function, and implicates a role for *ABCA7* in additional neurodegenerative diseases [63].

ABCA7 has previously been shown to be associated with AD, with increased levels of *ABCA7* correlating to increased plaque burden and more rapid cognitive decline [30, 58]. Increased levels of ABCA7 increase microglial phagocytosis and Aβ clearance, which is believed to be regulated through the C1q complement pathway. Additionally, *ABCA7*$^{-/-}$ mice display increased Aβ deposition, suggesting that this protein is important for the appropriate clearance of Aβ aggregates by microglia [64]. It is possible that ABCA7 can affect AD through multiple pathways, given its multiple roles in transport and microglial function.

TREM2

Complete loss of function of TREM2 results in Nasu Hakola syndrome, a rare recessive disorder characterized by multifocal bone cysts and frontotemporal dementia. This is driven by loss of function in macrophages in many tissues, including microglia [65]. TREM2 is a transmembrane-glycoprotein that acts as a receptor on the surface of immune cells of myeloid origin, including microglia, and senses lipids that are exposed after cellular damage. Heterozygous rare variants of *TREM2* are associated with an increased risk of developing AD in European, African American and Asian populations [66–69]. The identified AD-risk SNPs in this region are likely to result in partial loss of function [70]. Evidence suggests that the same variants may increase risk for other neurodegenerative diseases including Parkinson's Disease (PD), amyotrophic lateral sclerosis (ALS), and frontotemporal lobar degeneration (FTLD) [16, 66, 67, 71]. However, meta-analysis of other diseases shows that data linking *TREM2* to these neurodegenerative diseases are far less compelling than in the AD studies [71].

TREM2 associates with its adaptor protein, TYROBP/DAP12, which is responsible for the propagation of downstream signaling through this receptor [65]. Network analysis of whole transcriptome gene expression data in healthy individuals identified *TREM2* as a central hub in five brain regions, suggesting that it can drive expression levels of its associated genes [72]. Many of the genes that associate with *TREM2* are immune genes, and others have previously been associated with AD risk [72]. *TREM2* expression is increased in AD, which may be a compensatory mechanism, as AD-associated *TREM2* mutations are partial loss of function and can affect receptor binding of TREM2 to its associated ligands [73, 74].

Activation of TREM2 through ligand-receptor binding stimulates macrophage and microglia phagocytosis, survival, and mobilization, whereas absence of TREM2 in microglia impedes their ability to phagocytose and alters their gene expression signatures [75]. TREM2 has been shown to bind apolipoproteins, including APOE and APOJ/CLU, and disease variants of TREM2 showed lower binding to these AD-associated ligands [76]. *Trem2*$^{-/-}$ mice bred to an accelerated AD mouse model (5XFAD transgenic mice) show significant Aß accumulation in hippocampal regions and an increase in insoluble Aß [77]. These mice also show defects in microglial reactivity, Aß plaque clearance, and survival [77, 78]. The selective expression of *TREM2* in microglia, the association of *TREM2* with other immune genes, and the impaired function of *TREM2* mutant microglia suggest that this cell type is a key player in the development in LOAD.

Additional plausible microglial genes

CD33

GWAS studies in multiple ethnic populations have identified variants within the *CD33* locus, located on chromosome 19q13.33, that are associated with AD. These loci were genome-wide significant in early studies, but fell short of genome-wide significance in large meta-analyses [23, 49]. The variant rs3865444 is associated with *CD33* exon 2 splicing [27] and with a reduction in *CD33* expression [79]. Fine-mapping studies have shown that rs12459419, a SNP in high LD with rs3865444, likely mediates the altered splicing [27]. Both variants are associated with chromatin marks signifying low/repressed transcription in brain tissues, but is closely associated with active transcription start sites in myeloid cells. Introduction of rs12459419 into microglial BV2 cells modulates exon 2 splicing efficiency and microglial activation [27].

CD33, a member of the sialic acid-binding Ig-like family, is a myeloid cell receptor that is exclusively expressed by microglia and macrophages in the brain. Increased *CD33* expression is seen in AD brain and is associated with increased plaque burden, advanced cognitive decline, and disease severity [30, 80]. *Cd33*$^{-/-}$ mouse models indicate that knocking out CD33 results in lower Aß levels and reduced amyloid plaque burden in brain [79]. However, these mice do not exhibit altered APP processing, suggesting that it may be Aß clearance mechanism of microglia that is responsible for this phenotype.

INPP5D/SHIP1 and CD2AP

GWAS have also identified common variants in the locus that codes for phosphatidylinositol-3,4,5-trisphosphate-5-phosphatase 1, also known as SHIP1, which is encoded by the gene *INPP5D*. The AD-risk variant rs35349669 is associated with high gene expression in myeloid cells, and weak expression in brain tissues and neurons. It is near another gene *CD2AP*, which was also identified in GWAS by the SNP rs10948363. However, this SNP is associated with low transcription in both brain and myeloid cells.

INPP5D and *CD2AP* are both expressed in macrophages and microglia within the brain. SHIP1 is linked to another major AD risk gene TREM2, and inhibits TREM2 signaling through the necessary adaptor DAP12 [81]. *INPP5D* has also been identified as associated with AD in network analysis, providing additional support for its involvement in AD [41]. These data suggest that *INPP5D* may be playing a relevant role in microglia in AD.

Gene expression networks in AD

Insights as to the contribution of microglia in AD have been uncovered through gene expression network analysis. By comparing gene expression changes between healthy and AD samples, we can identify quantifiable internal cellular changes, assess the contributions of these genes, and hypothesize functional interactions. There are two methods by which we can approach gene expression analysis to understand AD etiology; the first is through a candidate gene approach, by identifying genes of interest and looking at their co-expression partners. The second is by constructing network modules based on functional associations between genes and looking for enrichment of these modules in disease states.

Most AD-associated risk variants identified through GWAS have not been related to gene expression changes in brain whole brain tissue [82]. That is, most of these risk loci do not overlap with brain eQTLs. In many cases, AD-risk genes identified through GWAS are expressed at very low levels in brain samples [82], which limits our ability to study these genes further. These low expression signatures may be because the heterogeneous population of brain cells sampled for these studies dilutes cell-specific signatures of small populations of cells, including microglia. By looking at co-expression networks and cell-specific signatures, we can compensate for the low expression of microglial genes in brain (as compared to the gene expression seen in other brain cell types) and gain insight as to the roles of these genes to determine their contribution to AD pathology.

Gene expression data networks can be used to identify a gene's interaction partners and subsequently, the cellular systems that are dysregulated in disease. Building these networks will teach us more about their normal function and identify targets for future therapies. Previous work in whole-brain gene expression datasets has narrowed down network signatures to identify microglial dysfunction as a key element of AD [41, 72, 83]. These analyses revealed AD-associated networks as involved in innate and adaptive immunity, providing support for the role of microglia and/or brain infiltrating peripheral myeloid cells in AD.

Interaction of key AD drivers in healthy controls

One such method for conducting network analysis is to perform weighted gene co-expression network analysis (WGCNA), which groups genes into association modules in an unsupervised manner, such that genes within these modules are co-expressed and co-regulated. The shared regulation of these genes suggests that they are also functionally related. Forabosco et al. conducted a WGCNA, in which they analyzed microarray gene expression data from ten brain regions of 101 pathologically normal individuals [72]. They then grouped genes into association modules, focusing on *TREM2*, a major risk factor for LOAD that has also been identified in GWAS [84]. They discovered that *TREM2* is a central and highly connected gene within its expression module, suggesting that it is a hub that drives module function. The *TREM2* module shares a significant number of genes with another microglial module, and is enriched for genes of the innate immune system and adaptive immune system, such as the microglial-specific genes *CX3CR1, ITGAM, AIF1, FCER1G,* and *CD68*. The authors then looked at a number of other genes that have previously been associated with AD through additional studies, including GWAS. Strikingly, the *TREM2* module is also enriched for genes implicated in AD, suggesting that under normal physiological conditions AD-risk genes interact to promote normal function of microglia.

As network analysis evolves, newer and improved techniques such as multiscale embedded gene co-expression network analysis (MEGENA) can also be used to verify these findings [85].

Co-expression networks in brains of AD-affected individuals

Zhang et al., conducted a similar analysis with case and control samples from three brain areas in 376 LOAD patients and 173 non-demented controls [83]. They then constructed multi-tissue co-expression networks to investigate the differences in these modules between case and control samples. The number of modules differed between cases and controls, and new modules were created (described as "gain of connectivity") and existing modules were disrupted (described as "loss of connectivity") in AD. They then ranked the modules through an integrative network-based approach that looked at module disease association, based on clinical and neuropathological findings and network properties. In such a ranking, the highest ranked module would contain genes most highly associated with disease. Highest ranked was the immune/microglia module, which was a gain of connectivity module that showed the most functional enrichment in this analysis. It is possible that the decreased rank of neuronal modules and increased rank of glial modules may be due to the depletion of neurons within AD brains. However, the role of an immune component in AD was supported by further interrogation of this module. *TYROBP*, also known as DAP12, and the key adaptor protein for the function of TREM2, was determined to be a key driver in this module. Together, these data support the role of *TREM2* and its associated immune-related signaling partners in AD.

Epigenetic signals in AD suggest immune component

Previous gene expression network papers have highlighted the important role of *TREM2* and its associated immune networks as seen through expression network analysis. However, these investigations did not look closely at epigenetic regulation of gene expression. Gjoneska et al. sought to investigate the contribution of epigenetic factors to neurodegeneration using an AD mouse model (CK-p25) at early and late stages of disease, as well as postmortem brain samples from 22 AD patients [41]. In their transcriptome analysis, they observed consistent enrichments in immune-related genes, similar to what was seen in previous experiments. In their epigenome analysis, they used ChIP-seq to profile seven chromatin marks associated with both activation and repression of transcription. They identified molecular signatures associated with AD, including depletion of neuronal promoters and enhancers, and an enrichment of AD-associated loci in enhancer regions. They also identified a putative therapeutic target, PU.1 (coded for by the gene *SPI1)* a transcription factor that is associated with microglial activation and immune function, and whose binding motif was enriched in their analysis. As with previous network analyses, it is possible that the enrichment of these epigenome marks associated with microglia could reflect the increased presence of microglia and fewer neurons (as a result of neurodegeneration) in AD brains, rather than changes within the cell. However, follow-up functional studies support the role of immune-related genes, including *SPI1*, in AD [26].

Together, these network analyses from brain tissue suggest that AD-associated genes are co-expressed and co-regulated under normal conditions to support the normal function of microglia in the brain. Under disease conditions, these networks can be disrupted and expanded, and such disruptions are correlated to the presence and severity of AD. Through looking at additional factors such as gene regulation, we can validate the contribution of important gene targets such as *TREM2* and *SPI1*, as well as identify novel targets associated with AD.

Conclusion

Modeling microglial involvement in AD

Genes identified by GWAS and sequencing, as well as expression network analyses support the involvement of microglia in the development and progression of AD. However, it is still not understood how all of these genes functionally interact to promote disease pathology and whether or how they contribute to the prevailing amyloid cascade hypothesis.

The majority of studies of microglial involvement in AD have focused on one particular function: microglial clearance of Aß plaques. It is suggested that when the natural mechanisms that regulate the phagocytic function of these cells are disrupted, Aß accumulates and activates the cascade that promotes subsequent neuronal degeneration [86]. This is supported by network analyses, which show that normal microglial networks are disrupted in AD. *CD33*, *ABCA7*, and *TREM2* have all been implicated in microglial phagocytosis. It is also supported by many functional studies, which show microglial clearance of Aß plaques is disrupted in AD mouse models.

However, while Aß plaques are a defining feature of AD, they are not the only feature, and it is possible that microglia have other underexplored related functions. Microglia display increased proliferation in LOAD, which is mediated by the receptor colony-stimulating factor 1 (CSF1R) [87]. Microglial proliferation correlates with disease severity in humans and in transgenic mouse models of AD [87]. Inhibiting CSF1R in AD mouse models (including APPswe [88], PSEN1dE9 [89], APP/PS1 [88], and 5xfAD mice [90]) decreases the proliferation of microglia and rescues behavioral deficits [87, 91].

However, the number of Aß plaques is not significantly changed, suggesting that their presence is not directly contributing to AD progression. This is in contrast to previous studies, which focus on microglial engulfment of Aß as a major indicator of disease impact [92]. The importance of microglial proliferation and activation is also supported by *APOE* isoform differences in microglial response and migration. This, in turn, can impact clearance of Aß or influence other functions [93, 94].

Microglia may also have other clearance targets beyond Aß plaques. The significance of *APOE* and *TREM2* on LOAD risk suggests that lipoproteins may be playing a larger role in this pathway than previously anticipated, and that lipid-sensing features of microglia contribute to disease. It is possible that microglia are specifically tagging similar lipid-rich cellular debris for phagocytosis. This theory is supported by initial reports of the disease made by Alois Alzheimer in 1907, who described the accumulation of "adipose saccules," or "lipid droplets," within glial cells. Lipid droplets are lipid-rich organelles that also contain cholesterol and triglycerides, and the accumulation of these droplets has been linked to cellular stress and neurodegenerative diseases including ALS and AD [95]. Mouse models of AD amyloidosis (Tg2576) show increased lipid peroxidation, which precedes amyloid plaque formation [96]. It is possible that accumulation of these lipids and associated oxidative damage contribute to AD pathology. Whether these lipid droplets are causative or reflective of abnormal glial function remains to be investigated.

The enrichment of immune pathways in AD is complemented by the enrichment of other pathways, including endocytosis and cholesterol metabolism. These three pathways involve many of the same genes, including (but not limited to) *APOE*, *TREM2*, and *ABCA7*. Combining these pathways together suggests a new model of microglial involvement in AD relating to microglial efferocytosis, or clearance of dying cells. The efferocytosis model reveals a functional role for microglia and support for the enrichment of immune genes in AD that has been revealed through gene network studies and disease genetics (Fig. 2). Many of these genes interact either directly (as with binding partners APOE and TREM2) or indirectly (as with PU.1 and its downstream gene targets). It is possible that these three pathways converge within microglia, which require an ability to respond, engulf, remove, and process cellular debris.

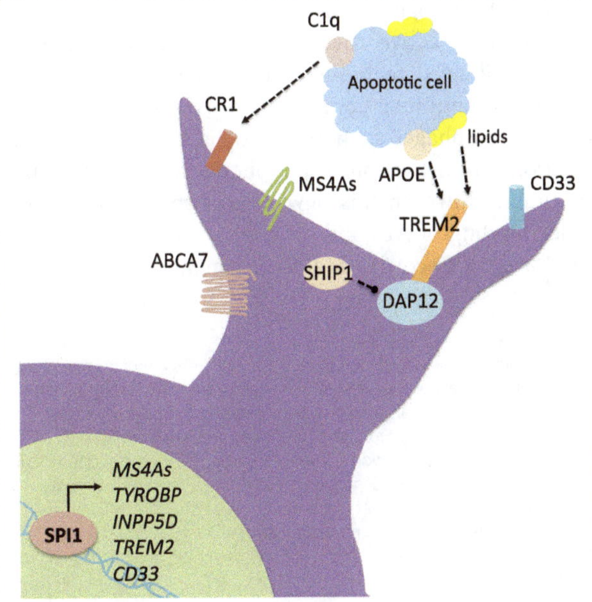

Fig. 2 Efferocytosis model of microglia in LOAD. Microglia contain multiple receptors that can recognize cellular distress signals and other ligands on apoptotic or necrotic cells, including lipids, C1q, and APOE. Propagation of downstream signals activate the transcription factor PU.1, which transcribes the majority of the genes involved in these pathways

What confers risk: endogenous microglia or invading peripheral immune cells?

As indicated previously, microglia share a similar developmental pattern, gene expression, and function with other immune cells. It is possible that other myeloid cells, such as monocytes and macrophages, could be contributing to the observed immune effect. The strong association between LOAD signals and myeloid cells provides evidence for the immune system's role in LOAD, and this relationship can be exploited to investigate genetic risk factors and potentially use peripheral immune cells as a source for easily accessible biomarkers to monitor, diagnose, and eventually treat LOAD. However, another interpretation of these data suggests that the relevant cell-types could be residing outside of the brain, and that the relationship between LOAD and the immune system is controlled by infiltrating peripheral cells [28].

Deciphering the exact contribution of resident microglia versus infiltrating peripheral immune cells in LOAD will be of utmost importance. There are unique molecular and functional signatures in microglia that are not retained in microglial cell lines and are not observed in monocytes that are recruited to the central nervous system, which will serve as a useful tool in determining the contribution of each [97]. Similarly, microglia and infiltrating monocytes have different functions. Monocyte-derived macrophages are highly phagocytic and inflammatory, and can initiate demyelination of neurons [98]. In contrast, microglia have a suppressed cellular metabolism and perform more surveying functions and clear debris [98]. It will take time to determine which of these pathways is contributing most to LOAD.

Genetic studies play an essential role in identifying the molecular mechanism of disease, particularly in highly heritable diseases such as AD. These studies, conducted in mouse models and human subjects, have uncovered the role of microglia in disease and suggest that this cell type plays an active role in AD pathogenesis. Further studies will need to be conducted in order to confirm whether the immune component of AD is from resident tissue macrophages such as microglia, or due to the infiltration and activation of peripheral immune cells into the brain. However, this new area of study updates our understanding of AD, and provides a wider range of targets for drug discovery and development.

Abbreviations

AD: Alzheimer's disease; ADAD: Autosomal dominant Alzheimer's disease; ALS: Amyotrophic lateral sclerosis; ChIP-seq: Chromatin immunoprecipitation and sequencing; EOAD: Early onset Alzheimer's disease; eQTL: expression quantitative trait loci; FTLD: Frontotemporal lobar degeneration; GWAS: Genome-wide association study; GWAX: Genome-wise association study by proxy; IGAP: International Genomics of Alzheimer's Project; LD: Linkage disequilibrium; LOAD: Late onset Alzheimer's disease; MEGENA: Multiscale embedded gene co-expression network analysis; PD: Parkinson's disease; SNP: Single nucleotide polymorphism; WGCNA: Weighted gene co-expression network analysis; WGS: Whole genome sequencing

Acknowledgements

We would like to thank Dr. Edoardo Marcora for his help in discussing the manuscript and Dr. Kathryn Bowles for her critical reading of the manuscript.

Funding

National Institutes of Health (U01AG049508; U01AG052411; RF1AG054011), JPB Foundation.

Authors' contributions

Both authors read and approved the final manuscript.

Authors' information

Not applicable.

Competing interests

A.M.G. is on the scientific advisory board for Denali Therapeutics and has served as a consultant for AbbVie and Cognition Therapeutics.

References

1. Alzheimer's Association. 2016 Alzheimer's Disease Facts and Figures. Alzheimers Dement. 2016;12(4).
2. Goate A, et al. Segregation of a missense mutation in the amyloid precursor protein. Lett to Nat. 1991;349:704–6.
3. Sherrington R, et al. Cloning of a gene bearing missense mutations in early-onset familial Alzheimer's disease. Nature. 1995;375:754–60.
4. Alzheimer's Disease Collaborative Group. The structure of the presenilin 1 (S182) gene and identification of six novel mutations in early onset AD families. Nat Genet. 1995;11:219–22.
5. Rogaev EI, et al. Familial Alzheimer's disease in kindreds with missense mutations in a gene on chromosome 1 related to the Alzheimer's disease type 3 gene. Nature. 1995;376:775–8.
6. Levy-lahad AE, et al. Candidate gene for the chromosome 1 familial Alzheimer's Disease Locus. Science. 1995;269:973–7.
7. Guerreiro RJ, Gustafson DR, Hardy J. The genetic architecture of Alzheimer's disease: Beyond APP, PSENS and APOE. Neurobiol Aging. 2012;33:437–56.
8. Hardy JA, Higgins GA. Alzheimer's Disease: The Amyloid Cascade Hypothesis. Science. 1992;256:3–5.
9. Corder EH, et al. Gene dose of apolipoprotein E type 4 allele and the risk of Alzheimer's disease in late onset families. Science. 1993;261:921–3.
10. Strittmatter WJ, et al. Binding of human apolipoprotein E to synthetic amyloid, B peptide: Isoform-specific effects and implications for late-onset Alzheimer disease. Med Sci. 1993;90:8098–102.
11. McKhann G, Drachman D, Folstein M, Katzman R. Views & reviews Clinical diagnosis of Alzheimer's disease. Neurology. 1984;34:939.
12. Mawuenyega KG, et al. Decreased clearance of CNS beta-amyloid in Alzheimer's disease. Science. 2010;330:1774.
13. Mosher KI, Wyss-Coray T. Microglial dysfunction in brain aging and Alzheimer's disease. Biochem Pharmacol. 2014;88:594–604.
14. Gold M, El Khoury J. β-amyloid, microglia, and the inflammasome in Alzheimer's disease. Semin Immunopathol. 2015;37:607–11.
15. Mhatre SD, Tsai CA, Rubin AJ, James ML, Andreasson KI. Microglial malfunction: the third rail in the development of Alzheimer's disease. Trends Neurosci. 2015; 38:621–36.
16. Karch CM, Goate AM. Alzheimer's disease risk genes and mechanisms of disease pathogenesis. Biol Psychiatry. 2015;77:43–51.
17. Reitz C, et al. Variants in the ATP-binding cassette and the risk of late-onset Alzheimer Disease. JAMA. 2013;309:1483–92.
18. Tishkoff SA, Williams SM. Genetic analysis of African populations: human evolution and complex disease. Nat Rev Genet. 2002;3:611–21.
19. Tosto G, Reitz C. Genome-wide association studies in Alzheimer's disease: a review topical collection on dementia. Curr Neurol Neurosci Rep. 2013;13:381.
20. Grupe A, et al. Evidence for novel susceptibility genes for late-onset Alzheimer's disease from a genome-wide association study of putative functional variants. Hum Mol Genet. 2007;16:865–73.
21. Lambert J-C, et al. Genome-wide association study identifies variants at CLU and CR1 associated with Alzheimer's disease. Nat Genet. 2009;41:1088–93.
22. Harold D, et al. Genome-wide association study identifies variants at CLU and PICALM associated with Alzheimer's disease. Nat Genet. 2009;41:1088–93.
23. Naj AC, et al. Common variants at MS4A4/MS4A6E, CD2AP, CD33 and EPHA1 are associated with late-onset Alzheimer's disease. Nat Genet. 2011;43:436–41.
24. Lambert JC, et al. Meta-analysis of 74,046 individuals identifies 11 new susceptibility loci for Alzheimer's disease. Nat Genet. 2013;45:1452–8.
25. Liu JZ, Erlich Y, Pickrell JK. Case – control association mapping by proxy using family history of disease. 2016. doi:10.1038/ng.3766.
26. Huang K, et al. A common allele lowers SPI1 expression in myeloid cells and delays age at onset for Alzheimer's disease. Nat Neurosci. 2017; in press.
27. Malik M, et al. CD33 Alzheimer's risk-altering polymorphism, CD33 expression, and exon 2 splicing. J Neurosci. 2013;33:13320–5.
28. Raj T, et al. Polarization of the effects of autoimmune and neurodegenerative risk alleles in leukocytes. Science. 2014;344:519–23.
29. Crehan H, et al. Complement receptor 1 (CR1) and Alzheimer's disease. Immunobiology. 2012;217:244–50.
30. Karch CM, et al. Expression of novel Alzheimer's disease risk genes in control and Alzheimer's disease brains. PLoS One. 2012;7:e50976.
31. Shen Y, Li R, McGeer EG, McGeer PL. Neuronal expression of mRNAs for complement proteins of the classical pathway in Alzheimer brain. Brain Res. 1997;769:391–5.
32. Pruim RJ, et al. LocusZoom: regional visualization of genome-wide association scan results. Bioinformatics. 2011;27:2336–7.
33. Boyle AP, et al. Annotation of functional variation in personal genomes using RegulomeDB. Genome Res. 2012;22:1790–7.
34. Iida BYK, Mornaghi R, Nussenzweig V. Complement receptor (CR1) deficiency in erythrocytes from patients with systemic lupus erythematosus. J Exp Med. 1982;155;1427–38.
35. Wu Y, Dissing-olesen L, Macvicar BA, Stevens B. Microglia: dynamic mediators of synapse development and plasticity. Trends Immunol. 2015;36:605–13.
36. Klickstein LB, Barbashov SF, Liu T, Jack RM, Nicholson-weller A. Complement Receptor Type 1 (CR1, CD35) Is a Receptor for C1q. 7. Immunity. 1997;345–55.
37. Jiang H, Burdick D, Glabe CC, Cotman CW, Tenner AJ. beta-Amyloid activates complement by binding to a specific region of the collagen-like domain of the C1q A chain. 2017.
38. Cribbs DH, Velazquez CAP, Soreghan B, Glabe CG, Tenner AJ. Complement activation by cross-linked truncated and chimeric full-length -amyloid. 1997;8:3457–62.
39. Velazquez P, Cribbs DH, Poulos TL, Tenner AJ. Aspartate residue 7 in amyloid [beta]-protein is critical for classical complement pathway activation: Implications for Alzheimer's disease pathogenesis. Nature. 1997;3:77-9.

40. Crehan H, Hardy J, Pocock J. Blockage of CR1 prevents activation of rodent microglia. Neurobiol Dis. 2013;54:139–49.
41. Gjoneska E, et al. Conserved epigenomic signals in mice and humans reveal immune basis of Alzheimer's disease. Nature. 2015;518:365–9.
42. Desikan RS, et al. Personalized genetic assessment of age-associated Alzheimer's disease risk; 2016. p. 1–29.
43. Bagger FO, et al. BloodSpot: a database of gene expression profiles and transcriptional programs for healthy and malignant haematopoiesis. Nucleic Acids Res. 2016;44:D917–24.
44. Zhang Y, et al. Purification and characterization of progenitor and mature human astrocytes reveals transcriptional and functional differences with mouse. Neuron. 2016;89:37–53.
45. Eon Kuek L, Leffler M, Mackay GA, Hulett MD. The MS4A family: counting past 1, 2 and 3. Immunol Cell Biol. 2016;94:11–23.
46. Liang Y, Buckley TR, Tu L, Langdon SD, Tedder TF. Structural organization of the human MS4A gene cluster on Chromosome 11q12. Immunogenetics. 2001;53:357–68.
47. Ma J, Yu JT, Tan L. MS4A Cluster in Alzheimer's Disease. Mol Neurobiol. 2014;1240–8. doi:10.1007/s12035-014-8800-z.
48. Antúnez C, et al. The membrane-spanning 4-domains, subfamily A (MS4A) gene cluster contains a common variant associated with Alzheimer's disease. Genome Med. 2011;3:33.
49. Hollingworth P, et al. Common variants at ABCA7, MS4A6A/MS4A4E, EPHA1, CD33 and CD2AP are associated with Alzheimer's disease. Nat Genet. 2011; 43:429–35.
50. Deng YL, et al. The prevalence of CD33 and MS4A6A variant in Chinese Han population with Alzheimer's disease. Hum Genet. 2012;131:1245–9.
51. Tan L, et al. Association of GWAS-linked loci with late-onset Alzheimer's disease in a northern Han Chinese population. Alzheimers Dement. 2013;9:546–53.
52. Cruse G, et al. The CD20 homologue MS4A4 directs trafficking of KIT toward clathrin-independent endocytosis pathways and thus regulates receptor signaling and recycling. Mol Biol Cell. 2015;26:1711–27.
53. Greer PL, et al. A Family of non-GPCR chemosensors defines an alternative logic for Mammalian Olfaction. Cell. 2016; doi:10.1016/j.cell.2016.05.001.
54. Jun G, et al. A novel Alzheimer disease locus located near the gene encoding tau protein. Mol Psychiatry. 2016;21:108–17.
55. Kaminski WE, et al. Identification of a novel human sterol-sensitive ATP-binding cassette transporter (ABCA7). Biochem Biophys Res Commun. 2000;273:532–8.
56. Wang N, et al. ATP-binding Cassette Transporter A7 (ABCA7) Binds Apolipoprotein A-I and Mediates Cellular Phospholipid but Not Cholesterol Efflux. J Biol Chem. 2003;278:42906–12.
57. Abe Dohmae S, et al. Human ABCA7 supports apolipoprotein-mediated release of cellular cholesterol and phospholipid to generate high density lipoprotein. J Biol Chem. 2004;279:604–11.
58. Vasquez JB, Fardo DW, Estus S. ABCA7 expression is associated with Alzheimer's disease polymorphism and disease status. Neurosci Lett. 2013; 556:58–62.
59. Steinberg S, et al. Loss-of-function variants in ABCA7 confer risk of Alzheimer's disease. Nat Genet. 2015;47:445–7.
60. Del-Aguila JL, et al. Role of ABCA7 loss-of-function variant in Alzheimer's disease: a replication study in European-Americans. Alzheimers Res Ther. 2015;7:73.
61. Cuyvers E, et al. Mutations in ABCA7 in a Belgian cohort of Alzheimer's disease patients: a targeted resequencing study. Lancet Neurol. 2015;14:814–22.
62. Guennec K, Le et al. ABCA7 rare variants and Alzheimer disease risk. Neurology. 2016;1–4. doi:10.1212/WNL.0000000000002627.
63. Allen M, et al. *ABCA7* loss-of-function variants, expression, and neurologic disease risk. Neurol Genet. 2017;3:e126.
64. Satoh K, Abe-Dohmae S, Yokoyama S, St. George-Hyslop P, Fraser PE. ATP-binding cassette transporter A7 (ABCA7) loss of function alters Alzheimer amyloid processing. J Biol Chem. 2015;290:24152–65.
65. Paloneva J, et al. Mutations in two genes encoding different subunits of a receptor signaling complex result in an identical disease phenotype. Am J Hum Genet. 2002;71:656–62.
66. Guerreiro R, et al. *TREM2* Variants in Alzheimer's Disease. N Engl J Med. 2013; 368:117–27.
67. Jonsson T, et al. Variant of TREM2 Associated with the Risk of Alzheimer's Disease. N Engl J Med. 121114152813005 (2012). doi:10.1056/NEJMoa1211103.
68. Jiang T, et al. A rare coding variant in TREM2 increases risk for Alzheimer's disease in Han Chinese. Neurobiol Aging. 2016;42:17.e1–217.e3.
69. Jin SC, et al. Coding variants in TREM2 increase risk for Alzheimer's disease. Hum Mol Genet. 2014;23:5838–46.
70. Kleinberger G, et al. TREM2 mutations implicated in neurodegeneration impair cell surface transport and phagocytosis. Sci Transl Med. 2014;6:243ra86.
71. Lill CM, et al. The role of TREM2 R47H as a risk factor for Alzheimer's disease, frontotemporal lobar degeneration, amyotrophic lateral sclerosis, and Parkinson's disease. Alzheimers Dement. 2015;11:1407–16.
72. Forabosco P, et al. Insights into TREM2 biology by network analysis of human brain gene expression data. Neurobiol Aging. 2013;34:2699–714.
73. Ma L, et al. Expression and processing analyses of wild type and p.R47H TREM2 variant in Alzheimer's disease brains. Mol Neurodegener. 2016;11:72.
74. Kober DL, et al. Neurodegenerative disease mutations in TREM2 reveal a functional surface and distinct loss-of-function mechanisms. elife. 2016;5:1–24.
75. Lue L, Schmitz C, Walker DG. What happens to microglial trem2 in alzheimer's disease: immunoregulatory turned into immunopathogenic? Neuroscience. 2015;302:138–50.
76. Yeh FL, Wang Y, Tom I, Gonzalez LC, Sheng M. TREM2 binds to apolipoproteins, including APOE and CLU/APOJ, and thereby facilitates uptake of amyloid-beta by microglia. Neuron. 2016;91:328–40.
77. Wang Y, et al. TREM2 lipid sensing sustains the microglial response in an Alzheimer's disease model. Cell. 2015;160:1061–71.
78. Wang Y, et al. TREM2-mediated early microglial response limits diffusion and toxicity of amyloid plaques. J Exp Med. 2016;213:667–75.
79. Griciuc A, et al. Alzheimer's disease risk gene cd33 inhibits microglial uptake of amyloid beta. Neuron. 2013;78:631–43.
80. Jiang T, et al. CD33 in alzheimer's disease. Mol Neurobiol. 2014;49:529–35.
81. Peng Q, et al. TREM2- and DAP12-dependent activation of PI3K requires DAP10 and is inhibited by SHIP1. Sci Signal. 2010;3:ra38.
82. GTEx Consortium, T. Gte. The Genotype-Tissue Expression (GTEx) project. Nat Genet. 2013;45:580–5.
83. Zhang B, et al. Integrated systems approach identifies genetic nodes and networks in late-onset Alzheimer's disease. Cell. 2013;153:707–20.
84. Colonna M, Wang Y. TREM2 variants: new keys to decipher Alzheimer disease pathogenesis. Nat Rev Neurosci. 2016;17:201–7.
85. Song WM, Zhang B. Multiscale embedded gene co-expression network analysis. PLoS Comput Biol. 2015;11:e1004574.
86. Murphy MP, LeVine H III. Alzheimer's disease and the beta-amyloid peptide. J Alzheimers Dis. 2010;19:1–17.
87. Olmos-Alonso A, et al. Pharmacological targeting of CSF1R inhibits microglial proliferation and prevents the progression of Alzheimer's-like pathology. Brain. 2016;139:891–907.
88. Jankowsky JL, et al. Co-expression of multiple transgenes in mouse CNS: a comparison of strategies. Biomol Eng. 2001;17:157–65.
89. Jankowsky JL, et al. Mutant presenilins specifically elevate the levels of the 42 residue beta-amyloid peptide in vivo: evidence for augmentation of a 42-specific gamma secretase. Hum Mol Genet. 2004;13:159–70.
90. Oakley H, et al. Intraneuronal β-Amyloid aggregates, neurodegeneration, and neuron loss in transgenic mice with five familial alzheimer's disease mutations: potential factors in amyloid plaque formation. J Neurosci. 2006; 26:10129–40.
91. Spangenberg EE, et al. Eliminating microglia in Alzheimer's mice prevents neuronal loss without modulating amyloid-β pathology. Brain. 2016;139:1265–81.
92. Gandy S, Heppner FL. Microglia as dynamic and essential components of the amyloid hypothesis. Neuron. 2013;78:575–7.
93. Cudaback E, Li X, Montine KS, Montine TJ, Keene CD. Apolipoprotein E isoform-dependent microglia migration. FASEB J. 2011;25:2082–91.
94. Rodriguez GA, Tai LM, LaDu MJ, Rebeck GW. Human APOE4 increases microglia reactivity at Abeta plaques in a mouse model of Abeta deposition. J Neuroinflammation. 2014;11:111.
95. Liu L, et al. Glial lipid droplets and ROS induced by mitochondrial defects promote neurodegeneration. Cell. 2015;160:177–90.

15

TRPA1 channels promote astrocytic Ca^{2+} hyperactivity and synaptic dysfunction mediated by oligomeric forms of amyloid-β peptide

Anthony Bosson[1,2], Adrien Paumier[1,2], Sylvie Boisseau[1,2], Muriel Jacquier-Sarlin[1,2], Alain Buisson[1,2†] and Mireille Albrieux[1,2*†]

Abstract

Background: Excessive synaptic loss is thought to be one of the earliest events in Alzheimer's disease (AD). However, the key mechanisms that maintain plasticity of synapses during adulthood or initiate synapse dysfunction in AD remain unknown. Recent studies suggest that astrocytes contribute to functional changes observed during synaptic plasticity and play a major role in synaptic dysfunction but astrocytes behavior and involvement in early phases of AD remained largely undefined.

Methods: We measure astrocytic calcium activity in mouse CA1 hippocampus *stratum radiatum* in both the global astrocytic population and at a single cell level, focusing in the highly compartmentalized astrocytic arbor. Concurrently, we measure excitatory post-synaptic currents in nearby pyramidal neurons.

Results: We find that application of soluble Aβ oligomers (Aβo) induced fast and widespread calcium hyperactivity in the astrocytic population and in the microdomains of the astrocyte arbor. We show that astrocyte hyperactivity is independent of neuronal activity and is repaired by transient receptor potential A1 (TRPA1) channels blockade. In return, this TRPA1 channels-dependent hyperactivity influences neighboring CA1 neurons triggering an increase in glutamatergic spontaneous activity. Interestingly, in an AD mouse model (APP/PS1-21 mouse), astrocyte calcium hyperactivity equally takes place at the beginning of Aβ production, depends on TRPA1 channels and is linked to CA1 neurons hyperactivity.

Conclusions: Our experiments demonstrate that astrocytes contribute to early Aβo toxicity exhibiting a global and local Ca^{2+} hyperactivity that involves TRPA1 channels and is related to neuronal hyperactivity. Together, our data suggest that astrocyte is a frontline target of Aβo and highlight a novel mechanism for the understanding of early synaptic dysregulation induced by soluble Aβo species.

Keywords: Astrocyte, Calcium, Alzheimer, Synapse, TRPA1, APP/PS1

* Correspondence: mireille.albrieux@univ-grenoble-alpes.fr
† Equal contributors
[1] University Grenoble Alpes, Grenoble Institut des Neurosciences, GIN, Chemin Fortuné Ferrini, BP170, F-38000 Grenoble, France
[2] Inserm, U1216, F-38000 Grenoble, France

Background

Formation of toxic amyloid-β (Aβ) species and their accumulation in plaques are key hallmarks in the pathogenesis of Alzheimer's disease (AD) but it has now been recognized that, far ahead of plaques formation, soluble Aβ oligomers (Aβo) are the pathology-triggering species [1]. More specifically, Aβo manage a progressive loss of synaptic connectivity leading to neurodegeneration. Astrocytes are important safeguards of synaptic function and it becomes increasingly evident that these cells accomplish a more important role in brain function than previously thought. The loss of synapses may reflect functional downfall of astrocytes. These cells possess receptors and signaling machinery for all known neurotransmitters thus sensing neuronal activity [2]. They also actively secrete gliotransmitters such as ATP, glutamate, D-serine hence modulating activity of neuronal receptors [3, 4]. Consequently, through their involvement in the tripartite synapse, they both sense and modulate synaptic output [5].

Unlike neurons, astrocytes are electrically non-excitable cells but they are equipped with numerous channels, receptors or exchangers triggering Ca^{2+} signals. Thus, astrocytic excitability is based on highly spatiotemporally coordinated fluctuations of intracellular Ca^{2+} concentration relying on plasmalemmal and intracellular channels [6]. Important progress has been made in studying astrocytes branches Ca^{2+} signaling since they are the primary sites for interactions with neurons [7–9]. Direct monitoring of Ca^{2+} dynamics in the processes of adult mouse hippocampal astrocytes has revealed intense local and compartmentalized activity that is dissociated from activity in the cell body [8]. However, until recently, it was difficult to specifically explore this astrocytic calcium activity since channels and receptors involved in astrocytic calcium signaling were commonly expressed in neurons. However, among the receptors involved in astrocytic calcium signaling, transient receptor potential A1 (TRPA1) channel seems to be specifically expressed in astrocytes and absent from neurons within hippocampus *stratum radiatum* [10, 11]. The discovery of TRPA1 channel as an important mediator of Ca^{2+} entry restricted to astrocytes in the mouse hippocampus provided new opportunity to explore astrocyte signaling in relation to neuron-astrocyte interaction particularly in case of synaptic dysregulation.

In late transgenic AD mouse models, i.e. in phases associated with plaques formation, it has been shown that astrocytic calcium activity dramatically increases, becomes synchronous nearby Aβ plaques and coordinates calcium signals at long distance [12]. Within somatosensory cortex, this astrocyte hyperactivity around plaques is mediated by purinergic signaling [13]. Surprisingly, astrocytes behavior and reactions in early phases of AD remained largely undefined despite their probable involvement in the progressive loss of synaptic connectivity and in the complex and critical cellular phase of AD [14]. We thus chose to study the impact of soluble Aβ oligomers on astrocytic function at the onset of early defensive cellular phase well before astrogliosis or inflammatory processes.

In this work, we monitored astrocytic calcium activity within the CA1 *stratum radiatum* region of the mouse hippocampus both at the astrocytic population level and at a single cell level, focusing in the astrocytic arbor. We characterized spontaneous Ca^{2+} signaling properties at these two related levels and showed that Aβo exposition induced at once a global and a local Ca^{2+} hyperactivity. We showed that this hyperactivity was independent of neuronal activity and was totally restored to physiological level by blocking TRPA1 channels. This TRPA1 channels-dependent influence of Aβo on astrocyte activity consequently impacted neighboring CA1 neurons, increasing glutamatergic spontaneous activity. In an AD mouse model, we showed that astrocyte hyperactivity was an early phenomenon setting up at the onset of Aβ production, being also related to neuronal hyperactivity and preceding TRPA1 channel overexpression. Overall, our data provide a novel mechanism for the understanding of early toxicity of soluble Aβo species.

Methods

Slice preparation

Coronal hippocampal slices (ranging from 300 to 350 μm thick) were prepared from Swiss mice (postnatal day 17–23; Janvier, Le Genest St Isle, France) or APP/PS1-21 transgenic mice [15] (postnatal day 19–28) together with control littermates. Mice were killed by decerebration and decapitated. The brain was rapidly removed and cut in ice-cold cutting ACSF containing (in mM): 2.5 KCl, 7 $MgCl_2$, 0.5 $CaCl_2$, 1.2 NaH_2PO_4, 25 $NaHCO_3$, 11 D-glucose and 234 sucrose bubbled with 95% O_2 and 5% CO_2, with a vibratome VT1200S (Leica, Wetzlar, Germany). Slices containing the hippocampus were placed in ACSF containing (in mM): 126 NaCl, 2.5 KCl, 1.2 $MgCl_2$, 2.5 $CaCl_2$, 1.2 NaH_2PO_4 bubbled with 95% O_2 and 5% CO_2 and supplemented with 1 mM sodium pyruvate at room temperature for a recovery period.

Slices bulk loading with Fluo-4 AM.

Briefly, 350 μm coronal slices were loaded with the calcium indicator dye Fluo-4 by immersion for 45 min at 35 °C in a bath containing 5 μM Fluo-4 AM (Life Technologies), 0.01% Pluronic acid F-127 (Molecular Probes), 0.005% Cremophor EL (Sigma-Aldrich) and 0.05% DMSO (dimethyl sulfoxide, Sigma-Aldrich) in

ACSF. The loading chamber was continuously oxygenated with 95% O_2 and 5% CO_2. Slices were then transferred into dye-free ACSF for at least 45 min prior to experiments. Mainly live astrocyte took up the fluorescent dye with these conditions [16, 17].

Single-astrocyte dye loading with Fluo-4

Coronal 300 μm slices were transferred to a chamber allowing constant perfusion with ACSF at room temperature, bubbled with 95% O_2 and 5% CO_2 on the stage of an upright compound microscope (Eclipse E600 FN, Nikon, Paris, France) equipped with a water immersion 60× objective (NA 1.0) and an infrared-differential interference contrast optics with CCD camera (Optronis VX45, Kehl, Germany). Glass pipettes 8–11 MΩ (Harvard apparatus) were filled with intracellular solution containing (in mM): 105 K-gluconate, 30 KCl, 10 phosphocreatine, 10 HEPES, 4 ATP-Mg, 0.3 GTP-Tris, 0.2 Fluo-4 pentapotassium salt (Life Technologies), adjusted to pH 7.2 with KOH. Signals were amplified by Axopatch 200B, sampled by a Digidata 1440A interface and recorded with pClamp8 software (Molecular Devices, Foster City, USA). Astrocytes were identified based on morphological, localization in the *stratum radiatum* and negative resting potential (between −70 and −80 mV). Input resistance was calculated by measuring current in response to a 10 mV pulse with 80 ms duration, near the end of the voltage command. Only passive astrocytes showing linear *I/V* relationship and low input resistance (~ 50 MΩ) were kept for dye loading. After achieving whole-cell configuration, access resistance was constantly monitored, and astrocytes were excluded from this study when this parameter varied >20% throughout the experiment. To allow sufficient diffusion of the dye and avoid astrocyte dialysis, the time in whole-cell configuration was limited to less than 5 min. Then, the patch pipette was carefully withdrawn to allow the astrocyte to recover. In order to maximize the diffusion of the dye into the astrocytic processes, we waited at least 15 min before calcium imaging [8, 18].

Calcium imaging

Bulk or single-astrocyte loaded slices were placed in a constantly perfused chamber on the stage of an upright compound microscope (Eclipse E600 FN, Nikon, Paris, France) equipped with a water immersion 40× (NA 0.8) or 60× (NA 1.0) objective and a confocal head (confocal C1 head, Nikon, Paris, France). Excitation was achieved with light at 488 nm and emission was filtered with a 515 ± 15 nm filter. Images were acquired with EZ-C1 software (Nikon, Paris, France) at 1.2 s intervals in a single confocal plane over a period of 5 min.

Bulk loading calcium imaging data analysis

Prior to analysis, raw images were stabilized (when needed if slight *x-y* drift occurred during recordings, z drifts were excluded) using ImageJ plugin Template Matching. *CalSignal* software was used to measured intracellular Ca^{2+} activity, analyzing the fluorescence signal F within each region of interest (ROI) corresponding to the cell body area of each astrocyte [19]. F_0 was calculated for each ROI on the recording period. Based on the $\Delta F/F_0$ ratios, significant fluorescence variations were detected and a Ca^{2+} event was defined as a significant and continuous signal increase larger than a fixed threshold followed by a significant and continuous signal decrease larger than the same threshold. Thus, cells were defined as active when fluorescence increased ≥2 standard deviations relative to baseline fluorescence. After peak detection, each Ca^{2+} transients were visually checked by the operator. The theoretical Poisson distribution was calculated by the method of least squares approximating λ until it most closely fits the observed frequency distribution.

Single astrocyte loading data analysis

Ca^{2+} transients were measured in two-dimensional images, in individual subregions matching the shape of the astrocyte structure. Manually selected ROIs (~1 μm^2) were placed along astrocytic processes lying in the focal plane [8] and a ROI was also selected in the soma if accessible. Prior to analysis, raw images were stabilized (when needed if slight *x-y* drift occurred during recordings, z drifts were excluded) using ImageJ plugins Template Matching and filtered with 3D Hybrid Median Filter [7]. *CalSignal* software was used to measure intracellular Ca^{2+} activity, analyzing the fluorescence signal F within each ROI. As described above, significant changes in fluorescence were detected on the basis of the calculated $\Delta F/F_0$ ratios. Each Ca^{2+} transients within ROI were visually checked by the operator and reported in a raster plot in order to discriminate focal activities from expanded ones (as described by [8]). At the end of each recording, z-stacks (0.5 μm steps) were performed to obtain tri-dimensional projections of astrocyte territories revealed by Fluo-4 loading. Images were then filtered with 3D Hybrid Median Filter plugin in ImageJ.

Electrophysiological recordings

Whole-cell recordings were made from the somata of visually identified CA1 pyramidal neurons. Patch pipettes (4–6 MΩ) were filled with an internal solution containing (in mM): 105 K-gluconate, 30 KCl, 10 phosphocreatine, 10 HEPES, 4 ATP-Mg, 0.3 GTP-Tris, 0.3 EGTA, adjusted to pH 7.2 with KOH. Spontaneous excitatory post-synaptic currents (sEPSCs) were collected at a membrane holding potential of −65 mV which is close to the reverse potential of GABA. All recordings were done at room temperature (22–24 °C) and only a single neuron was studied per slice. sEPSCs and their kinetics were analyzed in 5-min epochs within the time frame of the recordings. Each epoch was compared to the initial 5-min recording and sEPSCs frequencies were normalized to this initial value. Access resistance was constantly monitored and recordings were excluded from this study when this parameter varied >20% throughout the experiment. Recordings were analyzed using the Clampfit module of the pClamp8 software (Molecular Devices, Foster City, USA) with a threshold at −20 pA to exclude miniature EPSCs.

Aβ oligomerization, monomer purification and drug application

Recombinant $A\beta_{1-42}$ peptide (Bachem) was resuspended in 1,1,1,3,3,3-hexafluoro-2-propanol (HFIP) to 1 mM until complete resuspension as described previously [20]. Following HFIP evaporation, Aβ oligomers were prepared by diluting Aβ to 1 mM in DMSO, then to 100 μM in ice-cold ACSF with immediate vortexing and bath sonication, and then incubated at 4 °C for 24 h with mild agitation.

When appropriate, the Aβ monomer is purified on a C18 column (SPE-Chromabond-HRX C18 ec, 200 μl, 5 mg, Macherey-Nagel, France). The column was equilibrated with 0.1% trifluoroacetic acid (TFA) in water. Immediately after dilution in DMSO, the Aβ sample was loaded and the column was washed three times with 0.1% TFA. Then, a gradient of acetonitrile from 30 to 60% was applied (Additional file 1). Fractions (0.1 ml) were collected. The elution profile was determined by measuring the absorbance at 275 nm. The peak fraction was collected and the concentration of peptide was determined by absorbance at 275 nm using $\varepsilon_{275\ nm}$ = 1400 M^{-1} cm^{-1}. The peptide is then stored at −80 °C.

Aβo, Aβm, tetrodotoxin (TTX; Latoxan, Valence, France), Ca^{2+}-free solution (ACSF - 0 Ca^{2+} - 1 mM EGTA) and HC 030031 (Sigma-Aldrich) were bath applied at the appropriate concentration during 5 min before and during calcium imaging or electrophysiological recordings. Minocycline hydrochloride (Sigma-Aldrich) was bath applied during 15 min before and during calcium imaging recording.

Immunohistochemistry

Mice were deeply anesthetized with 10% chloral hydrate and perfused intracardially with 10 ml 0.9% NaCl followed by 35 ml 4% paraformaldehyde in 0.1 M PBS, pH 7.3. Brains were rapidly removed, post-fixed overnight at 4 °C in 4% paraformaldehyde, immersed in 20% sucrose in 0.1 M PBS, pH 7.5 overnight, frozen in cooled (−35 °C) isopentane and stored at −30 °C. Serial frontal sections (30 μm thick) were cut with a cryostat microtome (HM 500 M, Microm, Francheville, France). Sections were blocked by incubation with 3% bovine serum albumin in TBS-Tween-Triton (TBSTT) (0.1 M Tris Base, 0.15 M NaCl, 0.1% Tween, 0.1% Triton X-100) for 30 min (dilution/blocking buffer). Tissue sections were then incubated overnight at 4 °C with either an anti-NeuN antibody (AbCys, France, mouse monoclonal; 1:500), anti-GFAP antibody (Molecular Probes, USA, mouse monoclonal; 1:1000), anti-TRPA1 antibody (Novus, USA, rabbit polyclonal; 1:100) or anti-Iba-1 antibody (Wako, USA, rabbit polyclonal; 1:500). Tissue sections were washed in TBSTT and incubated for 2 h at room temperature with Cyanin 3- (Jackson Immuno Research Laboratories, USA; 1:1000) or Alexa 488-conjugated secondary antibodies (Life Tecchnology, USA; 1:1000). Sections were washed in TBSTT and mounted in Dako fluorescent mounting medium (Dako, USA).

When appropriate, amyloid-β deposits were stained using Thioflavine S [21]. Sections were re-hydrated in TBS buffer (0.1 M Tris Base, 0.15 M NaCl), incubated in filtered 1% aqueous Thioflavine S (Sigma, France) for 8 min at room temperature, in the dark and washed several times in TBS buffer.

Image acquisition

Sections were examined with a Zeiss LSM 710 confocal laser scanning microscope with a Plan Apochromat 20× objective (NA 0.8) or an oil immersion Plan Neofluor 40× objective (NA 1.3) and translating platform with motorized crossed roller stages. When appropriate, mosaics were acquired for each channel separately with "Zen" software, in a 12 bit format, using the tile scan function. For TRPA1 and GFAP co-staining, sections were also acquired with a Zeiss Airyscan module with an oil immersion Plan Apochromat 63× objective (NA 1.46) to improve lateral resolution (~140 nm) and signal-to-noise ratios. For illustration, images were merged with ImageJ software.

Immunoblotting

Dissected hippocampi from 1-month old APP/PS1–21 mice were homogenized in cold buffer containing 0.32 M sucrose and 10 mM HEPES, pH 7.4. Samples were maintained at 4 °C during all steps of the experiments. Homogenates were cleared at 1000 x g for 10 min to remove nuclei and large debris. Samples in loading buffer were boiled for 10 min and equal amounts of proteins (20 μg, quantified by micro-BCA assay (Pierce) in duplicate extracts) were resolved on a 4–20% gradient Bis-Tris polyacrylamide precast stain free gels (Bio-Rad) in denaturing conditions. Proteins were transferred to a polyvinylidene difluoride membrane (Millipore) for 30 min at 4 °C. Membranes were blocked with 3% dry milk in Tris-Buffered Saline (TBS: 10 mM Tris, 150 mM NaCl, pH 7.4) containing 0.1% Tween for 1 h at room temperature. Membranes were probed with anti-TRPA1 antibody (Novus, USA; 1:2000) and anti-GFAP antibody (Dako, USA, rabbit polyclonal; 1:100000) diluted in 3% dry milk in 0.1% Tween TBS overnight at 4 °C. Membranes were washed in 0.2% Tween TBS and probed with HRP-conjugated anti-rabbit IgG (Fab') (Interchim, France; 1:40,000) antibody for 45 min at room temperature. After washes, specific proteins were visualized with an enhanced chemiluminescence ECL Detection System (Bio-Rad) and the chemidoc system (Bio-Rad). Chemiluminescence signals were normalized to protein loading signals acquired using Stain-free pre-cast gels (Bio-Rad).

Statistical analysis

Data were analyzed using R (the R Project for Statistical Computing) [22]. Comparisons between two groups were conducted with the two-tailed Mann-Whitney test. Kruskal-Wallis test followed by Pairwise comparison using Wilcoxon rank sum test was used when needed for multiple comparisons. Proportions of hyperactive/active astrocyte and focal/expanded activities were compared with χ^2-test. Data were expressed as mean ± SEM accompanied by distribution of experimental points. Graphic significance levels were *, $p < 0.05$; **, $p < 0.01$ and ***, $p < 0.001$.

Results

Ca^{2+} activity in the astrocytic population and individual processes in mouse hippocampus

Ca^{2+} signals encoding is known to be different in astrocytic cell body versus processes and involves different calcium sources such as internal stores release or external entry. Spatio-temporal Ca^{2+} activity characteristics within astrocyte correlate to specific function associated with different territories. Astrocytes not only operate as individual cells but also take part in functional network through gap-junction coupling allowing remote communication in delimited functional brain area. We studied astrocytic Ca^{2+} activity at once in the global astrocytic population and in single cell microdomains on mouse hippocampal slices (P17-P23) by using two complementary imaging techniques: i) Fluo-4 AM bulk loading to record calcium activity in the astrocytic population and ii) whole-cell patch-clamp technique to load individual astrocytes with Fluo-4 dye giving access to single cell processes territory (Additional file 2).

We analyzed signals by positioning regions of interest (ROIs) either in each cell body of Fluo-4 AM loaded astrocytes (20.0 ± 1.3 ROIs by frame; n = 43 slices from 14 animals in physiological condition; Fig. 1a, b) or by subdividing the entire patch-clamp loaded territory into subregions of similar area (1 μm^2; 111.7 ± 7.3 ROIs by astrocyte; n = 7 astrocytes from 6 animals in physiological condition; Fig. 1e, f). These subregions corresponded to functional microdomains as previously defined by Di Castro et al. [8] since their size matched approximately the synaptic density in the neuropil region. We investigated some of the temporal properties of astrocytic Ca^{2+} signals (such as the proportion of active cells, the proportion of active microdomains, the frequency of events) and some of the spatial properties of Ca^{2+} signals within the astrocytic arbor (such as the events propagation).

In physiological condition, 49.1 ± 2.2% of bulk loaded astrocytes were spontaneously active during a 5 min recording period (n = 43 slices from 14 animals) with a mean frequency of 0.49 ± 0.01 event/min (n = 817 astrocytes; Fig. 1c). Frequency histograms revealed that the occurrence of Ca^{2+} events in the astrocyte population was similar to a Poisson distribution with $\lambda = 1.85$ suggesting that spontaneous Ca^{2+} event within *stratum radiatum* was a stochastic phenomenon (Fig. 1d). Based on an in vivo study performed in mouse cortical astrocytes [13], we classified astrocytes as inactive (0 event/min), active (0.2–0.6 event/min) and hyperactive (> 0.6 event/min). We observed a minority of hyperactive astrocytes (11%) within mouse hippocampus *stratum radiatum* in physiological condition (Fig. 1d). This spontaneous activity is independent of neuronal activity since TTX (500 nM) had no effect on either the proportion of active astrocytes or the frequency of calcium activity or the proportion of active/hyperactive astrocyte (Fig. 2a–c). This therefore confirmed that the global activity of the astrocytic population is totally autonomous within the mouse hippocampus *stratum radiatum* [18]. In single patch-clamp loaded astrocyte, we had access to Ca^{2+} activity in a two-dimensional acquisition plane representing on average 1945.3 ± 140.1 μm^2 (n = 7 astrocytes; Fig. 1e). We analyzed spatio-temporal encoding of Ca^{2+} signals in 111.7 ± 7.3 microdomains within the astrocytic arbor. In physiological condition, 57.9 ± 4.8% of these microdomains were active (i.e. at least 1 Ca^{2+} event; Fig. 1f, g) during a 5 min recording period with a mean activity frequency of 0.59 ± 0.01 event/min (n = 782 ROIs). As previously described in mouse dentate gyrus astrocytes [8], we identified two types of Ca^{2+} events: "focal events" that are confined to 1 to 4 microdomains and "expanded events" appearing in more than 4 contiguous subregions (Fig. 1h). An additional movie file shows these two types of events in more details (Additional file 3). Focal events were the large majority (67%) occurring randomly in all subregions. Expanded events arose less often (33%) and spread over 7.1 ± 0.4 μm^2. Within *stratum radiatum*, these two types of Ca^{2+} event were independent of neuronal activity since

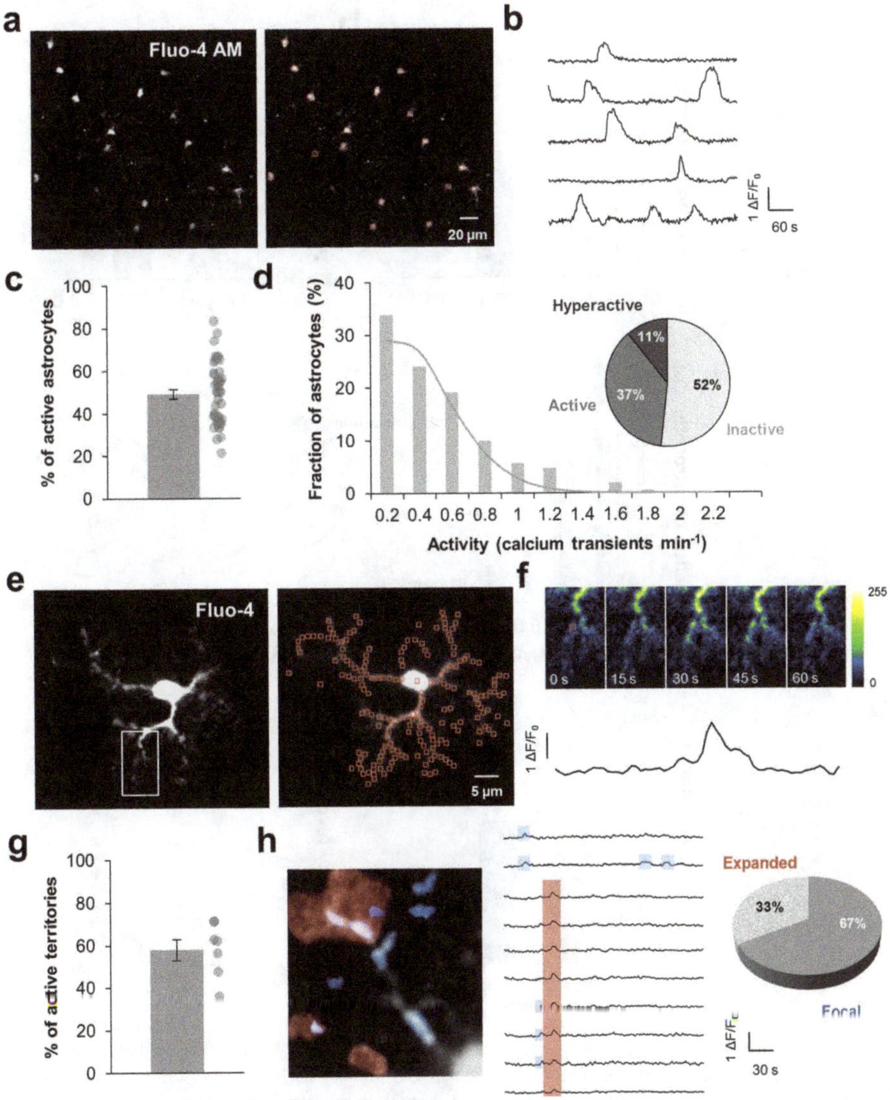

Fig. 1 Detection of global and compartmentalized Ca^{2+} events in astrocytes. **a** Fluo-4-loaded astrocytes in the *stratum radiatum* of a mouse coronal slice. Fluorescence variations were analyzed in astrocyte cell bodies (*red square*). **b** Example of typical fluorescence variations recorded in physiological condition. **c** Proportion of astrocytes displaying calcium activity during a 5-min recording. Each dot corresponds to individual value for each recorded slice ($n = 43$). **d** Frequency histogram showing the occurrence of Ca^{2+} events in the astrocyte population and the related theoretical Poisson distribution (*grey curve*). Pie chart representing inactive (0 event per min), active (0.2–0.6 event per min) and hyperactive (> 0.6 event per min) astrocytes in physiological condition. **e** Single patch-clamp Fluo-4-loaded astrocyte in the *stratum radiatum* of a mouse coronal slice. Fluorescence variations within processes were analyzed in subregions of ~1 μm^2 (*red square*) in a single z-plane. **f** Time-lapse Ca^{2+} imaging in an astrocyte process showing an example of Ca^{2+} event. Time between frames, 15 s. The *black curve* corresponded to the fluorescence signal recorded in a selected ROI (*red square*, first image). **g** Proportion of subregions displaying a calcium activity during a 5-min recording. Each dot corresponds to individual value for each recorded astrocyte ($n = 7$). **h** Artificial color superposition of focal Ca^{2+} events (1–4 contiguous subregions, *blue*) and expanded Ca^{2+} events (> 4 contiguous subregions, *red*) occurring during a 5-min recording in an astrocyte process, as defined by [8]. Traces showing occurrence of Ca^{2+} peaks in contiguous subregions with blue and red highlights identifying focal (*blue*) and expanded (*red*) Ca^{2+} events respectively. In physiological condition, focal events represent the major part of Ca^{2+} events within the astrocytic processes

TTX application didn't affect either the proportion or the frequency of focal and expanded events (Fig. 2d, e).

Astrocytic Ca^{2+} signaling involves both internal Ca^{2+} stores and external Ca^{2+} entry. Within the *stratum radiatum* astrocyte population, removal of external Ca^{2+} from the bath (ACSF - 0 Ca^{2+} - EGTA 1 mM) had no effect on the proportion of spontaneously active astrocytes (48.2 ± 2.7% in Ca^{2+}-free medium vs 49.1 ± 2.2% in ACSF; $n = 9$ slices from 5 animals; $p = 0.97$) but aborted approximately 35% of events within active cells

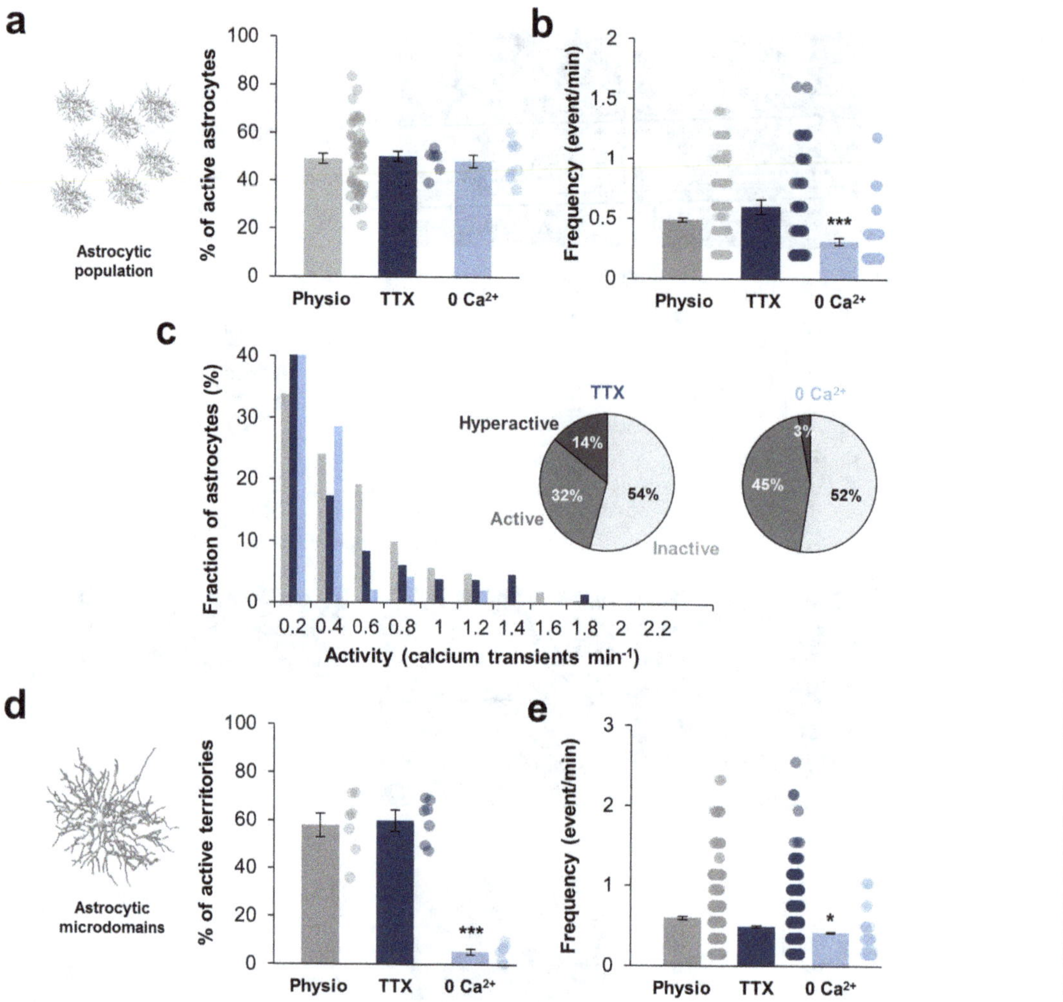

Fig. 2 Spontaneous astrocytic Ca^{2+} events are fully autonomous and partly depend on external Ca^{2+} entry. **a**, **b** Within the astrocytic population, proportion of astrocytes displaying calcium activity and frequency of astrocyte calcium activity in physiological condition (*grey*; $n = 43$), under 500 nM TTX application (*dark blue*; $n = 6$) or in Ca^{2+}-free medium (0 Ca; *light blue*; $n = 9$). Each dot corresponds to individual value for each recorded slice (proportion) or each recorded ROI (frequency). **c** Frequency histogram revealing that 500 nM TTX had no effect on the frequency distribution whereas significantly less astrocytes were hyperactive in Ca^{2+}-free medium (0 Ca^{2+}; *light blue*). **d**, **e** Within single astrocyte arbor, proportion of subregions displaying calcium activity and frequency of astrocyte calcium activity in physiological condition (*grey*; $n = 7$), under 500 nM TTX application (*dark blue*; $n = 7$) or in Ca^{2+}-free medium (0 Ca^{2+}; *light blue*; $n = 7$). Each dot corresponds to individual value for each recorded astrocyte (proportion) or each recorded ROI (frequency). Results are compared with the physiological condition with *, $p < 0.05$; **, $p < 0.01$ and ***, $p < 0.001$

(0.31 ± 0.02 event/min in Ca^{2+}-free medium vs 0.48 ± 0.01 in physiological condition; $n = 103$ astrocytes; $p < 0.0001$) meaning that one third of somatic Ca^{2+} events depended on a Ca^{2+} entry (Fig. 2a–c). Particularly, the proportion of hyperactive/active astrocytes was strongly affected (3% of hyperactive astrocytes versus 11% in physiological condition; $p < 0.001$). Yet, location of internal stores is not uniformly distributed in the astrocytic territory since they are concentrated in cell body and thick processes, thin astrocytic processes being practically devoid of Ca^{2+} stores [23]. Consistently, we observed that removing external Ca^{2+} suppressed nearly all the compartmentalized Ca^{2+} transients in the astrocytic arbor (5.1 ± 1.3% active territories vs 57.8 ± 4.8% in physiological condition; $n = 7$ astrocytes from 6 animals; $p = 0.0006$) and reduced the frequency of the residual signals (0.41 ± 0.01 event/min vs 0.59 ± 0.01 in physiological condition; $n = 687$ ROIs; $p = 0.04$) (Fig. 2d, e).

Astrocytes become hyperactive in presence of amyloid-β oligomers

To investigate the effect of soluble $A\beta_{1-42}$ oligomers (Aβo) on astrocytic calcium signaling, we perfused hippocampal slices with 100 nM of oligomeric forms of the peptide during 5 min before recording. In the global astrocytic population, application of Aβo resulted in a significant increase in the proportion of active astrocytes (69.7 ± 2.1% vs 49.1 ± 2.2% in physiological condition; n = 12 slices; $p < 0.0001$; Fig. 3a). Within active cells, the frequency of Ca^{2+} events also significantly rose (0.83 ± 0.04 event/min vs 0.48 ± 0.01 event/min in physiological condition; n = 237 astrocytes; $p < 0.0001$; Fig. 3b). Frequency histogram was switched to high frequency and developed differently from the basal Poisson distribution (λ = 4.39; Fig. 3c). This suggested that Ca^{2+} event was not anymore a stochastic phenomenon but was managed by Aβo. The fraction of hyperactive astrocyte (i.e. > 0.6 event/min) was significantly larger (41% in Aβo condition vs 11% in physiological condition; p = 0.012; Fig. 3c). Thus, under application of 100 nM Aβo, there is an increase in the population of hyperactive astrocytes at the expense of basal-active and -inactive astrocytes.

In individual patch-clamped astrocyte, application of Aβo induced a significant increase of the fraction of active territories (75.8 ± 2.5% vs 57.9 ± 4.8% in physiological condition; n = 13 astrocytes; p = 0.0055; Fig. 3f) with no effect on the frequency of Ca^{2+} events within these microdomains (0.54 ± 0.01 vs 0.59 ± 0.02 event/min; n = 1806 ROIs; p = 0.178; Fig. 3g). Both focal and expanded event numbers were increased and the ratio of expanded/focal Ca^{2+} events was not significantly affected by Aβo (41% of expanded events in Aβo condition vs 33% in physiological condition; p = 0.27; Additional file 4a). However, expanded events size significantly increased compared to physiological condition (9.2 ± 0.5 μm^2 vs 7.1 ± 0.4 μm^2; p = 0.045; Additional file 4c).

Application of monomeric forms of $A\beta_{1-42}$ (Aβm) had no effect on either the proportion of active cells or the Ca^{2+} signal properties within cells confirming that only

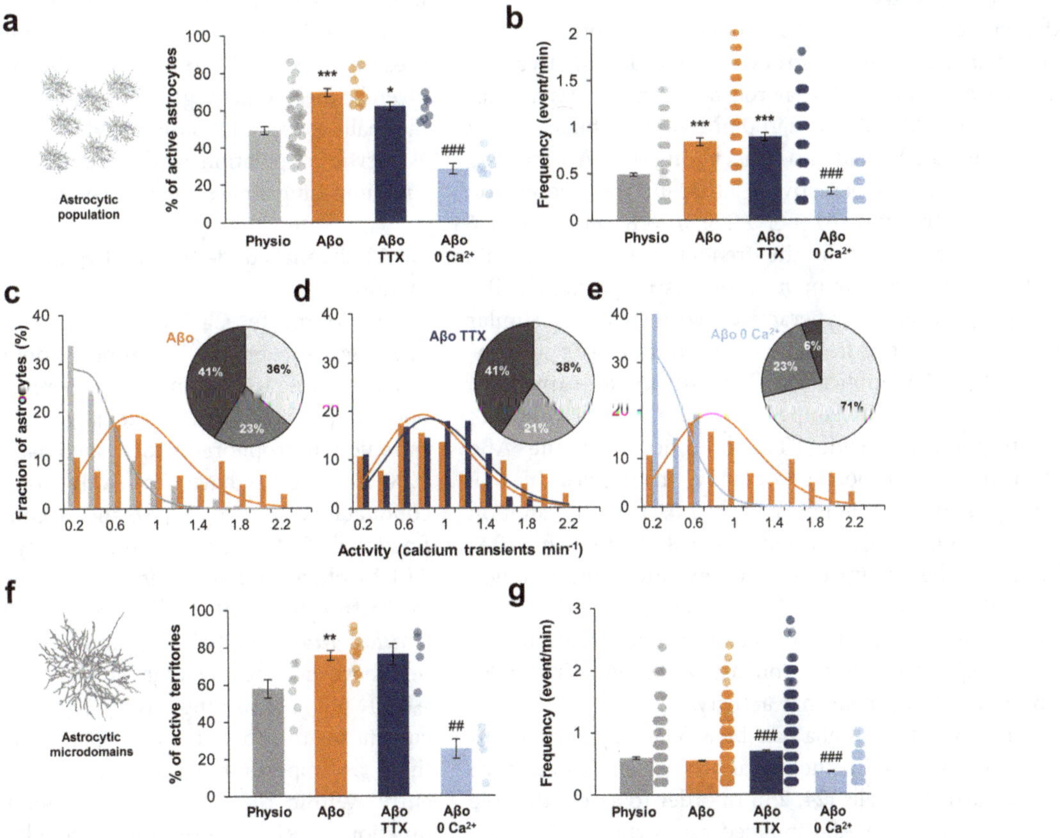

Fig. 3 Extracellular Aβo application induces astrocytes hyperactivity. **a**, **b**. Within the global astrocytic population, proportion of astrocytes displaying calcium activity and frequency of astrocyte calcium activity in physiological condition (*grey*; n = 43), under 100 nM Aβo application (*orange*; n = 12), 100 nM Aβo + 500 nM TTX co-application (*dark blue*; n = 8) and 100 nM Aβo in Ca^{2+}-free medium application (0 Ca^{2+}; *light blue*; n = 8). **c**, **d**, **e**. Frequency histogram revealing that significantly more astrocytes were hyperactive and less were inactive under 100 nM Aβo application or 100 nM Aβo + 500 nM TTX co-application. Aβo-induced hyperactivity is abolished in Ca^{2+}-free medium. Related theorctical Poisson distributions were shown accordingly. **f**, **g**. Within single astrocyte arbor, proportion of subregions displaying calcium activity and frequency of astrocyte calcium activity in physiological condition (*grey*; n = 7), under 100 nM Aβo application (*orange*; n = 13), 100 nM Aβo + 500 nM TTX co-application (*dark blue*; n = 5) and 100 nM Aβo in Ca^{2+}-free medium application (0 Ca^{2+}; *light blue*; n = 5). Results are compared with the physiological condition with *, $p < 0.05$; **, $p < 0.01$ and ***, $p < 0.001$ or the Aβo condition with #, $p < 0.05$; ##, $p < 0.01$ and ###, $p < 0.001$

oligomeric forms of Aβ were responsible for this Ca^{2+} hyperactivity (n = 14 slices from 4 animals; Additional file 1c). Major oligomers present in our samples were low-molecular weight oligomers (2- to 4- mers; Additional file 1a).

Thus, 100 nM Aβo triggered astrocytic calcium hyperactivity within the *stratum radiatum* as soon as 5 min in the global astrocytic population, manifested as an increase of the proportion of active cells along with an increase of the frequency of individual Ca^{2+} events. Interestingly, this global hyperactivity went along with a sustained increase of Ca^{2+} activity within astrocytic processes including an increase of the proportion of active microdomains together with an increase of the expanded events size in the astrocytic processes.

Aβo-induced astrocytic Ca^{2+} hyperactivity is independent of neuronal activity or microglia activation and involves external Ca^{2+} entry

Aβo could potentially affect directly and/or indirectly Ca^{2+} signaling within astrocytes. In order to ascertain the neuronal part in the astrocyte hyperactivity, we co-applied 500 nM TTX with 100 nM Aβo. In bulk loading condition, TTX had no effect on the Aβ-induced astrocytic Ca^{2+} hyperactivity either in the proportion of active astrocytes (61.9 ± 2.2%; n = 8 slices from 6 animals; Fig. 3a) or in the frequency of Ca^{2+} events (0.89 ± 0.04 event/min; n = 145 astrocytes; Fig. 3b). The proportion of hyperactive astrocytes was similar (p = 0.16) and the frequency distribution was not impacted by TTX application (Fig. 3d). In the same way, in individual patch-clamped astrocyte, the blockade of action potentials with TTX did not affect the Aβo effect on the proportion of active territories (n = 5 astrocytes from 4 animals; p = 1.0; Fig. 3f) and on the frequency of Ca^{2+} events (n = 870 ROIs; p = 0.9; Fig. 3g). The enlarged size of expanded events was not reduced with TTX (9.0 ± 0.5 μm^2; p = 0.68; Additional file 4c). These data suggested that, within 5 min, Aβo acts directly on astrocyte signaling independently of any neuronal activity.

Activation of microglia can be a relatively early event in the Aβ mediated pathological process and can in turn activate astroglia cells [24, 25]. In order to assess the role of microglia in the Aβo-induced astrocytic Ca^{2+} hyperactivity, we pretreated slices with minocycline, an inhibitor of microglia activation [24–26]. Minocycline 50 nM pre-incubated during 15 min did not prevent the ability of Aβo to trigger astrocytic Ca^{2+} hyperactivity increasing to the same extent the proportion of active astrocytes (61.0 ± 3.3%; n = 6 slices from 4 animals; p = 0.0043) and the frequency of Ca^{2+} events (0.79 ± 0.08 event/min; n = 69 astrocytes; p = 0.02; Additional file 5a). Thus, within 5 min, Aβo acts directly on astrocyte signaling independently of any microglia activation.

To investigate the external and/or internal origin of Ca^{2+} implicated in the Aβo-induced Ca^{2+} hyperactivity, we applied 100 nM Aβo in Ca^{2+}-free ACSF. Within the astrocytic population, we observed a 60% decrease of the proportion of active astrocytes (28.1 ± 2.7% active astrocytes in Ca^{2+}-free medium versus 69.7 ± 2.1% in ACSF; n = 8 slices from 6 animals; p = 0.0002; Fig. 3a). The Aβo-induced frequency increase of Ca^{2+} events was also strongly reduced in Ca^{2+}-free medium (0.30 ± 0.03 event/min; n = 73 astrocytes; p < 0.0001; Fig. 3b) and the proportion of hyperactive cells strongly declined (6% vs 41%; p < 0.0001; Fig. 3e). Within astrocytic processes, removing external Ca^{2+} avoided 1/3 of compartmentalized Aβo-induced Ca^{2+} hyperactivity (25.2 ± 5.2% of active territories; n = 5 astrocytes from 4 animals; p = 0.0016; Fig. 3f) and strongly reduced the frequency of the remaining signals (0.37 ± 0.01 event/min; n = 870 ROIs; p < 0.0001; Fig. 3g). The enlarged size of expanded events was however not significantly reduced in Ca^{2+}-free medium (7.7 ± 0.7 μm^2; p = 0.7; Additional file 4c). Overall, these data suggested that external Ca^{2+} entry is the main source of Aβo-induced Ca^{2+} hyperactivity in the astrocytic population and in the astrocytic processes, superimposing a new signal encoding.

TRPA1 channels underlie Ca^{2+} hyperactivity induced by Aβo

Within astrocyte, Ca^{2+} entry can occur through astrocytic ligand-gated Ca^{2+} channels (ionotropic receptors), transient receptor potential (TRP) receptors and reverse operation of Na^+/Ca^{2+} exchanger (NCX). Astrocytic cationic ionotropic receptors (such as AMPA, NMDA or P2X receptors) have relatively low single channel conductance (~1 to 3 pS) and accounted for ~4% of fractional Ca^{2+} current [6]. Among TRP receptors, TRPA1 channels have been recently involved in regulating astrocyte basal Ca^{2+} levels in the hippocampus *stratum radiatum* [10, 11]. Interestingly, TRPA1 channels have a relatively high single channel conductance (~110 pS) accounting for ~17% of fractional Ca^{2+} current for the constitutively open channel [27] referring them as important actors involved in astrocytic Ca^{2+} entry. Within the CA1 region of mouse hippocampus, functional TRPA1 were only detected in astrocytes [10]. Based on immunohistochemistry of fixed brain sections, we found that TRPA1 channels staining appeared as discrete punctates predominantly co-localized with astrocytes (GFAP-positive cells; Additional file 6). Higher-resolution images showed that TRPA1 channels were expressed in both cell body and thick processes of *stratum radiatum* astrocytes objectivized by the GFAP co-staining. Some staining also appeared in adjacent territories (Fig. 4a) continuous with GFAP-positive stem processes. An additional 3D–reconstruct movie file shows this in more details (Additional file 7) and suggested that TRPA1 channels were expressed in astrocyte thin processes. These observations agreed with immunogold electron microscopy studies performed in rat trigeminal caudal nucleus showing that TRPA1 channels are localized in astrocyte peripheral processes [28].

In physiological condition, incubation of slices with the selective TRPA1 blocker, HC 030031 (40 μM) [29], during 5 min had no effect on the proportion of spontaneous active astrocytes within the global astrocytic population (56.5 ± 3.5% active astrocytes; n = 7 slices from 3 animals; p = 0.17; Fig. 4b) but increased the frequency of Ca^{2+} events (0.56 ± 0.03 event/min; n = 167 astrocytes; p = 0.043; Fig. 4c). In patch-clamped cells, incubating 5 min slices with 40 μM HC 030031 had no impact on the proportion of active microdomains (62.8 ± 5.7%; n = 7 astrocytes from 4 animals; p = 0.71; Fig. 4e) or on Ca^{2+} signal frequency (0.50 ± 0.01 event/min; n = 919 ROIs; p = 0.19; Fig. 4f). Together, these data confirmed that TRPA1 does not massively

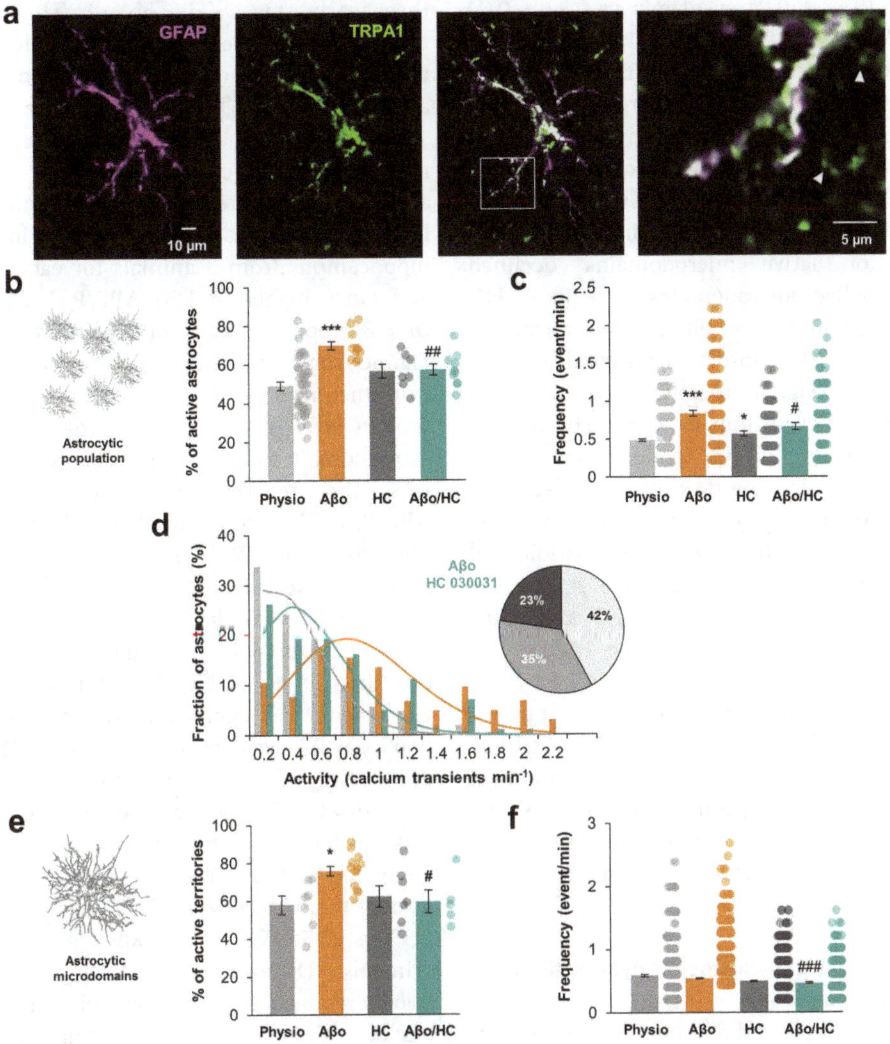

Fig. 4 TRPA1 channels mediate astrocytic hyperactivity. **a** Immunohistochemistry of mouse *stratum radiatum* astrocytes showing that TRPA1 channels expression (*green*) was located in GFAP-positive processes (*magenta*) but also went over in distal processes excluding GFAP staining (e.g. *white arrowheads*). **b**, **c**. Within the astrocytic population, proportion of astrocytes displaying calcium activity and frequency of astrocyte calcium activity in physiological condition (*light grey*; n = 43), under 100 nM Aβo application (*orange*; n = 12), 40 μM HC 030031 application (*dark grey*, n = 7) and 100 nM Aβo + 40 μM HC 030031 co-application (*cyan*; n = 10). **d** Frequency histogram revealing that Aβo-induced hyperactivity is reduced when HC 030031 is co-applied (*cyan*). Related theoretical Poisson distributions were shown accordingly. **e**, **f**. Within single astrocyte arbor, proportion of subregions displaying calcium activity and frequency of astrocyte calcium activity in physiological condition (*light grey*; n = 7), under 100 nM Aβo application (*orange*; n = 13), 40 μM HC 030031 application (*dark grey*; n = 7) and 100 nM Aβo + 40 μM HC 030031 co-application (*cyan*; n = 5). Results are compared with the physiological condition with *, $p < 0.05$; **, $p < 0.01$ and ***, $p < 0.001$ or the Aβo condition with #, $p < 0.05$; ##, $p < 0.01$ and ###, $p < 0.001$

contribute to spontaneous Ca^{2+} signaling in the astrocytic arbor territory of *stratum radiatum* astrocytes [11, 30].

Interestingly, when Aβo was applied in presence of HC 030031 (40 μM), the astrocytic Ca^{2+} hyperactivity was totally abolished and restored to basal levels either in the global astrocytic population or in the processes territory. In bulk loading condition, the proportion of active astrocytes decreased (57.1 ± 2.8% in Aβo + HC 030031 vs 69.7 ± 2.1% in Aβo condition; n = 10 slices from 3 animals; p = 0.0021; Fig. 4b) and was reversed to physiological condition level (49.1 ± 2.2%; p = 0.08). Frequency also decreased when HC 030031 was co-applied with Aβo (0.67 ± 0.04 event/min vs 0.83 ± 0.04 event/min in Aβo condition; n = 181 astrocytes; p = 0.013; Fig. 4c) but remained higher than in physiological condition (0.49 ± 0.01 event/min; p = 0.0002). Frequency distribution tended toward physiological distribution and the proportion of hyperactive astrocytes was reduced (23% in Aβo + HC 030031 vs 41% in Aβo condition; p = 0.023; Fig. 4d). Within individual cells, the proportion of active microdomains declined (59.4 ± 6.0% of active microdomains in Aβo + HC 030031 vs 75.8 ± 2.5% in Aβo condition; n = 5 astrocytes from 4 animals; p = 0.03) close to physiological value (57.9 ± 4.8%; p = 0.87; Fig. 4e) together with the events frequency (0.47 ± 0.09 event/min in Aβo + HC 030031 vs 0.54 ± 0.07 event/min in Aβo condition; n = 760 ROIs; p < 0.0001; Fig. 4f). The ratio of expanded/focal event decreased (30% of expanded event in Aβo + HC 030031 vs 41% in Aβo condition; p = 0.039; Additional file 4a) reaching physiological value (33%; p = 0.45). Expanded surface extension also shrank (7.2 ± 0.5 μm^2 vs 9.2 ± 0.5 μm^2; p = 0.017; Additional file 4c) close to physiological size (7.1 ± 0.4 μm^2).

Thus, while having a negligible impact on physiological spontaneous Ca^{2+} activity, blocking TRPA1 channels cancelled astrocyte Ca^{2+} hyperactivity induced by Aβo leading most of the spatiotemporal Ca^{2+} signal properties back to physiological state in either the astrocytic arbor microdomains or the global astrocytic population.

APP/PS1-21 mice display early astrocytic hyperactivity that involves TRPA1 channels

APP/PS1–21 mice co-express the human KM/67/671NL mutation in the amyloid precursor protein (APPswe) and the human L166P-mutated presenilin 1 (PS1) under the control of Thy1 promotor. These transgenic mice display high transgene expression with $A\beta_{1-42}$ levels being significant at 1 month and plaques appearing at 6 weeks of age in the neocortex and at 4–5 months in the CA1 hippocampus [15]. As external application of Aβo induced an immediate astrocytic hyperactivity in hippocampal healthy brain slices, we wonder about the effect of Aβ in APP/PS1–21 mice at the beginning of its secretion within the brain. Thy1 is known to be expressed from ~P14 in mouse CA1 hippocampus [31] thus $A\beta_{1-42}$ might be produced from this stage. However, while being present at this early stage [15], Aβ were not yet aggregated in plaques in APP/PS1–21 mice at 1-month-old (Fig. 5a) while Aβ plaques were present in the hippocampus at 6-month-old as testified with Thioflavin S labeling [21]. Likewise, astroglial marker such as GFAP showed a similar profile in WT versus APP/PS1–21 mice at 1-month-old confirming the lack of reactive astrogliosis in these early stages (Fig. 5b, d). Thus, studying astrocyte activity at these early stages allowed us to measure the impact of not aggregated Aβ on healthy astrocytes in an AD transgenic mice model.

We first investigated the expression of TRPA1 channels in the hippocampus of young APP/PS1–21 mice and their littermates (WT). We found that the protein level of TRPA1 channels was similar in P19 mice (n = 6 hippocampus from 3 animals for each; p = 0.9; Fig. 5c) and twice higher in P30 APP/PS1–21 than WT mice (n = 8 hippocampus from 4 animals for each; p = 0.02; Fig. 5c) suggesting an early upregulation of this channel from the onset of Aβ secretion. At the same time, GFAP protein level was stable (Fig. 5d) testifying the lack of astrogliosis in these early AD stages.

We then recorded astrocytic Ca^{2+} signals in young APP/PS1–21 mice (from P19 to P28) and compared to their littermates (WT). In bulk loaded slices, the proportion of active astrocytes within *stratum radiatum* was similar in both condition (45.4 ± 4.1% in APP/PS1–21 vs 47.1 ± 4.9% in WT; n = 8 slices from 5 animals in each condition; p = 0.8; Fig. 6a). However, the frequency of Ca^{2+} events was significantly higher in APP/PS1–21 cells (0.65 ± 0.07 event/min in APP/PS1–21 vs 0.33 ± 0.03 event/min in WT; n = 103 and 105 astrocytes respectively; p = 0.0013; Fig. 6a) and the frequency distribution was switched to higher frequency in APP/PS1–21 compared to WT mice (λ = 2.1 vs 1.21 in WT; Fig. 6b) leading to an increase of the fraction of hyperactive cells (21% vs 6% in WT; p = 0.0009; Fig. 6b).

In this AD mouse model, no signs of neuroinflammation were apparent in 1-month-old mice and microgliosis has been described to be concomitant with plaques appearance [15]. Indeed, at these early stages, microglia phenotype was not different in APP/PS1–21 mice from WT littermate (Iba-1 immunostaining; Additional file 5b). However, to confirm that microglia was not involved in these early astrocytic events, we pretreated slices with minocycline in order to inhibit potential microglia activation [24–26]. Minocycline 50 nM, pre-incubated during 15 min, had no effect on either the proportion of active cells or the frequency of astrocytic Ca^{2+} events within

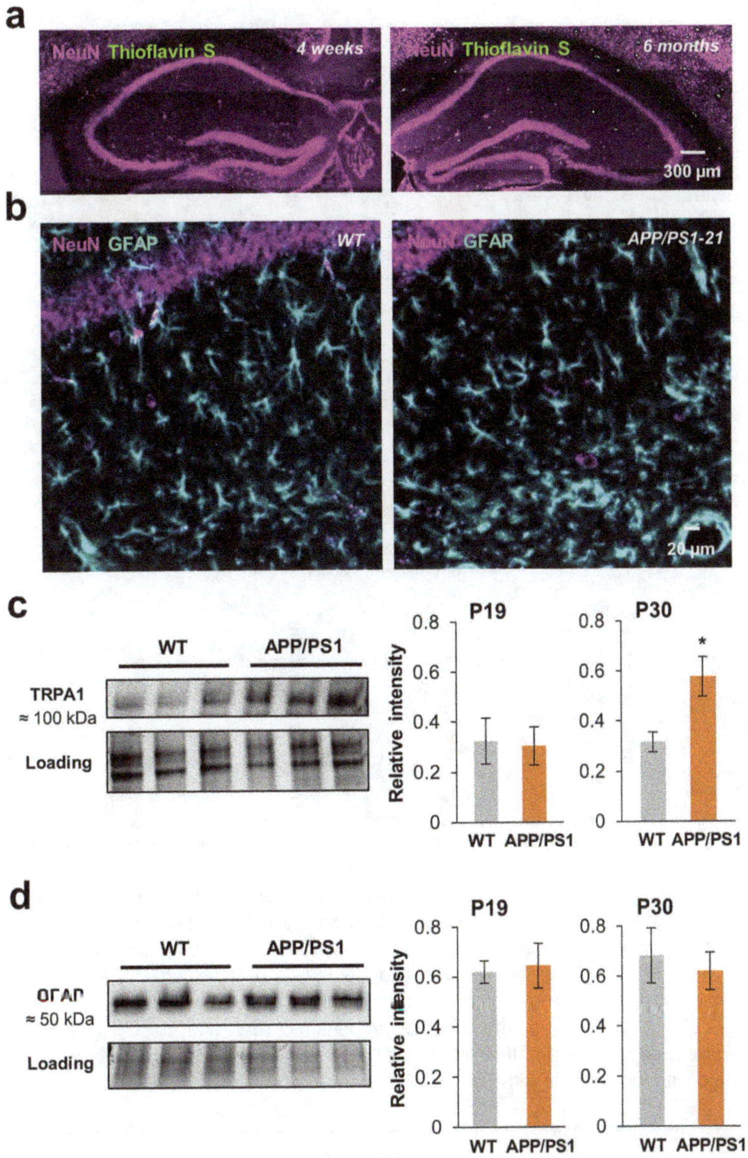

Fig. 5 Young APP/PS1–21 mice are devoid of amyloid deposit and reactive astrocyte whereas gradually overexpress TRPA1. **a** Thioflavin S staining for β-amyloid deposits (*green*) and NeuN immunostaining (*magenta*) in the hippocampus of 1-month-old (*left*) and 6-month-old (*right*) APP/PS1–21 mice showing the progression of the number of amyloid deposits. **b** GFAP (*cyan*) and NeuN (*magenta*) immunostainings in the *stratum radiatum* of a P30 WT (*left*) and APP/PS1–21 (*right*) mice. **c** Western-blot analysis of protein levels of TRPA1 channels in hippocampus extracts from P19 and P30 WT and APP/PS1–21 mice (3 different extracts of P30 WT and APP/PS1–21 mice are shown). Histogram showing quantification of TRPA1 channels expression normalized to protein loading levels ($n = 6$ hippocampus in each group at P19 and 8 hippocampus in each group at P30). **d** Western-blot analysis of protein levels of GFAP in hippocampus extracts from P19 and P30 WT and APP/PS1–21 mice (extracts of same P30 lysates depicted in c are shown). Histogram showing quantification of GFAP expression normalized to protein loading levels ($n = 7$ hippocampus in each group at P19 and P30). Results are compared with the WT mice with *, $p < 0.05$; **, $p < 0.01$ and ***, $p < 0.001$

APP/PS1–21 mice ($n = 6$ slices from 4 animals; $p = 0.88$ and 0.82 respectively; Additional file 5c) testifying that microglia activation was not involved in the astrocytic hyperactivity setting up at the beginning of Aβ secretion in this AD mouse model. In patch-clamp loaded astrocyte, the proportion of active microdomains increased in APP/PS1–21 mice (65.7 ± 2.0% vs 55.0 ± 4.8% in WT; $n = 4$ astrocytes from 4 animals for each; $p = 0.052$; Fig. 6c) together with the frequency of events within these microdomains (0.45 ± 0.02 event/min vs 0.40 ± 0.01 event/min in WT; $n = 255$ and 426 ROIs respectively; $p = 0.04$; Fig. 6c). The proportion of expanded/focal events was slightly affected in APP/PS1–21 mice in favor of expanded event and the size of expanded events was similar (6.8 ± 0.3 μm^2 in WT vs 6.7 ± 0.3 μm^2 in APP/PS1–21; $p = 0.42$; Additional

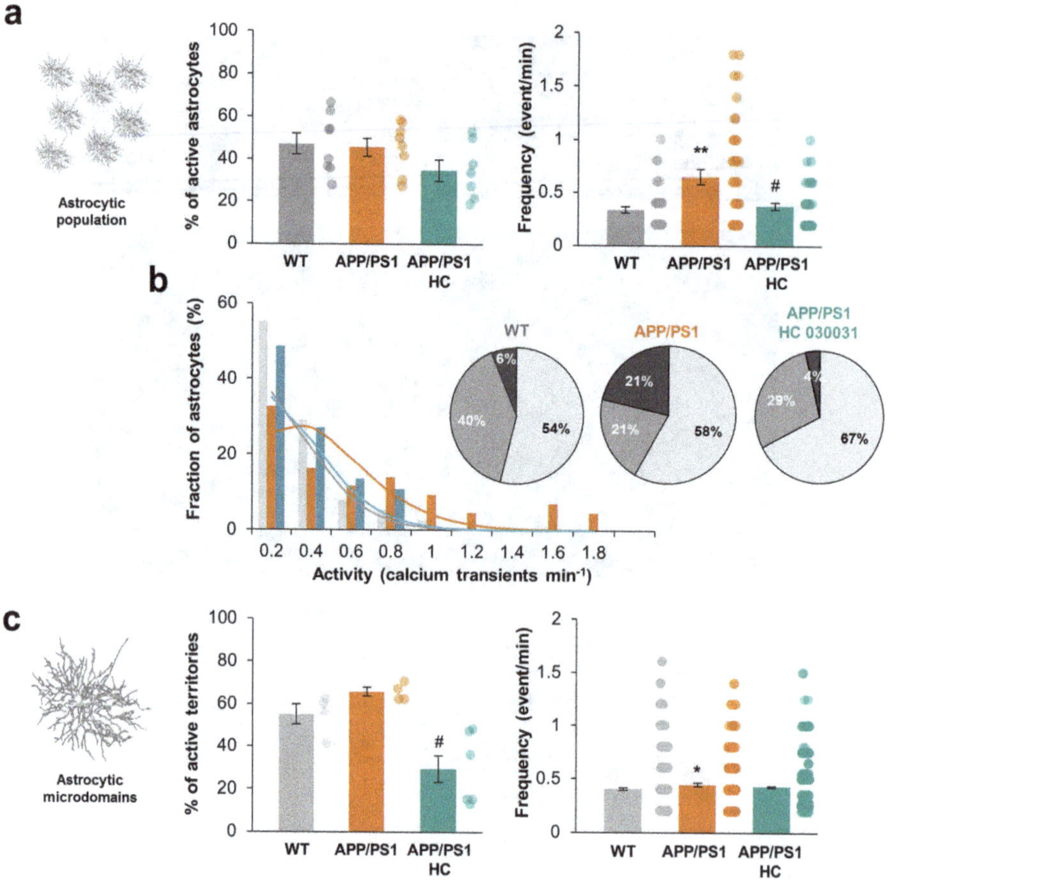

Fig. 6 Young APP/PS1–21 mice display an early global and compartmentalized astrocytic hyperactivity. **a** Within the global astrocytic population, proportion of astrocytes displaying calcium activity and frequency of calcium activity in APP/PS1–21 mice (*orange*; $n = 8$) and their littermates (WT, *grey*; $n = 8$) in physiological condition or with 40 μM HC 030031 (*cyan*, $n = 7$). **b** Frequency histogram showing the occurrence of Ca^{2+} events in the astrocyte population of APP/PS1–21 (*orange*), WT (*grey*) and APP/PS1–21 mice treated with 40 μM HC 030031 (*cyan*). Related theoretical Poisson distributions were shown accordingly. Pie chart representing inactive, active and hyperactive astrocytes in WT and APP/PS1–21 mice treated or not with HC 030031. **c** Within single astrocyte arbor, proportion of subregions displaying calcium activity and frequency of calcium activity in APP/PS1–21 mice (*orange*; $n = 4$) and their littermates (WT, *grey*; $n = 4$) in physiological condition or with 40 μM HC 030031 (*cyan*, $n = 7$). Results are compared with the WT mice with *, $p < 0.05$; **, $p < 0.01$ and ***, $p < 0.001$ or the APP/PS1–21 mice with #, $p < 0.05$; ##, $p < 0.01$ and ###, $p < 0.001$

file 4b, d). Thus, in young APP/PS1–21 mice, Ca^{2+} activity in the global astrocytic population and the compartmentalized activity within the astrocytic arbor started to be affected from the beginning of Aβ overproduction.

In these conditions, blocking TRPA1 channels with HC 030031 (40 μM) in APP/PS1–21 mice strongly decreased the frequency of Ca^{2+} events (0.37 ± 0.03 event/min with HC 030031 vs 0.64 ± 0.07; $n = 113$ astrocytes from 7 slices; $p = 0.013$; Fig. 6a) resulting in a clear redistribution of Ca^{2+} events frequency ($\lambda = 1.35$) and a decrease of the proportion of hyperactive cells that look alike the WT situation (4% in APP/PS1–21 + HC 030031 vs 21% in APP/PS1–21; $p = 0.0025$; Fig. 6b). In patch-clamp loaded astrocyte, HC 030031 induced a significant decrease of the proportion of active microdomains in APP/PS1–21 mice (29.3 ± 6.2%; $n = 7$ from 4 animals; $p = 0.01$; Fig. 6c) together with a restrained effect on the frequency (0.43 ± 0.06 event/min; $n = 1213$ and 1577 ROIs respectively; $p = 0.058$). The proportion of expanded/focal events was also reduced with HC 030031 treatment (Additional file 4b). Overall, these observations in young APP/PS1–21 mice matched the above related effect of Aβo application in healthy slices consistently with a TRPA1 channel involvement. Merely, they were more subtle and initially restrained to the astrocytic arbor.

Aβo-induced CA1 neurons hyperactivity is related to TRPA1 channels activation

Astrocytes are known to actively regulate synaptic activity and plasticity [4]. Given the time range of the Aβ-mediated impact on astrocyte excitability, we wonder about its consequences on basal synaptic activity. Thus, to explore the outcome of Aβo induced TRPA1-dependent astrocyte hyperexcitability on neighboring synapses, we recorded CA1 pyramidal neurons spontaneous excitatory post-synaptic currents (sEPSCs) performing whole-cell patch-clamp recordings on CA1 neurons cell bodies (Fig. 7a). The initial mean frequency of sEPSCs recorded from CA1 pyramidal neurons was 0.13 ± 0.03 Hz (n = 22 neurons from 17 animals) and was stable during a 30-min recording (Fig. 7b). The mean peak amplitude of sEPSCs recorded from CA1 pyramidal neurons was 31.1 ± 2.0 pA. Interestingly, application of 40 μM HC 030031 alone had no effect on sEPSCs frequency (74 ± 22% from 5 to 10 min; n = 5 cells from 3 animals; p = 0.6; Fig. 7b, c) suggesting that TRPA1 channels were not involved in physiological sEPSCs modulation. Application of 100 nM Aβo in the extracellular medium induced a rapid, strong and persistent increase of sEPSCs frequency (Fig. 7b; n = 7 cells from 6 animals) with no effect on the sEPSCs amplitude (32.4 ± 2.5 pA; p = 0.3). We confirmed that application of monomeric forms of $A\beta_{1-42}$ (Aβm) had no effect on sEPSCs frequency during the 30-min recording (n = 5; p = 0.78; Additional file 1d) settling that only oligomeric forms of $A\beta_{1-42}$ were active. Interestingly, the strong

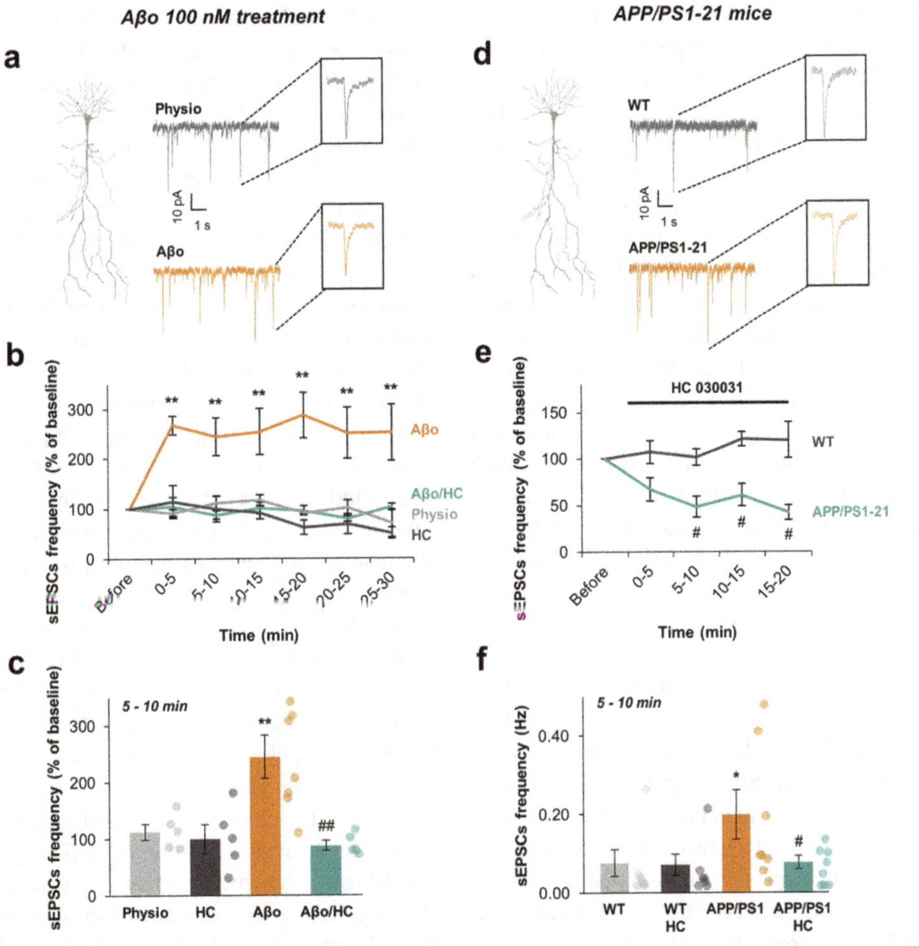

Fig. 7 Aβo increases the frequency of spontaneous excitatory post-synaptic currents (sEPSCs) from CA1 pyramidal neurons in a TRPA1 channels dependent manner. **a** Representative traces of voltage-clamp recordings from CA1 pyramidal cells held at −65 mV in physiological condition (*grey*) and under Aβo 100 nM application (*orange*). Examples of single EPSC with higher time resolution are shown in the corresponding insets. **b** Time course of the frequency of sEPSCs in physiological condition (*light grey*; n = 5), under application of 100 nM Aβo (*orange*; n = 7), 40 μM HC 030031 (*dark grey*; n = 5) or co-application of 100 nM Aβo + 40 μM HC 030031 (*cyan*; n = 4). **c** Histogram showing the sEPSCs frequency at a time matching the astrocyte calcium activity measurements (i.e. 5 to 10 min after drugs application). Results are compared with the physiological condition with *, $p < 0.05$; **, $p < 0.01$ and ***, $p < 0.001$ or the Aβo condition with #, $p < 0.05$; ##, $p < 0.01$ and ###, $p < 0.001$. **d** Representative traces of voltage-clamp recordings from CA1 pyramidal cells held at −65 mV in APP/PS1–21 mice (*orange*) and their WT littermates (*grey*). Examples of single EPSC with higher time resolution are shown in the corresponding insets. **e** Time course of the normalized frequency of sEPSCs in WT (*dark grey*; n = 7) and APP/PS1–21 mice (*cyan*; n = 8) under application of 40 μM HC 030031. **f** Histogram showing the sEPSCs frequency in basal condition in WT (*light grey*; n = 7), APP/PS1–21 mice (*orange*; n = 8) and 5 to 10 min after HC 030031 application (*dark grey* and *cyan* respectively). Results are compared to the WT basal activity with *, $p < 0.05$; **, $p < 0.01$ and ***, $p < 0.001$ or the APP/PS1–21 basal activity with #, $p < 0.05$; ##, $p < 0.01$ and ###, $p < 0.001$

and persistent increase of sEPSCs frequency induced by Aβo was time-concomitant with the setting up of astrocyte hyperexcitability (i.e. 5 to 10 min, 245 ± 38%; $p = 0.01$; Fig. 7c) and was fully abolished by a co-application of HC 030031 (40 μM) with Aβo (88 ± 8% from 5 to 10 min; $n = 5$ cells from 5 animals; $p = 0.005$; Fig. 7b, c). This suggests that TRPA1 channels-dependent astrocyte hyperactivity induced by Aβo directly influenced CA1 neurons activity and its blockade was enough to counteract the neuronal hyperactivity, at least in the short and medium term.

We then recorded spontaneous EPSCs in APP/PS1–21 mice at the onset of Aβ overproduction (P20-P28) and compared to their littermates (WT). We observed an increase of CA1 neurons sEPSCs frequency setting up at P20 in APP/PS1–21 mice (0.20 ± 0.06 Hz in APP/PS1–21 vs 0.08 ± 0.03 Hz in WT; $n = 8$ neurons from 6 animals in APP/PS1–21 and 7 neurons from 5 animals in WT; $p = 0.0271$; Fig. 7d, f) with no difference in their amplitude (33.7 ± 1.9 pA in APP/PS1–21 vs 33.0 ± 2.3 pA in WT; $p = 0.955$). These data confirmed that neuronal hyperexcitability is one of the earliest dysfunction in the pathophysiological cascade initiated by abnormal Aβ accumulation [32]. Application of HC 030031 (40 μM) strongly reduced sEPSCs frequency in APP/PS1–21 mice as soon as 5 min after its bath perfusion (0.08 ± 0.02 Hz; $n = 8$ neurons from 6 animals; $p = 0.0234$) while it had no effect on WT mice (0.07 ± 0.03 Hz; $n = 7$ neurons form 5 animals; $p = 0.854$; Fig. 7e, f). These data corroborate the highlighted precocious involvement of TRPA1 channel in AD pathogenesis.

Discussion

In this study, we investigated the contribution of astrocytes in early Aβo toxicity by studying calcium signaling in different parts of the whole astrocyte territory. We found that astroglia is a frontline target of Aβo exhibiting a global and local Ca^{2+} hyperactivity that involves TRPA1 channels. This TRPA1 channel-dependent astrocytic Ca^{2+} hyperactivity exerts regulatory influences on synaptic function and is linked to the glutamatergic synapse hyperactivity recorded in CA1 neurons. Concurrently to these acute Aβo-induced effects, astrocytes in young APP/PS1–21 mice hippocampus elicit a similar pattern of calcium hyperactivity in close relationship with the setting up of a precocious neuronal hyperactivity that are both reversed when TRPA1 channel is blocked. Moreover, the TRPA1 channel is gradually overexpressed at the onset of Aβ production in this AD mouse model.

Intracellular Ca^{2+} transients are considered as the primary signal by which astrocytes interact with each other and with neighboring neurons. Ca^{2+} has been extensively studied within the astrocytic cell body and thick branches. More recently, local Ca^{2+} dynamics in distal fine processes has been investigated emphasizing a highly compartmentalized signaling, interconnected with physiological transmission at neighboring synapses [8, 9]. Compartmentalization of astrocytic Ca^{2+} dynamics needs to be attentively considered in order to understand how astrocytes may contribute to brain information processing [8]. We thus chose to study both levels of information (i.e. global population signaling and local microdomain signaling) combining bulk loading and single cell astrocyte loading. Genetically encoded Ca^{2+} indicators (GECIs) have been recently used to study Ca^{2+} signals in distal thin processes [9]. Alternatively, patch pipette loading give access to the whole territory of a single astrocyte and, currently, Fluo-4 is far more sensitive than GECIs therefore enabling to track smaller signals [8]. Accordingly, we observed a similar and even better diffusion of Fluo-4 in a single astrocyte compared to SR101. We first characterized the physiological calcium activity of mouse CA1 *stratum radiatum* astrocytes and showed that this activity is fully autonomous, i.e. independent of neuronal activity, both at the astrocytic population level and at the microdomain level. This is in agreement with data obtained in mouse CA1 hippocampus [30, 33] but not with astrocyte behavior in the dentate gyrus where expanded Ca^{2+} events were partly dependent on neuronal activity [8]. Interestingly, external Ca^{2+} entry is the main source of Ca^{2+} within thin processes whereas it only partly contributes to somatic signaling. This discrepancy between Ca^{2+} sources in astrocyte soma and distal processes has already been described in brain slices [34]. This might be supported by the subcellular location of calcium stores that are concentrated in the cell body and thick processes but are almost absent from thin processes [23].

A central element of the pathogenesis of AD is the progressive accumulation of Aβo species, ultimately resulting in the formation of plaques. Yet, small soluble Aβ oligomers are sufficient to induce several features of the AD phenotype [1]. The paths by which Aβo leads to neurodegeneration are probably multifactorial but all converge all towards synaptic dysfunction. The major challenge of AD research is to understand the complex cellular reaction underlying the long prodromal phase of AD [14]. Astrocytes are an integral part of synaptic transmission and are therefore critical for the establishment and maintenance of neuronal health [5]. They contribute to neuronal dysfunction by being proinflammatory [35] but also play a protective role, e.g. through the release of gliotransmitters [36] and Aβ clearance [37, 38]. It is therefore of major importance to distinguish the beneficial from the deleterious impact of Aβo on astrocyte function. Aβo has already been involved as a direct effector on astrocytes in primary cultures [39], in hippocampal slices [40] and in vivo [12] but here we showed a peculiar rapid action on compartmentalized calcium activity, activating a membrane Ca^{2+} permeable channel. Indeed, Aβo application triggers global Ca^{2+} hyperactivity in CA1 hippocampus astroglial population together with an intensification of the compartmentalized Ca^{2+} activity in the astrocytic processes and a spatial extension of the size of the expanded Ca^{2+} events within microdomains. These effects are specific to oligomeric forms of Aβ since application of the monomeric form in the same conditions had no impact on astrocytic calcium activity. We reported that the effect of Aβo on astrocyte excitability is fully independent of neuronal activity since TTX application does not prevent the Aβo effect neither on the global hyperactivity nor on the compartmentalized hyperactivity in processes. Concurrently, microglia activation does not participate in this astrocytic hyperactivity, at least in the time scale studied, whereas longer applications of Aβ activate microglia together with astroglia [24]. Thus, astrocytes seem to express a distinctive precocious detector involved at the onset of Aβo appearance. Removal of external Ca^{2+} largely inhibits Aβo-induced astrocyte hyperactivity at the population level while it has no effect in physiological conditions. Removal of external Ca^{2+} also inhibits the majority of the compartmentalized Aβo-induced hyperactivity. Thus, transmembrane Ca^{2+} entry carries most of the Aβo-induced hyperactivity. Remarkably, we showed that both global and compartmentalized hyperactivities are driven by TRPA1-dependent Ca^{2+} entry since HC 030031, a specific TRPA1 channel inhibitor [29], strongly abolishes Aβo-induced astrocyte hyperexcitability and totally restores the spatiotemporal properties of Ca^{2+} events back to a physiological level.

The TRPA1 channel is a Ca^{2+} permeable non-selective cation channel initially known to be expressed in primary afferent nociceptive neurons [29]. In mouse CA1 hippocampus, TRPA1 channels are found to be preferentially expressed in astrocytes [10]. However, their involvement in physiological astrocytic Ca^{2+} signaling is highly debated. It has been shown that TRPA1 channels contribute to maintain basal Ca^{2+} levels and regulate ~20% of spontaneous Ca^{2+} signals within astrocyte branches [11] but in the end, poorly take part in basal astrocytic Ca^{2+} signaling [30, 33]. Our data assume that TRPA1 channels are only slightly involved in the astrocytic Ca^{2+} signaling in physiological conditions. However, we highlighted they are quickly and largely involved in case of Aβo presence. The absence of an obvious involvement of these channels in astrocyte physiological Ca^{2+} signaling is startling since we evidenced a TRPA1 channel expression in thick and in adjacent thin astrocytic processes. Thus, TRPA1 channels might only behave as an "aggression sensor". Indeed, TRPA1channel gating is particularly regulated by numerous electrophilic activators - such as reactive oxygen species, reactive nitrogen species or oxidized lipids - and also functions as a mechanosensor [27]. Hence, TRPA1 channels might be directly targeted by Aβo or might be secondarily activated through an Aβo-induced oxidative stress and/or through its mechanosensor properties if Aβo binds to the astrocytic cholesterol-rich plasma membrane [14].

Strikingly, in young APP/PS1–21 mice (~3–4 weeks), we observed a similar pattern of astrocytic hyperactivity starting at the beginning of Aβ overproduction in the hippocampus, long before its aggregation into plaques. These early repercussions in young APP/PS1–21 mice were restricted to the frequency of astrocytic Ca^{2+} events in either the astrocytic population and microdomains of astrocytic processes with fewer impacts on the proportion of active cells or microdomains. This suggests a gradual impact of surrounding Aβ on astrocyte signaling, increasing the frequency of compartmentalized Ca^{2+} events and, to a lesser extent, the proportion of active territories within the astrocytic processes. These impacts on astrocytic processes go along with a noteworthy redistribution of the frequency of Ca^{2+} events within the astrocytic population. Interestingly, blockade of TRPA1 channels with HC 030031 abolished the astrocyte Ca^{2+} hyperactivity. Overall, TRPA1 channel signaling seems to be at the frontline in mediating these Aβo progressive effects in early stages of AD. Data obtained in an advanced AD transgenic model showed an astrocyte network hyperactivity in cortical areas close to Aβ plaques and an involvement of metabotropic purinergic signaling in this astrocyte hyperactivity [13]. This suggests a differential evolution of astrocyte engagement in AD pathogenesis depending on the stage, the structure and the physiopathological state of the astrocyte. Likewise, it has been reported that the TRPA1 channels' protein level was increased in hippocampal astrocytes of 8 month-old APP/PS1 mice at where it mediated inflammation through astrocyte activation [41]. Here, we showed that TRPA1 channel expression in hippocampus is increased much earlier, as soon as 1 month of age, in a more aggressive AD mouse model (APP/PS1–21). These data point towards a TRPA1 channel contribution in early stages of pathophysiology, that is as soon as the Aβo level increases and long before the setting up of astrogliosis or inflammatory mechanisms.

Numerous laboratory studies in the past decade have shown that Aβo impairs synaptic function and synaptic structure [42]. However, how soluble Aβo initiates these effects remains to be determined. Each astrocyte deploys many fine processes to contact up to 140,000 synapses in the CA1 region [43]. As we highlighted an intense and early effect of Aβo on astrocyte Ca^{2+} activity within processes, we assessed the link with spontaneous neuronal activity. Indeed Aβo is also known to enhance spontaneous neuronal excitability in CA1 [32, 44, 45]. Consistently, we showed here that Aβo induces a rapid and strong increase of spontaneous EPSCs frequency in CA1 neurons. Strikingly, blocking TRPA1 channels totally prevents this Aβo neuronal impact. Yet, when we blocked neuronal activity with TTX, we did not affect the Aβo-induced astrocyte hyperactivity which would be partly the case if a neuronal TRPA1 was involved. This precocious Aβo impact thus seems to trigger a one-way communication from astrocyte to neuron related to TRPA1 activation. This TRPA1-dependent neuronal hyperactivity was similarly observed in APP/PS1−21 mice at the onset of Aβ overproduction testifying its physiopathological relevance in the AD initiation process. It has been shown that Aβ can increase astrocytic release of glutamate to the extrasynaptic space resulting in the activation of extrasynaptic NMDARs and the disruption of neuronal signaling [40, 46, 47]. Besides, astrocytes can regulate synaptic and extrasynaptic neurotransmitter concentrations, such as glutamate, in a Ca^{2+}-dependent manner e.g. via vesicular release, bidirectional transport or hemichannel opening [48]. We will further decipher pathways implemented by the Aβ-induced TRPA1-mediated Ca^{2+} entry that consequently affect neuronal transmission.

It has been demonstrated that soluble Aβo can affect astrocyte signaling properties in various ways in mouse hippocampal CA1 astrocytes [40, 49, 50]. To some extent, the involvement of TRPA1 channels superimposed to these effects, directly affecting local synaptic function in a distinctive precocious manner. This actor might thus contribute to the complex cellular phase of AD, upstream of symptomatic neurodegeneration [14].

Conclusions

In this work, we have shown that intricate global and compartmentalized astroglial Ca^{2+} signaling disturbances induced by Aβo are mediated by a TRPA1 channel-dependent Ca^{2+} signaling. This new highlighted mechanism is at work with both external supply of Aβo and at the onset of Aβ production in an AD transgenic mouse model. This astrocytic pathway is promptly implemented and involved in the well-known and characteristic Aβo-induced synaptic dysfunction. Blockade of TRPA1 channel, that appears to be preferentially expressed in astrocytes within the hippocampus [11], is sufficient to counteract the impact of Aβo on spontaneous neuronal activity. This suggests that astrocytes can be considered as a particularly precocious target in Aβo toxicity consequently affecting nearby synapses. Up until now, altered astrocyte activation was usually associated with late AD, i.e. when amyloid plaques are already developed, and the role of astrocytes in the initial toxic effect of Aβo was not yet evidenced. One of the major findings of our study is to suggest that astrocytes are implicated far before astrogliosis and inflammatory processes. Thus, focusing on this astrocyte involvement, for instance by modulating TRPA1 channel activity, may represent a novel target to hamper early dysfunction in AD.

Additional files

Additional file 1: Characterization and effects of Aβ oligomers and purified monomers. (**a**) SDS-PAGE analysis of Aβ oligomers examined by western-blot with 4G8 antibody. Aβo showed faintly monomers and abundant dimers and trimers. (**b**) SDS-PAGE analysis of Aβ monomers after purification on C18 column. All fractions were electrophoresed on 15% tris-glycine gel. Aβ monomer is mainly eluted at 30% acetonitrile. S, sample loaded; FT, flow through; peptides eluted at 30, 40, 50 and 60% acetonitrile. (**c**) Within the astrocytic population, proportion of astrocytes displaying calcium activity and frequency of astrocyte calcium activity in physiological condition (grey; $n = 43$), under 100 nM Aβo application (orange; $n = 12$) and under 100 nM Aβm application (light orange; $n = 7$). (**d**) Time course and histogram at 5–10 min of the frequency of sEPSCs in physiological condition (grey; $n = 5$), under application of 100 nM Aβo (orange; $n = 7$) or 100 nM Aβm (light orange; $n = 5$). In any case, Aβm was obtained from the 30% acetonitrile fraction purified in b. (TIFF 291 kb)

Additional file 2: Characterization of Fluo-4-loaded cells in the *stratum radiatum* of mouse coronal slice. (**a**) Confocal image of Fluo-4-loaded (cyan) and SR101-labeled (magenta) cells in the CA1 *stratum radiatum*. Merged image showing the proportion of loaded astrocytes (white), confirming that most of the loaded cells are astrocytes. One hour before slicing, animals were iv injected with SR101 as described previously [51]. Vessels are only labeled with SR101 (white arrow). (**b**) Z-stack projections of confocal images of a patched astrocyte loaded with Fluo-4 (cyan) and SR101 (magenta). Merged image showing the Fluo-4 diffusion in the whole astrocytic territory. (**c**) Example of a passive whole-cell current recorded in a *stratum radiatum* astrocyte. Cell was held at −70 mV and 10 mV hyper- and depolarizing voltage steps of 80 ms duration were applied (−110 to +80 mV). (TIFF 1907 kb)

Additional file 3: Expanded and focal Ca^{2+} events in astrocytic processes. Time-lapse imaging of calcium activity in Fluo-4 loaded astrocytic processes in a 5-min recording. Focal and expanded events were pseudo-colored in blue and red respectively (left panel). Raw data were shown in the right panel. (MP4 10286 kb)

Additional file 4: Spatial properties of compartmentalized calcium events in the astrocytic processes. (**a**) Proportion of expanded/focal events in physiological condition, under 100 nM Aβo application, 100 nM Aβo + 500 nM TTX co-application and 100 nM Aβo + 40 μM HC 030031 co-application. (**b**) Proportion of expanded/focal events in APP/PS1−21 mice and their littermates (WT) in physiological condition or under 40 μM HC 030031 treatment. (**c**) Mean size of expanded Ca^{2+} events in physiological condition (grey), under 100 nM Aβo application (orange), 100 nM Aβo + 500 nM TTX co-application (dark blue), 40 μM HC 030031 (dark grey), 100 nM Aβo in Ca^{2+}-free medium application (0 Ca; light blue) and 100 nM Aβo + 40 μM HC 030031 co-application (cyan). (**d**) Mean size of expanded Ca^{2+} events in APP/PS1−21 mice (orange) and their littermates (WT, light grey) in physiological condition or with 40 μM HC 030031 treatment (WT, dark grey and APP/PS1−21, cyan). Results are compared with the physiological condition with *, $p < 0.05$; **, $p < 0.01$ and ***, $p < 0.001$ or the Aβo condition with #, $p < 0.05$; ##, $p < 0.01$ and ###, $p < 0.001$. (TIFF 752 kb)

Additional file 5: Blockade of microglia activation with minocycline does not prevent the effect of Aβo on astrocyte Ca^{2+} activity. (**a**) Within the astrocytic population, proportion of astrocytes displaying calcium activity and frequency of astrocyte calcium activity in physiological condition (grey; $n = 43$), under 50 nM minocycline (dark grey; $n = 5$); 100 nM Aβo application (orange; $n = 12$) and under 50 nM minocycline +100 nM Aβo application (dark orange; $n = 6$). (**b**) Immunohistochemistry of mouse *stratum radiatum* microglia showing that Iba1-positive cells were not hypertrophic in one-month-old APP/PS1–21 mice when compared to WT littermates. Higher magnification of representative microglia is shown in the lower panels. (**c**) Proportion of astrocytes displaying calcium activity and frequency of astrocyte calcium activity in APP/PS1–21 mice (orange; $n = 8$), under 50 nM minocycline application (dark orange; $n = 6$) or in WT littermates (grey; $n = 8$). Minocycline is pre-incubated 15 min before recording. Results are compared with the physiological condition, with or without minocycline, or with the WT littermates with *, $p < 0.05$; **, $p < 0.01$ and ***, $p < 0.001$. (TIFF 1680 kb)

Additional file 6: TRPA1 is expressed in *stratum radiatum* astrocyte cell body and processes. (**a**) Immunohistochemistry of mouse *stratum radiatum* astrocytes showing that TRPA1 channels (green) are expressed within astrocytic domains certified by GFAP staining (magenta). (**b**) Merge image showing that most TRPA1 staining co-localized and surrounded GFAP-positive processes. (TIFF 2786 kb)

Additional file 7: TRPA1 channels expression is located in thick GFAP-positive processes and in adjacent thin processes lacking GFAP staining. 3D–recontsruct of astrocytic processes objectivized by GFAP staining (magenta) showing that TRPA1 channels (green) expression went over in contiguous processes excluding GFAP staining. Scale bar: 50 nm. (MP4 25.2 mb)

Abbreviations

AD: Alzheimer's disease; APP: Amyloid Precursor Protein; Aβ: Amyloid-β peptide; Aβm: Amyloid-β monomers; Aβo: Amyloid-β oligomers; Ca^{2+}: calcium; CA1: Cornu Ammonis 1; GFAP: Glial Fibrillary Acidic Protein; PS1: Presenilin 1; ROI: Regions Of Interest; sEPSC: spontaneous Excitatory PostSynaptic Current; TRPA1: Transient Receptor Potential A1 channel; TTX: tetrodotoxin

Acknowledgements

We gratefully acknowledge Fabien Mehr and Flore Rimet for their technical assistance in animal perfusion, Rebecca Powell for correcting the english, Yasmina Saoudi for her technical assistance in Airyscan image acquisition on PIC-GIN platform of Grenoble Institut des Neurosciences, Dr. Jean Claude Platel and Dr. Elodie Fino for stimulating scientific discussions.

Funding

This work was supported by INSERM and University Grenoble Alpes.

Authors' contributions

ABo performed the calcium imaging experiments. AP carried out the electrophysiological experiments and contributed to some calcium imaging experiments. SB performed the immunoblotting and immunohistochemistry experiments. MJ-S carried out purification of Aβ monomeric forms. ABo, ABu and MA designed the experiments. ABo, AP, SB and MA analyzed the data. ABo and MA wrote the manuscript. All authors discussed the results and commented on the manuscript at all stages. All authors read and approved the final manuscript.

Author's information

Not applicable.

Competing interests

The authors declare that they have no competing interests.

References

1. Haass C, Selkoe DJ. Soluble protein oligomers in neurodegeneration: lessons from the Alzheimer's amyloid beta-peptide. Nat Rev Mol Cell Biol. 2007;8:101–12.
2. Verkhratsky A, Steinhauser C. Ion channels in glial cells. Brain Res Brain Res Rev. 2000;32:380–412.
3. Panatier A, Theodosis DT, Mothet JP, Touquet B, Pollegioni L, Poulain DA, et al. Glia-derived D-serine controls NMDA receptor activity and synaptic memory. Cell. 2006;125:775–84.
4. Haydon PG. GLIA: listening and talking to the synapse. Nat Rev Neurosci. 2001;2:185–93.
5. Araque A, Parpura V, Sanzgiri RP, Haydon PG. Tripartite synapses: glia, the unacknowledged partner. Trends Neurosci. 1999;22:208–15.
6. Verkhratsky A, Reyes RC, Parpura V. TRP channels coordinate ion signalling in astroglia. Rev Physiol Biochem Pharmacol. 2014;166:1–22.
7. Haustein MD, Kracun S, Lu X-H, Shih T, Jackson-Weaver O, Tong X, et al. Conditions and constraints for astrocyte calcium signaling in the hippocampal mossy fiber pathway. Neuron. 2014;82:413–29.
8. Di Castro MA, Chuquet J, Liaudet N, Bhaukaurally K, Santello M, Bouvier D, et al. Local Ca2+ detection and modulation of synaptic release by astrocytes. Nat Neurosci. 2011;14:1276–84.
9. Shigetomi E, Bushong EA, Haustein MD, Tong X, Jackson-Weaver O, Kracun S, et al. Imaging calcium microdomains within entire astrocyte territories and endfeet with GCaMPs expressed using adeno-associated viruses. J Gen Physiol. 2013;141:633–47.
10. Shigetomi E, Tong X, Kwan KY, Corey DP, Khakh BS. TRPA1 channels regulate astrocyte resting calcium and inhibitory synapse efficacy through GAT-3. Nat Neurosci. 2012;15:70–80.
11. Shigetomi E, Jackson-Weaver O, Huckstepp RT, O'Dell TJ, Khakh BS. TRPA1 channels are regulators of astrocyte basal calcium levels and long-term potentiation via constitutive D-serine release. J Neurosci. 2013;33:10143–53.
12. Kuchibhotla K V, Lattarulo CR, Hyman BT, Bacskai BJ. Synchronous hyperactivity and intercellular calcium waves in astrocytes in Alzheimer mice. Science (80-.). 2009;323:1211–5.
13. Delekate A, Füchtemeier M, Schumacher T, Ulbrich C, Foddis M, Petzold GC. Metabotropic P2Y1 receptor signalling mediates astrocytic hyperactivity in vivo in an Alzheimer's disease mouse model. Nat Commun. 2014;5:5422.
14. De Strooper B, Karran E. The cellular phase of Alzheimer's disease. Cell. 2016;164:603–15.
15. Radde R, Bolmont T, Kaeser SA, Coomaraswamy J, Lindau D, Stoltze L, et al. Abeta42-driven cerebral amyloidosis in transgenic mice reveals early and robust pathology. EMBO Rep. 2006;7:940–6.
16. Barat E, Boisseau S, Bouyssières C, Appaix F, Savasta M, Albrieux M. Subthalamic nucleus electrical stimulation modulates calcium activity of nigral astrocytes. PLoS One. 2012;7:e41793.
17. Reeves AM, Shigetomi E, Khakh BS. Bulk loading of calcium indicator dyes to study astrocyte physiology: key limitations and improvements using morphological maps. J Neurosci. 2011;31:9353–8.
18. Nett WJ, Oloff SH, McCarthy KD. Hippocampal astrocytes in situ exhibit calcium oscillations that occur independent of neuronal activity. J Neurophysiol. 2002;87:528–37.
19. Platel J-C, Dupuis A, Boisseau S, Villaz M, Albrieux M, Brocard J. Synchrony of spontaneous calcium activity in mouse neocortex before synaptogenesis. Eur J Neurosci. 2007;25:920–8.
20. Stine WB, Dahlgren KN, Krafft GA, LaDu MJ. In vitro characterization of conditions for amyloid-beta peptide oligomerization and fibrillogenesis. J Biol Chem. 2003;278:11612–22.
21. Apelt J, Schliebs R. Beta-amyloid-induced glial expression of both pro- and anti-inflammatory cytokines in cerebral cortex of aged transgenic Tg2576 mice with Alzheimer plaque pathology. Brain Res. 2001;894:21–30.
22. R Development Core Team. R: A language and environment for statistical computing. R Foundation for Statistical Computing, Vienna, Austria. (2008). ISBN 3–900051–07-0. https://www.r-project.org/.
23. Patrushev I, Gavrilov N, Turlapov V, Semyanov A. Subcellular location of astrocytic calcium stores favors extrasynaptic neuron-astrocyte communication. Cell Calcium. 2013;54:343–9.
24. Orellana JA, Shoji KF, Abudara V, Ezan P, Amigou E, Sáez PJ, et al. Amyloid β-induced death in neurons involves glial and neuronal hemichannels. J Neurosci. 2011;31:4962–77.
25. Abudara V, Roux L, Dallérac G, Matias I, Dulong J, Mothet JP, et al. Activated microglia impairs neuroglial interaction by opening Cx43 hemichannels in hippocampal astrocytes. Glia. 2015;63:795–811
26. Familian A, Boshuizen RS, Eikelenboom P, Veerhuis R. Inhibitory effect of minocycline on amyloid β fibril formation and human microglial activation. Glia. 2006;53:233–40.
27. Nilius B, Appendino G, Owsianik G. The transient receptor potential channel TRPA1: from gene to pathophysiology. Pflügers Arch Eur J Physiol. 2012;464:425–58.

28. Lee SM, Cho YS, Kim TH, Jin MU, Ahn DK, Noguchi K, et al. An ultrastructural evidence for the expression of transient receptor potential ankyrin 1 (TRPA1) in astrocytes in the rat trigeminal caudal nucleus. J Chem Neuroanat. 2012;45:45–9.
29. McNamara CR, Mandel-Brehm J, Bautista DM, Siemens J, Deranian KL, Zhao M, et al. TRPA1 mediates formalin-induced pain. Proc Natl Acad Sci U S A. 2007;104:13525–30.
30. Rungta RL, Bernier L-P, Dissing-Olesen L, Groten CJ, LeDue JM, Ko R, et al. Ca(2+) transients in astrocyte fine processes occur via Ca(2+) influx in the adult mouse hippocampus. Glia. 2016;
31. Porrero C, Rubio-Garrido P, Avendaño C, Clascá F. Mapping of fluorescent protein-expressing neurons and axon pathways in adult and developing Thy1-eYFP-H transgenic mice. Brain Res. 2010;1345:59–72.
32. Busche MA, Konnerth A. Neuronal hyperactivity - a key defect in Alzheimer's disease? BioEssays. 2015;37:624–32.
33. Nakayama R, Sasaki T, Tanaka KF, Ikegaya Y. Subcellular calcium dynamics during juvenile development in mouse hippocampal astrocytes. Eur J Neurosci. 2016;43:923–32.
34. Srinivasan R, Huang BS, Venugopal S, Johnston AD, Chai H, Zeng H, et al. Ca2+ signaling in astrocytes from Ip3r2−/− mice in brain slices and during startle responses in vivo. Nat Neurosci. 2015;18:708–17.
35. Orre M, Kamphuis W, Osborn LM, Jansen AHP, Kooijman L, Bossers K, et al. Isolation of glia from Alzheimer's mice reveals inflammation and dysfunction. Neurobiol Aging. 2014;35:2746–60.
36. Jung ES, An K, Hong HS, Kim J-H, Mook-Jung I. Astrocyte-originated ATP protects Aβ(1-42)-induced impairment of synaptic plasticity. J Neurosci. 2012;32:3081–7.
37. Kraft AW, Hu X, Yoon H, Yan P, Xiao Q, Wang Y, et al. Attenuating astrocyte activation accelerates plaque pathogenesis in APP/PS1 mice. FASEB J. 2013;27:187–98.
38. Wyss-Coray T, Loike JD, Brionne TC, Lu E, Anankov R, Yan F, et al. Adult mouse astrocytes degrade amyloid-beta in vitro and in situ. Nat Med. 2003;9:453–7.
39. Grolla AA, Sim JA, Lim D, Rodriguez JJ, Genazzani AA, Verkhratsky A. Amyloid-beta and Alzheimer's disease type pathology differentially affects the calcium signalling toolkit in astrocytes from different brain regions. Cell Death Dis. 2013;4:e623.
40. Pirttimaki TM, Codadu NK, Awni A, Pratik P, Nagel DA, Hill EJ, et al. α7 nicotinic receptor-mediated astrocytic gliotransmitter release: Aβ effects in a preclinical Alzheimer's mouse model. PLoS One. 2013;8:e81828.
41. Lee K-I, Lee H-T, Lin H-C, Tsay H-J, Tsai F-C, Shyue S-K, et al. Role of transient receptor potential ankyrin 1 channels in Alzheimer's disease. J Neuroinflammation. 2016;13:92.
42. Mucke L, Selkoe DJ. Neurotoxicity of amyloid β-protein: synaptic and network dysfunction. Cold Spring Harb Perspect Med. 2012;2:a006338.
43. Bushong EA, Martone ME, Jones YZ, Ellisman MH. Protoplasmic astrocytes in CA1 stratum radiatum occupy separate anatomical domains. J Neurosci. 2002;22:183–92.
44. Varga E, Juhász G, Bozsó Z, Penke B, Fülöp L, Szegedi V. Abeta(1-42) enhances neuronal excitability in the CA1 via NR2B subunit-containing NMDA receptors. Neural Plast. 2014;2014:584314.
45. Lei M, Xu H, Li Z, Wang Z, O'Malley TT, Zhang D, et al. Soluble Aβ oligomers impair hippocampal LTP by disrupting glutamatergic/GABAergic balance. Neurobiol Dis. 2016;85:111–21.
46. Talantova M, Sanz-Blasco S, Zhang X, Xia P, Akhtar MW, Okamoto S, et al. Aβ induces astrocytic glutamate release, extrasynaptic NMDA receptor activation, and synaptic loss. Proc Natl Acad Sci U S A. 2013;110:E2518–27.
47. Kervern M, Angeli A, Nicole O, Leveille F, Parent B, Villette V, et al. Selective impairment of some forms of synaptic plasticity by oligomeric amyloid-beta peptide in the mouse hippocampus: implication of extrasynaptic NMDA receptors. J Alzheimers Dis. 2012;32:183–96.
48. Malarkey EB, Parpura V. Mechanisms of glutamate release from astrocytes. Neurochem Int. 2008;52:142–54.
49. Scimemi A, Meabon JS, Woltjer RL, Sullivan JM, Diamond JS, Cook DG. Amyloid-β1-42 slows clearance of synaptically released glutamate by mislocalizing astrocytic GLT-1. J Neurosci. 2013;33:5312–8.
50. Yi C, Mei X, Ezan P, Mato S, Matias I, Giaume C, et al. Astroglial connexin43 contributes to neuronal suffering in a mouse model of Alzheimer's disease. Cell Death Differ. 2016;7:1–11.
51. Girod S, Maurin M, van der Sanden B, Boisseau S, Appaix F, Guillemain I, et al. Specific in vivo staining of astrocytes in the whole brain after intravenous injection of sulforhodamine dyes. PLoS One. 2012;7:e35169.

Permissions

All chapters in this book were first published in MN, by BioMed Central; hereby published with permission under the Creative Commons Attribution License or equivalent. Every chapter published in this book has been scrutinized by our experts. Their significance has been extensively debated. The topics covered herein carry significant findings which will fuel the growth of the discipline. They may even be implemented as practical applications or may be referred to as a beginning point for another development.

The contributors of this book come from diverse backgrounds, making this book a truly international effort. This book will bring forth new frontiers with its revolutionizing research information and detailed analysis of the nascent developments around the world.

We would like to thank all the contributing authors for lending their expertise to make the book truly unique. They have played a crucial role in the development of this book. Without their invaluable contributions this book wouldn't have been possible. They have made vital efforts to compile up to date information on the varied aspects of this subject to make this book a valuable addition to the collection of many professionals and students.

This book was conceptualized with the vision of imparting up-to-date information and advanced data in this field. To ensure the same, a matchless editorial board was set up. Every individual on the board went through rigorous rounds of assessment to prove their worth. After which they invested a large part of their time researching and compiling the most relevant data for our readers.

The editorial board has been involved in producing this book since its inception. They have spent rigorous hours researching and exploring the diverse topics which have resulted in the successful publishing of this book. They have passed on their knowledge of decades through this book. To expedite this challenging task, the publisher supported the team at every step. A small team of assistant editors was also appointed to further simplify the editing procedure and attain best results for the readers.

Apart from the editorial board, the designing team has also invested a significant amount of their time in understanding the subject and creating the most relevant covers. They scrutinized every image to scout for the most suitable representation of the subject and create an appropriate cover for the book.

The publishing team has been an ardent support to the editorial, designing and production team. Their endless efforts to recruit the best for this project, has resulted in the accomplishment of this book. They are a veteran in the field of academics and their pool of knowledge is as vast as their experience in printing. Their expertise and guidance has proved useful at every step. Their uncompromising quality standards have made this book an exceptional effort. Their encouragement from time to time has been an inspiration for everyone.

The publisher and the editorial board hope that this book will prove to be a valuable piece of knowledge for researchers, students, practitioners and scholars across the globe.

List of Contributors

Ellis Patrick, Sathyapriya Rajagopal, Jishu Xu, Nathalie Pochet, Lori B. Chibnik and Philip L. De Jager
Departments of Neurology and Psychiatry, Brigham and Women's Hospital, Program in Translational NeuroPsychiatric Genomics, Institute for the Neurosciences, 77 Avenue Louis Pasteur, NRB 168C, Boston, MA 02115, USA
Harvard Medical School, Boston, MA, USA
Program in Medical and Population Genetics, Broad Institute, Cambridge, MA, USA

Anna Tang
Departments of Neurology and Psychiatry, Brigham and Women's Hospital, Program in Translational NeuroPsychiatric Genomics, Institute for the Neurosciences, 77 Avenue Louis Pasteur, NRB 168C, Boston, MA 02115, USA
Program in Medical and Population Genetics, Broad Institute, Cambridge, MA, USA

Cristin McCabe
Program in Medical and Population Genetics, Broad Institute, Cambridge, MA, USA

Julie A. Schneider and David A. Bennett
Rush Alzheimer's Disease Center, Rush University Medical Center, Chicago, IL, USA

Hon-Kit Andus Wong, Selina H. Imboywa and Anna M. Krichevsky
Departments of Neurology, Brigham and Women's Hospital, Boston, MA, USA

Philippe Hantraye
CEA, DSV, I2BM, MIRCen, Fontenay-aux-Roses 92265, France
INSERM UMS27, Fontenay-aux-Roses 92265, Université Paris-Sud, Université Paris-Saclay, Orsay 94100, France
CNRS UMR9199, Fontenay-aux-Roses 92265, Université Paris-Sud, Université Paris-Saclay, Orsay 94100, France

Nicole Déglon
Department of Clinical Neurosciences, Laboratory of Cellular and Molecular Neurotherapies, Lausanne University Hospital, Lausanne, Switzerland
Neuroscience Research Center, Laboratory of Cellular and Molecular Neurotherapies, Lausanne University Hospital, Lausanne, Switzerland

Katarzyna Marta Zoltowska, Masato Maesako, Shuko Takeda, Laura J. Keller, Bradley T. Hyman and Oksana Berezovska
Department of Neurology, MassGeneral Institute for Neurodegenerative Disease, Massachusetts General Hospital, Harvard Medical School, 114 16th Street, Rm. 2006, 02129 Charlestown, MA, USA

Iryna Lushnikova and Galina Skibo
Department of Cytology, Bogomoletz Institute of Physiology, National Academy of Sciences of Ukraine, 4 Bogomoletz Street, 01024 Kyiv, Ukraine

Gao-Shang Chai, Qiong Feng, Zhi-Hao Wang, Yu Hu, Dong-Sheng Sun, Xiao-Guang Li, Dan Ke and Hong-Lian Li
Department of Pathophysiology, School of Basic Medicine, Tongji Medical College, Huazhong University of Science and Technology, Wuhan 430030, China
the Collaborative Innovation Center for Brain Science, Key Laboratory of Ministry of Education of China for Neurological Disorders, Tongji Medical College, Huazhong University of Science and Technology, Wuhan 430030, China

Gong-Ping Liu and Jian-Zhi Wang
Department of Pathophysiology, School of Basic Medicine, Tongji Medical College, Huazhong University of Science and Technology, Wuhan 430030, China
The Collaborative Innovation Center for Brain Science, Key Laboratory of Ministry of Education of China for Neurological Disorders, Tongji Medical College, Huazhong University of Science and Technology, Wuhan 430030, China
Co-innovation Center of Neuroregeneration, Nantong University, Nantong, JS 226001, China

Anastasia G. Efthymiou and Alison M. Goate
Department of Neuroscience, Ronald M. Loeb Center for Alzheimer's disease, Icahn School of Medicine at Mount Sinai, 1425 Madison Ave, New York, NY 10029, USA

Mickael Audrain, Romain Fol and Marie-Anne Burlot
INSERM UMR1169, Université Paris-Sud, Université Paris-Saclay, Orsay 94100, France
Université Paris Descartes, Paris, France
CEA, DSV, I2BM, MIRCen, Fontenay-aux-Roses 92265, France

Sandro Alves, Gaelle Dufayet-Chaffaud, Nathalie Cartier and Jérome Braudeau
INSERM UMR1169, Université Paris-Sud, Université Paris-Saclay, Orsay 94100, France
CEA, DSV, I2BM, MIRCen, Fontenay-aux-Roses 92265, France

Patrick Dutar, Brigitte Potier and Jean-Marie Billard
INSERM UMR894, Centre de Psychiatrie et Neurosciences, Université Paris Descartes, Sorbonne Paris Cité, Paris, France

Julien Flament
CEA, DSV, I2BM, MIRCen, Fontenay-aux-Roses 92265, France
INSERM UMS27, Fontenay-aux-Roses 92265, Université Paris-Sud, Université Paris-Saclay, Orsay 94100, France

Alexis-Pierre Bemelmans and Julien Valette
CEA, DSV, I2BM, MIRCen, Fontenay-aux-Roses 92265, France
CNRS UMR9199, Fontenay-aux-Roses 92265, Université Paris-Sud, Université Paris-Saclay, Orsay 94100, France

Markus Britschgi
Department of Neurology and Neurological Sciences, Stanford University School of Medicine, Stanford, CA, USA
Roche Pharma Research and Early Development, NORD DTA, Roche Innovation, Center Basel, Basel, Switzerland

Aitana Sogorb-Esteve and Javier Sáez-Valero
Instituto de Neurociencias de Alicante, Universidad Miguel Hernández-CSIC, 03550, Av. Ramón y Cajal s/n, Sant Joan d'Alacant E-03550, Spain
Centro de Investigación Biomédica en Red sobre Enfermedades Neurodegenerativas (CIBERNED), Sant Joan d'Alacant & Barcelona, Spain

María-Salud García-Ayllón
Instituto de Neurociencias de Alicante, Universidad Miguel Hernández-CSIC, 03550, Av. Ramón y Cajal s/n, Sant Joan d'Alacant E-03550, Spain
Centro de Investigación Biomédica en Red sobre Enfermedades Neurodegenerativas (CIBERNED), Sant Joan d'Alacant & Barcelona, Spain
Unidad de Investigación, Hospital General Universitario de Elche, FISABIO, 03203 Elche, Spain

Alberto Lleó
Centro de Investigación Biomédica en Red sobre Enfermedades Neurodegenerativas (CIBERNED), Sant Joan d'Alacant & Barcelona, Spain
Memory Unit, Neurology Department, Hospital de la Santa Creu I Sant Pau, 08026 Barcelona, Spain

Juan Fortea
Centro de Investigación Biomédica en Red sobre Enfermedades Neurodegenerativas (CIBERNED), Sant Joan d'Alacant & Barcelona, Spain
Memory Unit, Neurology Department, Hospital de la Santa Creu I Sant Pau, 08026 Barcelona, Spain
Down Medical Center, Fundació Catalana Síndrome de Down, 08029 Barcelona, Spain

Raquel Sánchez-Valle and José-Luis Molinuevo
Alzheimer's Disease and Other Cognitive Disorders Unit, Neurology Service, Hospital Clinic; Institut d'Investigacions Biomèdiques Agust Pi i Sunyer, 08036 Barcelona, Spain

Katarina Willén and Gunnar K. Gouras
Department of Experimental Medical Science, Lund University, 221 84 Lund, Sweden

James R. Edgar
Cambridge Institute for Medical Research, University of Cambridge, Cambridge CB2 0XY, UK UCL Institute of Ophthalmology, London EC1V 9EL, UK

Clare E. Futter
UCL Institute of Ophthalmology, London EC1V 9EL, UK

Takafumi Hasegawa
Division of Neurology, Department of Neuroscience and Sensory Organs, Tohoku University Graduate School of Medicine, Sendai 980-8574, Japan

Nobuyuki Tanaka
Division of Cancer Biology and Therapeutics, Miyagi Cancer Center Research Institute, Natori 981-1293, Japan

Eric B. Dammer
Department of Human Genetics, Emory University School of Medicine, Atlanta, GA 30322, USA

Minghui Wang, Won-Min Song, Xianxiao Zhou, Yongzhong Zhao, Noam Beckmann, Pei Wang, Jun Zhu, Eric E. Schadt and Bin Zhang
Department of Genetics and Genomic Sciences, Icahn School of Medicine at Mount Sinai, One Gustave L. Levy Place, 1470 Madison Avenue, Room S8-111, New York, NY 10029, USA
Icahn Institute of Genomics and Multiscale Biology, Icahn School of Medicine at Mount Sinai, One Gustave L. Levy Place, New York, NY 10029, USA

Andrew T. McKenzie and Igor Katsyv
Department of Genetics and Genomic Sciences, Icahn School of Medicine at Mount Sinai, One Gustave L. Levy Place, 1470 Madison Avenue, Room S8-111, New York, NY 10029, USA
Icahn Institute of Genomics and Multiscale Biology, Icahn School of Medicine at Mount Sinai, One Gustave L. Levy Place, New York, NY 10029, USA
Medical Scientist Training Program, Icahn School of Medicine at Mount Sinai, One Gustave L. Levy Place, New York, NY 10029, USA

Sarah Moyon
Fishberg Department of Neuroscience and Friedman Brain Institute, Icahn School of Medicine at Mount Sinai, One Gustave L. Levy Place, New York, NY 10029, USA
Neuroscience Initiative, The City University of New York, Advanced Science Research Center, 85 St. Nicholas Terrace, New York, NY 10031, USA

Nicholas T. Seyfried
Department of Biochemistry, Emory University School of Medicine, Atlanta, GA 30322, USA
Integrated Proteomics Core Facility, Emory University School of Medicine, Atlanta, GA 30322, USA
Department of Neurology, Emory University School of Medicine, Atlanta, GA 30322, USA

Duc M. Duong
Department of Biochemistry, Emory University School of Medicine, Atlanta, GA 30322, USA
Integrated Proteomics Core Facility, Emory University School of Medicine, Atlanta, GA 30322, USA

Joshua Aaker and Brian Popko
Department of Neurology, The University of Chicago Pritzker School of Medicine, 5841 S. Maryland Avenue, Chicago, IL 60637, USA

Pavel Katsel
Department of Psychiatry, Icahn School of Medicine at Mount Sinai, New York, NY 10029, USA

James J. Lah and Allan I. Levey
Department of Neurology, Emory University School of Medicine, Atlanta, GA 30322, USA
Center for Neurodegenerative Disease, Emory University School of Medicine, Atlanta, GA 30322, USA

Vahram Haroutunian
Icahn Institute of Genomics and Multiscale Biology, Icahn School of Medicine at Mount Sinai, One Gustave L. Levy Place, New York, NY 10029, USA
Department of Psychiatry, Icahn School of Medicine at Mount Sinai, New York, NY 10029, USA
Mental Illness Research, Education, and Clinical Center (VISN 3), James J. Peters VA Medical Center, Bronx, NY 10468, USA

Patrizia Casaccia
Icahn Institute of Genomics and Multiscale Biology, Icahn School of Medicine at Mount Sinai, One Gustave L. Levy Place, New York, NY 10029, USA
Fishberg Department of Neuroscience and Friedman Brain Institute, Icahn School of Medicine at Mount Sinai, One Gustave L. Levy Place, New York, NY 10029, USA
Neuroscience Initiative, The City University of New York, Advanced Science Research Center, 85 St. Nicholas Terrace, New York, NY 10031, USA

Maitane Ortiz-Virumbrales
Department of Neurology, NFL Neurological Care Center, Icahn School of Medicine at Mount Sinai, New York, NY 10029, USA

Cesar L. Moreno and Sam Gandy
Department of Neurology, NFL Neurological Care Center, Icahn School of Medicine at Mount Sinai, New York, NY 10029, USA
Department of Psychiatry, Alzheimer's Disease Research Center, Icahn School of Medicine at Mount Sinai, 5 E 98th St, New York, NY 10029, USA

Lucio Della Guardia, Valeria Shnyder and Christoph Buettner
Department of Medicine, Diabetes, Obesity, and Metabolism Institute, Icahn School of Medicine at Mount Sinai, New York, NY 10029, USA

Ilya Kruglikov and Scott Noggle
New York Stem Cell Foundation Laboratories, New York, NY 10032, USA

Bin Zhang and Eric E. Schadt
Icahn Institute and Department of Genetics and Genomic Sciences, Icahn School of Medicine at Mount Sinai, New York, NY 10029, USA

Rudolph E. Tanzi
Genetics and Aging Unit, Harvard Medical School, Massachusetts General Hospital, 114 16th Street, Charlestown, MA 02129, USA

Maud Gratuze, Cheryl E. G. Leyns and David M. Holtzman
Department of Neurology, St. Louis, USA
Hope Center for Neurological Disorders, St. Louis, USA
Knight Alzheimer's Disease Research Center, Washington University School of Medicine, St. Louis, MO 63110, USA

Jia Luo, Sue H. Lee, Lawren Vande Vrede, Zhihui Qin and Gregory R. J. Thatcher
Department of Medicinal Chemistry and Pharmacognosy, College of Pharmacy, University of Illinois at Chicago, Chicago, IL, USA

Manel Ben Aissa
Department of Medicinal Chemistry and Pharmacognosy, College of Pharmacy, University of Illinois at Chicago, Chicago, IL, USA
Department of Anatomy and Cell Biology, College of Medicine, University of Illinois at Chicago, Chicago, IL, USA

John Larson
Department of Psychiatry, Neuropsychiatric Institute, University of Illinois at Chicago, Chicago, IL, USA

Andrew F. Teich and Ottavio Arancio
Department of Pathology, The Taub Institute for Research on Alzheimer's Disease and the Aging Brain, Columbia University, New York, NY, USA

Yohan D'Souza, Ahmed Elharram and Brian M. Bennett
Department of Biomedical & Molecular Sciences, Faculty of Health Sciences, Queen's University, Kingston, ON, Canada

Kevin Koster, Leon M. Tai and Mary Jo LaDu
Department of Anatomy and Cell Biology, College of Medicine, University of Illinois at Chicago, Chicago, IL, USA

Claudia Cicognola, Ulf Andreasson and Kaj Blennow
Institute of Neuroscience and Physiology, Department of Psychiatry and Neurochemistry, The Sahlgrenska Academy at University of Gothenburg, House V3, SU / Mölndal hospital, Göteborgsvägen 31, SE-431 80 Mölndal, Sweden
Clinical Neurochemistry Laboratory, Sahlgrenska University Hospital, SE-431 80 Mölndal, Sweden

Davide Chiasserini, Paolo Eusebi and Lucilla Parnetti
Section of Neurology, Department of Medicine, Center for Memory Disturbances, University of Perugia, Sant' Andrea delle Fratte, 06132 Perugia, Italy

Hugo Vanderstichele
ADx NeuroSciences, Gent, Belgium

Henrik Zetterberg
Institute of Neuroscience and Physiology, Department of Psychiatry and Neurochemistry, The Sahlgrenska Academy at University of Gothenburg, House V3, SU / Mölndal hospital, Göteborgsvägen 31, SE-431 80 Mölndal, Sweden
Clinical Neurochemistry Laboratory, Sahlgrenska University Hospital, SE-431 80 Mölndal, Sweden
UCL Institute of Neurology, Queen Square, London, UK

Jérôme Robert, Emily B. Button, Sophie Stukas, Guilaine K. Boyce, Megan Gilmour, Wai Hang Chung, Sonja K. Soo, Brian Yuen, Arvin Bahrabadi, Kevin Kang, Iva Kulic and Cheryl L. Wellington
Department of Pathology and Laboratory Medicine, University of British Columbia, Vancouver, BC V6T 1Z3, Canada
Djavad Mowafaghian Centre for Brain Health, University of British Columbia, 2215 Wesbrook Mall, Vancouver, BC V6T 1Z3, Canada

Ebrima Gibbs and Neil Cashman
Djavad Mowafaghian Centre for Brain Health, University of British Columbia, 2215 Wesbrook Mall, Vancouver, BC V6T 1Z3, Canada
Department of Neurology, University of British Columbia, Vancouver, BC V6T 2B5, Canada

Catherine M. Cowan
Department of Zoology, University of British Columbia, Vancouver, BC V6T 2B5, Canada

Gordon Francis
Department of Medicine, University of British Columbia, Vancouver, BC V6Z 1Y6, Canada

Elizabeth D. Kirby, Rachelle Abbey, Hudson Johns, Ramya Narasimhan, Suraj Pradhan and Chung-Huan Sun
Department of Neurology and Neurological Sciences, Stanford University School of Medicine, Stanford, CA, USA

Philipp A. Jaeger
Department of Neurology and Neurological Sciences, Stanford University School of Medicine, Stanford, CA, USA
Institute of Chemistry and Biochemistry, Free University Berlin, Berlin, Germany
Departments of Bioengineering and Medicine, University of California San Diego, La Jolla, CA, USA

Trey Ideker
Departments of Bioengineering and Medicine, University of California San Diego, La Jolla, CA, USA

Badri Vardarajan
Department of Medicine (Biomedical Genetics), Boston University Schools of Medicine, Boston, MA, USA

Ruochun Huang and Ruo-Pan Huang
RayBiotech, Guangzhou, China
RayBiotech, Norcrosse, GA, USA

Bradley F. Boeve, David S. Knopman and Ronald C. Petersen
Department of Neurology, Mayo Clinic, Rochester, MN, USA

Adam L. Boxer, Anna Karydas and Bruce L. Miller
Department of Neurology, University of California San Francisco, San Francisco, CA, USA

Lindsay A. Farrer
Department of Medicine (Biomedical Genetics), Boston University Schools of Medicine, Boston, MA, USA
Departments of Neurology, Ophthalmology, Genetics and Genomics, Epidemiology, and Biostatistics, Boston University Schools of Medicine and Public Health, Boston, MA, USA

NiCole Finch, Rosa Rademakers and Steven G. Younkin
Department of Neuroscience, Mayo Clinic, Jacksonville, FL, USA

Neill R. Graff-Radford
Department of Neurology, Mayo Clinic, Jacksonville, FL, USA

Elizabeth Head
Departments of Pharmacology and Nutritional Sciences and Sanders-Brown Center on Aging, University of Kentucky, Lexington, KY, USA

Matan Hofree
Department of Computer Science and Engineering, University of California San Diego, La Jolla, CA, USA

Andrey Loboda and Alexei Podtelezhnikov
Genetics and Pharmacogenomics, Merck Research Laboratories, West Point, PA, USA

Eliezer Masliah
Department of Pathology, University of California San Diego, La Jolla, CA, USA

Tony Wyss-Coray
Department of Neurology and Neurological Sciences, Stanford University School of Medicine, Stanford, CA, USA
Center for Tissue Regeneration, Repair and Restoration, VA Palo Alto Health Care System, Palo Alto, CA, USA

Kurt M. Lucin
Department of Neurology and Neurological Sciences, Stanford University School of Medicine, Stanford, CA, USA
Biology Department, Eastern Connecticut State University,Willimantic, CT, USA

Anthony Bosson, Adrien Paumier, Sylvie Boisseau, Muriel Jacquier-Sarlin, Alain Buisson and Mireille Albrieux
University Grenoble Alpes, Grenoble Institut des Neurosciences, GIN, Chemin Fortuné Ferrini, BP170, F-38000 Grenoble, France
Inserm, U1216, F-38000 Grenoble, France

Index

www.ingramcontent.com/pod-product-compliance
Lightning Source LLC
LaVergne TN
LVHW080735210926
848485LV00003B/565
9781639274352